Health Care Delivery and Clinical Science:

Concepts, Methodologies, Tools, and Applications

Information Resources Management Association
USA

Volume II

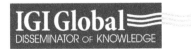

Published in the United States of America by
IGI Global
Medical Information Science Reference (an imprint of IGI Global)
701 E. Chocolate Avenue
Hershey PA, USA 17033
Tel: 717-533-8845
Fax: 717-533-8661
E-mail: cust@igi-global.com
Web site: http://www.igi-global.com

Library of Congress Cataloging-in-Publication Data

Names: Information Resources Management Association, editor.
Title: Health care delivery and clinical science : concepts, methodologies,
    tools, and applications / Information Resources Management Association,
    editor.
Description: Hershey PA : Medical Information Science Reference, [2018] |
    Includes bibliographical references.
Identifiers: LCCN 2017025957| ISBN 9781522539261 (hardcover) | ISBN
    9781522539278 (eISBN)
Subjects: | MESH: Medical Informatics | Education, Professional--methods |
    Health Literacy | Patient Participation | Patient-Centered Care
Classification: LCC R858.A2 | NLM W 26.5 | DDC 362.10285--dc23 LC record available at https://lccn.loc.
gov/2017025957

British Cataloguing in Publication Data
A Cataloguing in Publication record for this book is available from the British Library.

For electronic access to this publication, please contact: eresources@igi-global.com.

List of Contributors

Table of Contents

Volume I

Section 1
Fundamental Concepts and Theories

Section 3
Tools and Technologies

Volume II

Section 4
Utilization and Applications

Volume III

Section 5
Organizational and Social Implications

Section 6
Critical Issues and Challenges

Preface

The constantly changing landscape of Health Care Delivery and Clinical Science makes it challenging for experts and practitioners to stay informed of the field's most up-to-date research. That is why Medical Information Science Reference is pleased to offer this three-volume reference collection that will empower students, researchers, and academicians with a strong understanding of critical issues within Health Care Delivery and Clinical Science by providing both broad and detailed perspectives on cutting-edge theories and developments. This reference is designed to act as a single reference source on conceptual, methodological, technical, and managerial issues, as well as to provide insight into emerging trends and future opportunities within the discipline.

Health Care Delivery and Clinical Science: Concepts, Methodologies, Tools, and Applications is organized into six distinct sections that provide comprehensive coverage of important topics. The sections are:

1. Fundamental Concepts and Theories;
2. Development and Design Methodologies;
3. Tools and Technologies;
4. Utilization and Applications;
5. Organizational and Social Implications; and,
6. Critical Issues and Challenges.

The following paragraphs provide a summary of what to expect from this invaluable reference tool.

Section 1, "Fundamental Concepts and Theories," serves as a foundation for this extensive reference tool by addressing crucial theories essential to the understanding of Health Care Delivery and Clinical Science. Introducing the book is "A Relational Perspective on Patient Engagement: Suggestions From Couple-Based Research and Intervention" by Silvia Donato, a great foundation laying the groundwork for the basic concepts and theories that will be discussed throughout the rest of the book. Section 1 concludes and leads into the following portion of the book with a nice segue chapter, "Application of SMAC Technology" by Manu Venugopal.

Section 2, "Development and Design Methodologies," presents in-depth coverage of the conceptual design and architecture of Health Care Delivery and Clinical Science. Opening the section is "Managing Knowledge Towards Enabling Healthcare Service Delivery" by Tiko Iyamu and Sharol Sibongile Mkhomazi. Through case studies, this section lays excellent groundwork for later sections that will get into present and future applications for Health Care Delivery and Clinical Science. The section concludes with an excellent work by Ignace Djitog, Hamzat Olanrewaju Aliyu, and Mamadou Kaba Traoré, "Multi-Perspective Modeling of Healthcare Systems."

Section 3, "Tools and Technologies," presents extensive coverage of the various tools and technologies used in the implementation of Health Care Delivery and Clinical Science. The first chapter, "Hospital Social Media Strategies: Patient or Organization Centric?" by Fay Cobb Payton and Natasha Pinto, lays a framework for the types of works that can be found in this section. The section concludes with "RFID in Health Care: Building Smart Hospitals for Quality Healthcare" by Amir Manzoor. Where Section 3 described specific tools and technologies at the disposal of practitioners, Section 4 describes the use and applications of the tools and frameworks discussed in previous sections.

Section 4, "Utilization and Applications," describes how the broad range of Health Care Delivery and Clinical Science efforts has been utilized and offers insight on and important lessons for their applications and impact. The first chapter in the section is "Utilisation of Health Information Systems for Service Delivery in the Namibian Environment" written by Ronald Karon. This section includes the widest range of topics because it describes case studies, research, methodologies, frameworks, architectures, theory, analysis, and guides for implementation. The breadth of topics covered in the section is also reflected in the diversity of its authors, from countries all over the globe. The section concludes with "The Power of Words: Deliberation Dialogue as a Model to Favor Patient Engagement in Chronic Care" by Sarah Bigi and Giulia Lamiani, a great transition chapter into the next section.

Section 5, "Organizational and Social Implications," includes chapters discussing the organizational and social impact of Health Care Delivery and Clinical Science. The section opens with "Management of Tacit Knowledge and the Issue of Empowerment of Patients and Stakeholders in the Health Care Sector" by Marc Jacquinet, Henrique Curado, Ângela Lacerda Nobre, Maria José Sousa, Marco Arraya, Rui Pimenta, and António Eduardo Martins. This section focuses exclusively on how these technologies affect human lives, either through the way they interact with each other or through how they affect behavioral/workplace situations. The section concludes with "Patient Privacy and Security in E-Health" by Güney Gürsel.

Section 6, "Critical Issues and Challenges," presents coverage of academic and research perspectives on Health Care Delivery and Clinical Science tools and applications. The section begins with "The Administrative Policy Quandary in Canada's Health Service Organizations" by Grace I. Paterson, Jacqueline M. MacDonald, and Naomi Nonnekes Mensink. Chapters in this section will look into theoretical approaches and offer alternatives to crucial questions on the subject of Health Care Delivery and Clinical Science. The section concludes with "Smart Medication Management, Current Technologies, and Future Directions" by Seyed Ali Rokni, Hassan Ghasemzadeh, and Niloofar Hezarjaribi.

Although the primary organization of the contents in this multi-volume work is based on its six sections, offering a progression of coverage of the important concepts, methodologies, technologies, applications, social issues, and emerging trends, the reader can also identify specific contents by utilizing the extensive indexing system listed at the end of each volume. As a comprehensive collection of research on the latest findings related to using technology to providing various services, *Health Care Delivery and Clinical Science: Concepts, Methodologies, Tools, and Applications* provides researchers, administrators, and all audiences with a complete understanding of the development of applications and concepts in Health Care Delivery and Clinical Science. Given the vast number of issues concerning usage, failure, success, policies, strategies, and applications of Health Care Delivery and Clinical Science in countries around the world, *Health Care Delivery and Clinical Science: Concepts, Methodologies, Tools, and Applications* addresses the demand for a resource that encompasses the most pertinent research in technologies being employed to globally bolster the knowledge and applications of Health Care Delivery and Clinical Science.

Chapter 27
Intelligent Medication Adherence Monitoring System

Athanasios Anastasiou
National Technical University of Athens, Greece

Kostas Giokas
National Technical University of Athens, Greece

Georgia Koutsouri
National Technical University of Athens, Greece

Dimitra Iliopoulou
National Technical University of Athens, Greece

ABSTRACT

This chapter presents the architecture and implementation of an automatic medication dispenser specifically for users who take medications without close professional supervision. By relieving the users from the error-prone tasks of interpreting medication directions and administrating medications accordingly, the device can improve the required level in compliance and prevent serious medication errors. By taking advantage of the scheduling flexibility provided by medication directions, the device makes the user's medication schedule easy to adhere and tolerant to tardiness whenever possible. This work is done collaboratively by the medication scheduler and dispenser controller in an action-oriented manner. An advantage of the action-oriented interface between the components is extensibility, as new functions can be added and existing ones removed with little or no need to modify the dispenser control structure. This chapter first describes the action-oriented design, major components and hardware structures of the smart device. It then provides an overview of the heuristic algorithms used by the medication scheduler and their relative merits. The different available user options will be presented depicting the user-specific operating modes of the device/service. The scope of this chapter is to describe the development of a smart electronic drug dispenser unit for the pharmaceutical adherence of patients.

DOI: 10.4018/978-1-5225-3926-1.ch027

INTRODUCTION

Thanks to years of advances in medical and pharmaceutical technologies, more and more drugs can cure or control, previously fatal diseases and help people live actively for decades longer. The benefits of the drugs would be even more wondrous were it not for the high rate of preventable medication errors (Veacez, 2006; Lisby et al., 2005; Law et al., 2003; Wertheimer, 2003). Medication errors are known to occur throughout the medication use process of ordering, transcription, dispensing, and administration. They lead to many hundred thousands of serious adverse drug events, thousands of deaths and billions of Euros in hospital cost each year. These alarming statistics have motivated numerous efforts in research, development and deployment of information technology systems and tools for prevention of medication errors (Kuperman et al.,2007 ; Baron et al.,2005).

Medication adherence usually refers to whether patients take their medications as prescribed, as well as whether they continue to take a prescribed medication. Medication nonadherence is a growing concern to clinicians, healthcare systems, and other stakeholders because of mounting evidence that it is prevalent and associated with adverse outcomes and higher costs of care. To date, measurement of patient medication adherence and use of interventions to improve adherence are rare in routine clinical practice. The proposed solution aims to develop a medication adherence monitoring system, comprising of a portable medication dispenser with communication capabilities and a software platform allowing monitoring by medical personnel and/or carer. The patient data recorded by the dispenser (rate of medication intake) will be collected and will be transmitted in real-time to the hospital (via any Internet link), where it will be analyzed, and any alerts will be raised.

This will enable the doctors to:

- Monitor the progress of the patient and intervene in the case of an anomaly.
- Monitor treatment compliance of the patient.

On the other hand, it will also enable the carer to:

- Monitor the depletion of one or more medication.

Our system addresses the needs of patients with chronic illnesses that require encouragement and supervision with their medication. Monitoring is achieved through the use of a medication dispenser, which collects information about the patients' medication adherence. The dispenser will contain electronics that record automatically the time and date the dispenser is accessed. These data will be transmitted via an Internet connection to the clinical team base.

BACKGROUND

According to the International Society for Pharmacoeconomics and Outcome Research (ISPOR), adherence is "the extent to which a patient acts, in accordance with the prescribed interval, and a dose of a dosing regimen." Medication nonadherence can affect patient health adversely, negatively impact a patient's relationship with his/her care provider, skew results of therapy clinical trials, and increase health resource consumption. Medication nonadherence remains a common health care problem. Poor adherence causes approximately 33% to 69% of medication-related hospitalizations and accounts for $100 billion in annual health care costs. Irrespective of disease, medication complexity, or how adherence is measured, the average adherence rate to chronic medication therapy is approximately 50%. Adherence monitoring should be performed routinely to ensure therapeutic efficacy, avoid unnecessary dose and regimen changes, contain health care costs, and in certain cases, prevent resistance to therapy from emerging.

Medication adherence is a growing concern to clinicians, healthcare systems, and other stakeholders because of mounting evidence that nonadherence is prevalent and associated with adverse outcomes and higher costs of care. Medication nonadherence is likely to grow as the EU population ages and as patients take more medications to treat chronic conditions. Moreover, the rise of performance measures that reward quality based on the attainment of treatment targets such as blood pressure and low-density lipoprotein (LDL) levels or outcomes such as 1-year mortality after hospitalization for conditions like acute myocardial infarction reinforces the import of longitudinal medication adherence. Unlike other quality measures that are under the more direct control of care providers and healthcare systems (e.g., prescribing medications at discharge), the achievement of longer-term therapeutic and outcome goals requires a partnership with patients. To date, measurement of patient medication adherence and use of interventions to improve adherence are rare in routine clinical practice. (Cutler, D. et.al 2005).

Methods to measure adherence, including patient self-reports, pill counts, refill rates, biological monitoring, and electronic monitoring, have limitations and are only proxy measures. Patient self-reports rely on memory and are prone to inaccuracies and recall bias. Pill counts are unreliable if patients fail to return bottles or dump pills before the count. Biological monitoring (e.g., sampling blood, urine) is either impractical, invasive, or intrusive and does not measure adherence unless the time and dose administered before sampling are verified. Refill rates or electronic monitoring cannot determine whether patients actually take the medication. Although the process of cap removal does not necessarily reflect dose ingestion, medication electronic monitoring systems are useful for calculating adherence rates for dose taking and dose timing and often are viewed as the best method to measure adherence. Nonetheless, despite their limitations, all of these methods are adequate for documenting nonadherence, but in general, only self-report methods can distinguish among the various types of nonadherence described below. (Davis, 2005).

The cause of medication nonadherence varies among patients and is broadly categorized as unintentional or intentional. Unintentional nonadherence involves intending to take medication as instructed but failing to do so for some reason (e.g., forgetfulness, carelessness). Unintentional nonadherence is influenced by patient characteristics, treatment factors, and patient–provider issues. In contrast, intentional nonadherence involves making a reasoned decision not to take medication as instructed based on perceptions, feelings, or beliefs. Intentional nonadherence reflects a rational decision-making process by the patient whereby the benefits of treatment are weighed against any adverse effects of the treatment. Broadly characterizing nonadherence may oversimplify the complexities involved with nonadherence, but it is practical and illustrates that mitigating nonadherence requires different interventions.

Most medication adherence models are based on several social cognition models, including the health belief model, social cognitive theory, and theory of planned behavior. These models are similar, and all assume that beliefs developed by individuals shape how they interpret information and experiences and ultimately influence their behavior. Accordingly, health behavior (e.g., medication taking) results from rational decisions based on all available information.

Many methods to improve medication adherence have been studied. Most methods attempt to change patient behavior by using reminders, counseling, reinforcement, education, dosage simplification, or a combination of these methods. Generally, adherence interventions are categorized as behavioral, educational, or organizational based on modifying the patient's environment or incentives, providing more information, or lifting barriers associated with medication complexity and communication with care providers (Durso, 2001).

Most studies on improving adherence involve behavioral interventions (Yeh, H. et. al., 2006) Data suggest that patient education is one of the best methods for improving adherence, especially for those simultaneously managing more than six medications. Depending on the type of nonadherence and patient characteristics, using a combination of tailored interventions such as patient education, patient self-monitoring of specialized care, and stimuli to take medications have the greatest potential for improving adherence (Anastasiou, et.al., 2015).

MAIN FOCUS OF THE CHAPTER

Methodology

In order to acquire the most of our system, the proposed solution consists of four basic components:

1. **Medication Dispenser:** A dispenser that will provide the patient with the prescribed medication and will be able to record whether the drug has been taken. The patient's doctor or the pharmacist will provide the dispenser together with the right dosage of drugs needed by the patient. They will then insert the right amount of drugs dosage in each compartment of the dispenser according to the medication prescribed to each patient. The medication dispensers will be integrated with a communications device, which will transmit the patient's data to the clinic for monitoring. The data will be transmitted from the dispensers to the clinic for monitoring by the medical staff via cloud-based services. The dispenser will alarm the doctor, nurse or any other relatives of the patient that the patient has taken his drug and at which time of the day. The doctor will define the threshold values describing the patients' compliance to the treatment and when these values are reached, an alarm will be triggered letting the doctor know that the patients' compliance is not satisfactory (Tsai, P. et. al., 2008).

2. **Telematics Infrastructure:** The recordings from each medical dispenser will be transmitted to the clinic immediately. This will allow the clinic to monitor the patient in real-time and take action in the case of an anomaly. It is envisaged that the dispenser will transmit the patient's data (i.e. if he took a medicine and what dosage of medicine he received) to the server at the clinic. From this point of view, our system is non-obtrusive to the everyday life of the patient and his/her family, since it will not even use their telephone line. Concerning security issues, the system will incorporate 128-bit cryptography – a virtual private network will be set up during data transfer between the patient's home and the server at the clinic. Besides, the patient is only known by a code stored in our system. One would have to cross-check the code with the clinic's records, which are locally held at the clinic, in order to reveal the identity of the patient.

3. **Datastore with Patient Records:** This already exists in the electronic form in clinics around Europe. The proposed solution will develop a flexible interface for the integration of the system to the patient datastore.

4. **User Interface (UI) for the Medical Staff and Patients:** From the side of the clinic, the UI will enable complete control of the system by the operator, be that a doctor or a nurse. It is envisaged that different privileges will be given in order to access/write/modify the content of the system, according to the authority of the operator. From the side of the patient and, indeed, his family and carers, his record will be accessible via the Internet, using a password provided by the clinic. The patient/family/carer will also have access to an information library, which will assist them to assess the state of the patient and take action (i.e. call the doctor) if needed.

Clinicians will be able to connect to the System's web app. The web app will include the following data:

1. A list of personal details.
2. The current patient thresholds and alert types.
3. Each patient's medication prescription and historical data.
4. Medication dispensers' identification numbers.
5. Adherence events and alerts generated by the medication dispenser.

The hospital doctors will also be able to connect to the System's web app. This database will include the following elements:

- Personal information for the patient.
- The predetermined limits for the particular patient and various types of signals of danger
- The pharmaceutical education of patient.
- Unique code-number for the medical dispenser allocated to the specific patient.
- The compliance of the patient to the regime and the alerts that the dispenser has transmitted.

Among these systems, it is important that we use HL7 messages. Before discussing HL7, it is critical to understand that each healthcare establishment is radically different in terms of politics, business relationships, payment structures, data collected, database structures, and software systems. That means every hospital, clinical lab, imaging center, outpatient surgery center, podiatrist's office, and acupuncture center have unique requirements for interacting with data and patients (Smalling, J., et.al 2005).

If we multiply the uniqueness of each healthcare setting by the number of countries or political settings where care will be delivered we can expect the result to be an almost infinite number of unique requirements that like English, Spanish, and German are close in terms of their needs but not exactly the same.

It is in this hazardous arena where all care settings and users of clinical systems are different that HL7 attempts to establish a single, flexible, worldwide standard for the representation/movement of clinical data. Hospitals and other healthcare provider organizations typically have many different computer systems used for everything from billing records to patient tracking. All of these are based on the HL7 Reference Information Model (RIM) and the HL7 Version 3 Data Types. The CDA specifies that the content of the document consists of a mandatory textual part and optional structured parts. The structured part relies on coding systems (such as from SNOMED and LOINC) to represent concepts (Wan, D. 1999).

The service of our system begins when a supplier of medical services (e.g. a pharmacist or a nurse) programs the dispenser with the satisfactory doses for a determined period, which is bigger than the time interval that intervenes up to the visit for the next supply. As soon as the dispenser is provided with the medication, the electronic operations of the distributor as autonomous "sensor" will record various data with first and most important the time when the dispenser will open and close. All the above will shape the personal profile of the patient with regards to the continuous observation of his pharmaceutical adherence. The omissions of doses are characterized as alerts when they take place systematically for a time period and not as isolated incidents. Moreover, if one patient loses at least 50% of one week's doses an alert for the direct attention of the supplier responsible for the medical service is provided. Each time the patient will use each unique medical compartment, there will be a direct connection between his profile and his medical record according to the HL7 standards, and the latter will be updated thus letting know both sides if any changes are required.

The adoption of the HL7 standard is allowing for the creation of better tools with which to transfer critical information. This will make every aspect of healthcare more efficient and dynamic and will lessen the opportunity for mistakes (Kuperman, et al.. 2007).

These days, a patient's visit to a clinic or a doctor's office goes like this: A nurse measures a patient's weight, which is electronically populated into his or her medical record. The nurse then takes the patient's blood pressure, and the result is also electronically populated into the medical record. Next, the doctor selects criteria for a lab order, and the lab receives it electronically almost instantly. The lab performs the order and electronically populates the patient's medical record with the results (Governo, et.al. 2003).

HL7 certainly doesn't make these types of technological advancements happen, but the adoption and implementation of the HL7 message standard certainly help make them possible among different systems.

State of the Art

Our proposed platform is innovative both in the use of the technology (state of the art electro-mechanics, latest telecommunication standards, sophisticated interface features) but also in the business concept, as a medication adherence monitoring application. It is a truly innovative solution that reduces the cost of treatment and the hospitalization period while at the same time drastically improves the monitoring of the post-surgery or chronically ill patient enabling him to enjoy lower hospitalization costs and improved quality of life.

It introduces a ground-breaking communication channel between doctor and patient through a simple but intelligent device. The bi-directional communication offers the grounds for an effective reminder-compliance process. Also, through the series of features, the system possesses, critical, top-quality information is provided to the monitoring doctor at real-time. The device itself is highly sophisticated, with electromechanical features that provide highly efficient and secure medication management (compartment locking, intelligent medication allowance, remote dosage update, etc.). Also, being wireless and fully portable it offers ubiquitous service and ultimate efficiency. This device, coupled with the sophisticated supporting platform constitutes a pioneering application for widespread health home-monitoring.

The mechanical part of our system features an advanced design since it is able to accept changes in medication dosage and apply them in an ad-hoc manner. Likewise, it has the ability not only to increase or reduce (through doctors' specific online prescription) the dosage of a specific drug, but it can also implement an increase or a reduction in the time intervals between the dosages. It offers the ability to have different drugs at different times of day (as long as it is preloaded with these drugs). (Fulton, M. 2005).

If the dispenser is coupled with the innovative platform through the web interface, it becomes an innovative integrated solution for monitoring chronic patients.

SYSTEM ARCHITECTURE

In this section, the overall architecture of the proposed platform and how the various components will be connected to each other, are depicted. The main components of the system can be seen in Figure 1, and are described in the successive sections in greater detail.

Health Record Database (HRD)

These databases already exist in numerous hospitals around Europe and contain patients' medical records that contain comprehensive information relating to the patient and his medical state. The proposed system will develop a flexible interface for the integration of the health record database (HRD) in order to acquire patient's information. This will enable the platform's server to query and enter/ retrieve information to/ from the hospital health record database.

Central Server

The central server is the heart of the system and is composed of several modules, responsible for the integrity as well as the performance of the system:

Figure 1. System architecture

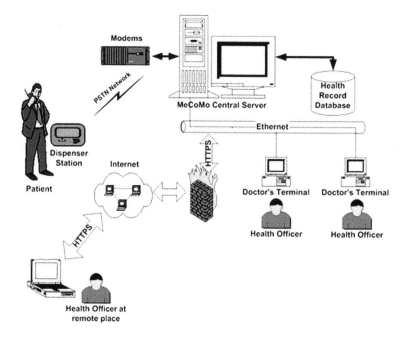

1. **Monitoring Module:** This is the main management system of the patient. The control functions on the server-side relate to continuous automatic monitoring of the dispenser's malfunctioning as well as patient's medication adherence. According to the specific medical scenario monitored, the dispenser will provide as input to the monitoring module a range of parameters, which will depend on the patient's case and the choices of the treating doctor.
2. **Presentation Module:** This module is responsible for producing adherence medication diagrams proving the medical staff with a brief and comprehensive view of the patient's medication adherence status. These diagrams will be customized according to doctor's preferences and patient parameters.
3. **Administration Module:** This module handles the requests for addition/removal/modification of patients, medical staff, and medication data. This module also audits user privilege and protects the system from any user errors.

Clinic User Interface (CUI)

At the side of the clinic, the CUI will enable complete control of the system by the operator, be that a doctor or a nurse. It is envisaged that different privileges will be given in order to access/write/modify the content of the system, according to the authority of the operator. All functions of the Control Module will be managed by the CUI. The CUI will be developed as a user-friendly Windows environment; it will be accessed through the clinic LAN and/or via a web server.

Medication Dispenser

As mentioned above, the medication dispenser will be a user-friendly device, capable of monitoring patient's medication adherence. The dispenser will provide the patient with the prescribed medication and record whether and when this has been taken. The doctor is able to program the medication dispenser according to medication prescription remotely. The medication dispenser records the timestamp of accessing a medication and conveys the recorded data to the hospital central server over a GPRS link. A detailed description of the medication dispenser's functionality and design requirements is given in the respective section.

Patient User Interface (PUI)

From the side of the patient and his family and carers, the patient record, including the system's readings, will be accessible via the Internet. The patient/ family/ carer will also have access to an information library, which will assist them to assess the state of the patient and take action (i.e. call the doctor) if needed.

HARDWARE COMPONENTS DESCRIPTION

Dispenser Components

The medication dispenser will be of the shape of a computer hard disk drive with a detachable rotating Carousel. It will enclose rechargeable batteries, the necessary GPRS modem, and respective antenna, an alarm bell, as well as the user interface for medication dispensing (LCD, buttons, etc).

The carousel will be doughnut-shaped, with a hole in the middle to couple with the base unit. It will contain a number of compartments, one for each dose. Considering that each dose usually does not exceed 4 pills, each compartment will be sized accordingly. It will have a single opening door, which should be locked when the carousel is not coupled so that the medication is not accessible by the patients or children. When coupled, the carousel door will open only when the patient chooses to take his medication (see Figure 2).

Dispenser Operation

The two modules (carousel and base unit) will couple together in an easy and fault tolerant way, with no need of external aid (e.g. keys). Attention will be given to make the door opening mechanism as tamperproof as possible. Medication will be provided only when requested by the patient and allowed by the logic, which will be programmable by the supervising doctor.

Specific Technical Requirements

The dispenser will be portable, and thus:

- **Wireless:** The only cable connection should be the power cable for recharging the battery. Normal operation will be with the dispenser being entirely wireless.
- **Ubiquitous:** This concerns the use of the GPRS networks for the communication purposes of the dispenser. Roaming will be supported for use in more than one country.
- **Of Limited Size and Weight:** The dispenser will be carried around by the patient, so it should even fit a pocket if possible.

Figure 2. Medication dispenser (carousel)

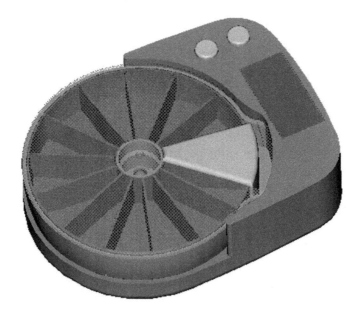

- **Autonomous:** In terms of power consumption. It should have battery autonomy of at least two weeks of normal operation. Rechargeable batteries should be used.

After being filled with the right dosage of the drug, the dispenser will be locked so that the patient does not have direct access to more than the daily dosage. Following the above, the dispenser:

- Must be tamperproof– in terms of design and materials used in its manufacture. This means that it will not be possible for the patient to access its whole contents at once. Also, if it is opened by force, a notification must be sent to the monitoring server.
- An alarm, reminding the patient to take the prescribed dosage is also desirable. It will be activated according to the desire of the patient, and the programming will be done through the PC interface and data link. The patient will be able to deactivate the alarm.
- There will be an indicator warning for signal loss, low battery or system malfunction, showing blocking of the dispenser, errors in the logic circuit, etc.
- The dispenser will be robust, built so that it withstands being occasionally dropped. For this reason, high-quality materials shall be used. Furthermore, the design should be attractive and without sharp corners.
- The dispenser should be intuitive to use. Special skills will not be required for its use. Patients will be given a set of simple instructions for the use of the dispenser. This will include advice not to open the dispenser unless they plan to take their medication at that time, to remove the prescribed dose only when opening the dispenser and to close it immediately after removing the dose and should be sufficient for the complete understanding of the dispenser operation.
- The operation of the dispenser should not be intrusive to the patient's life. This means that the patient should not need to change any of his/her habits concerning the acquisition of medication.
- The dispenser will be childproof as it concerns access to the medication. To ensure that, coordinated action will be needed to access the dosage. This could be achieved by the use of a button that needs rotating before pushing or a door that opens only when a button is kept pressed, etc.

OPERATIONAL SCENARIO

This section describes the medication adherence monitoring procedure, focusing on points important for decisions to be made concerning the design of the system:

1. The doctor prescribes medication for a patient, who is then registered with the platform's service. The timing and frequency of taking medication are specified (the frequency of medication is estimated to be up to 4 times a day).
2. The patient is given a medication dispenser by the hospital pharmacist (or nurse). The dispenser contains the correct amount of medication that will be sufficient until the patient's medication is next reviewed by the doctor and a new prescription is issued (either a repeat or a change in medication). The system can handle any interval between medication reviews.
3. The pharmacist will program the dispenser on his PC terminal – the commands will be transmitted to the dispenser over the GPRS link (this task should be simplified as much as possible).

4. The dispenser should lock, i.e. in a single day, it should not allow the patient to take more medication than that prescribed on that specific day. This is a precaution against accidental access to medicine by children or other individuals and also a safeguard against accidental or deliberate overdose by the patient. Additionally, at any given dispensing time the patient has access only to the medication in the relevant compartment and not to the entire supply of medicines in the dispenser.

5. The patient uses the dispenser to take his/her medication. This should be made as simple as possible: e.g. by pressing just one button. Every time the patient accesses the dispenser for taking his medication, the system's monitoring server should be notified by the dispenser automatically. It is, of course, impossible to know if the patient actually took his or her medication just based on a single recording (although one can infer this from the pattern of accessing over a period of a few days). However, the dispenser may "sense" whether the patient tipped it over to remove the tablet.

6. Medical Staff is interested in knowing how many times per day and the exact time the patient accesses his medications. Therefore timestamp recording of the access events is important – this will also be addressed in the presentation module.

7. The notification messages arriving at the central monitoring server are compared to the profile of the respective patients. If they indicate a wrongful medication pattern (e.g. omission of more than 50% of dosages for a week), an alert is generated and sent to two members of the medical staff responsible for the concerned patient. The alerts can be sent by the "preferred" means, as chosen by the receiver – this can be SMS, email, recorded telephone call, etc.

8. The nurse (or doctor) can review the patients' access to medication record from a terminal at the hospital or even online. They can generate a patient profile that they can discuss with the patient at regular medication reviews. Alternatively, the nurse or doctor can log on to the system after they have received specific alert messages regarding medication non-adherence. They should log on to the system's server via a terminal at the hospital (Internet access is also available), acknowledge the receipt of the alert and take any necessary action (phone call to the patient, schedule a visit at the patient's home, etc). Logging on to the system, the members of the medical staff will be able to edit/browse through the patients' details, log files showing messages arriving from the dispensers and edit the thresholds for the generation of alerts for each patient as well as the medication patterns that should be followed. The user interface of the system should be very user-friendly, minimizing the time spent on it.

RESULTS

Results are grouped according to five themes: Ease of Use, Reliability, Medication Management Assistance, Routine Task Performance, and Acceptability.

1. **Ease of Use**: On a scale of 1 to 5, where 1 indicated "very difficult" and 5 indicated "very easy", 94% (90 of 96) participants rated the medication dispenser as "very easy" to use and 2% (2 of 96) rated it "very difficult". In addition, 3% (3 of 96) of participants rated it a "4" and 1% (1 of 96) rated it a "3" on this same scale. Five participants commented on the need for the nurses' help if they were to continue to use the machine due to difficulty with pill set up.

2. **Reliability**: On a scale of 1 to 5, where 1 indicated "very reliable" and 5 indicated "very unreliable", 95% (91 of 96) participants rated the medication dispenser as "very reliable" and 1% (1 of 96) rated it "very unreliable". In addition, 3% (3 of 96) of participants rated it a "4" and 1% (1 of 96) rated it a "3" on this same scale.

3. **Medication Management Assistance**: Ninety-nine percent (95 of 96) of participants responded "yes" that the medication dispenser helped them manage their medications. According to one participant, the dispenser "does not let you forget".

4. **Routine Task Performance**: Ninety percent (86 of 96) of participants indicated that the dispenser did not affect their ability to do things for themselves. Ninety-two percent (88 of 96) of participants indicated that the dispenser did not affect their ability to get around or leave the house. Ninety-eight percent (94 of 96) of participants indicated that the medication dispenser did not affect their ability to talk with or reach their nurse. Ninety-nine percent (95 of 96) of participants indicated that the dispenser did not interfere with their other activities.

5. **Acceptability**: Ninety-five percent (91 of 96) of participants responded positively that the dispenser gave them peace of mind. Eighty-four percent (81 of 96) of participants indicated that they would like to use the medication dispenser in the future.

The results show that nearly all participants perceived the medication dispensing device as very easy to use, very reliable and helpful in the management of their medications. In addition, nearly all participants reported that the machine did not interfere with other activities or the ability to reach their nurses. To a lesser degree, most participants reported that the device did not interfere with their independence or their ability to get around or leave the house. Many participants were initially not comfortable with the machine. However, as the study progressed, their comfort increased. For some participants, the machines became a key part of their home environment

CONCLUSION

Previous sections described the design and operations of a smart medication dispenser. Except for setting up operation and retrieval of individual doses from medication containers, the dispenser would be fully automatic. By monitoring the user's actions during set up, the dispenser prevents errors in medication identification. By automating the choices of dose sizes, the dispenser relieves the user from the burden of interpreting medication directions and special administration instructions and thus prevents the common errors due to misinterpretation.

By using algorithms that can take advantage of the scheduling flexibility provided by the sizable ranges of dosage parameters of modern medications, the scheduler can often adjust dose times of medications to keep compliance when the user is tardy. The bulk of the critical work in medication administration is done collaboratively by the dispenser controller and medication scheduler.

The medication dispensing device was designed to simplify the complex task of medication management with the aim of reducing medication errors and improving communication with providers. Medication error reduction and better communication are important to reach the larger goals of improved outcomes in older adult health status, rates of hospitalization, rates of nursing home admission, total costs of care and costs per quality-adjusted life year.

Older adults in this study accepted the medication dispensing device as reliable, easy to use and useful in coordinating personal medication management. These results indicate that technology-enhanced medication dispensers can be acceptable tools for older adults to help manage their care in collaboration with home care nurses. These results are encouraging because acceptance of technology-enhanced medication management is a requirement for improved monitoring of unpredictable responses to drug therapy in older adults.

The design is an iterative process, and implementations in a real-world context often reveal opportunities for better design. With older adults, it is particularly important to match personal abilities to device controls for medication management activities.

Future research should include:

1. Design studies for medication management devices
2. Research into new cost models that enable better access to medication management devices
3. Comparison of medication management devices with and without home services and
4. Integration studies of medication management interventions and data bundled with other informatics interventions for holistic support of older adults.

Last but not least, a challenge would be how to dispense the correct dose size of each medication given that medications can come in arbitrary shapes and forms. Our system answers the need for cost-effectiveness, fast-response, ubiquitous patient monitoring, focusing on the adherence medication area. Offering such an innovative solution, it brings itself ahead of the competition, setting the pace of the fast-moving healthcare technology area.

This research was previously published in Design, Development, and Integration of Reliable Electronic Healthcare Platforms edited by Anastasius Moumtzoglou, pages 72-85, copyright year 2017 by Medical Information Science Reference (an imprint of IGI Global).

REFERENCES

Anastasiou, A., Giokas, K., Koutsouris, D. (2015). Monitoring of compliance on an individual treatment through mobile innovations. *EMBC*, 7320-7323.

Baron, R. J., Fabens, E. L., Schiffman, M., & Wolf, E. (2005). Electronic health records: Just around the corner? Or over the cliff? *Annals of Internal Medicine*, *143*(3), 222–226. doi:10.7326/0003-4819-143-3-200508020-00008 PMID:16061920

Cutler, D. M., Feldman, N. E., & Horwitz, J. R. (2005). U. S. Adoption of Computerized Physician Order Entry Systems. *Health Affairs*, *24*(6), 1654–1663. doi:10.1377/hlthaff.24.6.1654 PMID:16284040

Davis, R. L. (2005). Computerized Physician Order Entry Systems: The Coming of Age for Outpatient Medicine. *PLoS Medicine*, *2*(9), e290. doi:10.1371/journal.pmed.0020290 PMID:16173835

Durso, S. C. (2001). Technological advances for improving medication adherence in the elderly. *Annals of Long Term Care: Clinical Care and Aging, 9*, 43–48.

Fulton, M. M., & Riley Allen, E. (2005). Polypharmacy in the elderly: A literature review. *Journal of the American Academy of Nurse Practitioners, 17*(4), 123–132. doi:10.1111/j.1041-2972.2005.0020.x PMID:15819637

Governo, M., Riva, V., Fiorini, P., & Nugent, P. P. (2003). *MEDICATE Teleassistance System.* The 11th International Conference on Advance Robotics.

Kuperman, G. J., Bobb, A., Payne, T. H., Avery, A. J., Gandhi, T. K., Burns, G., & Bates, D. W. et al. (2007). Medication related clinical decision support in computerized provider order entry systems: A Review. *Journal of the American Medical Informatics Association, 14*(1), 29–40. doi:10.1197/jamia. M2170 PMID:17068355

Law, A. V., Ray, M. D., Knapp, K. K., & Balesh, K. K. (2003). Unmet needs in medication use process: Perceptions of physician, pharmacists, and patients. *Journal of the American Pharmaceutical Association, 43*(3), 394–402. doi:10.1331/154434503321831111 PMID:12836790

Lisby, M., Nielsen, L. P., & Mainz, J. (2005). Errors in the medication process: Frequency, type, and potential clinical consequences. *International Journal for Quality in Health Care, 17*(1), 15–22. doi:10.1093/intqhc/mzi015 PMID:15668306

Smaling, J., & Holt, M. A. (2005, April). Integration and automation transform medication administration safety. *Health Care Management Technology.*

Tsai, P. H., Shih, C. S., & Yu, C. Y. (2008). *Smart Medication Dispenser Design, Architecture and Implementation* (Technical Report TR-IIS-08-010). Institute of Information Science, Academia Sinica.

Veacez, P. J. (2006). An individual based framework for a study on medical error. *International Journal for Quality in Health Care, 18*(4), 314–319. doi:10.1093/intqhc/mzl011 PMID:16672255

Wan, D. (1999). Magic Medicaine Cabinet: A situated portal for consumer healthcare. *Proceedings of First International Symposium on Handheld and Ubiquitous Computing (HUC '99).* doi:10.1007/3-540-48157-5_44

Wertheimer, A. I., & Santella, T. M. (2003). Medication compliance research. *Journal of Applied Research in Clinical and Experimental Therapeutics, 3*(3), 254–261.

Yeh, H. C., Hsiu, P. C. C., Shih, S., Tsai, P. H., & Liu, J. W. S. (2006). APAMAT: A Prescription Algebra for Medication Authoring Tool. *Proceedings of IEEE International Conference on Systems, Man and Cybernetics.* doi:10.1109/ICSMC.2006.384807

KEY TERMS AND DEFINITIONS

Compliance: Compliance describes the degree to which a patient correctly follows medical advice.

Hardware Design: Allows hardware designers to understand how their components fit into system architecture and provides to software component designers important information needed for software development and integration.

Medical Dispensers: Items which release medication at specified times. Their purpose is to help senior citizens and other people who may suffer from impaired ability to adhere to their prescribed medication regime.

M-Health: A general term for the use of mobile phones and other wireless technology in medical care.

Software Design: The process of implementing *software* solutions to one or more sets of problems.

This research was previously published in Health Information Systems and the Advancement of Medical Practice in Developing Countries edited by Kgomotso H. Moahi, Kelvin Joseph Bwalya, and Peter Mazebe II Sebina, pages 93-114, copyright year 2017 by Medical Information Science Reference (an imprint of IGI Global).

Chapter 28
Achieving E-Health Success:
The Key Role for ANT

Nilmini Wickramasinghe
Epworth Healthcare, Australia & RMIT University, Australia

Arthur Tatnall
Victoria University, Australia

ABSTRACT

Healthcare delivery continues to be challenged in all OECD countries. To address these challenges, most are turning their attention to e-health as the panacea. Indeed, it is true that in today's global and networked world, e-health should be the answer for ensuring pertinent information, relevant data, and germane knowledge anywhere anytime so that clinicians can deliver superior healthcare. Sadly, healthcare has yet to realize the full potential of e-health, which is in stark contrast to other e-business initiatives such as e-government and e-education, e-finance, or e-commerce. This chapter asserts that it is only by embracing a rich theoretical lens of analysis that the full potential of e-health can be harnessed, and thus, it proffers Actor-Network Theory (ANT) as such a lens.

INTRODUCTION

Superior access, quality and value of healthcare services have become a global priority for healthcare to combat the exponentially increasing costs of healthcare expenditure. E-Health in its many forms and possibilities appears to offer a panacea for facilitating the necessary transformation for healthcare. While a plethora of e-health initiatives keep mushrooming both nationally and globally, there exists to date no unified system to evaluate these respective initiatives and assess their relative strengths and deficiencies in realizing superior access, quality and value of healthcare services. Our research serves to address this void. Specifically, we focus on three key components namely: 1) understanding the web of players (regulators, payers, providers, healthcare organizations, suppliers and last but not least patients) and how e-health can modify the interactions between these players as well as create added value healthcare services. 2) the development of an e-health preparedness grid that provides a universal assessment tool

DOI: 10.4018/978-1-5225-3926-1.ch028

for all e-health initiatives and 3) the development of an e-health manifesto, a declaration of policy, intent and the necessary components of successful e-health initiative. Taken together and applied systematically this will then enable a critical assessment of the areas that e-health initiatives should best target as well as the necessary steps and key success factors that must be addressed such as technological, infrastructure, education or policy elements. However, the paper goes further and notes that simply being e-health prepared is a necessary but not sufficient condition. It identifies the need to incorporate a rich theoretical lens of actor-network theory (ANT) in order to truly uncover all key issues and thereby ensure successful realization of the full potential of any e-health solution.

HEALTHCARE

Healthcare is a growing industry. Between 1960 and 1997 the percentage of Gross Domestic Product (GDP) spent on healthcare by 29 members of the Organization for Economic Cooperation and Development (OECD) nearly doubled from 3.9 to 7.6% while the growth between 1995-2005 was on average 4% with the US spending the most (nearly 2.5 times more than any other country) and this is expected to reach 19.5% GDP by 2017[1]. Since 2000, total spending on healthcare in these countries has been rising faster than economic growth, which has resulted in an average ratio of health spending to GDP of 9.0% in 2008 (OECD, 2010). Hence, reducing this expenditure as well as offering effective and efficient quality healthcare treatment is becoming a priority globally as is reflected in the fact that all OEDC countries are looking seriously into healthcare reform and especially the role for e-health solutions (OECD, 2010). Technology and automation have the potential to reduce these costs (Ghani et al., 2010; America Institute of Medicine, 2001; Wickramasinghe, 2000); thus, e-health, specifically the adoption and adaptation of web based technologies and advancements through Web 2.0, appears to be a powerful force of change for the healthcare industry worldwide.

Such external environmental forces are translating into numerous changes with regard to the role of technology for healthcare delivery at the organizational level. So much so that we are witnessing, healthcare providers grasping at many opportunities, especially in response to legislative mandates, to incorporate IT(information technology) and telecommunications with web based strategies to improve service and cost effectiveness to their key stakeholders; most notably patients. Many such e-initiatives including the e-medical record which in some form or other is currently being implemented in various countries. However these do not seem to represent a coherent and universal adoption of e-health.

To date, healthcare has been shaped by each nation's own set of cultures, traditions, payment mechanisms and patient expectations. Therefore, when looking at health systems throughout the world, it is useful to position them on a continuum (Figure 1) ranging from high (essentially 100%) government involvement (i. e. a public healthcare system as can be seen in the UK or Canada) at one extreme to little (essentially 0%) government involvement (i. e., private healthcare system as can be seen in the US) at the other extreme with many variations of a two tier system (i. e. mix of private and public as can be seen in countries like Australia and Germany) in between. However, given the common problem of exponentially increasing costs facing healthcare globally, irrespective of the particular health system one examines, the future of the healthcare industry will be partially shaped by commonalties such as this key unifying problem and the common forces of change including: i) empowered consumers, ii) e-health adoption and adaptability and iii) shift to focus on the practice of preventative versus cure

Figure 1. Continuum of healthcare systems

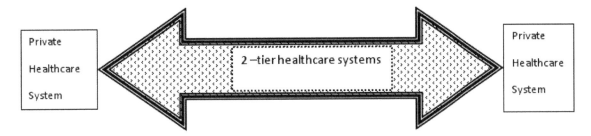

driven medicine, as well as four key implications, including: i) health insurance changes, ii) workforce changes and changes in the roles of stakeholders within the health system, iii) organizational changes and standardization and iv) the need for healthcare providers and administrators to make difficult, yet necessary choices regarding practice management.

E-HEALTH

E-health is a very broad term that encompasses various activities related to the use of many e-commerce technologies and infrastructures most notably the Internet for facilitating healthcare practice. The World Health Organization (WHO, 2005) defines e-health as "a new term used to describe the combined use of electronic communication and information technology in the health sector" or "as the use, in the health sector, of digital data-transmitted, stored and retrieved electronically-for clinical, educational and administrative purposes, both at the local site and at a distance". What is significant to note from this definition is that e-health entails the delivery of health services and health information enhanced through the Internet and other related e-commerce technologies. Moreover, the term characterizes not only a technical development, but also a paradigm shift to focus on networked, global thinking, to improve healthcare locally, regionally, and globally by using information and communication technologies which impact a web of players as depicted in Figure 2. E-health then is an emerging field at confluence of medical informatics, technology, public health and business.

In addition to the definition of e-health, we believe it is important when examining e-health initiatives to focus beyond the "electronic: component of the "e" in e-health and in fact think about this in a broader manner; i.e. to think of the 8 "e's" in e-health (i.e. efficiency, enhancing quality, evidence-based, empowerment, education, extending the scope, ethics and equity)(Eysenbach, 2001; Wickramasinghe et al, 2005; Wickramasinghe & Schaffer, 2010). Table 1 serves to summarize these important "e's" of e-health.

BEING E-HEALTH PREPARED

In order for successful e-health solutions to ensure a necessary first step is for a state of e-health preparedness to be achieved (Wickramasinghe et al., 2012; Wickramasinghe and Schaffer, 2010). An appropriate level of preparedness can only be achieved through the assessment and analysis of broadly-based knowledge and key facts (Wickramasinghe and Schaffer, 2010; Wickramasinghe et al., 2012).

Figure 2. Web of healthcare players (adapted from Wickramasinghe and Schaffer, 2010)

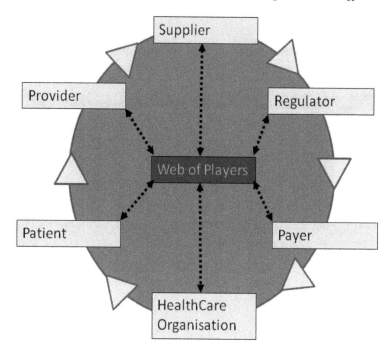

Table 1. Summary of the "e's" in e-health (Eysenbach, 2001; Wickramasinghe et al, 2005; Wickrama-singhe & Schaffer, 2010)

E's in E-Health	Description
Efficiency	Support cost effective healthcare delivery
Enhancing quality	Reduce medical errors
Evidence based	Support evidence based medicine
Empowerment	Help patients to be more active and informed in their healthcare decisions and treatments
Education	Help physicians and patients understand the latest techniques and healthcare issues
Extending the scope	Do not limit healthcare treatment to conventional boundaries
Ethics	Including but not limited to privacy and security concerns
Equity	Decrease rather than increase the gap between "haves" and "have nots"

Thus, development of appropriate preparedness is predominantly a strategic task that requires intimate knowledge of several aspects of the environment.

By taking into consideration all the e's of e-health and after a thorough analysis of various e-health initiatives as well as an in depth assessment of critical success factors necessary to effect successful e-health projects work by Wickramasinghe et al. (2005; Wickramasinghe and Schaffer, 2010) has resulted in the development of a framework to assess the e-health potential and preparedness of a country with regard to its e-health initiatives (Figure 3). In particular, the framework highlights the key elements that are required for successful e-health initiatives and therefore provides an elegant tool that allows analysis beyond the quantifiable data into a systematic synthesis of the major impacts and pre-requisites.

Figure 3. A framework for assessing a country's/region's e-health potential (adapted from Wickramas-inghe et al. 2005; Wickramasinghe and Schaffer, 2010)

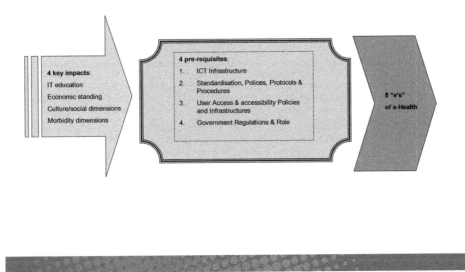

Moreover, the framework contains four main pre-requisites, four main impacts, and the implications of these parameters to the eight e's of e-health. Tables 2 and 3 serve to summarize the four pre-requisites and impacts respectively. By examining both the pre-requisites and the impacts, not only is it possible to assess the potential of a country and its preparedness for e-health but it is also possible to assess its ability to maximize the eight "e's" of e-health.

In assessing ones level of preparedness for any e-health initiative, a good first is to examine ones standing with respect to the four pre-requisites and four impacts discussed above and from this then evaluate if it will be possible to evaluate to move forward successfully (ref). In the following section, we will attempt to provide a guideline that will facilitate such an evaluation. A systematic way to do this is via the e-health preparedness grid.

THE E-HEALTH PREPAREDNESS GRID

By taking the four main pre-requisites as well as the four major impacts identified in the e-health frame-work in Figure 3; namely, the information communication technology infrastructure, the standardization policies, protocols and procedures, the user access and accessibility policies and infrastructures, gov-ernmental regulations and role as well as the impact of IT education, the impact of morbidity rate, the impact of world economic standing and the impact of cultural/social dimensions, it is possible to develop a grid for assessing e-health preparedness (Figure 4; Wickramasinghe et al., 2005; Wickramasinghe and Schaffer, 2010). The grid consists of four quadrants that represent the possible states of preparedness with respect to the key parameters for e-health success. The low preparedness quadrant identifies situa-tions that are low with respect to all four pre-requisites for e-health potential. The medium preparedness quadrant identifies two symmetric situations; namely, a combination of high and low positioning with respect to the four pre-requisites for e-health potential. Finally, the high preparedness quadrant identifies

Table 2. Pre-requisites for e-health (adapted from Wickramasinghe et al., 2005; Wickramasinghe and Schaffer, 2010)

Pre-Requisite	Description
ICT Infrastructure	A typical ICT infrastructure is envisaged to include a combination of the following: phone lines, fibre trunks and submarine cables, T1, T3 and OC-xx, ISDN, DSL other high-speed services used by businesses as well as satellites, earth stations and teleports. A sound technical infrastructure is an essential ingredient to the undertaking of e-health initiatives by any nation. Such infrastructures should also include telecommunications, electricity, access to computers, number of Internet hosts, number of ISP's (Internet Service Providers) and available bandwidth and broadband access. To offer a good multimedia content and thus provide a rich e-health experience, one would require a high bandwidth. ICT considerations are undoubtedly one of the most fundamental infrastructure requirements (Samiee, 1988).
Standardization Policies, Protocols and Procedures	As e-Health spans many parties and geographic dimensions, to enable such a far reaching coverage, significant amounts of document exchange and information flows must be accommodated. Standardization is the key for this. Hence, standardization polices, protocols and procedures must be developed at the outset to ensure the full realization of the eight e's of e-health. The standardization polices, protocols and procedures play a significant role in the adoption of e-health and the reduction of many structural impediments (Samiee, 1998).
User Access and Accessibility Policies and Infrastructure	Access to e-commerce is defined by the WTO (World Trade Organization) as consisting of two critical components 1) access to Internet services and 2) access to e-services (Panagariya, 2000). The user infrastructure includes a number of Internet hosts and number of web sites, web users as a percent of the population as well as ISP(internet service providers) availability and costs for consumers, PC penetration level etc.
Governmental Regulation and Control	The key challenges regarding e-health use include; 1) cost effectiveness; i.e. less costly than traditional healthcare delivery, 2) functionality and ease of use, i.e., they should enable and facilitate many uses for physicians and other healthcare users by combining various types and forms of data as well as be easy to use; and 3) they must be secure. One of the most significant legislative regulations in the US is the Health Insurance Portability and Accountability Act (HIPPA, 2001). Given the nature of healthcare and the sensitivity of healthcare data and information, it is incumbent on governments not only to mandate regulations that will facilitate the exchange of healthcare documents between the various healthcare stakeholders but also to provide protection of privacy and the rights of patients (Samiee, 1998; Goff, 1992; Gupta, 1992). Irrespective of the type of healthcare system; i.e., whether 100% government driven, 100% private or a combination thereof, it is clear that some governmental role is required to facilitate successful e-health initiatives.

Table 3. Key impacts for e-health (adapted from Wickramasinghe et al., 2005; Wickramasinghe and Schaffer, 2010)

Impacts	Description
IT Education	A sophisticated, well educated population boosts competition and hastens innovation. According to Michael Porter, one of the key factors to a country's strength in an industry is strong customer support (Porter, 1990). Thus, a strong domestic market leads to the growth of competition which leads to innovation and the adoption of technology enabled solutions to provide more effective and efficient services such as e-health and telemedicine. As the health consumer is the key driving force in pushing e-health initiatives, a more IT educated healthcare consumer would then provide stronger impetus for e-health adoption.
Morbidity Rate	There is a direct relationship between health education and awareness and the overall health standing of a country. Therefore, a more health conscious society, which tends to coincide with a society that has a lower morbidity rate, is more likely to embrace any e-health initiatives. Furthermore, higher morbidity rates tend to indicate the existence of more basic health needs (WHO, 2003) and hence treatment is more urgent than the practice of preventative medicine and thus e-health could be considered an unrealistic luxury and in some instances such as when a significant percentage of a population is suffering from malnutrition related diseases is even likely to be irrelevant at least in the short term. Thus, the modifying impact of morbidity rate is to prioritize the level of spending on e-health versus other basic healthcare needs.
Cultural/Social Dimensions	Healthcare has been shaped by each nation's own set of cultures, traditions, payment mechanisms and patient expectations. While the adoption of e-health, to a great extent, dilutes this cultural impact, social and cultural dimensions will still be a moderating influence on any countries e-health initiatives. Another aspect of the cultural/social dimension relates to the presentation language of the content of the e-health repositories. The entire world does not speak English so the e-health solutions have to be offered in many other languages. The e-health supporting content in web servers/ sites must be offered in local languages, supported by pictures and universal icons. This becomes a particularly important consideration when we look at the adoption and diffusion of evidence-based medicine as it will mean that much of the available evidence and case study data will not be easily accessible globally due to language barriers.
World Economic Standing	Economies of the future will be built around the Internet. All governments are very aware of the importance and critical role that the Internet will play on a country's economy. This makes it critical that appropriate funding levels and budgetary allocations become a key component of governmental fiscal policies so that such initiatives will form the bridge between a traditional healthcare present and a promising e-health future. Thus, the result of which would determine success of effective e-health implementations and consequently have the potential to enhance a country's economy and future growth.

Figure 4. E-Health preparedness grid (adapted from Wickramasinghe et al., 2005)

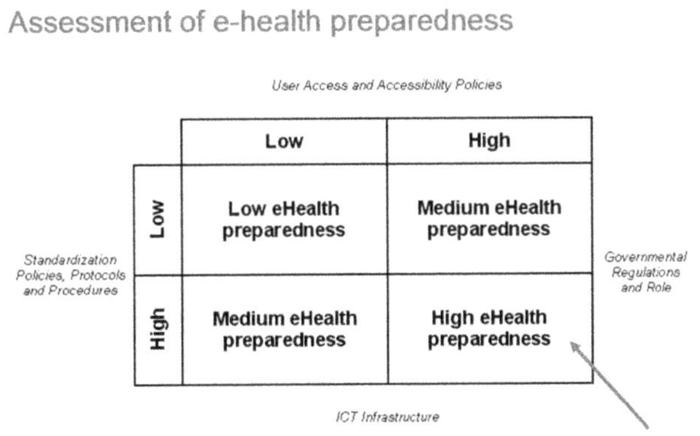

Assessment of e-health preparedness

User Access and Accessibility Policies

	Low	High
Low	Low eHealth preparedness	Medium eHealth preparedness
High	Medium eHealth preparedness	High eHealth preparedness

Standardization Policies, Protocols and Procedures

Governmental Regulations and Role

ICT Infrastructure

situations that are high with respect to all four pre-requisites for e-health potential. This grid not only shows the possible positioning of a given e-health initiative with respect to its e-health preparedness (i. e. low, medium or high) but also the path that should be taken, and more specifically the pre-requisite factors must be focused on, to migrate to the ideal state of preparedness.

However, being prepared is only the first necessary step. It is also essential to be ready for an up-coming-health initiative. Readiness must be based on germane knowledge. Furthermore it requires the background of germane knowledge that will dictate the nature of the subsequent response. Readiness is therefore context dependent. Readiness is thus a most essential tool in response to the embracement of a new e-health initiative. While intuitively obvious, the practical development of readiness is not an easy task. Possession of knowledge is not equivalent to the ability to employ it under the stress of less-than-routine circumstances. Thus to establish an appropriate level of readiness the first step is to assess the situation and key aspects through an appropriately robust and rich theoretical lens. We believe actor-network theory because of its ability to blend and combine social and technical perspectives is a most suitable lens.

ACTOR-NETWORK THEORY

Actor-Network Theory (ANT) is based on a recursive philosophy (Latour 1992). Its fundamental stand is that technologies and people are linked in a network. ANT tries to bridge the gap between a socio-technical divide by denying the existence of purely social or technical relations. In doing so it takes a very radical stand and assumes that each entity (such as technologies, organization) are actors therefore have the potential to transform and mediate social relationships (Cresswell et al. 2010). It also empha-sizes the concept of heterogeneous networks because of the non-similar nature of elements and their relationship in network makes these networks open and evolving systems (Hanseth 2007). Therefore Actor- networks are highly dynamic and inherently unstable in their nature; and a better understanding of how alignment between people, technology, their roles, routines, values, training and incentives as well as understanding of the role of technology that how it can facilitate or negatively impact the work processes and tasks in an organization can stabilize these network to some extent (Greenhalgh & Stones 2010; Wickramasinghe et al. 2011). For this reason, ANT can be a material-semiotic approach and can provide an appropriate lens to study the ordering of scientific, technological, social, and organizational processes and events (Wickramasinghe et al. 2011). To realize the importance of the application of ANT it is important to understand the key concepts of ANT and then map them to the critical issues concerning e-health initiatives.

Key Stages of ANT

In addition to the key concepts of ANT described in Table 4, there are also three critical stages of ANT which need to be considered as discussed in turn below.

Stage 1: Inscription

A process of creating technical text and communication artifacts to protect actor's interests in a network is described as an inscription (Leila 2009; Wickramasinghe & Bali 2009; Latour 2005). This is a term used for all texts and communications in different mediums including but not limited to journal articles, conference papers and presentations, grants proposals and patents. The idea of Inscription also relates to the notion of durability; for instance a general discussion would be less durable as compared to a recorded meeting. Therefore, the idea behind Inscription is to enhance the durability of the network by associating them with durable material. Actors can use Inscription as a path to gain credibility in enrolment and the co-optation process during translation.

Stage 2: Translation

Translation is a very important and vital concept in ANT. This term is used to explain the process of creation of Actor-Networks and the formation of ordering effects (Callon 1986; Law 1992). This stage can help researchers in providing the insight into how the software system can be integrated into the very complex environment of healthcare. The process of Translation can also be called the process of negotiation because after the creation of the network in the presence of many actors a strong or primary actor would translate interests of other actors into his/her own by negotiating with them. At this stage all actors decide to be part of network if it is worthwhile to build it (Wickramasinghe & Bali 2009).

The process of Translation of Actors/Actants is achieved through a series of four moments of translations (Callon, 1986). Figure 3 depicts the key ANT concepts along with these four moments of Translation.

Stage 3: Framing

Framing is an operation that can help to define actors and distinguish different actors and goods from each other (Callon, 1986). This last and final stage in the ANT process can help network to stabilize. At this stage key issues occurred throughout the e-health adoption /implementation should already have been negotiated within the network and technologies can become more stable over time (Wickramasinghe & Bali 2009).

Table 4. Key ANT concepts and their mapping to e-health initiatives

Key Constructs of ANT	Mapping to E-Health Initiatives
Actor/Actant: Actors are the web of participants in the network including all human and non-human entities. Because of the strong biased interpretation of the word actor towards human; a word actant is commonly used to refer both human and non-human actors.(Wickramasinghe et al. 2011).	In any e-health context Actors/Actants include different stakeholders in healthcare delivery settings such as Technology (Web 2.0, Databases, Graphical User Interfaces and different Computer hardware and Software) and People (service providers, healthcare funders, healthcare service recipients, healthcare organizations, suppliers and private health insurers) as well as clinical administrative technologies, work process and health records in the form of paper or electronic.
Heterogeneous Network: is a network of aligned interests formed by the actors. This is a network of materially heterogeneous actors that is achieved by a great deal of work that both shapes those various social and non-social elements, and "disciplines" them so that they work together, instead of "making off on their own" (Latour, 1996, Latour, 2005; Wickramasinghe et al. 2011).	The specific technology clearly forms the main network of different applications in this context. But it is important to understand that the heterogeneous network in ANT requires conceptualizing the network as aligned interest including people, organizations, standards and protocols and their interaction with technology.
Tokens/Quasi Objects: are created through the successful interaction of actors/actants in a network and are passed between actors within the network. As the token is increasingly transmitted or passed through the network, it becomes increasingly punctualized and also increasingly reified. When the token is decreasingly transmitted, or when an actor fails to transmit the token, punctualization and reification are decreased as well (Wickramasinghe et al. 2011).	In e-health contexts this translates to successful cost effective and efficient healthcare delivery. It is important to understand that to maintain the integrity of the network at all times is very important because if wrong information is passed through the network, the errors would be devastating and can propagate quickly and will multiply.
Punctualization: Within the domain of ANT every actor in the web of relations is connected to others and as a whole it will be considered as a single object or concept same as the concept of abstraction is treated in Object Oriented Programming. These sub-actors are sometime hidden from the normal view and only can be viewed in case of the network break-down; this concept is often referred as a depunctulization. Because ANT require all actors or sections of network to perform required tasks and therefore maintain the web of relations. In case of any actor cease to operate or maintain link the entire Actor-Network would break down resulting in ending the punctualization. Punctualization is a process and cannot be achieved indefinitely rather is a relational effect and is recursive that can reproduce itself (Law 1997)	For example, a computer on which one is working would be treated as a single block or unit. Only when it breaks down and one needs help with spare parts can reveal the hidden chain of network consist of different actors made up of (People, Computer parts and organizations). Similarly in an e-health context, uploading the health record of a patient is in reality a consequence of the interaction and coordination of many sub-tasks. This will only reveal itself if some kind of breakdown at this point occurs and depunctualization of the network happens and all sub-tasks then would need to be carefully examined.
Obligatory Passage Point (OPP): broadly refers to a situation that has to occur in order for all the actors to satisfy the interests that have been attributed to them by the focal actor. The focal actor defines the OPP through which the other actors must pass through and by which the focal actor becomes indispensable (Callon, 1986).	In e-health contexts, we can illustrate this by taking the example of access and user rights. The interface of the system is developed in a way that no service can access any record without using secure logins, which in this case constitute an obligatory passage point through which they have to pass for their everyday activities.
Irreversibility: Callon (1986, p. 159) states that the degree of irreversibility depends on (i) the extent to which it is subsequently impossible to go back to a point where that translation was only one amongst others and (ii) the extent to which it shapes and determines subsequent translations.	In the context of the very complex nature of healthcare operations, irreversibility is less likely to occur and would be more dependent on social networks and the nature of the interaction between human and non-human actors in the network. Here it is important to remember though the chain of events needs to be monitored carefully so the future events can be addressed in the best possible manners.

DISCUSSION

ANT is considered an appropriate choice to facilitate a state of readiness in the context of e-health initiatives because it can identify and acknowledge any impact of human and non-human social or policy issues within the healthcare setting (Latour et al. 1996). Moreover, it is robust enough to accurately capture all the complexities, nuances and richness of healthcare operations. In so doing, it can also help to investigate and theorize the question of why and how networks come into existence, what sort of associations and impact they can have on each other, how they move and change their position in a network, how they enrol and leave the network and most importantly how these networks can achieve stability (Doolin & Lowe 2002; Callon 1986; McLean & Hassard 2004). ANT's assumption is that if any new actor is enrolled in the network or an old actor leaves the network it would affect whole network (Cresswell et al. 2010; Doolin & Lowe 2002). These considerations are naturally most relevant in the context of any e-health scenario.

In addition, ANT also can help to understand the active role of objects in shaping social realities by challenging assumptions of the separation between non-human and human worlds (Walsham 1997; Greenhalgh & Stones 2010; Tobler 2008; Law & Hassard 1999; Rydin 2010). This helps researchers to study the complexities of the relationships between human and non-human actors, the sustainability of power relationships between human actors and what kind of influence artifacts can have on human actors relationships in transforming healthcare (Cresswell et al. 2010).

The rationale to choose ANT to assess the state of readiness for any e-health initiative is thus connected with the strength of ANT to identify and explore the real and perceived complexities involved in the healthcare service delivery sector. Indeed several scholars have noted the benefits of ANT and it has been applied in the implementation and adoption of different healthcare innovation studies (Berg, 2001; Cresswell et al. 2010; Cresswell et al. 2011; Bossen, 2007; Hall, 2005). To date it has yet to be embraced as a tool to facilitate a macro level analysis of e-health readiness as we have suggested in the proceeding discussion.

CONCLUSION

E-commerce, as noted by the UN Secretary General's address, is an important aspect of business in today's 21st century. No longer then is it a luxury for nations, rather it is a strategic necessity in order for countries to achieve economic and business prosperity as well as social viability. One of the major areas within e-commerce that has yet to reach its full potential is e-health. This is due to the fact that healthcare generally has been slow in adopting information technologies. In addition most e-health initiatives to date have been less than successful. Not only is there a shortage of robust normative frameworks that may be used as guidelines for assessing e-health preparedness and identifying the key areas and deficiencies that need to be addressed in order for successful e-heath initiatives to ensue, but also there is a lack of appropriate analytic frameworks to address the level of readiness. Moreover, e-health is more than a technological initiative; rather it also requires a major paradigm shift in healthcare delivery, practice and thinking. We have attempted to address this gap by discussing the need to be both prepared and ready. To address the needs of preparedness we have discussed the importance of – and presented a useful framework to- assessing e-health preparedness and thereby, facilitating the focus of efforts and resources on the relevant issues that must be addressed in order that successful e-health initiatives follow (i. e., the eight e's of e-health are in fact realized). For readiness, we have presented ANT as an appropriate, robust and rich, theoretical framework. The first step in the development of any viable e-health strategy is to make an assessment of the current state of e-health preparedness and then how to either move to a state of higher preparedness (i. e., the high quadrant) or focus on maintaining a current high quadrant status – both of these will be possible through the use of our framework and thus its value. It is advised that next an assessment of readiness is made which by definition must be context dependent. We believe that taken together the assessments of preparedness and readiness will enable a comprehensive assessment for e-health initiatives, that to date has been lacking. More importantly such a comprehensive assessment will ensure that successful outcomes and the full potential of the e-health solution is indeed realized.

REFERENCES

America Institute of Medicine. (2001). *Crossing the Quality Chasm - A New Health System for the 21st Century Committee on Quality of Health Care*. National Academy Press.

Eysenbach, G. (2001). What is e-health? *Journal of Medical Internet Research*, *3*(2). doi:10.2196/jmir.3.2.e20

Ghani, M., Bali, R., & Naguib, I., Marshall, & Wickramasinghe, N. (2010). Critical issues for implementing a Lifetime Health Record in the Malaysian Public Health System. [IJHTM]. *International Journal of Healthcare Technology and Management*, *11*(1/2), 113–130. doi:10.1504/IJHTM.2010.033279

Goff, L. (1992). Patchwork of Laws Slows EC data Flow. *Computerworld*, *26*(15), 80.

Gupta, U. (1992). Global Networks: Promises and Challenges. *Information Systems Management*, *9*(4), 28–32. doi:10.1080/10580539208906896

Health Insurance Portability and Accountability Act (HIPPA). (2001, May). *Privacy Compliance Executive Summary*. Protegrity Inc.

OECD. (2010). *OECD health data 2010*. Retrieved from http://stats.oecd.org/Index.aspx?DatasetCode=HEALTH World Health Organization (WHO). (2005). *What is e-health?* Retrieved from http://www.emro.who.int/his/ehealth/AboutEhealth.htm

Panagariya, A. (2000). E-commerce, WTO and developing countries. *World Economy*, *23*(8), 959–978. doi:10.1111/1467-9701.00313

Porter, M. (1990). *The Competitive advantage of Nations*. New York: Free Press.

PricewaterhouseCoopers Healthcare Practice. (n.d.). Retrieved from www.pwchealth.com

Samiee, S. (1998). The Internet and International Marketing: Is There a Fit? *Journal of Interactive Marketing*, *12*(4), 5–21. doi:10.1002/(SICI)1520-6653(199823)12:4<5::AID-DIR2>3.0.CO;2-5

United Nations Conference on trade and Development. (2002). Retrieved from http://r0.unctad.org/ecommerce/ecommerce_en

Wickramasinghe, N. (2000). IS/IT as a Tool to Achieve Goal Alignment: A theoretical framework. *International Journal of Healthcare Technology and Management*, *2*(1-4), 163–180. doi:10.1504/IJHTM.2000.001089

Wickramasinghe, N., Bali, R., Kirn, S., & Sumoi, R. (2012). *Critical Issues for the Development of Sustainable E-health Solutions*. New York: Springer. doi:10.1007/978-1-4614-1536-7

Wickramasinghe, N., Fadllala, A. M. A., Geisler, E., & Schaffer, J. L. (2005). A framework for assessing e-health preparedness. *International Journal e-Health, 1* (3), 316-334.

Wickramasinghe, N., & Schaffer, J. (2010). *Realzing Value Driven e-health Solutions.* Washington, DC: IBM Center for the Business of Government.

World Health Organization (WHO). (2003). Retrieved February 23, 2010 from http://www.emro.who.int/ehealth/

KEY TERMS AND DEFINITIONS

E-Health: The use of computer and web based technologies to provide healthcare delivery.

E-Health Potential: The initial ability and structures that an entity possesses before implementing an e-health solution. The better suited the underlying structure is and the better skilled the key stakeholders are regarding e-health the more prepared the entity is said to be.

Healthcare Challenges: Key areas that are impacting the ease of healthcare delivery e.g. escalating financial pressures, rapid increase of technology solutions, an aging population and the growth of chronic diseases.

Preparedness: Is predominantly a strategic task that requires intimate knowledge of several aspects of the environment.

Readiness: Is based on germane knowledge and it requires the background of germane knowledge that will dictate the nature of the subsequent response. Readiness is therefore context dependent.

ENDNOTE

[1]   OECD Health Data 2009.

This research was previously published in Technological Advancements and the Impact of Actor-Network Theory edited by Arthur Tatnall, pages 209-221, copyright year 2014 by Information Science Reference (an imprint of IGI Global).

Chapter 29
Health Apps by Design:
A Reference Architecture for Mobile Engagement

Pannel Chindalo
InfoClin, Toronto, Canada

Arsalan Karim
InfoClin, Toronto, Canada

Ronak Brahmbhatt
InfoClin, Toronto, Canada

Nishita Saha
InfoClin, Toronto, Canada

Karim Keshavjee
InfoClin, Toronto, Canada

ABSTRACT

The mobile health (mhealth) app market continues to grow rapidly. However, with the exception of fitness apps and a few isolated cases, most mhealth apps have not gained traction. The barriers preventing patients and care providers from using these apps include: for patients, information that contradicts health care provider advice, manual data entry procedures and poor fit with their treatment plan; for providers, distrust in unknown apps, lack of congruence with workflow, inability to integrate app data into their medical record system and challenges to analyze and visualize information effectively. In this article, the authors build upon previous work to define design requirements for quality mhealth apps and a framework for patient engagement to propose a new reference architecture for the next generation of healthcare mobile apps that increase the likelihood of being useful for and used by patients and health care providers alike.

DOI: 10.4018/978-1-5225-3926-1.ch029

INTRODUCTION

The popularity and usage of mobile technology continues to boom (Research2guidance, 2015). Increasingly, people are inclined to seek guidance from smartphones than from other persons (Elias, 2015). Smartphones' ascendance to this level is highly associated to its practicality in communicating, information resourcefulness, portability and flexible costs for most people, regardless of their economic status (Silow-Carroll & Smith, 2013). Mobile health (mhealth) care applications are seeing a similar boom. Of the millions of apps in circulation, about 45,000 are mhealth apps (Research2guidance, 2015). More than half of these mhealth apps are new on the market. Thirteen percent of these apps were introduced in the first quarter of 2015. However, most mhealth apps are not used in healthcare despite their growing popularity (in terms of downloads) and potential medical purposes (Research2guidance, 2015).

Researchers from various backgrounds have proposed ways that consumers can select useful mhealth apps for their health and health information needs (Albrecht, 2013; Boudreaux, 2014; Powell, 2014; Kumar, 2013). Several studies have identified hurdles that challenge wide usage, including poor user interface designs, differing user literacy levels, implementation issues and organizational structures (Bailey, 2014, Boudreaux 2014; Brown 2013; Caburnay, 2015; McMillan, 2015; McCurdie, 2012). These efforts have so far not been successful at wooing patients and care providers to greater use of mhealth apps. Health app developers are caught in a dilemma of not knowing how to overcome these hurdles.

In this paper, we build upon Albrecht et al.'s "synopsis for apps" in health care (Albrecht, 2014) to propose a novel reference architecture for mhealth apps that can overcome current barriers. Albrecht et al provide a comprehensive framework for mhealth app publishers to describe their compliance with a variety of pragmatic and evidence-informed criteria that are worth considering when evaluating apps. We found their framework useful as a scaffold for considering important elements of an app during the design process.

We also build upon the patient engagement framework developed by Balouchi et al. that describes an enabling environment for engagement and communication between patients and providers (Balouchi, 2014). We propose a refined approach for engaged communication between patients and care providers. This approach focuses on the patient and care provider relationship as the starting place to add value that is likely to grow exponentially in ways we can only now imagine. Our approach considers the constraints identified by the studies cited above in order to identify the critical functions that can elevate how apps can deliver added value. Further, we propose an architecture for mhealth apps that arranges the critical functions identified in order to accomplish the following: (a) capture, validate and communicate data about the processes and outcomes of a disease; and (b) enable on-going communication during treatment to enhance the patient-care provider relationship and ensure patients get the support they need to implement the advice and interventions prescribed by their health care provider.

METHODS

We conducted a literature search in PubMed and Google Scholar to identify articles that described methods to evaluate mobile apps. We utilized the related articles feature to find additional articles. We also identified articles on mhealth architecture and patient engagement with apps. We conducted a narrative synthesis of the studies we identified and applied a critical analysis by way of identifying common hurdles that restrict wide usage of mhealth apps. Our process of deliberation comprised distributing the studies we identified as critical to the research topic. We had three workings sessions: one concept development meeting which led to designating responsibilities for drafting the study's sections; a rethinking and refinement session and a final interdisciplinary discussion to finalize the story arc of the study. We also utilized Google Drive file sharing to coordinate our communication.

We used a gap analysis that drew on philosophy, data science, education, life science and business analyses methods to develop a concept that would overcome the constraints and meet the goals identified in the introduction. Through analysis, discussion and iteration, we arrived at a proposed architecture that is evidence-informed, uses validated tools effectively and is situated in a philosophy that puts a high value on the patient-physician relationship.

RESULTS

Other than fitness tracker apps and some tethered apps provided by insurance companies and by integrated delivery systems, most mhealth apps in app stores have not gained much traction (Research-2guidance, 2015). We hypothesize that this is due to multiple factors: a) apps may provide information that conflicts with information received from health care providers (Bierbrier, Lo & Wu, 2014); b) the language and terminology of the app may not be compatible with the patient's health literacy (Caburnay, 2015); c) the patient has to enter the data himself or herself (Gruman, 2013); d) the patient has no way to use the information in a meaningful way; e.g., they cannot order diagnostic testing for or prescribe medications to themselves; e) daily use of the app is not required for most diseases and therefore the patient does not get into the habit of using it; f) lack of incentives to use, such as cost savings or social approval; g) providers may not value or use the data collected by patients in apps downloaded from an app store whose provenance and pedigree is not known or established (Terry, 2015); h) there is no way for providers to consume (i.e., visualize, analyze, derive meaning from) the large amounts of data that are collected in apps (Terry, 2015) and i) there is no way for providers to integrate the app data into their own electronic medical record system (EMR) for analysis or follow-up or share the data in their EMR with their patient's apps (Abebe, 2013).

In our search, we identified authors who are pioneering a paradigm that is supportive of a scientific validation process and a technology convenient platform. The Open mHealth group (Chen, 2012) has developed some sophisticated tools to assist app publishers in designing and developing useful mhealth apps. Their open source tools allow developers to obtain standardized data from other systems and display them in high quality visualizations. However, the "architecture" they present is focused entirely on an information technology view. There is no proposed business architecture or information architecture. Thus, developers are left to their own devices on how they will connect the various pieces of technology to create a viable technology. Silow-Carroll and Smith (Silow-Carroll, 2013) describe apps that have had some success in healthcare. They point to several features which have gained some success, including having apps prescribed by health care providers who monitor their use and patient outcomes. These exemplars are mostly found in leading health care systems like Geisinger and Kaiser Permanente. However, they do not propose a comprehensive architecture that can be used by mhealth developers as a reference architecture.

Our approach, illustrated in Figure 1, is an adaptation of Balouchi et al.'s "enabling environment" for patient engagement. Successful use of mhealth apps is predicated on having an enabling environment, including the functions shown in the margins of the diagram (Balouchi, 2014). To this enabling

Figure 1. Patient-Health provider centered approach (Adapted from Balouchi)

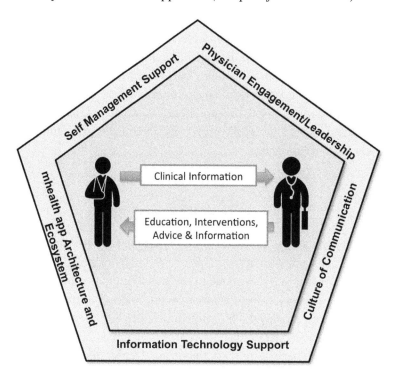

environment, we propose that mhealth apps must, in addition, provide useful functions to have value for health care providers and patients. At a high level, this means that the app must be able to capture clinical information about the patient that providers can use for their clinical decision-making and treatment recommendations. And, the app must also be able to communicate advice, education, information and treatment recommendations from providers to the patient. This simple architecture, if applied correctly, can be a powerful driver of change through on-going feedback, accountability and congruence between patient and provider; something that is sorely missing in current mhealth apps.

As previously mentioned, some of the leading health systems in the US, such as Geisinger and Kaiser Permanente, have already started along this path. Other care models such as the Accountable Care Organizations (ACOs), the Patient Centred Medical Homes (PCMH) and the Ontario Family Health Teams (FHTs) are all care models that have elements of the enabling environment in place for chronic disease management. Health care providers working within these organizations already have the infrastructure and the reimbursement model (salaried or capitation funding) to facilitate use of mhealth apps within their practice offerings.

Context for Patient Engagement

Patients and healthcare providers have for centuries operated in a relationship that demonstrates trust, skills, dependence and knowledge. Yet, most mhealth apps try to avoid getting entangled in this relationship. It would be helpful to introduce mhealth apps into the patient and health provider relationship (Edelman & Singer, 2015).

Most commercial mhealth apps do not take into consideration the critical role of the patient-healthcare provider relationship. A patient and health provider relationship is important for patients to understand the difference between a gadget for entertainment and a tool for improving health. In order to understand how seemingly this small difference can have an outsize impact, we have to see it from patients' and healthcare providers' viewpoints. On the one hand, a patient's perspective is informed by a culture of excitement for hi-tech gadgets that has become part of daily life experiences. Consumers have developed an insatiable appetite for hi-tech gadgets that compete for their attention. This high expectation not only drives business, but it also reduces the shelf-life of hi-tech gadgets. This cultural expectation could explain the lack of retention of mhealth apps. On the other hand, a healthcare provider's perspective on hi-tech is very different when it comes to professional practice. A health provider makes a clear distinction between a gadget for entertainment and how to evaluate its use in a professional environment. There are a lot of apps that give health information for personal use, but this type of information may not be credible for a licensed healthcare provider to use when advising a patient in a healthcare binding relationship. A licensed healthcare provider is trained to advise patients by using information that is acceptable by a professional code of standards as they evaluate a patient's condition and a patient's overall health story. An evidence-based assessment that a health provider performs before advising a patient requires an understanding of approved evidence-based knowledge about the problem, transforming this knowledge in view of the patient's condition based on clinical experience and arriving at a final treatment decision based on discussion with the patient about their values and preferences. For our discussion purpose, it means that both the patient and the healthcare provider do not consider standalone mhealth apps as credible resources in their healthcare relationship. In practice, it simply means that an app fails a reality-test to patients and health providers for reasons of entertainment and unreliable measurements respectively. In order to gain acceptance, mhealth apps need to be designed to enter, meet, and enhance the patient and the health provider relationship. A patient and a health provider relationship is based on trust and skills, as such apps should be designed in a way that they could become valuable resources that fill-in the gaps in knowledge and support in a patient-provider relationship.

The task of advising patients to perceive apps as a form of "prescription" in order to enhance treatment and communicate a sense of accountability depends on the health providers' willingness to use apps. Patients are likely to associate an mhealth app as a treatment plan when health providers introduce to it to them in that way. Educating healthcare providers about how an app meets the scientific standards of measurements and demonstrating how user-friendly designs account for their diverse clientele's educational levels and age groups is crucial to their acceptance. User-friendly designs, ability to capture important information between visits, ability to monitor follow-throughs on patients, reduced time pressure during encounters and higher productivity are likely to self-advertise apps into the patient and healthcare provider relationship. Licensed health providers have considerable moral and psychological influence within the patient-provider relationship to rebrand and introduce mhealth apps as critical communication devices during monitoring or treatment phases.

Complying with Scientific Standards

Many apps are proving that useful algorithms can be generated without a scientific validating process. So why do we need a scientific validating process for mhealth apps? We use an illustration from the sporting industry. It is intriguing to observe how excited people become after a major sporting event like tennis or soccer. In excitement, people go to soccer fields and tennis courts to emulate the skills they watched on television. Soon, most fans realize that it requires above average skills and body conditioning to perform like conditioned athletes. Technology has a way of exciting people who don't understand it to think big but are soon disappointed by their lack of skills. Just because an app can take a blood pressure measurement and produce information about our bodies does not make patients experts in healthcare. Scales and measurements used for assessing and treating patients should be left to the experts.

Human ailments are diverse and specializations in health have developed validated ways of measuring and assessing diseases. mHealth apps could customize these scales and make them available for patients and healthcare providers. Success in patient treatment has depended on healthcare providers and patients as "managers" of treatment plans. It makes sense that this relationship be supplied with first class resources. The expediency of technology could enable treatment resources with an added value of communicating, monitoring and encouraging the patient in real-time from any location.

It is important to realize that the worth of specialized scales comes to make sense only when a patient's information is aligned with it to enable interpretation. The need to make precise interpretation about a patient's condition by using verifiable measurements that have been scientifically validated is critical for making a diagnosis and individualizing a treatment plan to the unique needs of each patient. The ease of appearance that technology gives healthcare makes it appear flatteringly simple, but the disciplined body of knowledge it takes to diagnose and set a treatment plan is complex. Figure 2 describes in further detail the types of information required for appropriate management of a patient in the context of the patient-provider relationship. More description is provided in the section entitled, Process and Outcomes.

Empowering the Patient

Inherent within the patient-provider relationship, there is a power and information asymmetry. Physicians have access to and control access to information generated by the health system, such as laboratory results, specialist reports, imaging reports and other health care data. Introducing mhealth apps in this relationship could empower patients and health providers in ways that could improve health care systems. The current structure positions the patient in a subservient role. The reasons are obvious, the patient describes the problem, and the expert interprets what it means according to the patient's medical history. In practice a healthcare provider may request tests in order to identify the cause of the problem. As expected the healthcare provider informs and advises a patient about a diagnosis. In most cases patients have little or superficial knowledge about their diagnosis. When patients are given an opportunity to ask questions, they are still at a disadvantage of lacking knowledge to ask informative questions.

Figure 2. Communicating process and outcomes in mHealth apps

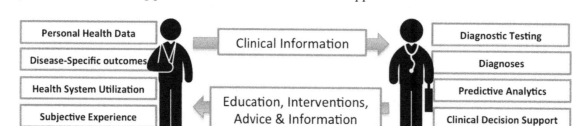

Many healthcare providers are well trained in delivering diagnosis news and proceeding further into treatment plans. In summary patients' dependence on healthcare providers is necessitated by a structure that limits patients and healthcare providers to spaces in buildings. There are many ways that apps would elevate the nature of this relationship. The potential of apps to collect information from patients during treatment is critical for empowering patients to speak about their experiences in real-time. This process can lead to collecting data based on patients' experiences and treatment outcomes in order to improve quality, patient awareness and professionalism.

Measuring Process and Outcomes

A trusted structure or framework speaks to the idea that content of apps need to be evidence-based (Albrecht, 2014). It is well-known that information technology exerts its effect through automating work flows and work processes; it is not a magic wand. An app is unlikely to provide valuable information without a defined process on how information should flow.

A validated evidence-based process requires a purposive procedure for ensuring the accuracy of patient information that is collected. For example, Coleman (2009) provides a chronic disease model that exemplifies a process of collecting information on a chronic disease.

Figure 2 describes a simple, but powerful information and business workflow that is centered on the patient-provider relationship. A mhealth app that meets evidence-based content and process requirements would embody the following properties:

1. It would explicitly identify the patient's diagnosis to ensure that the patient is eligible for guideline or other evidence-based content. Further, the physician should make the diagnosis and the app should be 'prescribed' by the physician as part of a course of treatment for the patient (see Figure 3). The app should interoperate with the EMR to allow this prescription functionality to activate it only when authorized by a licensed provider.

2. It would identify and track the process and proxy metrics for that disease (e.g., frequency of visits required for monitoring the disease, the biomarkers and/or patient questionnaires used to monitor disease severity for a particular disease such as HbA1c, blood pressure, PHQ9 scores, pain scores, etc.). Modern apps and Big Data approaches require as much data as possible to monitor and evaluate a patient's progress. Gamification data and other user behavior data is useful to an extent where its metric is assessed within a context of other validated metrics that correlate with the disease.

3. Identify and track important outcome measures. This includes clinical outcomes such as heart attacks, specialist consultations, medical procedures, hospitalization, strokes and death, which will come from the EMR. Patient reported outcome measures (PROMs) of all types need to be captured for comprehending patient specific patient health profile and data collection. Patient reported experience measures (PREMs) are also necessary to understand patient's subjective experiences that may have relevance to treatment adherence or goals. Any and all of the above outcome measures may be relevant for a particular disease and predictable based on process and proxy measures collected as described above. These need to be part of the mHealth app, since they are unlikely to be made available by the EMR vendor.

Figure 3. Sequence of Interactions between provider and patient in an mHealth app

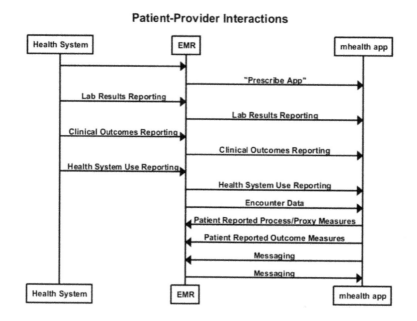

The concepts described above fit very nicely into Albrecht et al.'s framework (Albrecht 2014) into Item 4 Validity and Reliability, creating new Sub Items which we would label 4.3 Process and Proxy Measures and 4.4 Outcomes and Outcome Measures.

It is important to understand why this functionality must come from the mHealth app and not from the EMR. Most EMR vendors do not have the clinical knowledge or expertise to develop the type of functionality required for the mHealth apps described in this paper. mHealth app developers need to understand the entire value chain for the management of a particular disease and then make that available to patients and providers in their respective ehealth platforms –the PHR and the EMR.

EMR and App Interoperability

In order to ensure credibility of the data, which is critical for patient follow-up, the *provenance* of information (i.e., where it originates) is very important. For example, a physician should enter a diagnosis. A patient entered diagnosis, although useful, could be a sign that the physician lacks commitment to patient engagement, patient self-management and field professionalism. It could also be erroneously interpreted or understood by the patient. This means that the health care provider should activate the app to ensure that it is part of a "prescribed" intervention.

The app also needs to have interoperability with EMRs. This would provide the patient with important information that is recorded in the EMR by a clinician during a patient encounter or that is reported by various health care organizations to the physicians EMR (Figure 4). Interoperability is also required for patients to report important information such as process measures and self-monitoring information back to the physician or their designate for action or to update their records. There are an increasing number of interoperability platforms available to support this, including Open mHealth (Open mHealth, 2015), SMART Health IT (Smart Health IT, 2015) and the Apple HealthKit.

Figure 4. Reference architecture for mHealth app integration with EMRs

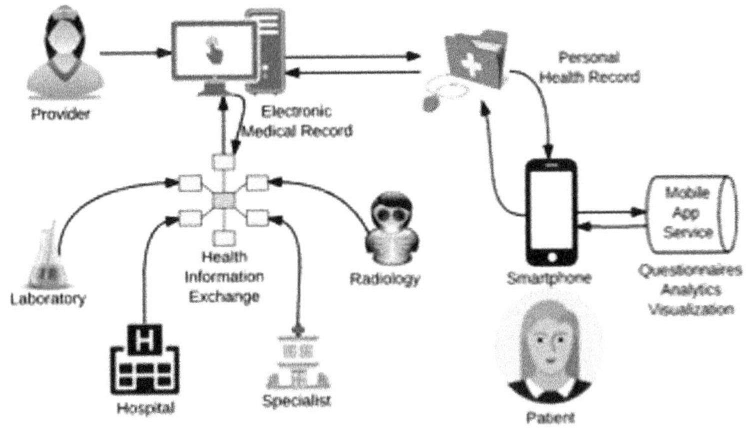

For the patient to be able to get appropriate support for questions about new information received or new symptoms or issues that arise from time to time, the app should allow for messaging back to the physician or their designate. The app should also allow the provider to communicate important updates and disease relevant information to the patient (Figure 3).

The concepts described in this section also fit well into Albrecht et al.'s (Albrecht, 2015) framework as additions to Item 5 Data requisitioning and management as new Sub Item 5.2 EMR-App Interoperability and 5.3 App-EMR Messaging.

CONCLUSION

This paper discusses a novel, interoperable architecture that can help mhealth apps become widely used as an asset for the enhancement of health care by strengthening the patient-provider relationship. The paper presents the difficulties that are impeding the acceptance of apps in health care. Although the hurdles for apps usage in health care are several, the paper focused on introducing apps into the patient and healthcare provider relationship because of the respect it commands among patients. By introducing mhealth into the patient and healthcare provider structure, especially physicians, it would communicate the importance apps can bring to healthcare. It is possible that patients and culture could eventually woo healthcare practitioners into accepting mhealth apps but the risks of this approach would require more work. In contrast, most healthcare providers are likely to be persuaded if apps were to embrace age-old cultural norms and values of the patient-provider relationship, core scientific methods of using validated measures in order to have confidence in the measurements that apps generate and interoperability that ensures two way communications. In an effort to differentiate our approach from providers 'prescribing' mhealth apps from the app store, we incorporate validating capabilities, communication and interoperability as keystones to facilitate patient empowerment, engagement and follow-up within the context of the patient-provider relationship.

REFERENCES

Abebe, N. A., Capozza, K. L., Des Jardins, T. R., Kulick, D. A., Rein, A. L., Schachter, A. A., & Turske, S. A. (2013). Considerations for community-based initiatives: Insights from three Beacon Communities. *Journal of Medical Internet Research*, *15*(10), e221. doi:10.2196/jmir.2803 PMID:24128406

Albrecht, U. V. (2013). Transparency of health-apps for trust and decision making. *Journal of Medical Internet Research*, *15*(12), e277. doi:10.2196/jmir.2981 PMID:24449711

Albrecht, U. V., Pramann, O., & von Jan, U. (2014). *Synopsis for health apps–transparency for trust and decision making. In Social Media and Mobile Technologies for Healthcare*. Hershey, PA, USA: IGI Global.

Bailey, S. C., Belter, L. T., Pandit, A. U., Carpenter, D. M., Carlos, E., & Wolf, M. S. (2014). The availability, functionality, and quality of mobile applications supporting medication self-management. *Journal of the American Medical Informatics Association*, *21*(3), 542–546. doi:10.1136/amiajnl-2013-002232 PMID:24163156

Balouchi, S., Keshavjee, K., Zbib, A., Vassanji, K., & Toor, J. (2014). Creating a Supportive Environment for Self-Management in Healthcare via Patient Electronic Tools. *Social Media and Mobile Technologies for Healthcare*, 109.

Bierbrier, R., Lo, V., & Wu, R. C. (2014). Evaluation of the accuracy of smartphone medical calculation apps. *Journal of Medical Internet Research*, *16*(2), e32. doi:10.2196/jmir.3062 PMID:24491911

Boudreaux, E. D., Waring, M. E., Hayes, R. B., Sadasivam, R. S., Mullen, S., & Pagoto, S. (2014). Evaluating and selecting mobile health apps: Strategies for healthcare providers and healthcare organizations. *Translational Behavioral Medicine*, *4*(4), 363–371. doi:10.1007/s13142-014-0293-9 PMID:25584085

Brown, W. III, Yen, P. Y., Rojas, M., & Schnall, R. (2013). Assessment of the Health IT Usability Evaluation Model (Health-ITUEM) for evaluating mobile health technology. *Journal of Biomedical Informatics*, *46*(6), 1080–1087. doi:10.1016/j.jbi.2013.08.001 PMID:23973872

Caburnay, C. A. (2015). Evaluating diabetes mobile applications for health literate designs and functionality, 2014. *Preventing Chronic Disease*, 12. PMID:25950568

Chen, C., Haddad, D., Selsky, J., Hoffman, J. E., Kravitz, R. L., Estrin, D. E., & Sim, I. (2012). Making sense of mobile health data: An open architecture to improve individual-and population-level health. *Journal of Medical Internet Research*, *14*(4), e112. doi:10.2196/jmir.2152 PMID:22875563

Coleman, K., Austin, B. T., Brach, C., & Wagner, E. H. (2009). Evidence on the Chronic Care Model in the new millennium. *Health Affairs*, *28*(1), 75–85. doi:10.1377/hlthaff.28.1.75 PMID:19124857

Edelman, D., & Singer, M. (2015). Competing on customer journeys. *HBR.org*. Retrieved from https://hbr.org/product/competing-on-customer-journeys/R1511E-PDF-ENG

Elias, J. (2015). In 2016, Users Will Trust Health Apps More Than Their Doctors. *Forbes*. Retrieved from http://www.forbes.com/sites/jenniferelias/2015/12/31/in-2016-users-will-trust-health-apps-more-than-their-doctors/

Grumman, J. (2013). What Patients Want from Mobile Apps. Retrieved from http://www.kevinmd.com/blog/2013/04/patients-mobile-apps.html

HONcode. (n. d.). Operational definition of the HONcode principles. Retrieved from http://www.hon.ch/HONcode/Webmasters/Guidelines/guidelines.html

Kumar, S., Nilsen, W. J., Abernethy, A., Atienza, A., Patrick, K., Pavel, M., & Hedeker, D. et al. (2013). Mobile health technology evaluation: The evidence workshop. *American Journal of Preventive Medicine*, *45*(2), 228–236. doi:10.1016/j.amepre.2013.03.017 PMID:23867031

McCurdie, T., Taneva, S., Casselman, M., Yeung, M., McDaniel, C., Ho, W., & Cafazzo, J. (2012). consumer apps: The case for user-centered design. *Biomedical Instrumentation & Technology*, *46*(Suppl. 2), 49–56. doi:10.2345/0899-8205-46.s2.49 PMID:23039777

McMillan, B., Hickey, E., Patel, M.G., & Mitchell, C. (2015). Quality assessment of a sample of mobile app-based health behavior change interventions using a tool based on the National Institute of Health and Care Excellence behavior change guidance. *Patient education and counseling*. Open mHealth. Retrieved from http://www.openmhealth.org/

Peeples, M. M., Iyer, A. K., & Cohen, J. L. (2013). Integration of a mobile-integrated therapy with electronic health records: Lessons learned. *Journal of Diabetes Science and Technology*, *7*(3), 602–611. doi:10.1177/193229681300700304 PMID:23759392

Powell, A. C., Landman, A. B., & Bates, D. W. (2014). In search of a few good apps. *Journal of the American Medical Association*, *311*(18), 1851–1852. doi:10.1001/jama.2014.2564 PMID:24664278

Pruitt, J., & Grudin, J. (2003, June 5-7). Personas: practice and theory. *Proceedings of the conference on Designing for User Experiences DUX '03*, San Francisco, CA, USA. doi:10.1145/997078.997089

Research2guidance. (2015). App Developer Economics 2015. Retrieved from http://research2guidance.com/r2g/r2g--App-Developer-Economics-2015.pdf

Silow-Carroll, S., & Smith, B. (2013). Clinical management apps: creating partnerships between providers and patients. *Commonwealth Fund Issue Brief*. SMART Health IT. Retrieved from http://smarthealthit.org/

SMART Health IT. (n. d.). Retrieved from http://smarthealthit.org/

Terry, K. (2015). Prescribing mobile apps: What to consider. Retrieved from http://medicaleconomics.modernmedicine.com/medical-economics/news/prescribing-mobile-apps-what-consider?page=full

This research was previously published in the International Journal of Handheld Computing Research (IJHCR), 7(2); edited by Wen-Chen Hu, pages 34-43, copyright year 2016 by IGI Publishing (an imprint of IGI Global).

Chapter 30
Expanding Role of Telephone Systems in Healthcare:
Developments and Opportunities

Jing Shi
North Dakota State University, USA

Ergin Erdem
North Dakota State University, USA

Heping Liu
North Dakota State University, USA

ABSTRACT

The telephone systems in healthcare settings serve as a viable tool for improving the quality of service provided to patients, decreasing the cost, and improving the patient satisfaction. It can play a pivotal role for transformation of the healthcare delivery for embracing personalized and patient centered care. This chapter presents a systematic review of new developments of healthcare telephone system operations in various areas such as tele-health. Current research on topics such as tele-diagnosis, tele-nursing, tele-consultation is outlined. Specific issues associated with the emerging applications such as under-referral, legal issues, patient acceptance, on-call physician are discussed. Meanwhile, the architecture and underlying technologies for healthcare telephone systems are introduced, and the performance metrics for measuring the system operations are provided. In addition, challenges and opportunities related with improving the healthcare telephone systems are identified, and the potential opportunities of optimizing these systems are pointed out.

1. INTRODUCTION

Telephone systems are an indispensible part of healthcare units. Coile (1999) indicated that the conventional call centers in various healthcare settings could enhance their means for 275 million health consumers to receive better health service. The telephone systems guide the patients to receive the care,

DOI: 10.4018/978-1-5225-3926-1.ch030

education, or related information. As such, the systems can be often considered as the entry gate for patients and other users of healthcare systems, and they present an immense opportunity to improve healthcare delivery, such as the efficient communication services for health care delivery especially in the laboratory medicine (Coiera, 2006), and supporting the functions of information technology for providing better care service (Schweiger et al., 2007).

The telephone systems in healthcare units usually involve the interaction and information exchange between the patients or their important ones and the customer service agents, nurses, or providers, with the help of telecommunication technologies. The systems can provide a variety of services such as scheduling an appointment, heath consultation, medication refills and renewals, enrollment, and co-pay. Stier (1999) indicated that the telephone systems provide substantial benefits for stakeholders in healthcare systems. Individuals who are looking for medical information to address their future health related problems or who are joining new healthcare insurance plans and would like to acquaint themselves with providers might reap substantial benefits by using those systems. In addition, hospital associates for arranging the transfer of patients within and between healthcare centers may also obtain timely and accurate information using the telephone systems. With the help of the telephone systems, the quality and efficiency of healthcare delivery systems can be significantly enhanced.

From the perspective of improving service quality and operation efficiency, this chapter reviews the new developments on telephone systems for healthcare delivery and identifies the challenges that the systems face and the potential opportunities for improvement and optimization. The organization of this chapter is as follows. In the second section, the architecture and functions of telephone systems for healthcare delivery are briefly introduced. In the third section, the indices for measuring the system performance are summarized. In the fourth section, the research progress and the expanding role of telephone systems for healthcare delivery are presented. In the fifth section, the challenges in optimizing the healthcare telephone systems are specified and analyzed. In the sixth section, the potential opportunities to improve service quality and operations efficiency are demonstrated. Finally, conclusive remarks are provided.

2. TELEPHONE SYSTEMS OPERATIONS AND TELE-HEALTH

Figure 1 illustrates the operations and activities of a typical healthcare telephone system. The schematic chart shows how a telephone system guides patients to communicate with clerks, nurses, physicians, or health counselors to obtain services. The data and education information flow is between the patients and the various units in the system. To cite an instance, a patient might provide his/her preferences on appointment date/time, and based on the data fetched from the database, a clerk/scheduler can provide the patient an appointment date/time that considers the patient preferences and the availability of clinic resources. On the other hand, the healthcare telephone systems might also be considered as a medium for dispensing information/education to the patients. For example, based on the triage algorithms implemented in the system, a nurse can decide whether the patient should be referred to another hospital. The services that can be obtained by the patients range from simple operations such as scheduling an appointment and medication refills, to complicated operations such as tele-nursing. In the telephone systems, more components such as tele-nursing, tele-counseling, tele-triage, computer telephony and computerized expert systems have been added (Mohan et al., 2004). In general, these components are also within the domain of tele-health. While the telemedicine and tele-health terms are used interchangeably in some cases (American Telemedicine Association, 2009), many believe that tele-health extends beyond the

Figure 1. Typical Operations of a Healthcare Telephone System

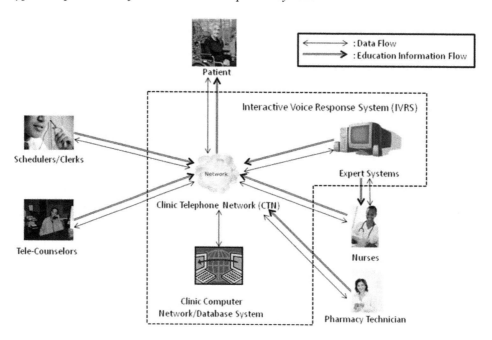

concept of telemedicine to encompass the non clinical applications which include, but are not limited to, home tele-health, remote patient monitoring, and the patient outreach programs (Darkins & Cary, 2000). New telehealth applications that aim to improve clinical outcomes associated with chronic disease management (Cassimatis & Kavanagh, 2012), and serious mental health problems (Pratt et al., 2014) are being developed. Also, recent advances in the electronics especially in sensor technology, miniaturization, and proliferation of the smart phones foster implementation of the tele-health approaches and contribute to the accessibility of the tele-health solutions (Boulos et al., 2011).

Hill and Powell (2009) indicated that medical errors cause the death of about 98,000 people per year, and the telephone systems can help significantly reduce the medical errors. The accessibility to adequate healthcare is an urgent issue for many countries. With tele-health, the geographic isolation, the scarcity of physicians and hospitals, and the difficulties of travel to medical facilities can be effectively addressed, and the patients do not need to physically visit clinics or hospitals but are able to receive proper care (Stamm & Pearce, 1995). Furthermore, tele-health can allow information to be readily communicated and shared among healthcare providers, and help curb healthcare costs over the long term. Tele-health applications cover a wide variety of application areas for diagnostics and treatment. One application area is audiology which includes audiometry, video-otoscopy, oto-acoustic emissions, and auditory brainstem response. The intervention strategies such as hearing aid verification, counseling, and Internet-based treatment for tinnitus can also be incorporated in tele-health applications (Swanepoel & Hall III, 2010). In addition, the advent of smart phone technology paves new ways for developing new tele-health applications. In that regard, Gregoski et al. (2012) proposed a tele-health application that features photoplethysmographic acquisition and heart rate measurement. It was shown that smart phones might offer some advantages and ease of use because of the lack of electrode patches or wireless sensor telemetric straps. The tele-health applications might also be used for offering care for diseases in advanced stages. Kidd et al. (2010) discussed the applications of tele-health for providing palliative care in oncology such as out-of-hours telephone support, advice services for palliative care patients, carers and health professionals, videoconferencing for interactive case discussions, consultations and assessments, and training and education of palliative care and other health-care staff. Anderson et al. (1996) discussed how the telephone and video conferencing can be used for clinic monitoring and technician recertification for the optic neuritis research. It was shown that tele-health can be an effective cost cutting tool, and also help to attain a high visit completion rate among the patients attending the clinical trials.

Tele-health projects have been reported in many countries and districts. Suleiman (2001) demonstrated that Malaysia's tele-health initiative under the Multimedia Super Corridor project can help realize the country's health vision and goals, and meet future health challenges. Mohan and Yaacob (2004) showed that the integration of information, telecommunication, and human—machine interface technologies can assist in healthcare delivery, promote the heath status of the people. Adewale (2004) developed an Internet-based telemedicine environment for Nigeria. It supports consultations among remotely placed patients, rural health workers and specialists in the urban cities and provides a secure access to remote patient records. Barlow et al. (2006) explored the interaction among project complexity, organizational context, and project management approach during the planning and implementation phase. It was pointed out that although the organizational context would deter the researchers from drawing some general conclusions, individuals in the organizations play a vital role in the overall success of the tele-health projects. Hsu et al. (2010) illustrated the tele-health pilot project in Taiwan which uses healthcare information technology to address high healthcare costs and the shortage of healthcare providers. The project includes the home-care, community-care, and residential care models and can assist the elders in the pursuit of better healthcare and quality of life. National telehealth applications are especially important in low-income countries for improving the access of the population to the healthcare resources where there are inequitable distribution of expertise, equipment and knowledge. Setting specific goals and developing corresponding solution might help proper implementation and facilitate the access to the corresponding resources and help dissemination of the medical knowledge to the clinicians. However, significant barriers exist and the involvement of the key personnel in this endeavor is a key requirement for successful implementation as demonstrated in Zambia (Chanda & Shaw, 2010).

The adoption of tele-health will change the structures of traditional telephone systems. Hamill and Lorri (1998) showed how the clinical call centers can provide a reliable and safe homecare service for the elderly patients, and emphasized the importance of standards to ensure the efficacy of homecare related services. Koch (2006) indicated that although stand alone applications such as blood sugar monitoring, tele-cardiography have been finding wide attention, a holistic approach that assesses the effect of tele-health on the current model of healthcare delivery systems has not been taken yet. It was noted that further research is needed to address the impacts and benefits of potential solutions and overcome a number of restrictions. The restrictions include the lack of standards to combine incompatible information systems, the lack of an evaluation framework considering legal, ethical, organizational, clinical, usability and technical aspects, and the lack of proper guidelines for practical implementation of home tele-health solutions.

The continuous adoption of information technology in telephone systems has been playing a crucial role for operation improvement. As a result, tele-health has proliferated, which reflects the convergence of scientific, technological, economic and social factors (Grigsby & Sanders, 1998). Ball and Lillis (2001) demonstrated that the consumers' interest in and demand for online administrative processes, information rich Internet health portals, and access to physician web pages and e-mail has introduced a new dimension to maintain wellness and treat diseases. It was shown that these activities are redefining the relationship of physicians and patients, improving clinical decision-making, increasing efficiency, and strengthening communication between physicians and patients. Nowadays, the comprehensive tele-health applications are being integrated into the Internet health portals through personal health record for developing patient-centric healthcare model, enhancing access to care, and ensuring the responsiveness of such technologies to the preferences and circumstances of patients. Such an approach is recently implemented in the Veteran Affairs healthcare system (Hogan et al., 2011)

Prince and Herrin (2007) documented the development of a patient-centric call process using real-time, rules-based task assignment and tracking software, which enhances healthcare communications, efficiency and patient safety, guides personalized and timely response to the needs of individual patients, and allows data mining for outcome analysis. Lenz and Reichert (2007) elaborated the potential and essential limitations of IT support for healthcare processes. A broad socio-technical perspective based on scientific literature and personal experience was adopted to illustrate that the huge potential of IT to improve healthcare quality has not been fully explored by the current solutions. Tsiknakis and Kouroubali (2009) presented an application of the "Fit between Individuals, Task and Technology" framework to analyze the socio-organizational-technical factors that influence IT adoption in the healthcare domain. Lee et al. (2009) investigated the efficacy of a ubiquitous healthcare service using Zigbee and mobile phone for elderly patients with diabetes mellitus or heart diseases. It was believed that ZigBee technology could become a key component for wireless ubiquitous healthcare systems due to its advantages of lower power consumption. Adler Milstein and Bates (2010) discussed the role of IT for revolutionizing healthcare industry. It was shown how IT can be effectively used for a paperless system and how medical information can be electronically shared among various parties. Hill and Powell (2009) showed that a national electronic healthcare network is one of the most important keys to resolving this crisis, but it is underappreciated and under-exploited, and faces several formidable barriers to implementation. Recent study suggested that electronic healthcare records play a viable role for the best clinical outcomes through the clinical decision support systems. Standardization and integration of the healthcare records to the existing information systems help develop efficient and effective approaches for improving the existing clinical decision support systems, which guide the clinicians to provide the required care based on the clinical guidelines (Romano and Stafford, 2011). Electronic healthcare records are also important input for developing genomics based medicine which is a very important milestone for developing personalized healthcare solutions (Gottesman et al., 2013).

3. PERFORMANCE METRICS FOR TELEPHONE SYSTEMS

Measuring the performance of a healthcare telephone system is a critical task. By using certain metrics, the current operations can be benchmarked against the baseline and the results directly indicate if an improvement plan is needed. A number of approaches have been developed in the literature for evaluating the performance of a telephone system. Stier (1999) identified eight factors that have a significant impact on the profitability of call centers and the quality of services. The eight factors are financial viability; shared outcome requirements, a three-year migration plan, cross discipline tasking, market alignment, system integration, process redesign, leveraging high margin services and quantified outcomes, and they have universal means in the context of healthcare settings. Jack at al. (2006) developed an embedded framework to identify the trade-offs encountered during the management of a telephone system. In order to improve the performance of a telephone system, four aspects should be taken into consideration and they are the efficient deployment and use of labor, the effective use of technology, capacity management, and demand management.

Miciak and Desmarais (2001) pointed out that managers of telephone systems can use a number of performance metrics, but the metrics for measuring customer satisfaction have been lacking. It was further stated that the metrics should be based on three different facets, namely, operational characteristics, employee/customer service representative (CSR) opinions on workplace issues, and customer opinions on service quality experience. Overall, the acquisition/retention ratio, percent of total customer relationship, calls answered with live voice, call centers with unionized representatives, and average number of call center representatives constitute the metrics related with the call center operating characteristics. On the other hand, service level (percentage of the calls answered in 20 seconds or less), average length of calls, average wrap-up time, and first call resolution are the indices associated with the individual call characteristics.

Tables 1 and 2 show the performance indices widely adopted in literature. These indices are generally applicable to any general telephone system in healthcare, but they are not necessarily exhaustive considering the variations among healthcare settings. For healthcare telephone systems, some of these indices are particularly important such as abandon rates, patient waiting time, rates of mismatches, first call resolution, and average and maximum queue length of calls from patients.

4. NEW DEVELOPMENTS OF HEALTHCARE TELEPHONE SYSTEMS

A number of unique new developments have been witnessed in healthcare telephone systems to expand the role of nurses/providers, improve patient-centered care, and facilitate the delivery of care. The new operation developments can be categorized into the forms of tele-counseling, tele-nursing, tele-triage, tele-diagnosis, computer telephony, interactive voice response systems (IVRS), on-call physicians, and operations of outgoing calls. In addition, national level healthcare telephone systems (call centers) are also included.

4.1 Tele-Nursing and Counseling

In recent years there has been a trend to increase the use of telephone nursing and consultation, which effectively reduce the workload of general practitioners (GPs) as well as emergency departments. Stirewalt et al. (1982) studied whether a specialized telephone service could cut down on unscheduled visits to ambulatory care and improve satisfaction with care. The results show that the telephone service, which provides a triage system for referrals as well as a source of central contact for scheduling or for complaints, helped to improve patient satisfaction and reduce the number of unscheduled visits. Similarly, McKinstry et al. (2002) showed that the use of telephone consultations for same-day appointments was associated with time saving, and did not result in lower scores of Patient Enablement Instrument which can measure patient perceptions and be used to report the willingness to use telephone consultations in the future. The possible reason is that this short-term saving is offset by higher re-consultation and less use of opportunistic health promotion. Kamei et al. (2014) conducted a meta-analysis of the existing research and showed that tele-home monitoring based tele-nursing in Chronic Obstructive Pulmonary Disease may affect the use of the healthcare services. The structure of counseling center is an important aspect for smooth operations of the tele-health applications. Russell (2012) indicated that organizing

Table 1. Performance Indices of Telephone Systems

	Metric	Reference
Call Center Related	Acquisition/retention ratio (%)	(Miciak and Desmarais, 2001)
	Percentage of total customer relationship at call center	(Miciak and Desmarais, 2001)
	Calls answered with live voice (%)	(Miciak and Desmarais, 2001)
	Average number of CSRs at call center	(Miciak and Desmarais, 2001)
	Service level (Percentage of calls answered within a given time frame)	(Miciak and Desmarais, 2001), (Ertogral and Bamuqabel, 2008), (Deslauriers et al., 2007)
	The number of touch-tones necessary to reach the most common transaction in the voice response system (VRU)	(Evenson et al., 1999)
	The percentage of incoming calls that are entirely handled by VRU (%)	(Evenson et al., 1999)
	Rate of outbound calls	(Deslauriers et al., 2007)
	Rate of mismatches	(Deslauriers et al., 2007)
Call Related	Average length of call in minutes	(Miciak and Desmarais, 2001)
	Average wrap-up time in minutes	(Miciak and Desmarais, 2001), (Jack et al., 2006), (Federspiel et al., 2004)
	First call resolution (%)	(Miciak and Desmarais, 2001), (Jack et al., 2006)
Customer Related	Customer waiting time	(Jack et al., 2006), (Duder and Rosenwein, 2001)
	Issue resolution time	(Jack et al., 2006)
	Customer abandon rate	(Jack et al., 2006), (Duder and Rosenwein, 2001), (Deslauriers et al., 2007)
	Short abandonment index	(Jouni et al., 2013)
	Frequency and manner the company chooses to elicit customer response	(Evenson et al., 1999)
	Average queue length of calls	(Garnet et al., 2002)
	Maximum queue length of calls	(Artelajo et al. 2007)
	Customer satisfaction rate	(Robinson and Morley, 2006)

tele-counseling centers as a professional call center might pose some challenges. For instance, ambiguities over the use of skills in a system that incorporates the deployment of computer algorithms might lead to the conflicts for monitoring performance evaluation and the use of time. Tele-counseling along with the other intervention strategies might be implemented on the mobile platforms and accessed by the users using the mobile phones for different approaches for supporting preventive medicine functions such as smoking cessation (Ghorai et al., 2014).

Dale et al. (1998) reported on the evaluation of an off-hour telephone triage in general practice. A computer-based decision support tool was used to guide nurses in the assessment of patients and outcome for calls. It was found that the nurses were able to handle just over half the calls received by giving advice alone. The service was remarkably consistent in the decisions taken by nurses. Gilmour (2001) presented approaches for developing a telephone system to manage disaster and trauma, and found that

Table 2. Evaluation Criteria of Staffing and Training

Metric	Reference
Call center with unionized CSRs (%)	(Miciak and Desmarais, 2001)
Average number of CSRs per supervisor	(Miciak and Desmarais, 2001)
CSRs with college degree	(Miciak and Desmarais, 2001)
CSRs with technical degree or some college	(Miciak and Desmarais, 2001)
Ratio of CSRs trained generalist/specialist	(Miciak and Desmarais, 2001), (Evenson et al., 1999)
More than 25 days of new-hire training	(Miciak and Desmarais, 2001)
More than 6 days annual ongoing training	(Miciak and Desmarais, 2001)
CSR salary	(Miciak and Desmarais, 2001)
Supervisor salary	(Miciak and Desmarais, 2001)
Total cost of new-hire CSR	(Miciak and Desmarais, 2001)
Turnover rate (the ratio of the average number of CSR leave an organization to total number of CSR in the company	(Evenson et al., 1999)
The average number of years CSR are employed in the call center	(Evenson et al., 1999)
Not utilized time (i.e. the amount of time CSR spends at work while not answering calls, training, or doing paperwork)	(Evenson et al., 1999), Deslauriers et al. (2007)
Average talk time	(Duder and Rosenwein, 2001), (Heschong Mashone Group, 2003), (Federspiel et al., 2004), (Tham and Willem, 2004), (Tham, 2004), (Wargocki et al., 2004)
Number of calls handled by CSR per unit time	(Witt, 2004)
Customer service quality (1-5 Likert scale) (self evaluation and supervisor evaluation)	(Witt, 2004), (Mcnall and Roch, 2009)
The amount of freedom given to CSR to handle calls that concern a threat to consumer defection	(Evenson et al., 1999)

without the physical contact, it is often easier to establish a closeness on telephone since the connection occurs without the initial distraction of physical cues. The perceived anonymity of callers contributes to the service quality. Callers are more open to the discussion of related matters with counselors. Bunn et al. (2005) reviewed the effects of telephone consultation on safety, service use, and patient satisfaction by using randomized controlled trials, controlled studies, controlled before/after studies, and interrupted time series of telephone consultation or triage in a general healthcare setting. The review supports that the telephone consultation and triage reduce the number of general patients visit, and at least 50% of calls can be handled by telephone advice. Zanaboni et al. (2009) studied the effect of tele-consultation on the reduction of the use of clinic resources and on the potential savings. In addition, tele-counseling applications have been developed for reducing the health risks associated with obesity through the mobile health platforms (Castelnuovo et al., 2011). Tele-counseling is also proposed as a viable method for providing follow-up psychological support for cancer survivors in the rural areas of Canada (Fuchsia et al., 2014).

4.2 Tele-Triage

A number of studies have been conducted to address the efficacy of tele-triage decisions. Telephone triage is a systematic process where the nurse screens existing symptoms for urgency, and provides the advice on whether existing symptoms require clinical center visit (Briggs, 2007) If a visit to clinic center is required, a nurse can also provide suggestions on the timing based on the urgency status. Crouch et al. (1996) indicated the importance of tele-triage even in densely populated urban centers. Devore (1999) examined the tele-triage from a perspective of midwife, pointed out the inherent difficulties of tele-triage, and provided suggestions and guidelines for improving the quality of tele-triage. A historical perspective on the development of telephone triage is presented by Breslin and Denison (2002), in which the ethical and legal implications of telephone triage are stressed, and the importance of procedures and nursing-time efficient allocation is discussed. Bunik et al. (2007) incorporated the cost concepts into tele-triage decisions by drawing the link between costs and compliance rates. Cost savings under different scenarios were discussed. Beaulieu and Humphreys (2008) conducted an observational study to assess the patient satisfaction with a nurse managed health center. It was confirmed that tele-triage might significantly reduce the number of visits made to emergency departments. The trust of the patients on the tele-triage applications is also an important factor for ensuring the efficiency and effectiveness of the service. Williams et al. (2012) showed that the users of the tele-triage services with greater self-efficacy and satisfaction with the nurse interaction are more likely to adhere to the advices for self-care. Similarly, a survey study was conducted among the patients using the tele-triage services. About 85% of the respondents indicated that they adhere to the recommendations and do not visit to the medical center. The adherence to the suggestions might reduce associated healthcare cost if the patients follow recommendations provided by the tele-triage services (Rimner et al., 2011). Mobile health platforms also contribute to the access to the healthcare resources through tele-triage functions especially for the population living in the rural areas in the developing nations (Burney et al., 2014). Tele-triage forms the backbone of the dispatch protocols and considerably improves the efficiency and effectiveness of providing medical emergency services (Alizadeh et al., 2012). Some researchers have expanded the function of tele-triage to offer the proactive care in the home-care setting. Associated with this approach, it might form the frontline for the healthcare provider network (Arnaert & Macfarlane, 2011).

Underreferral indicates the situation that nurses or providers assess the healthcare condition of callers as less serious compared to what it is. It significantly degrades the quality of healthcare delivery and puts patients at risk. Lee et al (2003b) and Kempe et al. (2003) presented studies that estimate the underreferral rate for pediatric patients. Kempe et al. (2006) used data mining techniques to sort and analyze a large collection of data to estimate the underreferral rate after hours. The findings show that the triage decisions after 11pm are more likely considered as underreferral, and adolescents and infants run the higher risks of being underreferred. Hirsh et al. (2007) calculated the underreferral rate for the patients receiving tele-triage decisions. Besides underreferral, overreferral is another important research topic about the efficiency of tele-triage decisions. Poole et al. (1993), Kempe et al. (2000b) and Hirsh et al. (2004) all indicated that healthcare call centers usually tended to overrefer patients for urgent disposition.

4.3 Tele-Diagnosis

Telephone can be used by nurses, physicians and consultants to diagnose and manage many common conditions in order to control costs, reduce appointments and visits, and maximize efficiency for patient visits. Revicki et al. (1997) evaluated the correspondence between in-person and telephone interview-derived data on affective symptoms, health-related quality of life, disability days, and medication compliance in patients with bipolar disorder. The results showed good to excellent agreement between telephone and in-person interviews. It was believed that telephone interviews are feasible and reliable for collecting data on psychiatric and other health-related outcomes in bipolar disorder patients. Feldman-Naim et al. (1997) examined the reliability and level of agreement between the telephone and face-to-face administration of two mood-rating scales in patients with rapid cycling bipolar disorder (RCBD). The results support the use of phone-administered mood ratings as a reliable and convenient method to monitor patients with RCBD. Rohde et al. (1997) examined the comparability of data obtained by telephone and face-to-face interviews for diagnosing axis I and II disorders. The agreement between telephone and face-to-face assessment was excellent for anxiety disorders, major depressive disorder, and alcohol use disorders. The findings provided qualified justification for the use of telephone interviews to collect axis I and II data. Based on an empirical research on the assessment of vulvovaginal complaints, Allen-Davis et al. (2002) examined the agreement between telephone and office management of vulvovaginal complaints and assessed the accuracy of diagnosis of vulvovaginitis. Prospective structured telephone nurse interviews of all patients with vulvovaginal complaints were conducted. The particular study challenges the notion that the telephone is an effective tool to diagnose and treat vulvovaginal complaints. Telephone systems might also support the tele-diagnosis applications for relaying the output. Muir et al. (2012) demonstrated the setting where the diagnosis obtained based on tele-dignosis applications are relayed to the medical center via telephone. It was found that the results obtained by the tele-diagnosis and face-to face diagnosis actually agree most of the time. Moreover, the agreement rate between tele-diagnosis and the final clinical diagnosis is strikingly higher (i.e., about 98%). Thomas and Kumar (2013) indicated that the telephone networks might be useful for relaying the voice, fax and data transmissions for the tele-dermatology applications. Ganapathy and Ravindra (2011) also suggested that telephone networks might play a supporting role for the tele-health applications and strongly affect the associated costs for the healthcare operations especially in the emerging economies. Novel tele-diagnosis approaches that use the existing telephone network have been developed. To cite an instance, Sakar and Kursun (2010) use the measurement of dysphonia for diagnosing the Parkinson's disease in earlier stages. Tele-diagnosis is also expanded for providing tele-dentistry functions to improve the assessment of oral health (Marino et al., 2015). Santana et al., (2012) develop a semi-automatic approach for tele-diagnosing the vascular problems. The proposed system in the first step aim to capture the relevant data using Echo-Doppler images, and the second step features the distributed tool for the collaborative diagnosis for those particular health problems.

Kathryn et al. (2003) presented a study identifying the efficacy of diagnosing the depression in outpatients. Most of the patients expressed interest in the tele-diagnosis of depression due to the various factors such as convenience and privacy. It showed that tele-diagnosis is a feasible alternative to face-to-face interviews for diagnosing the depression among cancer patients. Remschmidt et al. (2003) investigated the reliability and validity of data gathered in telephone interviews. The results indicated good reliability and underscored the validity of the collected data. Saraux et al. (2004) evaluated the agreement between a rheumatologist visit and a telephone interview, and the agreement between the two sources of data turned out to be poor for the classification criteria but satisfactory for the diagnosis. Standardized telephone interviews can accurately identify the diagnosis made by rheumatologists based on a physical examination and medical record review, whereas the agreement is poor regarding classification criteria for rheumatoid arthritis or spondyloarthropathy. Haghighat et al. (2007) demonstrated the efficiency of the tele-diagnosis system for evaluating the breast cancer related cases. The study indicated that consultants may diagnose and manage the cases successfully over a phone by using some well established diagnostic criteria, and that most of the time the findings are parallel with the findings of the specialists evaluating patients face to face.

4.4 Computer Telephony

Computer telephony is basically an integrated system combining telephone with computers to receive, transmit and process information (Edgar, 1992). It overlaps with the telephone based healthcare and tele-health (McBride & Rimer, 1999; Balas et al., 1997). The application of computer telephony dates back the late 1960's (Allen, 1969). Biem et al. (2003) conducted an exhaustive literature review by searching MEDLINE (1966-April 2003), CINAHL (1982-April 2003) and the Cochrane Central Register of Controlled Trials to identify the evidence for the medical applications of computer telephony system. The computer telephony systems, for some applications, make health care delivery more efficient by improving scheduling, communication and health information. For instance, computer telephony has been used for tracking the diet and obtaining feedback of the patients to increase the nutrition (Delichatsios et al., 2002). It has been used for evaluating the patient satisfaction (Isenberg et al., 2001). An education program based on the voice mail was developed to help the nurses for collecting administrative data (Narayan, 2001). Studies suggest that computer telephony system can actually help to improve the immunization rates (Dini, 2000) and facilitate the medical care of chronic diseases such as chronic lung diseases (Young et al., 2001) and diabetes (Piette, 2000). However, the effectiveness of computer telephony system-based management intervention is not certain. For some computer telephony applications, the controlled trials on the effectiveness based on randomized controlled trials might not be possible (Biem et al., 2004). In most of the studies, the sample size is not large enough to infer statistical conclusions or lacking follow-up studies, and the effects of computer telephony in the long run has not been fully established (Pinto et al., 2002; Rask et al., 2000). Computer telephony might also be used with the clinical longitudinal follow up studies. In that regard, Stewart et al. (2012) indicated that automated telephone contacts or web based questionnaire might be used with collecting follow-up data. It was reported that among the cohort of patients who are elderly and chronically ill, providing input using automated telephone contacts finds acceptance and might be used for longitudinal follow up studies. In addition, van der Marck et al. (2011) conducted a study in which computer telephony might be used in conjunction of reporting the falls for the elderly patients living in community-dwelling homes. It was shown that computer telephony is a suitable way of conveying the information regarding the falls for the patients. Computer telephony can be also used for providing the necessary e-coaching services for the patients that require complex care. Such approaches are very important for continuity of care for the patients suffering from serious chronic diseases (Ritchie et al., 2012), Systems that incorporate computer telephony have been proposed for various clinical settings such as the appointment reminders in clinics (Suomi et al., 2010), and reducing impulsivity among violent forensic outpatients and probationers (Berman et al., 2012).

4.5 Interactive Voice Response Systems (IVRS)

Interactive Voice Response System (IVRS) has been gaining attention in the recent years due to the ease of implementation, cost effectiveness and various other considerations. In an IVRS, a human operator is replaced by the high-quality recorded script, and the people using IVRS can be directed to various branches based on the answers provided to the system. IVRS offers advantages as compared to the human operated telephone systems. IVRS can be utilized to reach the hard-to-reach groups such as homeless people, sex workers (Alemagno et al., 1996). There is no operator bias, and human errors are eliminated. The cost per interview is likely to be small, and the detailed information using IVRS can be collected.

IVRS differs from Computer Assisted Telephone Interview (CATI) systems, although they share some technical similarities (Nicholls, 1988). In CATI, there is no person reading the questions and entering the responses into the system. Corkrey and Parkinson (2002) identified that the health related information services of IVRS in the literature are smoking cessation, depression screening, hepatitis B screening, and providing pediatric clinic information. IVRS can be used as reminder calls and handle the outbound calls for cardiac and the diabetic patients. IVRS is associated with the higher childhood immunization rates, and appointment and treatment compliance. Corkrey and Parkinson (2002) further pointed out the physical, psychological, and technical influences of voice in IVRS. For example, the soft speaker might be interpreted as less assured, the faster speaking pace might be perceived as the more convincing as compared to the slower speaking pace, the scripts recorded at the lower voice quality might hamper the intended outcome of IVRS, and the male or female voice in the scripts may have different effects.

Lee et al. (2003a) discussed the applications of (IVRS) in healthcare. It was demonstrated that the patients who interact with an IVRS through automated messages behave in a more honest manner. Combined with expert triage systems, IVRS can help healthcare providers to expand customer contracts, increase access to healthcare resources, reduce operating expenses, and increase staff efficiency. O'Brien et al. (2003) discussed the resource utilization during the clinical trial of the Viozan™ for chronic obstructive pulmonary disease. The authors indicated that IVRS can be effectively implemented to collect the resource utilization data and thus help reduce the clinical trial costs. Stritzke et al. (2005) showed that IVRS can be used to obtain daily reports of attitudes toward alcohol and tobacco use among children 9–13 years of age. Mundt et al. (2006) compared the reliability and validity of the self reported sadness and the pessimistic thought of participants in their study. A group of 60 participants were assessed using both the computer based and clinician administered versions of the Montgomery-Asberg Depression Rating Scale (MADRS). Two results turned out to be statistically insignificant. Abu-Hasaballah et al. (2007) discussed the use of IVRS as an electronic data capture tool in the clinical and behavioral research. They described how IVRS works, the advantages and pitfalls of IVRS, and some of the lessons learned from administering a number of clinical studies using IVRS. Kim et al. (2007) investigated the use of IVRS system for clinic screening of the depression along the low income, disadvantaged, urban pregnant women. It was indicated that IVRS can be a very suitable tool for prescreening and screening for the low income pregnant urban women. Compared to visiting the clinics physically, IVRS is a less costly alternative. Horton et al. (2008) discussed the compliance rate of the patients using IVRS for creating their own electronic diaries. The electronic medical diaries are considered to be a valuable tool for assessing the quantitative and qualitative mental health parameters. However, it is revealed that the excessive use of IVRS for handling outgoing calls might decrease the usefulness of IVRS. Heyworth et al. (2014) compared the interactive voice response system, patient mailing, and the mailed registry for encouraging screening for ostreoposis. It was discovered that IVRS is effective for increasing the response rate, and it remains the viable strategy for incorporating the population screening interventions. The IVRS might also be complemented with the prize based approaches. Lindsay et al. (2014) discussed enhancing the compliance of using IVRS for the cocaine addiction treatment and showed that augmenting IVRS with the prize based contingency management might produce more positive outcomes in terms of abstinence achievement. Similarly, Graham et al. (2012) found that IVRS in conjunction with the Geisinger Monitoring Program significantly reduces the 30-day readmission by 44% for the case managed Medicare population. IVRS might also be used for improving the treatment adherence for the HIV/AIDS setting in a resource limited setting for the developing countries. It is suggested that controlling access to the telephone system by providing a personal pin number might be used as an appropriate security measure for providing healthcare services for HIV/AIDS patients (Joshi et al., 2014). Telephone systems based on IVRS can also be used for collecting information regarding the patient feedback for the post clinical visits (Berner et al., 2014). The demographics of the users might have an effect on the usability of the IVRS systems. Auger et al. (2013) indicated that older users might have difficulties with using IVRS systems. Interestingly, the authors also pointed out that the education level of the users might be associated with more unsuccessful calls and lower reported usefulness.

In order to promote the acceptability for the IVRS systems especially among the elder population, the consideration of adjusting the system according to the user needs should be given. In the survey conducted among the elder population, it was discovered that the adaptive algorithms for changing the structure of the IVRS system, rather than prompting the user to adjust his/her input, is more viable method of obtaining the input of the population and gaining acceptance (Miller et al., 2011).

4.6 On-Call Physicians

On-call physicians provide services to the emergency departments, and usually screen and stabilize urgent medical conditions which require specific medical expertise and knowledge. Pike (2003) investigated the number of on-call physicians required for healthcare call centers to facilitate the smooth flow of operations. It was concluded that usually the on-call physicians are called for the house staff on the average once per night mostly on the medication type problems, and the importance of continuing medical education was emphasized to improve the effectiveness of the on-call system. Morton et al. (2004) assessed the on-call activity by performing a time-motion study of resident on-call activity at a university medical center and an urban affiliate hospital and pointed out that 25% of the total call time is spent with evaluating patients, but direct contact with patients comprised only 7% of the call night duties. Sleep deprivations, and frequent interruptions in activity are common aspects the on-call physicians and residents face during their call nights. Rudkin et al. (2004) used a mailed anonymous survey to assess the scope of problems with on-call physicians in California. It was discovered that on-call problems were more acute at night or on weekends, and patient insurance negatively affected willingness of on-call physicians to consult for at least a quarter of patients. Mohanty et al. (2006) presented a study to identify the link between the response time of on-call physicians and various factors such as the neighborhood, the type of emergency department facility and the income of corresponding healthcare facility. It was discovered that when the income of neighborhood and the corresponding healthcare facility increase, the physician response time generally decreases. McConnell et al. (2007) surveyed Oregon hospitals about the prevalence and magnitude of stipends for taking emergency call and assessed the ways in which hospitals are limiting services. The results showed that the problems with on-call coverage are prevalent in Oregon and affect hospital financing and delivery of services. Rudkin et al. (2009) reassessed the problems with on-call physician coverage in California by repeating the anonymous survey and the results showed the on-call situation in California worsened substantially. The main reasons for declining service were identified to be related to the service time (e.g., day/night of the day, whether it is a weekend coverage), and the complexity of the injury (Cantu et al., 2012). It has been reported that recent legislative changes in the on-call requirement changes contribute to the shortage of the on-call specialists. Under the Emergency Medical Treatment and Labor Act (EMTALA), the on-call physicians will be permitted to be on call simultaneously at more than one hospital. Moreover, they have the latitude of scheduling elective surgeries or other medical procedures. Additionally, hospitals have greater discretion on developing their on-call specialist list (Moran, 2014). The shortage of the on-call physicians are also confirmed with other studies as well. According to the survey among emergency department managers, about three-fourths responded that there are problems with the on-call coverage problems and sixty percent indicated that they lost around the clock 24/7 coverage for at least one specialty in the past and one-quarter reported unreliability issues (Rao et al., 2010). The level of care provided by on-call physician is also under question. Petersen et al. (2014) indicated that on-call physicians provide adequate care in 49% of the unanticipated intensive care cases. Although the sample size is small, there are similar studies confirming the worsening of on-call physician coverage. Increasing the availability of the on-call physician and improving the associated service are an important task that should be addressed promptly and carefully.

4.7 Operations of Outgoing Calls

Besides incoming calls, healthcare telephone systems can handle outgoing calls. Korcz and Moreland (1998) presented a study which utilizes a healthcare telephone system to prescreen cancer patients visiting the oncology clinic. Two clinic social workers were in charge of contacting cancer patients by telephone for prescreening purposes. The telephone prescreening can help patients/families adapt to clinic or hospital systems. It was reported that the efficiency as well as the patient satisfaction levels significantly increased after the prescreening implementation. In a similar vein, Reardon et al. (1988) discussed the effect of preadmission prescreening to access the elder people on the elective surgery list in Mt. Sinai Hospital in New York. It showed the efficiency and success of the outreach program and reported that the patients responded well and were highly satisfied with the effort to address their needs before surgery.

One more operation change in healthcare telephone systems is that a patient response platform is built to serve within a health care facility as opposed to a call center addressing the needs of outside callers. A patient response platform is essentially a computerized tool that can streamline patient care, support workflow efficiency, and enhance clinical communication and patient safety. Prince and Herrin (2007) showed that a patient response platform facilitates a 23% decrease in administration delay and it benefits the efficiency of targeted communication calls. Although the system is intended to address the request of inpatients, it can be adopted to manage the requests of outside callers. Clinic related outgoing calls is an important part of the specialty care physician trainees. For instance, a study shows that the trainee made 33 calls, each of which last 1.7 minutes on the average (Prasad et al., 2012). This indicated that a significant amount of time is spent on making outgoing calls in the clinic settings.

4.8 National Healthcare Telephone Systems

National healthcare information centers such as poisons information centers are open for inquiries from health service and the public. One of the primary tasks of the national healthcare information centers is the telephone advisory service. Hall et al. (2006) used the interview and inquires to study the structure and process of the drug information centers and the drug information services in Costa Rica. The drug information centers were designed to improve communication and offer additional information. Andrew (2006) reported the organization and functions of the poison centers located throughout Europe. Pohja-noksa-Mantyla et al. (2008) analyzed and described the utilization of a community pharmacy operated national drug information call center in Finland. The special focus was on calls concerning prescription drugs. Toverud et al. (2009) conducted a similar study to find caller satisfaction levels for people using the nation-wide poison center located in Norway, to provide the cost justification for the national call center and to evaluate the benefits to the public.

Hill and Powell (2009) pointed out the current status of the U.S. national healthcare system and il-lustrated how the e-health movement can help with providing a relief to the existing healthcare crisis. It was indicated that managing the electronic medical and personal health records play a key role in the implementation of the successful e-health projects. Hsu et al. (2010) discussed about how national pilot tele-health projects can have a positive impact on the hospital readmission rate, hospital visit rate, medi-cation non-adherence rate. In addition, nosocomial infection rate and adverse drug event incident rate are also decreased by the national tele-health project. Leydon et al. (2013) indicated that for identifying the racial information and ethnic monitoring, it is worthwhile to standardize the questions by providing the list of expected answers. This approach might be useful for increasing the overall efficiency of the system. Recently national telehealth services make extensive use of technology. A national telehealth center is founded in Taiwan to battle for the hypertension that is called "Citizen Telecare Service System (CTCS)" (Lin et al., 2014). The system integrates several important features of hardware and software infrastructure, such as biometric measurement, hypertension risk assessment and clinic appointment service, etc. The national telehealth system shows significant benefits such as reducing the percentage of participants with systolic blood pressure (SBP) above 140 mmHg from 36.38% to 27.24%, and a drop in the prevalence of SBP above 120mmHg from 75.05% to 71.24.

5. CHALLENGES AND OPPORTUNITIES

5.1 High Patient Expectations

Customers' expectations for high quality services increase the operation scale and scope of healthcare telephone systems. The new developments of telephone systems discussed above may experience dif-ficulties during routine work. Wahlberg et al. (2003) identified the major problem areas of tele-triage implementation, which include the insufficiency of healthcare resources, no physical interaction with patients, callers overstating or understating the health status of patients, and the language problems es-pecially related with immigrants. Also, Snooks et al. (2008) pointed out that nurses have disagreement between the job functions and the required skill sets of tele-nurses. The nurses assuming more traditional roles generally question the job functions of tele-nurses, and believe that the tight management style and computerized decision making systems cause erosion on the loss of nursing skills. Additionally, because of the high expectations of the callers, and the very nature of the healthcare delivery processes, the language choices that are realized in lexicogrammar play an indispensable role for successful development of medical telephone support (Wan, 2012). On the other hand, telemedicine might also change the relationship between the patients and the healthcare provider (Ekeland et al., 2010). This might create additional challenges in terms of satisfying the expectations of the patients.

As pointed out, one of the inherent difficulties in tele-counseling and tele-nursing is the lack of physical presence between callers and counselors (or nurses). A possible solution is that counselors and nurses can develop necessary skills to analyze the cues by listening to the voice of callers, and the e-mail based communication schemes can be implemented to follow up nursing and counseling services to improve the quality of services. Furthermore, telephone systems can become multi-channel communication centers where several new technologies can be used to provide a wide variety of services to patients. For example, fax, phone, internet, e-mail and web chat can all be used extensively to maximize opportunities of contacting with patients. Web services offer patients a non-obtrusive and easy way to get answers to their questions and patients do not need to wait in a call queue. The Internet has enabled healthcare telephone systems to yield more control to patients for the level of service desired and it can effectively reduce the cost of operations. Healthcare telephone systems have made great strides in the area of e-mail support. If patients are able to e-mail a question and get a quick reply, patients can have a very positive experience. In addition, the e-mail-based service is not real-time and it is unnecessary to staff for peak demand periods of calls, which can lead to the significant savings. Another promising technology is instant messaging that allows patients to contact nurses or doctors without waiting in phone queues.

5.2 Consistency and Efficiency of Services

The services provided need be consistent and reliable especially for national healthcare telephone systems, and the response time of healthcare telephone switchboards need to be short. Girling (2000) showed that National Health Service (NHS) of the U.K. was criticized on the grounds that the services provided to patients were inconsistent and that there were some issues with the reliability of services. Silvestro and Silvestro (2003) argued that NHS cannot bring consistency to the overall system due to the highly decentralized nature of system. With the increased complexity and reduced flexibility, aligning the decentralized call centers with each other to provide consistent and reliable services throughout the U.K. becomes increasingly difficult and the corresponding costs are increasing. The response time of hospital switchboards is critical for the quality of services. Shokrollahi et al. (2008) studied the response time of various NHS hospital switchboards and demonstrated that a maximum threshold response time of 20 seconds is deemed to be satisfactory. It was noted that automated response systems usually cannot perform well in terms of the total response time. Instead, they delay callers talking to representatives and add the expense of callers with no significant gains. Meanwhile, in the literature, Ekeland pointed out that a significant number of studies (19 out of 80) found that some evidence on the effectiveness of telemedicine exists but additional research is required. Moreover, many studies indicate that although significant benefits of the telemedicine exist, full realization of those benefits is a complex tax due to nature of complex environment and unpredictable processes associated with the telemedicine (Ekeland et al., 2010). Additional action should be taken regarding establishing licensing requirements across the states and development of standards of care associated with the tele-health applications (Martin et al., 2013).

There are some initiatives that are being taken to decrease the variation in the quality of healthcare services provided to the patients nationwide. NHS is decentralized in terms of key service design characteristics. In order to provide a consistent yet reliable service throughout the nation, the standardization of design and implementation is important. Streamlining call center operations is an effective method to improve the overall telephone systems. Silvestro and Silvestro (2003) illustrated that some necessary steps should be taken to standardize the services provided to callers. Standardization is also a way to solve the capacity management of calls. If the operations of call centers are standardized, the calls from the centers with excessive load can be transferred to the other centers with less call demand. In addition, standardization can ensure the smooth flow of operations.

5.3 Incorporating Human Factors

Incorporating human factors into a healthcare telephone system is a natural consideration. Many operations in a telephone system such as arrivals, services and abandonment reflect human behaviors. The design of telephone systems requires an integrated view of both operational and psychological considerations. Routing decisions affect customer abandonment from queue, and impatience is a psychological process. The perception from a patient of service depends on his or her interaction with a customer service representative. Therefore, operating design must be based on a proper understanding of the patient psychology and the social interactions. The operations management with the incorporation of human factors opens up a vast agenda for optimizing the operations of healthcare telephone systems. Grosjean and De Weerdt (2005) presented an ergonomic evaluation for the effect of organizational control on operators' well-being in two call centers. Mahesh and Kasturi (2006) analyzed the important aspects of the call center agents' job and the relationships between these aspects and agent effectiveness as perceived by agents' supervisors. Their study can help managers to improve the agents' performance. Croidieu et al. (2008) sought to describe call-center working conditions and call-handlers' subjective experience of their work, and confirmed the high rate of psychosocial constraints for call-handlers. Weir and Waddington (2008) investigated the emotion work in an NHS call centre in the U.K. from the perspectives of organizational psychology and sociology. Black et al. (2009) conducted a customer satisfaction survey of verbal responses provided by a pharmaceutical company's third-party medical information (MI) call center. The completeness and understanding of the medical responses were rated high, and the callers were treated in the courteous manner. The working conditions are strongly associated with the quality level of the service provided to the patients in the clinical call center. Roing and Holmstrom (2015), based on an interview with the employees and managers, noted that stress, shiftwork, fatigue, multitasking, understaffing, and factors embedded in the system affect the malpractice claims in Swedish telenursing centers. The study indicates the importance of the overall organizational commitment for improving the level of the care for telehealth applications. Those organizational approaches and improvement programs are also important for creating conductive environment for the employees.

5.4 Operation Management Tools

The qualitative and quantitative approaches in the domains of operation management, industrial engineering, and engineering management are useful to improve the efficiency of healthcare telephone systems. Simulation and analytical modeling approaches such as queuing models have been widely adopted for call center operations, and the lean principles have been introduced to re-design the healthcare telephone systems as well. A simulation model can be used to generate the operation results under "what-if" scenarios. Comparison between the simulation results and actual operation can yield valuable information which may be used to identify the system inefficiencies. Simulation may also provide a solution to analyzing the integration of human factors and operations models. Green (2006) discussed about the queuing applications that might be used in healthcare settings especially in the call center for healthcare institutions. Anton et al. (2000) elaborated the role of simulation in the call center settings and argued that healthcare call centers might benefit from improving the operations. The concept of "lean" can be introduced to healthcare telephone systems. The primary goal of lean thinking is to eliminate wastes. Despite the fact that Lean concept is originally developed for the automotive industry where the production volume is high, it has been adopted and customized by other manufacturing companies as well as service organizations (Lander & Liker 2007). Waste of money, time, supplies, or goods will negatively influence the quality of services. The applications of lean thinking in healthcare telephone systems are demonstrating a positive impact on the timely delivery of services via telephones. Needless to say, improper lean implementation may result in poorer services (Sinaiko, 1999). The warning signs include inaccurate billing and medical records, patient complaints on the service received, and low employee morality. Kim et al. (2006) consider the cultural issue as a critical important challenge in lean health care. The individually functioning units and silos in a healthcare organization should cooperate to enhance the entire process flow, and the big improvements are obtainable through continuous small changes (Spears, 2005). Applying the operations management principles in the form of re-engineering also benefits the improvement of the existing services of the telephone response systems. In that vein, Rateb et al. (2011) documented that the effect of the re-engineering in the selected check-up centers for pre-employment purposes. Six randomly selected centers were evaluated for this purpose with the re-engineering activities focusing on three main areas, namely, structure, process and outcome. The authors indicated that significant improvements (around 65% reduction) in the cycle time, and amount of the delay per customer were realized. Similarly, discrete event simulation and process improvement can also help increase patient service performance. Rohleder et al. (2013) indicated that their improvement project in the medical call center led to significant reductions in the average answering-speed (ASA) and average abandonment rate (AAR). However, the authors cautioned that the major difficulty lies with the evaluating true impact of the improvement projects because there is no control group that can be benchmarked with for evaluating the true effect of the improvement projects. Shi et al. (2014) applied the approach of discrete event simulation to improve the performance of a mini call center at a Veterans Affairs medical center. The resource pooling scenarios were proposed, and they were verified to outperform the current operations by reducing abandonment rate and balancing the resource utilizations.

5.5 Outsourcing

The potential outsourcing of calls in a healthcare telephone system is one important aspect to increase the capacity of healthcare telephone systems. The outsourcing of operations in call centers to foreign locations has been attractive (Aron et al., 2005) although the outsourcing trend brings some concerns for customer retention and loyalty. For example, advanced telecommunications systems have enabled companies such as Microsoft, Oracle, Bank of America, American Express to outsource their customers support centers to off-shore locations such as India and Philippines. Similarly, there exists the possibility to outsource the operations of healthcare telephone systems to other locations or companies (or departments). Barr (1997) discussed the role of outsourcing as part of the vision for expansion and suggested that outsourcing some functions can improve the healthcare operations and provide additional growth opportunities. Poster (2007) discussed the reasons behind the "national identity management" in outsourcing decisions where the employees are asked to subsume different national identities as part of their work. The authors indicated that this approach might be the result of various reasons such as being a tool for easing the tension between customer-agent relationship or a deliberate attempt for controlling the customers of the call center. No matter what the actual reason is, the outlined policy might be seen as a consequence of easing the tension that might stem from cultural and language differences that would be inevitably encountered during the process of receiving the service in a transnational call center.

5.6 Performance Metrics

Developing performance metrics for tele-health are of great importance. Various researchers have employed different measures to evaluate the effectiveness of the tele-health and telephone response systems. George et al. (2008) and Hirsch et al. (2007) discussed the tele-nursing from the overreferral and underreferral rates. Both underreferral and overreferral deteriorate the quality of the healthcare delivery systems, put the callers into healthcare risks, and increase the burden on the emergency departments. They should be incorporated to assess the effectiveness of the tele-nursing. Meanwhile, some studies are directed to establishing the computer telephony from cost perspective (Franzini et al., 2001). Others investigated the effect of computer telephony on the no-show rates (Piette and Schilinger, 2007), drug treatment services (Alemi et. al., 1997), medication adherence (Friedman et al, 1997), vaccination rates (Oake et al., 2009), accuracy of tele-diagnosis practices (Oztas et. al, 2007), the response rate of the clinical study (Stewart et al., 2012) The effect of tele-consultation on the reduction of the use of clinic resources and potential savings are also studied (Zanaboni et al., 2009) as well as the duration of the time to speak a live agent in emergency departments (Shokrollahi et al., 2008).

However, since tele-health is an umbrella term for a variety of different functions, developing overall performance metrics for tele-health is extremely challenging if not technically impossible. However, it should be noted that there is a substantial need for developing more comprehensive index for assessing the quality of the healthcare services delivered by the telephone systems. For this purpose, some of the performance metrics discussed in Section 3 might be borrowed and combined with the performance measures that are described in this section to construct composite indices to reflect the efficiency and effectiveness of telephone systems from a larger perspective. To cite an instance, the caller waiting time might be combined with the under referral rate for a tele-nursing applications to assess the quality of the service. Not only it would furnish the system designers, developers and analysts a powerful tool for assessing the limitations and strengths of a telephone system, but also at the same time, it would promote the transparency and accountability in the telephone response system.

6. CONCLUSIVE REMARKS

The healthcare industry faces enormous challenges of curbing costs, improving the service quality and operation efficiency. From the perspective of improving service quality and operation efficiency, it should be noted that telephone operations might provide the way for enhancing the activities of the hospital operations and might provide the base for the cost reductions during the delivery of the healthcare services. The paper in that sense systematically reviews the research progress of healthcare telephone systems and analyzes the related challenges and opportunities.

It is noted that besides traditional operations, healthcare telephone systems are being expanded to include some advanced functions, such as tele-counseling, tele-nursing, and tele-triage. These functions might be associated with improving the service of the operations, and provide the ways for bringing cost effective solutions that might be used for streamlining the patients and corresponding activities. However, the difficulties in optimizing healthcare telephone systems are also evident as the functions and complexity of these systems keep increasing. The major challenges are the high patient expectations, the potential legal issues that might arise with the remote tele-health applications. Consistency and efficiency of the services, incorporating the human factors in the telephone systems are of great importance. The chapter addresses the challenges and identifies the opportunities to improve the telephone systems in healthcare. It is expected that in the future healthcare telephone systems can serve as a better communication tool to help patients access more resources, and to assist nurses and providers to provide quality services. The lean concepts might be further applied for improving the telephone related services. The telephone system might provide a supporting role for transforming the healthcare institutions for embracing the new concepts such as the patient centered medical home and personalized care.

The recent advances in the sensor technology, miniaturization of the electronic devices, information technology, and the mobile health platforms are immensely affecting and reshaping the role of telephone systems in the healthcare industry. The telephone systems rather than being obsolete in the face of changing paradigms, play more supportive roles, and should be considered an indispensable tool for improving the access of the patients for healthcare services, and increasing the quality of the care. However, the seamless integration of the telephone systems with the rapidly developing information technology is far from being complete and additional research is called for. The telephone systems is also benefitting from the advances in related software and hardware. Those tools are viable for enriching the communication with patients due to the nature of the service and the unique expectation and needs of patients.

REFERENCES

Abu-Hasaballah, K., James, A., & Aseltine, R. H. Jr. (2007). Lessons and pitfalls of interactive voice response in medical research. *Contemporary Clinical Trials*, *28*(5), 593–602. doi:10.1016/j.cct.2007.02.007 PMID:17400520

Adewale, O. S. (2004). An Internet-based telemedicine system in Nigeria. *International Journal of Information Management*, *24*(3), 221–234. doi:10.1016/j.ijinfomgt.2003.12.014

Adler-Milstein, J., & Bates, D. W. (2010). Paperless healthcare: Progress and challenges of an IT-enabled healthcare system. *Business Horizons*, *53*(2), 119–130. doi:10.1016/j.bushor.2009.10.004

Alemagno, S. A., Cochran, D., Feucht, T. E., Stephens, R. C., Butts, J. M., & Wolfe, S. A. (1996). Assessing substance abuse treatment needs among the homeless: A telephone-based interactive voice response system. *American Journal of Public Health*, *86*(11), 1626–1628. doi:10.2105/AJPH.86.11.1626 PMID:8916533

Alemi, F., Stephens, R. C., Javalghi, R. G., Dyches, H., Butts, J., & Ghadiri, A. (1996). A randomized trial of a telecommunications network for pregnant women who use cocaine. *Medical Care, 34*(suppl 10), OS10–OS20. doi:10.1097/00005650-199610003-00002 PMID:8843933

Alizadeh, R., Panahi, F., Saghafinia, M., Alizadeh, K., Barakati, N., & Khaje-Daloee, M. (2012). Impact of Trauma Dispatch Algorithm Software on the Rate of Missions of Emergency Medical Services. *Trauma Monthly, 17*(3), 319–322. doi:10.5812/traumamon.6341 PMID:24350116

Allen, S. I. (1969). The telephone as a computer input-output terminal for medical information. *Journal of the American Medical Association, 208*(4), 673–679. doi:10.1001/jama.1969.03160040081012 PMID:5818568

Allen-Davis, J. T., Beck, A., Parker, R., Ellis, J. L., & Polley, D. (2002). Assessment of vulvovaginal complaints: Accuracy of telephone triage and in-office diagnosis. *Obstetrics and Gynecology, 99*(1), 18–22. doi:10.1016/S0029-7844(01)01670-2 PMID:11777504

American Telemedicine Association. (n.d.). *What is Telemedicine & Telehealth*. Retrieved from; http://www.americantelemed.org/files/public/abouttelemedicine/What_Is_Telemedicine.pdf

Anderson, M. M., Boly, L. D., & Deck, R. W. (1996). Remote clinic/patient monitoring for multicenter trials. *Controlled Clinical Trials, 17*(5), 407–414. doi:10.1016/S0197-2456(96)00021-9 PMID:8932973

Anton, J. (2000). The past, present and future of customer access centers. *International Journal of Service Industry Management, 11*(2), 120–130. doi:10.1108/09564230010323534

Arnaert, A., & Macfarlane, F. (2011). Telehealth Nursing in Canada: Opportunities for Nurses to Shape the Future. In Telenursing (pp. 29-45). Springer London.

Aron, R., Clemons, E. K., & Reddi, S. (2005). Just right outsourcing: Understanding and managing risk. *Journal of Management Information Systems, 22*(2), 37–55.

Artalejo, J. R., Economou, A., & Corral, A. G. (2007). Applications of Maximum Queue Length for Call Center Management. *Computers & Operations Research, 34*(4), 983–996. doi:10.1016/j.cor.2005.05.020

Auger, C., Forster, A. J., Oake, N., & Tamblyn, R. (2013). Usability of a computerised drug monitoring programme to detect adverse drug events and non-compliance in outpatient ambulatory care. *BMJ Quality & Safety, 22*(4), 306–316. doi:10.1136/bmjqs-2012-001492 PMID:23396853

Balas, E. A., Jaffrey, F., Kuperman, G. J., Boren, S. A., Brown, G. D., Pinciroli, F., & Mitchell, J. A. (1997). Electronic communication with patients. Evaluation of distance medicine technology. *Journal of the American Medical Association, 278*(2), 152–159. doi:10.1001/jama.1997.03550020084043 PMID:9214532

Ball, M. J., & Lillis, J. (2001). E-health: transforming the physician: patient relationship. *International Journal of Medical Informatics, 61*(1), 1–10. doi:10.1016/S1386-5056(00)00130-1 PMID:11248599

Barlow, J., Bayer, S., & Curry, R. (2006). Implementing complex innovations in fluid multi-stakeholder environments: Experiences of 'telecare'. *Technovation, 26*(3), 396–406. doi:10.1016/j.technovation.2005.06.010

Barr, J. L., Laufenberg, S., & Sieckman, B. L. (1997). Creating a vision for your medical call center. *Healthcare Information Management: Journal of the Healthcare Information and Management Systems Society of the American Hospital Association, 12*(2), 71-85.

Beaulieu, R., & Humphreys, J. (2008). Evaluation of a telephone advice nurse in a nursing faculty managed pediatric community clinic. *Journal of Pediatric Health Care, 22*(3), 175–181. doi:10.1016/j.pedhc.2007.05.006 PMID:18455066

Berman, A. H., Farzanfar, R., Kristiansson, M., Carlbring, P., & Friedman, R. H. (2012). Design and development of a telephone-linked care (TLC) system to reduce impulsivity among violent forensic outpatients and probationers. *Journal of Medical Systems, 36*(3), 1031–1042. doi:10.1007/s10916-010-9565-1 PMID:20721686

Berner, E. S., Ray, M. N., Panjamapirom, A., Maisiak, R. S., Willig, J. H., English, T. M., & Schiff, G. D. et al. (2014). Exploration of an automated approach for receiving feedback after outpatient acute care visits. *Journal of General Internal Medicine, 29*(8), 1105–1112. doi:10.1007/s11606-014-2783-3 PMID:24610308

Biem, H. J., Klimaszewski, A., & Florence, C. (2004). Computer Telephony in Healthcare. *ElectronicHealthcare, 3*(2), 80–86. PMID:15540408

Biem, H. J., Turnell, R. W., & D'Arcy, C. (2003). Computer telephony: Automated calls for medical care. *Canadian Medical Association, 26*(5), 259–268. PMID:14596488

Black, P., Marsh, C., & Ashworth, L. (2009). Assessment of customer satisfaction with verbal responses provided by a pharmaceutical company's third-party medical information call center. *Drug Information Journal, 43*(3), 263–271.

Boulos, M. N., Wheeler, S., Tavares, C., & Jones, R. (2011). How smartphones are changing the face of mobile and participatory healthcare: An overview, with example from eCAALYX. *Biomedical Engineering Online, 10*(1), 24. PMID:21466669

Breslin, E., & Denison, J. (2002). The development of telephone triage: Historical, professional and personal perspectives. *Journal of Orthopaedic Nursing, 6*(4), 191–197. doi:10.1016/S1361-3111(02)00070-5

Briggs, J. K. (2007). *Telephone triage practices for nurses.* Lippincott Williams & Wilkins.

Bunik, M., Glazner, J. E., Chandramouli, V., Emsermann, C. B., Hegarty, T., & Kempe, A. (2007). Pediatric Telephone Call Centers: How do they affect health care use and costs? *Pediatrics, 119*(2), 305–313. doi:10.1542/peds.2006-1511 PMID:17272593

Bunn, F., Byrne, G., & Kendall, S. (2005). The effects of telephone consultation and triage on healthcare use and patient satisfaction: A systematic review. *The British Journal of General Practice, 55*(521), 956–961. PMID:16378566

Burney, A., Abbas, Z., Mahmood, N., & Arifeen, Q. U. (2013). Prospects for mobile health in Pakistan and other developing countries. *Advances in Internet of Things, 3*(022A), 27–32. doi:10.4236/ait.2013.32A004

Cantu, R. V., Bell, J. E., Padula, W. V., Nahikian, K. R., & Pober, D. M. (2012). How do emergency department physicians rate their orthopaedic on-call coverage? *Journal of Orthopaedic Trauma, 26*(1), 54–56. doi:10.1097/BOT.0b013e31821d7a81 PMID:21904223

Cassimatis, M., & Kavanagh, D. J. (2012). Effects of type 2 diabetes behavioural telehealth interventions on glycaemic control and adherence: A systematic review. *Journal of Telemedicine and Telecare, 18*(8), 447–450. doi:10.1258/jtt.2012.GTH105 PMID:23209266

Castelnuovo, G., Manzoni, G. M., Corti, S., Cuzziol, P., Villa, V., & Molinari, E. (2011). Clinical psychology and medicine for the treatment of obesity in out-patient settings: the TECNOB project. *Telemedicine Techniques and Applications*, 257-268.

Chanda, K. L., & Shaw, J. G. (2010). The development of telehealth as a strategy to improve health care services in Zambia. *Health Information and Libraries Journal, 27*(2), 133–139. doi:10.1111/j.1471-1842.2010.00876.x PMID:20565554

Coiera, E. (2006). Communication systems in healthcare. *The Clinical Biochemist. Reviews / Australian Association of Clinical Biochemists, 27*(2), 89. PMID:17077879

Coile, R. C. Jr. (1999). Call centers: Phone lines, protocols, and patient care management in the 21st century. *Russ Coile's Health Trends, 11*(5), 1–4. PMID:10351310

Corkrey, R., & Parkinson, L. (2002). Interactive voice response: Review of studies 1989–2000. *Behavior Research Methods, Instruments, & Computers, 34*(3), 342–353. doi:10.3758/BF03195462 PMID:12395550

Croidieu, S., Charbotel, B., Vohito, M., Renaud, L., Jaussaud, J., Bourboul, C., & Bergeret, A. et al. (2008). Call-handlers' working conditions and their subjective experience of work: A transversal study. *International Archives of Occupational and Environmental Health, 82*(1), 67–77. doi:10.1007/s00420-008-0308-2 PMID:18320205

Crouch, R., Patel, A., & Dale, J. (1996). Paediatric calls to inner city accident and emergency department: Service demand and advice given. *Accident and Emergency Nursing, 4*(4), 170–174. doi:10.1016/S0965-2302(96)90072-7 PMID:8981836

Dale, J., Crouch, R., & Lloyd, D. (1998). Primary care: Nurse-led telephone triage and advice out of hours. *Nursing Standard, 12*(47), 41–45. doi:10.7748/ns1998.08.12.47.39.c2520 PMID:9752159

Darkins, A. W., & Carry, M. A. (2000). *Telemedicine and telehealth. Principles, policies, performance and pitfalls*. Springer Publishing Company.

Delichatsios, H. K., Friedman, R. H., Glanz, K., Tennstedt, S., Smigelski, C., Pinto, B. M., & Killman, M. W. et al. (2001). Randomized trial of a talking computer to improve adults eating habits. *American Journal of Health Promotion, 15*(4), 215–224. doi:10.4278/0890-1171-15.4.215 PMID:11349340

Deslauriers, A., L'Ecuyer, P., Pichitlamken, J., Ingolfsson, A., & Avramidis, A. N. (2007). Markov chain models of a telephone call center with call blending. *Computers & Operations Research, 34*(6), 1616–1645. doi:10.1016/j.cor.2005.06.019

DeVore, N. E. (1999). Telephone triage: A challenge for practicing midwives. *Journal of Nurse-Midwifery, 44*(5), 471–479. doi:10.1016/S0091-2182(99)00087-7 PMID:10540521

Dini, E. F., Wilkins, R. W., & Sigafoos, J. (2000). The impact of computer-generated messages on childhood immunization coverage. *American Journal of Preventive Medicine, 18*(2), 132–139. doi:10.1016/S0749-3797(99)00086-0 PMID:10698243

Duder, J. C., & Rosenwein, M. B. (2001). Towards "zero abandonments" in call center performance. *European Journal of Operational Research, 135*(1), 50–56. doi:10.1016/S0377-2217(00)00289-7

Ekeland, A. G., Bowes, A., & Flottorp, S. (2010). Effectiveness of telemedicine: A systematic review of reviews. *International Journal of Medical Informatics, 79*(11), 736–771. doi:10.1016/j.ijmedinf.2010.08.006 PMID:20884286

Ertogral, K., & Bamuqabel, B. (2008). Developing staff schedules for a bilingual telecommunication call center with flexible workers. *Computers & Industrial Engineering, 54*(1), 118–127. doi:10.1016/j.cie.2007.06.040

Evenson, A., Harker, P. T., & Frei, F. X. (1999). *Effective Call Center Management: Evidence from Financial Services*. Working Paper 9925B. Wharton Financial Institutions Center.

Executive, N. H. S. (1999). Quality and Performance in the NHS: Clinical Indicators. Author.

Federspiel, C. C., Fisk, W. J., Price, P. N., Liu, G., Faulkner, D., Dibartolemeo, D. L., & Lahiff, M. et al. (2004). Worker performance and ventilation in a call center: Analyses of work performance data for registered nurses. *Indoor Air, 14*(s8), 41–50. doi:10.1111/j.1600-0668.2004.00299.x PMID:15663459

Feldman-Naim, S., Myers, F. S., Clark, C. H., Turner, E. H., & Leibenluft, E. (1997). Agreement between face-to-face and telephone-administered mood ratings in patients with rapid cycling bipolar disorder. *Psychological Research, 71*, 129–132. PMID:9255857

Franzini, L., Rosenthal, J., Spears, W., Martin, H. S., Balderas, L., Brown, M., & Hanson, C. et al. (2000). Cost effectiveness of childhood immunization reminder/recall systems in urban private practices. *Pediatrics, 166*, 177–183. PMID:10888689

Friedman, R. H., Kazis, L. E., & Jette, A. (1996). A telecommunications system with monitoring and counseling patients with hypertension. Impact on medication adherence and blood pressure control. *American Journal of Hypertension, 9*(4 pt 1), 285–292. doi:10.1016/0895-7061(95)00353-3 PMID:8722429

Fuchsia Howard, A., Smillie, K., Turnbull, K., Zirul, C., Munroe, D., Ward, A., & Olson, R. et al. (2014). Access to Medical and Supportive Care for Rural and Remote Cancer Survivors in Northern British Columbia. *The Journal of Rural Health, 30*(3), 311–321. doi:10.1111/jrh.12064 PMID:24483272

Ganapathy, K., & Ravindra, A. (2011). Telenursing in an emerging economy: An overview. In Telenursing (pp. 47-59). Springer London.

Garnet, O., Mandelbaum, A., & Reiman, M. (2002). Designing a call center with impatient customers. *Manufacturing & Service Operations Management, 4*(3), 208–227. doi:10.1287/msom.4.3.208.7753

George, I. S. T., Cullen, M., Gardiner, L., Karabatsos, G., Ng, J. Y.-K., Patterson, A., & Wilson, A. (2007). Universal telenursing triage in Australia and New Zealand. *Australian Family Physician, 37*(6), 476–479. PMID:18523705

Ghorai, K., Akter, S., Khatun, F., & Ray, P. (2014). mHealth for Smoking Cessation Programs: A Systematic Review. *Journal of Personalized Medicine, 4*(3), 412–423. doi:10.3390/jpm4030412 PMID:25563359

Gilmour, M. B. (2001). A model for a telephone response system to disaster and trauma. *Traumatology, 6*(3), 120–125. doi:10.1177/153476560100700304

Girling, D. (2000). Important issues in planning and conducting multi-centre randomised trials in cancer and publishing their results. *Critical Reviews in Oncology/Hematology, 36*(1), 13–25. doi:10.1016/S1040-8428(00)00095-0 PMID:10996520

Gottesman, O., Kuivaniemi, H., Tromp, G., Faucett, W. A., Li, R., Manolio, T. A., & …, eMERGE Network, T. (2013). The Electronic Medical Records and Genomics (eMERGE) network: Past, present, and future. *Genetics in Medicine, 15*(10), 761–771. PMID:23743551

Graham, J., Tomcavage, J., Salek, D., Sciandra, J., Davis, D. E., & Stewart, W. F. (2012). Postdischarge monitoring using interactive voice response system reduces 30-day readmission rates in a case-managed Medicare population. *Medical Care, 50*(1), 50–57. doi:10.1097/MLR.0b013e318229433e PMID:21822152

Green, L. (2006). Queueing analysis in healthcare. In Patient flow: Reducing delay in healthcare delivery (pp. 281-307). Springer US. doi:10.1007/978-0-387-33636-7_10

Gregoski, M. J., Mueller, M., Vertegel, A., Shaporev, A., Jackson, B. B., Frenzel, R. M., & Treiber, F. A. et al. (2012). Development and validation of a smartphone heart rate acquisition application for health promotion and wellness telehealth applications. *International Journal of Telemedicine and Applications, 2012*, 696324. PMID:22272197

Grigsby, J., & Sanders, J. H. (1998). Telemedicine: Where it is and where it's going. *Annals of Internal Medicine, 129*(2), 123–127. doi:10.7326/0003-4819-129-2-199807150-00012 PMID:9669971

Grosjean, V., & De Weerdt, C. R. V. (2005). Towards a psycho-ergonomics study of wellbeing and emotions: The effects of organisational control in call centers. *Le Travail Humain, 68*(4), 355–378. doi:10.3917/th.684.0355

Haghighat, S., Yunesian, M., Akbari, M. E., Ansari, M., & Montezari, A. (2007). Telephone and face-to-face consultation in breast cancer diagnosis: A comparative study. *Patient Education and Counseling, 67*(1-2), 39–43. doi:10.1016/j.pec.2007.01.015 PMID:17467949

Hall, V., Gomez, C., & Fernandez-Llimos, F. (2006). Situation of drug information centers and services in Costa Rica. *Pharmacy Practice, 4*(2), 83–87. PMID:25246999

Hamill, C. T., & Lorri, H.-S. (1998). 24-hour call centers and home health care. *Home Care Provider, 3*(6), 324–325. doi:10.1016/S1084-628X(98)90012-0 PMID:10030213

Heschong Mahone Group. (2003). *Windows and offices: A study of office workers performance and the indoor environment.* California Energy Commission. Retrieved from http://www.ecw.org/sites/default/files/HMG_Windows_Offices.pdf

Heyworth, L., Kleinman, K., Oddleifson, S., Bernstein, L., Frampton, J., Lehrer, M., & Connelly, M. (2014). Comparison of interactive voice response, patient mailing, and mailed registry to encourage screening for osteoporosis: A randomized controlled trial. *Osteoporosis International, 25*(5), 1519–1526. doi:10.1007/s00198-014-2629-1 PMID:24566584

Hill, J. W., & Powell, P. (2009). The national healthcare crisis: Is eHealth a key solution? *Business Horizons, 52*(3), 265–277. doi:10.1016/j.bushor.2009.01.006

Hirsh, D. A., Massey, R., Simon, J., & Simon, H. (2004). Does use of a pediatric telephone triage system lead to appropriate pediatric ED utilization? *Pediatric Research, 55*, 120A.

Hirsh, D. A., Simon, H. K., Massey, R., Thomton, L., & Simon, J. E. (2007). The Host Hospital 24-Hour Underreferral Rate: An Automated Measure of Call-Center Safety. *Pediatrics, 119*(6), 1139–1144. doi:10.1542/peds.2006-1986 PMID:17545381

Hogan, T. P., Wakefield, B., Nazi, K. M., Houston, T. K., & Weaver, F. M. (2011). Promoting access through complementary eHealth technologies: Recommendations for VA's Home Telehealth and personal health record programs. *Journal of General Internal Medicine, 26*(2), 628–635. doi:10.1007/s11606-011-1765-y PMID:21989614

Horton, R. C., Minniti, A., Mireylees, S., & McEntegart, D. (2008). A randomized trial to determine the impact on compliance of a psychophysical peripheral cue based on the Elaboration Likelihood Model. *Contemporary Clinical Trials, 29*(6), 823–828. doi:10.1016/j.cct.2008.08.005 PMID:18805509

Hsu, M. H., Chu, T. B., Yen, J. C., Chiu, W. T., Yeh, G. C., Chen, T. J., & Li, Y. C. J. (2010). Development and implementation of a national telehealth project for long-term care: A preliminary study. *Computer Methods and Programs in Biomedicine, 97*(3), 286–292. doi:10.1016/j.cmpb.2009.12.008 PMID:20092907

Hyman, D. J., Ho, K. S., Dunn, J. K., & Simons-Morton, D. (1998). Dietary intervention for cholesterol reduction in public clinic patients. *American Journal of Preventive Medicine, 15*(2), 139–145. doi:10.1016/S0749-3797(98)00038-5 PMID:9713670

Isenberg, S. F., Davis, C. L., Adams, C. E., Isenberg, J. S., & Isenberg, M. A. (2001). Incentivized Digital Outcomes Collection. *American Journal of Medical Quality, 16*(6), 202–211. doi:10.1177/106286060101600604 PMID:11816851

Jack, E. P., Bedics, T. A., & McCary, C. E. (2006). Operational challenges in the call center industry: A case study and resource-based framework. *Managing Service Quality, 16*(5), 477–500. doi:10.1108/09604520610686142

Joshi, A., Rane, M., Roy, D., Emmadi, N., Srinivasan, P., Kumarasamy, N., & Rutten, R. et al. (2014, April). Supporting treatment of people living with HIV/AIDS in resource limited settings with IVRs. In *Proceedings of the 32nd annual ACM conference on Human Factors in Computing Systems* (pp. 1595-1604). ACM. doi:10.1145/2556288.2557236

Jouini, O., Koole, G., & Roubos, A. (2013). Performance indicators for call centers with impatient customers. *IIE Transactions*, *45*(3), 341–354. doi:10.1080/0740817X.2012.712241

Kamei, T., Yamamoto, Y., Kajii, F., Nakayama, Y., & Kawakami, C. (2013). Systematic review and meta-analysis of studies involving telehome monitoring-based telenursing for patients with chronic obstructive pulmonary disease. *Japan Journal of Nursing Science*, *10*(2), 180–192. doi:10.1111/j.1742-7924.2012.00228.x PMID:24373441

Kathryn, A., Cull, A., & Sharpe, M. (2003). Diagnosing medical depression in medical outpatient: Acceptability of telephone interviews. *Journal of Psychosomatic Research*, *55*(4), 385–387. doi:10.1016/S0022-3999(02)00637-2 PMID:14507551

Kempe, A., Bunik, M., Ellis, J., Magid, D., Hegarty, T., Dickinson, L. M., & Steiner, J. F. (2006). How safe is triage by an after-hours telephone call center? *Pediatrics*, *118*(2), 457–463. doi:10.1542/peds.2005-3073 PMID:16882795

Kempe, A., Dempsey, C., Hegarty, T., Frei, N., Chandramouli, V., & Poole, S. R. (2000a). Reducing after-hours referrals by an after-hours call center with second-level physician triage. *Pediatrics*, *106*(1), 226–230. PMID:10888697

Kempe, A., Dempsey, C., Whitefield, C., Bothner, T., Mackenzie, T., & Poole, S. (2000b). Appropriateness of urgent referrals by nurses at a hospital-based pediatric call center. *Archives of Pediatrics & Adolescent Medicine*, *154*(4), 355–360. doi:10.1001/archpedi.154.4.355 PMID:10768672

Kempe, A., Luberti, A. A., Hertz, A. R., Sherman, H. B., Amin, H. B., Dempsey, C., & Hegarthy, T. W. et al. (2001). Delivery of pediatric after-hours care by call centers: A multicenter study of parental perceptions and compliance. *Pediatrics*, *108*(6), 111–117. doi:10.1542/peds.108.6.e111 PMID:11731638

Khamis, A.-H., James, A., & Aseltine, R. H. (2007). Lessons and pitfalls of interactive voice response in medical research. *Contemporary Clinical Trials*, *28*(5), 593–602. doi:10.1016/j.cct.2007.02.007 PMID:17400520

Kidd, L., Cayless, S., Johnston, B., & Wengstrom, Y. (2010). Telehealth in palliative care in the UK: A review of the evidence. *Journal of Telemedicine and Telecare*, *16*(7), 394–402. PMID:20813893

Kim, C. S., Spahlinger, D. A., Kin, J. M., & Billi, J. E. (2006). Lean health care: What can hospitals learn from a world-class automaker? *Journal of Hospital Medicine*, *1*(3), 191–199. doi:10.1002/jhm.68 PMID:17219493

Kim, H., Bracha, A., & Tipnis, A. (2007). Automated depression screening in disadvantaged pregnant women in an urban obstetric clinic. *Archives of Women's Mental Health*, *10*(4), 163–169. doi:10.1007/s00737-007-0189-5 PMID:17593320

Koch, S. (2006). Home telehealth-Current state and future trends. *International Journal of Medical Informatics*, *75*(8), 565–576. doi:10.1016/j.ijmedinf.2005.09.002 PMID:16298545

Korcz, I. P., & Moreland, S. (1998). Telephone prescreening: Enhancing a model for proactive healthcare practice. *Cancer Practice*, *6*(5), 270–275. doi:10.1046/j.1523-5394.1998.00021.x PMID:9767345

Kwan, S. K., Davis, M. M., & Greenwood, A. G. (1988). A simulation model for determining variable worker requirements in a service operation with time-dependent customer demand. *Queueing Systems*, *3*(3), 265–276. doi:10.1007/BF01161218

Lander, E., & Liker, J. K. (2007). The Toyota production system and art: Making highly customized and creative products the Toyota way. *International Journal of Production Research*, *45*(16), 3681–3698. doi:10.1080/00207540701223519

Lee, H., Friedman, M. E., Cukor, P., & Ahern, D. (2003). Interactive Voice Response System (IVRS) in Health Care Services. *Nursing Outlook*, *51*(6), 277–283. doi:10.1016/S0029-6554(03)00161-1 PMID:14688763

Lee, H. J., Lee, S. H., Ha, K.-S., Jang, H. C., Chung, H. C., Kim, H. C., & Yoo, D. H. et al. (2009). Ubiquitous healthcare service using Zigbee and mobile phone for elderly patients. *International Journal of Medical Informatics*, *78*(3), 193–198. doi:10.1016/j.ijmedinf.2008.07.005 PMID:18760959

Lee, T. J., Baraff, L. J., Guzy, J., Johnson, D., & Woo, H. (2003b). Does telephone triage delay significant medical treatment? *Archives of Pediatrics & Adolescent Medicine*, *157*(7), 635–641. doi:10.1001/archpedi.157.7.635 PMID:12860783

Lenz, R., & Manfred, R. (2006). IT support for healthcare processes– premises, challenges, perspectives. *Data & Knowledge Engineering*, *61*(1), 39–58. doi:10.1016/j.datak.2006.04.007

Leydon, G. M., Ekberg, K., Kelly, M., & Drew, P. (2013). Improving ethnic monitoring for telephone-based healthcare: A conversation analytic study. *BMJ Open*, *3*(6e002676), 1–7. doi:10.1136/bmjopen-2013-002676 PMID:23811170

Lin, C. W., Pan, C. J., Paranjape, K., Yu, C., & Feng, P. (2014). Taipei Citizen Telecare Service System for Hypertension Management in Elders. In *2014 Annual SRII Global Conference (SRII)* (pp. 157-180). IEEE.

Lindsay, J. A., Minard, C. G., Hudson, S., Green, C. E., & Schmitz, J. M. (2014). Using prize-based incentives to enhance daily interactive voice response (IVR) compliance: A feasibility study. *Journal of Substance Abuse Treatment*, *46*(1), 74–77. doi:10.1016/j.jsat.2013.08.003 PMID:24029622

Mahesh, V. S., & Kasturi, A. (2006). Improving call centre agent performance - A UK-India study based on the agents' point of view. *International Journal of Service Industry Management*, *17*(2), 136–157. doi:10.1108/09564230610656971

Mariño, R., Clarke, K., Manton, D. J., Stranieri, A., Collmann, R., Kellet, H., & Borda, A. (2015). Teleconsultation and Telediagnosis for Oral Health Assessment: An Australian Perspective. In Teledentistry (pp. 101-112). Springer International Publishing.

Martin, A. C. (2013). Legal, clinical, and ethical issues in teletherapy.*Psychoanalysis Online: Mental Health, Teletherapy, and Training*, 75.

McBride, C. M., & Rimer, B. K. (1999). Using the telephone to improve health behavior and health service delivery. *Patient Education and Counseling*, *37*(1), 3–18. doi:10.1016/S0738-3991(98)00098-6 PMID:10640115

McConnell, K. J., Johnson, L. A., Arab, N., Richards, C. F., Newgard, C. D., & Edlund, T. (2007). The on-call crisis: A statewide assessment of the costs of providing on-call specialist coverage. *Annals of Emergency Medicine*, *49*(6), 727–733. doi:10.1016/j.annemergmed.2006.10.017 PMID:17210209

McDaniel, J. G. (1995). Discrete event simulation of a wide area health care network. *Journal of the American Medical Informatics Association*, *2*(4), 220–237. doi:10.1136/jamia.1995.96010391 PMID:7583646

McKinstry, B., Walker, J., Campbell, C., Heaney, D., & Wyke, S. (2002). Telephone consultations to manage requests for same-day appointments: A randomized controlled trial in two practices. *The British Journal of General Practice*, *52*(477), 306–310. PMID:11942448

McNall, L. A., & Roch, S. G. (2009). A social exchange model of employee reactions to electronic performance monitoring. *Human Performance*, *22*(3), 204–224. doi:10.1080/08959280902970385

McNemish, J., Lyle, D., McCowan, M., Emmerson, S., McAuley, S., & Reilly, J. (2007). Post-discharge surgical site infection surveillance by automated telephony. *Journal of Hospital Telephony*, *66*(3), 232–236. doi:10.1016/j.jhin.2007.04.003 PMID:17544545

Miciak, A., & Desmarais, M. (2001). Benchmarking service quality performance at business-to-business and business-to-consumer call centers. *Journal of Business and Industrial Marketing*, *16*(5), 340–353. doi:10.1108/08858620110400205

Miller, D. I., Bruce, H., Gagnon, M., Talbot, V., & Messier, C. (2011). Improving older adults' experience with interactive voice response systems. *Telemedicine Journal and e-Health*, *17*(6), 452–455. doi:10.1089/tmj.2010.0204 PMID:21631386

Mohan, J., Razali, R., & Yaacob, R. (2003). The Malaysian telehealth flagship application: A national approach to health data protection and utilisation and consumer rights. *International Journal of Medical Informatics*, *73*(3), 217–227. doi:10.1016/j.ijmedinf.2003.11.023 PMID:15066550

Mohanty, S. A., Donna, L., Washington, S., Lambe, S., Fink, A., & Asch, S. M. (2006). Predictors of on-call specialist response times in California emergency departments. *Academic Emergency Medicine*, *13*(5), 505–512. doi:10.1111/j.1553-2712.2006.tb01000.x PMID:16609102

Moran, M. (2014). Rule change on emergency care could reduce specialty coverage. *Psychiatr News, 38*, 10-28. Retrieved from http://pn.psychiatryonline.org/cgi/content/full/38/22/10?etoc

Morrissey, J. (1999). FHS hooks up with Access Health Group. Calif. HMO will outsource its telephone medical advice services to Colo. Company. *Modern Healthcare*, *29*(4), 36. PMID:10345464

Morton, J. M., Baker, C. C., Farrell, T. M., Yohe, M. H., Kimple, R. J., Herman, D. C., & Meyer, A. et al. (2004). What do surgery residents do on their call nights? *American Journal of Surgery*, *188*(3), 225–229. doi:10.1016/j.amjsurg.2004.06.011 PMID:15450824

Muir, J., Xu, C., Paul, S., Staib, A., McNeill, I., Singh, P., & Sinnott, M. (2011). Incorporating teledermatology into emergency medicine. *Emergency Medicine Australasia*, *23*(5), 562–568. doi:10.1111/j.1742-6723.2011.01443.x PMID:21995470

Mundt, J. C., Katzelnick, D. J., Kennedy, S. H., Eisfeld, B. S., Bouffard, B. B., & Greist, J. H. (2006). Validation of an IVRS version of the MADRS. *Journal of Psychiatric Research*, *40*(3), 243–246. doi:10.1016/j.jpsychires.2005.05.002 PMID:15979643

Narayan, M. C. (2001). Oasis Voice Mailbox InServices. *Home Healthcare Nurse*, *19*(9), 542–548. doi:10.1097/00004045-200109000-00011 PMID:11982193

Nicholls, W. L. (1988). Computer-assisted telephone interviewing: A general introduction. In R. M. Groves, P. P. Biemer, L. E. Lyberg, J. T. Massey, W. L. Nicholls, & J. Waksberg (Eds.), *Telephone Survey Methodology* (pp. 377–385). New York: Wiley.

O'Brien, J. A., Ward, A. J., Jones, M. K. C., McMillan, C., & Lordan, L. (2003). Utilization of health care services by patients with chronic obstructive pulmonary disease. *Respiratory Medicine*, *97*(S1), S53–S58. doi:10.1016/S0954-6111(03)80015-X PMID:12564611

Oake, N., Jennings, A., van Walrayen, C., & Forster, A. J. (2009). Interactive Voice Response Systems for Improving Delivery of Ambulatory Care. *The American Journal of Managed Care*, *15*(6), 283–291. PMID:19514804

Oztas, M. O., Calikoglu, E., Baz, K., Birol, A., Onder, M., Calikoglu, T., & Kitapci, M. T. (2004). Reliability of Web-based teledermatology consultations. *Journal of Telemedicine and Telecare*, *10*(1), 25–28. doi:10.1258/135763304322764158 PMID:15006212

Petersen, J. A., Mackel, R., Antonsen, K., & Rasmussen, L. S. (2014). Serious adverse events in a hospital using *early warning score*–What went wrong? *Resuscitation*, *85*(12), 1699–1703. doi:10.1016/j.resuscitation.2014.08.037 PMID:25238741

Piette, J. D. (2000). Perceived Access Problems among patients with diabetes in two public systems of care. *Journal of General Internal Medicine*, *15*(11), 797–804. doi:10.1046/j.1525-1497.2000.91107.x PMID:11119172

Piette, J. D., & Schilinger, D. (2007). *Medical management of vulnerable and underserved patients. Principles, practices and populations. Mc* Graw Hill Companies.

Pike, J. H. (2003). Nature of After-Hours Calls at a Tertiary-Level Rehabilitation Center. *Archives of Physical Medicine and Rehabilitation*, *84*(7), 1039–1042. doi:10.1016/S0003-9993(03)00028-5 PMID:12881831

Pinto, B. M., Friedman, R., Marcus, B. H., Kelley, H., Tennstedt, S., & Gillman, M. W. (2002). Effects of a computer based telephone-counseling system on physical activity. *American Journal of Preventive Medicine*, *23*(2), 113–120. doi:10.1016/S0749-3797(02)00441-5 PMID:12121799

Pohjanoksa-Mantyla, M. K., Antila, J., Eerikainen, S., Enakoski, M., Hannuksela, O., Pietila, K., & Airaksinen, M. (2008). Utilization of a community pharmacy-operated national drug information call center in Finland. *Research in Social & Administrative Pharmacy*, *4*(2), 144–152. doi:10.1016/j.sapharm.2007.05.001 PMID:18555967

Poole, S. R., Schmitt, B. D., Carruth, T., Peterson-Smith, A., & Slusarski, M. (1993). After-hours telephone coverage: The application of an area-wide telephone triage and advice system for pediatric practices. *Pediatrics*, *92*(5), 670–679. PMID:8414853

Poster, W. R. (2007). Who's On the Line? Indian Call Center Agents Pose as Americans for US-Outsourced Firms. *Industrial Relations*, *46*(2), 271–304. doi:10.1111/j.1468-232X.2007.00468.x

Prasad, M. K. S., Mahmood, S., Gregson, B. A., & Mitchell, P. (2012). Telephone logs of neurosurgery specialty trainees: A time study. *British Journal of Neurosurgery*, *26*(2), 195–198. doi:10.3109/026886 97.2011.633643 PMID:22149539

Pratt, S. I., Naslund, J. A., Wolfe, R. S., Santos, M., & Bartels, S. J. (2014). Automated telehealth for managing psychiatric instability in people with serious mental illness. *Journal of Mental Health*, 1-5.

Prince, S. B., & Herrin, D. M. (2007). The role of information technology in healthcare communications, efficiency, and patient safety. *The Journal of Nursing Administration*, *37*(4), 184–187. doi:10.1097/01. NNA.0000266841.46684.50 PMID:17415105

Rao, M. B., Lerro, C., & Gross, C. P. (2010). The Shortage of On-call Surgical Specialist Coverage: A National Survey of Emergency Department Directors. *Academic Emergency Medicine*, *17*(12), 1374–1382. doi:10.1111/j.1553-2712.2010.00927.x PMID:21091822

Rask, K. J., LeBaron, C. W., & Starnes, D. M. (2001). The Cost of Registry-Based Immunization Based Interventions. *American Journal of Preventive Medicine*, *21*(4), 267–271. doi:10.1016/S0749-3797(01)00370-1 PMID:11701296

Rateb, S. A. H., El Nouman, A. A. R., Rateb, M. A. H., Asar, M. N., El Amin, A. M., & Mohamed, M. S. E. (2011). Re-engineering pre-employment check-up systems: A model for improving health services. *International Journal of Health Care Quality Assurance*, *24*(6), 484–497. doi:10.1108/09526861111150734 PMID:21916149

Reardon, G. T., Blumenfield, S., Weissman, A., & Rosenberg, G. (1988). Findings and implications from preadmission screening of elderly patients waiting for elective surgery. *Social Work in Health Care*, *13*(3), 51–63. doi:10.1300/J010v13n03_05 PMID:2852851

Remschmidt, H., Hirsch, O., & Mattejat, F. (2003). Reliability and validity of evaluation data collected by telephone. *Zeitschrift fur Kinder- und Jugendpsychiatrie und Psychotherapie*, *31*(1), 35–49. doi:10.1024/1422-4917.31.1.35 PMID:12616747

Revicki, D. A., Tohen, M., Gyulai, L., Thompson, C., Pike, S., Davis-Vogel, A., & Zarate, C. (1997). Telephone versus in-person clinical and health assessment interviews in patients with bipolar disorder. *Harvard Review of Psychiatry*, *5*(2), 75–81. doi:10.3109/10673229709034730 PMID:9385024

Rimner, T., Blozik, E., Begley, C., Grandchamp, C., & von Overbeck, J. (2011). Patient adherence to recommendations after teleconsultation: Survey of patients from a telemedicine centre in Switzerland. *Journal of Telemedicine and Telecare*, *17*(5), 235–239. doi:10.1258/jtt.2011.101013 PMID:21565847

Ritchie, C., Richman, J., Sobko, H., Bodner, E., Phillips, B., & Houston, T. (2012). The E-Coach transition support computer telephony implementation study: Protocol of a randomized trial. *Contemporary Clinical Trials*, *33*(6), 1172–1179. doi:10.1016/j.cct.2012.08.007 PMID:22922245

Robinson, G., & Morley, C. (2006). Call centre management: Responsibilities and performance. *International Journal of Service Industry Management*, *17*(3), 284–300. doi:10.1108/09564230610667122

Rohde, P., Lewinsohn, P. M., & Seeley, J. R. (1997). Comparability of telephone and face-to-face interviews in assessing axis I and II disorders. *The American Journal of Psychiatry*, *154*(11), 1593–1598. doi:10.1176/ajp.154.11.1593 PMID:9356570

Rohleder, T., Bailey, B., Crum, B., Faber, T., Johnson, B., Montgomery, L., & Pringnitz, R. (2013). Improving a patient appointment call center at Mayo Clinic. *International Journal of Health Care Quality Assurance*, *26*(8), 714–728. doi:10.1108/IJHCQA-11-2011-0068 PMID:24422261

Röing, M., & Holmström, I. K. (2015). Malpractice Claims in Swedish Telenursing: Lessons Learned From Interviews With Telenurses and Managers. *Nursing Research*, *64*(1), 35–43. doi:10.1097/NNR.0000000000000063 PMID:25502059

Romano, M. J., & Stafford, R. S. (2011). Electronic health records and clinical decision support systems: Impact on national ambulatory care quality. *Archives of Internal Medicine*, *171*(10), 897–903. doi:10.1001/archinternmed.2010.527 PMID:21263077

Rudkin, S. E., Langdorf, M. I., Oman, J. A., Kahn, C. A., White, H., & Anderson, C. L. (2009). The worsening of ED on-call coverage in California: 6-year trend. *The American Journal of Emergency Medicine*, *27*(7), 785–791. doi:10.1016/j.ajem.2008.06.012 PMID:19683105

Rudkin, S. E., Oman, J., Langdorf, M. I., Hill, M., Bauche, J., Kivela, P., & Johnson, L. (2004). The state of ED on-call coverage in California. *The American Journal of Emergency Medicine*, *22*(7), 578–581. doi:10.1016/j.ajem.2004.08.001 PMID:15666264

Russell, B. (2012). Professional call centres, professional workers and the paradox of the algorithm: The case of telenursing. *Work, Employment and Society*, *26*(2), 195–210. doi:10.1177/0950017011433155

Sakar, C. O., & Kursun, O. (2010). Telediagnosis of Parkinson's disease using measurements of dysphonia. *Journal of Medical Systems*, *34*(4), 591–599. doi:10.1007/s10916-009-9272-y PMID:20703913

Santana, M. A. S., Aupet, J. B., Betbeder, M. L., Lapayre, J. C., & Ibarrola, J. A. C. (2012). Adaptive collaborative environment for vascular problems telediagnosis. In *Ambient Assisted Living and Home Care* (pp. 1–8). Springer Berlin Heidelberg. doi:10.1007/978-3-642-35395-6_1

Saraux, A., Guillemin, F., Fardellone, P., Guggenbuhl, P., Behier, J. M., Cantagrel, A., & Coste, J. et al. (2004). Agreement between rheumatologist visit and lay interviewer telephone survey for screening for rheumatoid arthritis and spondyloarthropathy. *Joint, Bone, Spine*, *71*(1), 44–50. doi:10.1016/S1297-319X(03)00092-7 PMID:14769520

Schweiger, A., Sunyaev, A., Leimeister, J. M., & Krcmar, H. (2007). Information systems and healthcare XX: Toward seamless healthcare with software agents. *Communications of the Association for Information Systems*, *19*(1), 33.

Shi, J., Peng, Y., Erdem, E., & Woodbridge, P. (2014, September). Simulation analysis on patient visit efficiency of a typical VA primary care clinic with complex characteristics. *Simulation Modelling Practice and Theory, 47,* 165–181. doi:10.1016/j.simpat.2014.06.003

Shokrollahi, K., Tadiparthi, S., & Jayagopal, S. (2008). How fast is fast enough? An audit and league table of response times of acute hospital NHS Trust switchboards in England. *Journal of the Royal Society of Medicine, 101*(7), 364–371. doi:10.1258/jrsm.2008.080006 PMID:18591690

Silvestro, R., & Silvestro, C. (2003). New service design in NHS: An evaluation of the strategic alignment of NHS Direct. *International Journal of Operations & Production Management, 23*(4), 401–417. doi:10.1108/01443570310467320

Sinaiko, J. E. (1999). The danger of being too lean. Warning signs that your health care organization has cut too much. *Cost & Quality: CQ, 5*(4), 29–31. PMID:11066613

Snooks, H. A., Williams, A. M., Griffiths, L. J., Peconi, J., Rance, J., Snelgrove, S., & Cheung, W. Y. et al. (2008). Real nursing? The development of telenursing. *Journal of Advanced Nursing, 62*(6), 631–640. doi:10.1111/j.1365-2648.2007.04546.x PMID:18302604

Spear, S. J. (2005). Fixing health care from inside. *Harvard Business Review, 83*(9), 78–91. PMID:16171213

Stanberry, B. (2001). Legal and Ethical Issues in Telemedicine. *Computer Methods and Programs in Telemedicine, 64*(3), 225–233. doi:10.1016/S0169-2607(00)00142-5 PMID:11226620

Stewart, J. I., Moyle, S., Criner, G. J., Wilson, C., Tanner, R., Bowler, R. P., & Regan, E. A et al.. (2012). Automated telecommunication to obtain longitudinal follow-up in a multicenter cross-sectional COPD study. *COPD: Journal of Chronic Obstructive Pulmonary Disease, 9*(5), 466–472. doi:10.3109/15412 555.2012.690010 PMID:22676387

Stier, R. D. (1999). The medical call center. *Marketing Health Services, 19*(2), 25–28. PMID:10557751

Stirewalt, C. F., Linn, M. W., Godoy, G., Knopka, F., & Linn, B. S. (1982). Effectiveness of an ambulatory care telephone service in reducing drop-in visits and improving satisfaction with care. *Medical Care, 20*(7), 739–748. doi:10.1097/00005650-198207000-00009 PMID:7121093

Stritzke, W. G. K., Dandy, J., Durkin, K., & Houghton, S. (2005). Use of interactive voice response (IVR) technology in health research with children. *Behavior Research Methods, 37*(1), 119–126. doi:10.3758/ BF03206405 PMID:16097351

Suleiman, A. B. (2001). The untapped potential of tele-health. *International Journal of Medical Informatics, 61*(2-3), 103–112. doi:10.1016/S1386-5056(01)00132-0 PMID:11311664

Suomi, R., Serkkola, A., & Mikkonen, M. (2010). Automated Telephone Services in Dentist Appointment Management. *Informatics in Oral Medicine: Advanced Techniques in Clinical and Diagnostic Technologies,* 269-276.

Swanepoel, D. W., & Hall, J. W. III. (2010). A systematic review of telehealth applications in audiology. *Telemedicine Journal and e-Health, 16*(2), 181–200. doi:10.1089/tmj.2009.0111 PMID:20187743

Tham, K. W. (2004). Effects of temperature and outdoor air supply rate on the performance of call center operators in the tropics. *Indoor Air, 14*(s7), 119–125. doi:10.1111/j.1600-0668.2004.00280.x PMID:15330779

Tham, K. W., & Willem, H. C. (2004). *Effects of reported neurobehavioral symptoms on call center operator performance in the tropics.* In RoomVentilation Conference, Coimbra, Portugal

Thomas, J., & Kumar, P. (2013). The scope of teledermatology in India. *Indian Dermatology Online Journal, 4*(2), 82. doi:10.4103/2229-5178.110579 PMID:23741661

Toverud, E. L., Pike, E., & Walloe, E. (2009). The national poison center in Norway: User satisfaction and health economic evaluation. *European Journal of Clinical Pharmacology, 65*(9), 935–940. doi:10.1007/s00228-009-0693-9 PMID:19590863

Tsiknakis, M., & Kouroubali, A. (2009). Organizational factors affecting successful adoption of innovative eHealth services: A case study employing the FITT framework. *International Journal of Medical Informatics, 78*(1), 39–52. doi:10.1016/j.ijmedinf.2008.07.001 PMID:18723389

van der Marck, M. A., Overeem, S., Klok, P., Bloem, B. R., & Munneke, M. (2011). Evaluation of the falls telephone: An automated system for enduring assessment of falls. *Journal of the American Geriatrics Society, 59*(2), 340–344. doi:10.1111/j.1532-5415.2010.03263.x PMID:21314652

Wahlberg, A., Anna, C., Cedersund, E., & Wredling, R. (2003). Telephone nurses' experience of problems with telephone advice in Sweden. *Journal of Clinical Nursing, 12*(1), 37–45. doi:10.1046/j.1365-2702.2003.00702.x PMID:12519248

Wan, Y. N. (2012). *Call centre communication: an analysis of interpersonal meaning.* (Master's thesis). The Hong Kong Polytechnic University.

Wargocki, P., Wyon, D. P., & Fanger, P. O. (2004). The performance and subjective responses of call-center operators with new and used supply air filters at two outdoor air supply rates. *Indoor Air, 14*(s8Suppl. 8), 7–16. doi:10.1111/j.1600-0668.2004.00304.x PMID:15663456

Weir, H., & Waddington, K. (2008). Continuities in caring? Emotion work in a NHS Direct call centre. *Nursing Inquiry, 15*(1), 67–77. doi:10.1111/j.1440-1800.2008.00391.x PMID:18271792

Williams, B., Warren, S., McKim, R., & Janzen, W. (2012). Caller self-care decisions following teletriage advice. *Journal of Clinical Nursing, 21*(7-8), 1041–1050. doi:10.1111/j.1365-2702.2011.03986.x PMID:22283747

Witt, L. A., Andrews, M. C., & Carlson, D. S. (2004). When conscientiousness isn't enough: Emotional exhaustion and performance among call center customer service representatives. *Journal of Management, 30*(1), 149–160. doi:10.1016/j.jm.2003.01.007

Young, M., Sparrow, D., Gottlieb, D., Selim, A., & Friedman, R. (2001). A telephone linked computer system for COPD care. *Chest, 119*(5), 1565–1575. doi:10.1378/chest.119.5.1565 PMID:11348968

Zanaboni, P., Scalvini, S., Bernocchi, P., Borghi, G., Tridico, C., & Masella, C. (2009). Teleconsultation service to improve healthcare in rural areas: Acceptance, organizational impact and appropriateness. *BMC Health Services Research, 9*(1), 238. doi:10.1186/1472-6963-9-238 PMID:20021651

KEY TERMS AND DEFINITIONS

Healthcare Telephone System: Part of the healthcare system that is intended for providing service to the callers/patients over various clinical and non-clinical matters.

IVRS: Telecommunication system that is based on Interactive Voice Response technology to interact with the callers by using the voice and the dual tone multi frequency signaling.

On-Call Physician: The physician, who according to the current practices, is supposed to provide the healthcare service in pre-specified amount of time after he/she is contacted or paged.

Tele-Diagnosis: The diagnosis of the related healthcare problems, symptoms, issues over a distance using the telecommunication technologies.

Tele-Health: Method of delivery for the health related services via various telecommunication technologies.

Telephone-Triage: It is a nursing service that is intended to provide the service of prioritizing the patient's treatments based on person's health condition over distance using the telecommunication technologies.

Underreferral: A situation where medical situation, problem, or symptom is deemed less important than it is.

This research was previously published in Reshaping Medical Practice and Care with Health Information Systems edited by Ashish Dwivedi, pages 87-131, copyright year 2016 by Medical Information Science Reference (an imprint of IGI Global).

Chapter 31
How the Rich Lens of ANT Can Help Us to Understand the Advantages of Mobile Solutions

Nilmini Wickramasinghe
Epworth Healthcare, Australia & RMIT University, Australia

Arthur Tatnall
Victoria University, Australia

Steve Goldberg
INET International Inc., Canada

ABSTRACT

The WHO has labelled diabetes the silent epidemic. This is because the instances of diabetes worldwide continue to grow exponentially. In fact, by 2030 it is expected that there will be a 54% global increase. Thus, it behooves all to focus on solutions that can result in superior management of this disease. Hence, this chapter presents findings from a longitudinal exploratory case study that examined the application of a pervasive technology solution, a mobile phone to provide superior diabetes self-care. Notably, the benefits of a pervasive technology solution for supporting superior self-care in the context of chronic disease are made especially apparent when viewed through the rich lens of Actor-Network Theory (ANT), and thus, the chapter underscores the importance of using ANT in such contexts to facilitate a deeper understanding of all potential advantages.

INTRODUCTION

In today's Information Technology Age one area that has yet to embrace the full benefits of ICT (Information Communication Technologies) to facilitate superior operations is healthcare. Yet slowly, this bastion is beginning to be besieged by numerous tools and solutions which at the surface at least appear to offer a panacea to the current challenges of escalating costs and poor quality.

DOI: 10.4018/978-1-5225-3926-1.ch031

In such a context then, it becomes important to have an appropriate and rich theoretical lens of analysis so that it is possible to judge and evaluate the true advantages of these potential ICT solutions. The following section serves to proffer that ANT (Actor-Network Theory) is indeed such a lens.

ACTOR-NETWORK THEORY (ANT)

Actor-network theory (ANT) provides a rich and dynamic lens of analysis for many socio-technical situations. Essentially, it embraces the idea of an organisational identity and assumes that organisations, much like humans, possess and exhibit specific traits (Brown, 1997). Although labelled a 'theory', ANT is more of a framework based upon the principle of generalised symmetry, which rules that human and non-human objects/subjects are treated with the same vocabulary. Both the human and non-human counterparts are integrated into the same conceptual framework.

ANT was developed by two French social sciences and technology scholars Bruno Latour and Michel Callon and British sociologist John Law (Latour, 1987, 2005; Law and Hassard, 1999; Law, 1992, 1987; Callon, 1986). It is an interdisciplinary approach that tries to facilitate an understanding of the role of technology in specific settings, including how technology might facilitate, mediate or even negatively impact organisational activities and tasks performed. Hence, ANT is a material-semiotic approach for describing the ordering of scientific, technological, social, and organisational processes or events.

Key Concepts of Actor Network Theory

Central to ANT and relevant for this specific context are the six key concepts as follows:

1. **Actor/Actant:** Typically actors are the participants in the network which include both the human and non-human objects and/or subjects. However, in order to avoid the strong bias towards human interpretation of Actor, the neologism Actant is commonly used to refer to both human and non-human actors. Examples include nurses, doctors, thermometers, electronic instruments, technical artifacts and graphical representations.
2. **Heterogeneous Network:** Is a network of aligned interests formed by the actors. This is a network of materially heterogeneous actors that is achieved by a great deal of work that both shapes those various social and non-social elements, and 'disciplines' them so that they work together, instead of 'making off on their own' (Latour, 2005).
3. **Tokens/Quasi Objects:** Are essentially the success outcomes or functioning of the Actors which are passed onto the other actors within the network. As the token is increasingly transmitted or passed through the network, it becomes increasingly punctualised and also increasingly reified. When the token is decreasingly transmitted, or when an actor fails to transmit the token (e.g., the broadband connection breaks), punctualisation and reification are decreased as well.
4. **Punctualisation:** Is similar to the concept of abstraction in Object Oriented Programming. A combination of actors can together be viewed as one single actor. These sub-actors are hidden from the normal view. This concept is referred to as Punctualisation. An incorrect or failure of passage of a token to an actor will result in the breakdown of a network. When the network breaks down the result is the breakdown of punctualisation and the viewers will then not be able to view the sub-actors making up the actor. This concept can be referred to as depunctualisation.

5. **Obligatory Passage Point (OOP):** Broadly refers to a situation that has to occur in order for all the actors to satisfy the interests that have been attributed to them by the focal actor. The focal actor defines the OPP through which the other actors must pass through and by which the focal actor becomes indispensable (Callon, 1986).

6. **Irreversibility:** Callon (1986) states that the degree of irreversibility depends on
   a. The extent to which it is subsequently impossible to go back to a point where that translation was only one amongst others; and
   b. The extent to which it shapes and determines subsequent translations.

In order to apply these to the context of diabetes self-care it is first necessary to provide a brief background on the current healthcare environment and the application of ICT for supporting diabetes self-care.

THE HEALTHCARE ENVIRONMENT BACKGROUND

Healthcare delivery for all OECD countries is experiencing exponentially increasing costs (OECD 2010a-c). This is of great concern to all and many believe information technology (IT) offers the promise of cost effective healthcare delivery (Geisler and Wickramasinghe, 2009). One area that appears to be particular problematic in this regard is connected with chronic diseases such as diabetes and hypertension, not only because they consume a disproportionate slice of healthcare services but also because there is no foreseeable cure and hence these cost pressures will continue for the life of the patient. Moreover, they are likely to increase, because if the chronic disease is poorly managed secondary complications will inevitably develop (Wickramasinghe and Goldberg, 2003).

Diabetes is one of the five major chronic diseases. It afflicts over twenty million people in the United States and accounts for almost $100 billion in medical costs (Geisler and Wickramasinghe, 2009). Diabetes is also one of the leading chronic diseases affecting Australians and its prevalence continues to rise. The total number of diabetes patients worldwide is estimated to rise from 171 million in 2000 to 366 million in 2030 (Wild et al., 2004). With increasingly growing prevalence this means that an estimated 275 Australians are developing diabetes daily (DiabetesAustralia, 2008). Given these alarming trends not only in Australia and the United States but worldwide diabetes has been termed as the silent epidemic by the WHO. Table 1 shows the increases for diabetes in various regions throughout the world.

Table 1. Prevalence of diabetes throughout the world

Region	2010 (Millions)	2030 (Millions)	% Increase
North America	33.9	53.2	42%
South America	18	29.6	65%
Africa	12.1	23.9	98%
Europe	55.2	66.2	20%
Middle East	26	51.5	94%
S.E Asia	58.7	101.0	72%
World	**284.6**	**438.4**	**54%**

Source: IDF, 2009 (http://www.idf.org) accessed January 2011

Given that technology may play a role in contributing to a more efficient and effective delivery of care that may also assist in controlling costs, the following examines the possible potential use of wireless technology in the monitoring of diabetic patients. Specifically, this paper provides insights from a longitudinal exploratory case study that investigated the major research question "how can technology support superior self-care for sufferers of chronic disease"? To understand the role for technology it is first necessary to understand critical issues regarding diabetes self-care.

DIABETES SELF-CARE

Diabetes is a chronic disease that occurs when there is too much glucose in the blood because the body is not producing insulin or not using insulin properly (DA, 2007).

Diabetes management involves a combination of both medical and non-medical approaches with the overall goal for the patient to enjoy a life which is as normal as possible (AIHW, 2008; AIHW, 2007). Critical to this management regimen is the systematic monitoring of blood sugar levels. However, as there is no cure for diabetes, achieving this goal can be challenging because it requires effective lifestyle management and careful and meticulous attention and monitoring by both the patient and health professionals (Britt, 2007). In particular, to be totally successful, this requires patients to be both informed and actively participate in their treatment regimen.

The Role for Technology to Facilitate Superior Chronic Disease Management

Simply stated, the research goal of this project was to design and develop a mobile (wireless) Internet environment to improve patient outcomes with immediate access to patient data and to provide the best available clinical evidence at the point of care. To do this, INET International Inc's research (Goldberg, 2002a-e; Wickramasinghe and Goldberg, 2003, 2004) started with a 30-day e-business acceleration assessment in collaboration with many key actors in hospitals (such as clinicians, medical units, administration, and IT departments). From this it was possible to design a robust and rigorous web-based business model: the INET web-based business model (figure 1). The business model brings together all the vital considerations and in turn provides the necessary components to enable the delivery framework to be positioned in the best possible manner so it can indeed facilitate and support superior chronic disease management. From this business model then the INET mobile solution was developed.

Thus the INET solution represents a pervasive technology enabled solution, which, while not exorbitantly expensive, can facilitate the superior monitoring of diabetes. The proposed solution (Figure 2) enables patient empowerment by way of enhancing self-management. This is a desirable objective because it allows patients to become more like partners with their clinicians in the management of their own healthcare (Radin, 2006; Mirza et al. 2008) by enhancing the traditional clinical-patient interactions (Opie 1998). The process steps in monitoring diabetes using this approach are outlined below (and depicted in Figure 2).

Each patient receives a blood glucose measurement unit.

1.   The patient conducts the blood glucose test and enters the blood glucose information into a handheld wireless device.

Figure 1. INET-web-based-business model. (Adapted from Wickramasinghe and Goldberg, 2004).

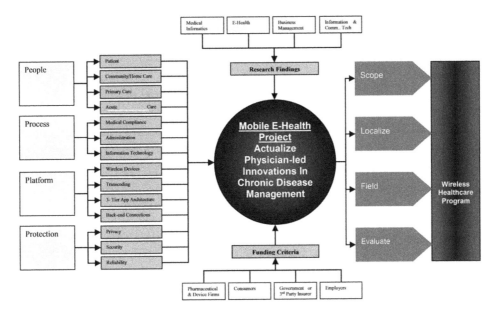

2. The blood glucose information is transmitted to specialised database servers that store patient data. The patient's hand-held device uniquely identifies the patient for recording the blood glucose data. Thus no patient information such as their name, ethnicity or date of birth is transmitted to the clinic.
3. The patient's blood glucose data is then stored/integrated with the clinic's electronic medical record (EMR) system.

Figure 2. The Wireless Enabled Solution for Diabetes Self-Care. (Reproduced with the permission of INET).

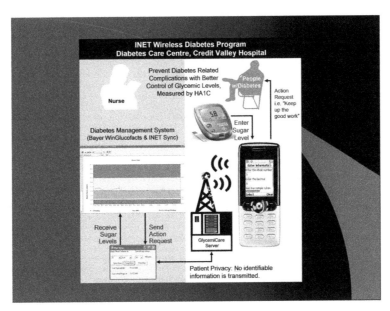

4.   An alert is generated for the clinical staff with the patient's blood glucose information.

5.   The blood glucose information of the patient is reviewed by the clinical staff (physician/nurse).

6.   Feedback on glucose levels is transmitted back to the patient's hand-held device. Feedback examples include complimenting the patient when glucose levels are normal or asking the patient to come for a follow-up appointment when the levels are out of norm.

7.   Monitor trends in diabetes management for patients over a period of time.

At face value this solution appears simple and trivial; however to fully understand the full and far reaching benefits of employing wireless technology solutions in this context it is necessary to view the solution through a combined lens of Social Network analysis and Actor-Network Theory as is presented in the following sections.

THE APPLICATION ON ANT TO RESEARCHING THE DIABETES SELF-CARE MODEL

To fully appreciate the application of ANT to the diabetes self-care model it is first necessary to map the key concepts of ANT to the critical issues in the diabetes self-care model just presented. This mapping is provided and summarised in Table 2.

Table 2. Key concepts of ANT

Concept	Relevance to Diabetes Self-Care
Actor/Actant: Typically actors are the participants in the network which include both the human and non-human objects and/or subjects. However, in order to avoid the strong bias towards human interpretation of Actor, the neologism 'Actant' is commonly used to refer to both human and non-human actors. Examples include humans, electronic instruments, technical artifacts, or graphical representations.	In the diabetes self-care model this includes the web of healthcare players such as providers, healthcare organisations, regulators, payers, suppliers and the patient as well as the clinical, wireless and administrative technologies that support and facilitate healthcare delivery.
Heterogeneous Network: is a network of aligned interests formed by the actors. This is a network of materially heterogeneous actors that is achieved by a great deal of work that both shapes those various social and non-social elements, and 'disciplines' them so that they work together, instead of 'making off on their own' (Latour, 2005).	The wireless technology combined with the specific application is clearly the technology network in this context. However it is important to conceptualise the heterogeneous network not as the technology alone but as the aligning of the actors through the various interactions with the technology so that it is possible to represent all interests and thereby provide the patient with superior healthcare delivery. The key is to carefully align goals so that healthcare delivery is truly patient centric at all times.
Tokens/Quasi Objects: are essentially the success outcomes or functioning of the Actors which are passed onto the other actors within the network. As the token is increasingly transmitted or passed through the network, it becomes increasingly punctualised and also increasingly reified. When the token is decreasingly transmitted, or when an actor fails to transmit the token (e.g., the broadband connection breaks), punctualisation and reification are decreased as well.	In the diabetes self-care model this translates to successful healthcare delivery, such as treating a patient in a remote location by having the capability to access critical information to enable the correct decisions to be made. Conversely, and importantly, if incorrect information is passed throughout the network errors will multiply and propagate quickly hence it is a critical success factor that the integrity of the network is maintained at all times.
Punctualisation: is similar to the concept of abstraction in object oriented programming. A combination of actors can together be viewed as one single actor. These sub actors are hidden from the normal view. This concept is referred to as punctualisation. An incorrect or failure of passage of a token to an actor will result in the breakdown of a network. When the network breaks down, it results in breakdown of punctualisation and the viewers will now be able to view the sub-actors of the actor. This concept is often referred to as depunctualisation.	For example, an automobile is often referred to as a single unit. Only when it breaks down, is it seen as a combination of several machine parts. Or in the diabetes self-care model the uploading task of one key actor, be it a provider or a patient is in reality a consequence of the interaction and co-ordination of several sub-tasks. This only becomes visible when a breakdown at this point occurs and special attention is given to analyse why and how the problem resulted and hence all sub-tasks must be examined carefully.
Obligatory Passage Point (OOP): broadly refers to a situation that has to occur in order for all the actors to satisfy the interests that have been attributed to them by the focal actor. The focal actor defines the OPP through which the other actors must pass through and by which the focal actor becomes indispensable (Callon, 1986).	In the diabetes self-care model we can illustrate this by examining the occurrence of the diabetes or secondary complications that have resulted because of the primary disease. Such incidents form the catalyst for developing shared goals and united focus of effort so necessary to affect superior healthcare delivery.
Irreversibility: Callon (1986) states that the degree of irreversibility depends on (i) the extent to which it is subsequently impossible to go back to a point where that translation was only one amongst others and (ii) the extent to which it shapes and determines subsequent translations.	Given the very complex nature of healthcare operations (von Lubitz and Wickramasinghe, 2006b-e) irreversibility is generally not likely to occur. However it is vital that chains of events are continuously analysed in order that future events can be addressed as effectively and efficiently as possible.

In applying ANT to the diabetes self-care model it is necessary to identify and trace the specific healthcare events and networks to "follow the actors" (Latour, 1996) and investigate all the relevant leads each new actor suggests. The first step then is to identify these actors (or actants), remembering that an actor is someone or something that can make its presence individually felt and can make a difference to the situation under investigation. Thus, in healthcare contexts the actors would include: medical practitioners, nurses, medical instruments, healthcare organisations, regulators, patients, equipment suppliers, medical administrators, administrative computer systems, medical researchers, and so on. In a particular operation (or event) it is important to identify all relevant actors before proceeding further.

The next step is to 'interview' the actors. With human actors this is, of course, quite straightforward, but with non-humans it is necessary to find someone (or something) to speak on their behalf. For an item of medical technology this might be its designer or user, or it might just be the instruction manual. The aim of this step is to see how these actors relate to each other and the associations they create – to identify how they interact, how they negotiate, and how they form alliances and networks with each other. These 'heterogeneous networks' consists of the aligned interests held by each of the actors.

Human actors, such as medical practitioners, can 'negotiate' with non-human actors such as X-Ray or dialysis machines by seeing what these machines can do for them, how easy they are to use, what they cost to use, and how flexible they are in performing the tasks required. If negotiations are successfully completed then an association between the medical practitioner and the machine is created and the machine is used to advantage – the network has become durable. If the negotiations are unsuccessful then the machine is either not used at all, or at least not used to full advantage.

Once this is developed it is then important to apply the techniques of ANT to map the flows of pertinent information and germane knowledge throughout this network and thereby not only enhancing the metacognition of the system but also the ability to rapidly extract and utilise the critical knowledge to support prudent decision making. In this way, it will be possible to be at all times in a state of being prepared and ready (Wickramasinghe and von Lubitz, 2007; von Lubitz and Wickramasinghe, 2006 a,f).

One of the main advantages of an ANT approach in considering the diabetes self-care model is in being able to identify and explore the real complexity involved. Other approaches to technological innovation, Innovation Diffusion for example, put much stress on the properties of the technology or organisation themselves, at the expense of looking at how these interact. Unfortunately in doing this they often tend to oversimplify very complex situations and so miss out on a real understanding. The ANT approach of investigating networks and associations provides a useful means to identify and explain these complexities as well as to track germane knowledge and pertinent information. This is paramount if the doctrine of network-centric healthcare is to be successfully realised.

Borrowing ideas from innovation translation in actor-network theory (Latour, 1996; 1986; 1999; Law, 1991) we will argue that, rather than just the technology, *people* are very important, as they may either accept an innovation in its present form, modify it to a form where it becomes acceptable, or reject it completely. "If we know one thing about innovation and reform, it is that it cannot be done successfully *to* others" (Fullan, 1991 pp xiv). An innovation translation approach has been shown to be useful in considering ICT (information and communications technology) innovation in small business (Tatnall and Davey, 2002) and in education (Tatnall, 2000; Tatnall and Davey, 2001; Bigum, 1998; Busch, 1997).

The innovation translation approach to innovation originates in actor-network theory (ANT) and draws on its sociology of translations. In ANT, translation (Law, 1992) can be defined as: "... the means by which one entity gives a role to others" (Singleton and Michael, 1993 pp. 229). Using an innovation translation approach to consider how the adoption of mobile medical technology occurs, it is necessary to examine the interactions of all the actors involved (Tatnall and Davey, 2003b).

DISCUSSION

The longitudinal exploratory case study that we embarked upon started with an examination of the technology solution to facilitate communication of blood sugars between patient and provider, to an assessment of the delivery framework and business model developed by INET to an analysis of the data from trials and pilot studies conducted. Based on rigorous thematic analysis of interview data, gathered following the techniques prescribed by Yin (1994), Kavale (1996) and Boyatsis (1998), triangulated with data from internal documents, reports and medical records as well as our own observations not only was proof of concept attained; ie using the pervasive technology solution did facilitate better self-care and resulted in a decrease in blood sugar, but all patients in the study reported only positive comments about the solution as the following quote highlights:

I loved the solution. It was like an answer to a pray. I could control my sugars more easily and have confidence and peace of mind to enjoy my life.

This serves to underscore the benefits of such an approach.

In the current context, healthcare delivery, especially in the US, is in need of fundamental re-design (Porter and Tiesberg, 2006). The focus on cost containment also necessitates a shift to prevention rather than cure. This is particularly important in the case of chronic diseases such as diabetes thereby making any solution that has the potential to enable cost effective quality care a strategic necessity.

Diabetes is the fifth-deadliest disease in the United States. Since 1987, the death rate due to diabetes has increased by 45 percent, while the death rates due to heart disease, stroke, and cancer have declined. The total annual economic cost of diabetes in 2002 was estimated to be $132 billion. Direct medical expenditures totalled $92 billion and comprised $23.2 billion for diabetes care, $24.6 billion for chronic diabetes-related complications, and $44.1 billion for excess prevalence of general medical conditions. Indirect costs resulting from lost workdays, restricted activity days, mortality, and permanent disability due to diabetes totalled $40.8 billion. The per capita annual costs of health care for people with diabetes rose from $10,071 in 1997 to $13,243 in 2002, an increase of more than 30%. Further, in 2010 alone the total cost of diabetes was $174 billion with approximately $116 billion direct medical costs and at least $58 billion in indirect costs (Wickramasinghe, 2010).

Without a doubt the costs in the United States are alarming, however it should also be noted that evidence also shows that diabetes and its complications incur significant costs for the health system in Australia and elsewhere. These costs include costs incurred by carers, government, and the entire health system (DiabCostAustralia, 2002). For instance, in 2004-05 direct healthcare expenditure on diabetes was A$907 million which constituted approximately 2% of the allocatable recurrent health expenditure in that year (AIHW, 2008). In addition, further costs include societal costs that represent productivity losses for both patients and their carers (DiabCostAustralia, 2002).

CONCLUSION

Technological developments in ubiquitous and mobile computing offer possibilities to many aspects of healthcare and, due to their non-reliance on traditional communications infrastructure they also offer emerging countries an opportunity to jump ahead. Exactly how these technologies should best be used in diabetes treatment, however, is not completely clear at this time (Morel et al., 2005).

There has been a considerable amount of research into the impact and use of technology in healthcare delivery, but not much into explaining the uptake of this technology. We have argued that for research of this type, it is useful to consider this technology in terms of technological innovation and to make use of an approach based on innovation theory. Actor-network theory provides a perspective that can resolve the dilemma of how to handle both the human and non-human contributions to technological innovation, and also provides a useful explanatory system for doing so (Tatnall, 2009).

In the specific case of diabetes discussed in the proceeding sections, clearly stemming the cost pressure is important but of greater importance is providing sufferers of diabetes with a possibility to experience a better quality of life. Where it is possible to provide both a low cost as well as a superior patient-centric solution this would appear to be a very compelling case for the large scale adoption of pervasive wireless solutions to facilitate superior care not only for diabetes patients but for patients with all chronic diseases. Our analysis of this solution drawing upon Actor-network theory demonstrates that there are very important aspects that are being addressed by adopting a pervasive wireless solution and these need further investigation. We close by not only calling for more research which particularly focus on how to move from idea to realisation as rapidly as possible but also for further exploration into the incorporation of pervasive technology solutions in general for supporting superior patient-centric healthcare delivery and the embracement of ANT as an appropriate lens of analysis.

AUTHORS' NOTE

An earlier version of this paper appeared in the proceedings of the 2011 Pacific Asia Conference on Information Systems (PACIS) July 2011 Brisbane, Australia.

REFERENCES

AIHW. (2007). *National Indicators for Monitoring Diabetes: Report of the Diabetes Indicators Review Subcommittee of the National Diabetes Data Working*. AIHW.

AIHW. (2008). *Diabetes: Australian Facts 2008*. Canberra, Australia: Australian Institute of Health and Welfare.

Bigum, C. (1998). Solutions in Search of Educational Problems: Speaking for Computers in Schools. *Educational Policy*, *12*(5), 586–601. doi:10.1177/0895904898012005007

Boyatzis, R. (1998). *Transforming Qualitative Information Thematic analysis And Code Development*. Sage Publications.

Britt, H., Miller, G. C., Charles, J., Pan, Y., Valenti, L., Henderson, J., & Knox, S. (2007). *General Practice Activity in Australia 2005-06 (Cat. no. GEP 16)*. Canberra, Australia: AIHW.

Busch, K. V. (1997). Applying Actor Network Theory to Curricula Change in Medical Schools: Policy Strategies for Initiating and Sustaining Change. In *Proceedings of Midwest Research-to-Practice Conference in Adult, Continuing and Community Education Conference*. Michigan State University.

DA. (2007). *Diabetes Facts*. New South Wales, Australia: Diabetes Australia.

Diabcost Australia. (2002). *Assessing the Burden of Type 2 Diabetes in Australia*. Adelaide, Australia: DiabCost Australia.

Diabetes Australia. (2008). *Diabetes in Australia*. Author.

Frost and Sullivan Country Industry Forecast – European Union Healthcare Industry. (2004, May 11). Retrieved from http://www.news-medical.net/print_article.asp?id=1405

Fullan, M. G., & Stiegelbauer, S. (1991). *The New Meaning of Educational Change* (2nd ed.). New York: Teachers College Press.

Geisler, E., & Wickramasinghe, N. (2009). *The Role and Use of Wireless Technology in the Management and Monitoring of Chronic Disease IBM Report*. Retrieved from www.businessofgovernment.org

Goldberg, S., et al. (2002a). Building the Evidence For A Standardized Mobile Internet (wireless) Environment In Ontario, Canada, January Update, internal INET documentation. Academic Press.

Goldberg, S. et al. (2002b). *HTA Presentational Selection and Aggregation Component Summary, internal documentation*. Academic Press.

Goldberg, S. et al. (2002c). *Wireless POC Device Component Summary, internal INET documentation*. Academic Press.

Goldberg, S. et al. (2002d). *HTA Presentation Rendering Component Summary, internal INET documentation*. Academic Press.

Goldberg, S. et al. (2002e). *HTA Quality Assurance Component Summary, internal INET documentation*. Academic Press.

Kavale, S. (1996). Interviews, an introduction to Qualitative Research. *Sage (Atlanta, Ga.)*.

Kulkarni, R., & Nathanson, L. A. (2005). *Medical Informatics in medicine, E-Medicine*. Retrieved from http://www.emedicine.com/emerg/topic879.htm

Lacroix, A. (1999). International concerted action on collaboration in telemedicine: G8sub-project 4, Sted. *Health Technol. Inform.*, *64*, 12–19.

Latour, B. (1986). The Powers of Association. In *Power, Action and Belief: A new sociology of knowledge?* Routledge & Kegan Paul.

Latour, B. (1992). On Recalling ANT. In *Actor Network Theory and After*. Blackwell Publishers.

Latour, B. (1996). *Aramis or the Love of Technology*. Cambridge, MA: Harvard University Press.

Law, J. (Ed.). (1991). *A Sociology of Monsters: Essays on power, technology and domination*. London: Routledge.

Morel, R., Tatnall, A., Ketamo, H., Lainema, T., Koivisto, J., & Tatnall, B. (2005). *Mobility and Education. E-Training Practices for Professional Organizations*. Kluwer Academic Publishers.

OECD. (2010a). *Growing health spending puts pressure on government budgets*. Retrieved January 31st, 2011 from http://www.oecd.org/document/11/0,3343,en_2649_34631_45549771_1_1_1_37407,00.html

OECD. (2010b). *OECD-Gesundheitsdaten 2010: Deutschland im Vergleich*. Retrieved January 31st, 2011 from http://www.oecd.org/dataoecd/15/1/39001235.pdf

OECD. (2010c). *OECD health data 2010*. Retrieved January 31st, 2011 from http://stats.oecd.org/Index.aspx?DatasetCode=HEALTH

Porter, M., & Tiesberg, E. (2006). *Re-defining health care delivery*. Harvard Business Press.

Rachlis, M. (2006). *Key to sustainable healthcare system*. Retrieved from http:www.improveingchronic-care.org

Singleton, V., & Michael, M. (1993). Actor-Networks and Ambivalence: General Practitioners in the UK Cervical Screening Programme. *Social Studies of Science*, *23*, 227–264. doi:10.1177/030631293023002001

Tatnall, A. (2009). Web Portal Research Issues. In *Encyclopedia of Information Science and Technology* (2nd ed.). Hershey, PA: Idea Group Reference.

Tatnall, A. (20002). *Innovation and Change in the Information Systems Curriculum of an Australian University: A Socio-Technical Perspective*. (PhD thesis). Central Queensland University, Rockhampton, Australia.

Tatnall, A., & Davey, B. (2001). How Visual Basic Entered the Curriculum at an Australian University: An Account Informed by Innovation Translation. In *Challenges to Informing Clients: A Transdisciplinary Approach*. Krakow, Poland: Academic Press.

Tatnall, A., & Davey, B. (2002). Understanding the Process of Information Systems and ICT Curriculum Development: Three Models. In *Human Choice and Computers: Issues of Choice and Quality of Life in the Information Society*. Kluwer Academic Publishers. doi:10.1007/978-0-387-35609-9_23

Tatnall, A., & Davey, B. (2003b). Modelling the Adoption of Web-Based Mobile Learning - An Innovation Translation Approach. In *Advances in Web-Based Learning*. Springer Verlag. doi:10.1007/978-3-540-45200-3_40

Wickramasinghe, N. (2007). Fostering knowledge assets in healthcare with the KMI model. *International Journal of Management and Enterprise Development*, *4*(1), 52–65. doi:10.1504/IJMED.2007.011455

Wickramasinghe, N. (2010). *Christmas Carol for IBM*. Paper presented at IBM Healthcare Executives Dinner. New York, NY.

Wickramasinghe, N., & Bali, R. (2009). The S'ANT imperative for realizing the vision of healthcare network centric operations. *International Journal of Actor-Network Theory and Technological Innovation, 1*(1), 45–58. doi:10.4018/jantti.2009010103

Wickramasinghe, N., & Goldberg, S. (2003). The Wireless Panacea for Healthcare. In *Proceedings of the 36th Hawaii International Conference on System Sciences* (HICSS-35). IEEE.

Wickramasinghe, N., & Goldberg, S. (2004). How M=EC2 in Healthcare. *International Journal of Mobile Communications, 2*(2), 140–156. doi:10.1504/IJMC.2004.004664

Wickramasinghe, N., & Goldberg, S. (2007a). Adaptive mapping to realisation methodology (AMR) to facilitate mobile initiatives in healthcare. *International Journal of Mobile Communications, 5*(3), 300–318. doi:10.1504/IJMC.2007.012396

Wickramasinghe, N., Goldberg, S., & Bali, R. (2008). Enabling superior m-health project success: A tri-country validation. *International Journal of Services and Standards, 4*(1), 97–117. doi:10.1504/IJSS.2008.016087

Wickramasinghe, N., & Mills, G. (2001). MARS: The Electronic Medical Record System The Core of the Kaiser Galaxy. *International Journal of Healthcare Technology and Management, 3*(5/6), 406–423. doi:10.1504/IJHTM.2001.001119

Wickramasinghe, N., & Misra, S. (2004). A Wireless Trust Model for Healthcare. *International Journal of Electronic Healthcare, 1*(1), 60–77. doi:10.1504/IJEH.2004.004658 PMID:18048204

Wickramasinghe, N., & Schaffer, J. (2006). Creating Knowledge Driven Healthcare Processes With The Intelligence *Continuum. International Journal of Electronic Healthcare, 2*(2), 164–174. PMID:18048242

Wickramasinghe, N., Schaffer, J., & Geisler, E. (2005). Assessing e-health. In T. Spil & R. Schuring (Eds.), *E-Health Systems Diffusion and Use: The Innovation, The User and the User IT Model*. Hershey, PA: Idea Group Publishing. doi:10.4018/978-1-59140-423-1.ch017

Wickramasinghe, N., & Silvers, J. B. (2003). IS/IT The Prescription To Enable Medical Group Practices To Manage Managed Care. *Health Care Management Science, 6*, 75–86. doi:10.1023/A:1023376801767 PMID:12733611

Wild, S., Roglic, G., Green, A., Sicree, R., & King, H. (2004). Global prevalence of diabetes: Estimates for the year 2000 and projections for 2030. *Diabetes Care, 27*(5), 1047–1053. doi:10.2337/diacare.27.5.1047 PMID:15111519

Yin, R. (1994). *Case Study Research: Design and Methods* (2nd ed.). Sage Publications.

KEY TERMS AND DEFINITIONS

Chronic Disease: A disease that has no cure hence once an individually contracts this disease they typically have it for the rest of their life.

Diabetes: A chronic disease that is due to incorrect amounts of blood sugar in the body. There are 3 major types of diabetes Type 1, Type 2 and gestational.

Diabetes Management: This involves a combination of both medical and non-medical approaches with the overall goal for the patient to enjoy a life which is as normal as possible. Most focus is placed on keeping blood sugar at appropriate levels.

Epidemic: A wide spreading a widespread occurrence of a disease in a community at a particular time.

Self-Care: Enabling the patient to take ownership of their healthcare maintenance regimen and consult doctors and care teams as and when required.

This research was previously published in Technological Advancements and the Impact of Actor-Network Theory edited by Arthur Tatnall, pages 87-99, copyright year 2014 by Information Science Reference (an imprint of IGI Global).

Chapter 32
ICT Use and Multidisciplinary Healthcare Teams in the Age of E-Health

Bolanle A. Olaniran
Texas Tech University, USA

ABSTRACT

This paper explores ICTs in the medical field specifically in the Multidisciplinary teams (MDTMs) in healthcare settings. The discussion offers benefits and disadvantages of ICTs along with implications for teams' communication and interaction. The paper also provides a few formidable challenges facing MTDMs while offering suggestions on how to overcome them in an attempt to fully experience and utilize technologies in an effective manner. Finally the paper presents areas for future research given the fact that ICT use in MTDMs will only continue to grow as e-health becomes the norm in patients care and healthcare delivery. In an attempt to accomplish these goals, Retchin's (2008) conceptual framework for inter-professional and co-managed care will be used. Retchin's framework considers the impact of temporality, urgency of care, and structure of authority. Specifically, this framework focuses on how information communication technologies can impact overall patient health care and delivery. In conclusion, the author provides guidelines and recommendations for how physicians and other health practitioners can use technologies to work with each other are provided.

INTRODUCTION AND BACKGROUND

Information Communication Technologies (ICTs) have become prevalent in every aspect of human lives. The manifestation of computer-mediated communication (CMC), Internet and computer support collaborative work (CSCW) in organizations, e-learning, and virtual collaborations has been well documented over the past two decades (Olaniran, 2007). One of the advantages of ICTs has been in the potential to increase productivity and effectiveness while reducing costs in organizations. ICT use is especially applicable to physicians and non-physician health providers who collaborate across disciplinary lines (Scholl & Olaniran, 2013; Wright, Sparks, & O'Hair, 2008). The use of ICTs in healthcare delivery is

DOI: 10.4018/978-1-5225-3926-1.ch032

gaining ground as a way to coordinate caregiving for patients. Central to this paper is the need to explore the impacts of ICTs on interdisciplinary healthcare groups and teams. For instance, Health Informatics – which addresses the use of technology for information dissemination or ICTs in telemedicine and healthcare practices are a few of the tools helping to support multidisciplinary teams to provide integrated care. Germane to the interdisciplinary healthcare team approach is how providers target multiple issues in order to maximize ICT benefits and health outcomes. To accomplish this goal, team members must be able to communicate with one another, have realistic goals and expectations for coordinating group interaction, know how to resolve conflict, and make successful decisions (Cooley, 1994; Lefley, 1998; Scholl & Olaniran, 2013; Wright et al., 2008). Notwithstanding, interdisciplinary team members often fail to communicate effectively (Scholl & Olaniran, 2013; Thomas, Sexton, & Helmreich, 2003; Wright et al., 2008). For instance, minor disagreements can escalate and at times lead to staff turnover and litigation (van Servellen, 2009). Therefore, the focus of this paper is to address and evaluate ICT usage in multidisciplinary or collaborative care giving. Specifically, the aim is to explore how different professional or specialists use ICTs to collaborate in healthcare delivery to patients.

ICTS AND MULTIDISCIPLINARY HEALTHCARE TEAMS

Multidisciplinary care is defined as an integrated team approach to healthcare, where relevant health care professionals evaluate treatment options and jointly develop treatment plan for patients (Robertson, Li, O'Hara, & Hansen, 2010; Salerno, 2015; Scholl & Olaniran, 2013). The contribution of various individuals who exist within different locations makes the collaboration among different specialists possible and is often referred to as multidisciplinary team (MDTM) and integrated care. For example, multidisciplinary teams for cancer treatment can consist of surgeons, nutritionists, radiologists, pathologists, oncologists and social workers along with general practitioners. In other words, hospitals, physicians, and Nurses provide healthcare services either through office or home visits in collaboration with other healthcare providers including general practitioners with the aid of ICTs. These technologies allow for the transfer of recorded data back to hospital environment (Salerno, 2015). Thus, ICTs represent the tools for increasing cooperation between different health professions across different settings and institutions, which in a way help foster the active/interactive role by patients, caregivers and other entities in caregiving (Scholl & Olaniran, 2013; Stellato et al., 2015a, 2015b).

With ICTs, the delivery of healthcare from a range of professions and disciplinary specialists allows for exchange of information between different experts, agencies, and institutions in co-located (same location or hospital) or non-co-located (different geographic boundaries) environments. Thus, ICTs offer a way to meet the call for coordinating patient care giving in efficient and effective manners (Dwivedi, Bali, James, Naguib, & Johnston, 2002; Robertson, et al., 2010; Salerno, 2015). Furthermore, healthcare is now commonly practiced in a widely distributed environment and organizational network where patients and clinical data are sent back and forth between general practitioners and specialists in order to enable up-to-date care (at the right time and place). In comparison to previous periods, it is a fact that nowadays; individuals live longer and often suffer chronic ailments that need to be closely monitored by several practitioners that are located in different places (Salerno, 2015; Stellato et al., 2015a; Winthereik & Vikkelso, 2005). The dispersion of caregivers and the duration of patient care necessitate Computer Supported Cooperative Work (CSCW) which is facilitated by ICTs.

Perhaps, one of the most important achievements in health care is the digitization of medical records. Digitization occurs when images or signals are converted into digital code by using an analogue to digital conversion device. Therefore, these digitalized records are a result of the conversion of signals from an analog to a digital medium allowing for the transferability of information between providers without increased expense (i.e., cost of physical delivery of records) or errors common to oral transmission of information (Dwivedi, et al., 2002; Wallace, 1997). Digitization in healthcare makes it possible to obtain or access health related information or patients medical record and store it in computer via audio, text, graphics and video formats (Dwivedi, et al., 2002; Richardson, Abramson, Pfoh, Kaushal, & HITEC Investigators, 2012). Specifically, chronic illnesses require constant monitoring, and digitization of medical record is believed to help set certain warning signals or thresholds that when triggered, allowed care givers to activate the necessary plan of action (Stellato et al., 2015a). At the same time, the approach allows for patients to live longer and or become active in participating in their own care. Furthermore, the transmission infrastructure has developed from Copper cables to more of Fiber optic networks that make it possible for a significant or large data (Bandwidth) to be transmitted over communication networks. Consequently, this possibility in communication networks and technology is believed to have exponentially increased the bandwidth (the quantity of data that can be transmitted over a particular time span) (Wallace, 1997). In essence, multimedia capability has made it possible to exchange information in a different manner or even in multiple formats such that data can be packaged with audio and video cues. Moreover, the information can be presented in an interactive format.

The multimedia data capability enhances and facilitates CSCW in general and more importantly in healthcare settings. Therefore, the role of ICTs in healthcare settings is being played out in asymmetries in resources for communication in computer-mediated communication (e.g. Gaver 1992; Heath and Luff 1992, 1996; Luff et al. 2003; Robertson 1997, 2002; Voida, Voida, Greenberg, & Aihi, 2008). ICTs are also affecting how existing technologies shape and are shaping the way people collaborate or interact within specific settings (e.g. Balandin, Shabaev, & Stibe, 2014; Ciolfi, Fitzpatrick, & Bannon, 2008; Ellingsen & Monteiro 2006; Fitzpatrick, Kaplan, & Mansfield, 1996; Harrison & Dourish 1996; 2006; Harrison and Tatar 2008; Olaniran, 2007a, 2007b, 2010) . Furthermore, ICTs emphasize the importance of understanding the sociotechnical and organizational environments in which practices involving technology use are entrenched (e.g., Balka, Bjorn, & Wagner, 2008; Gärtner & Wagner 1996).

Different information technology applications such as clinical information systems, electronic patient records and telemedicine have been used successfully, thereby demonstrating their potential to greatly improve the standard of medical care and healthcare administration (Dwivedi, et al., 2002; Rao, 2001; Stellato et al., 2015a, 2015b). In recent years advances in information technology applications have resulted in fast innovations and significant changes in healthcare deliveries (Balandin et al., 2014; Johns, 1997, Stellato et al., 2015a). Telemedicine, in particular, represents a growing area (Crompton, 2001) and it consists of healthcare delivery that uses advanced video conferencing communication technologies to close the geographical gap that exists between the licensed caregivers and/or the care receiver, with the primary objective of providing medical diagnosis and treatment. At times, telemedicine offers a way to provide healthcare for people in rural region where major hospital facilities may not be readily available.

Various National governments such as UK, Canada and Malaysia have seized the opportunity to make substantial efforts to link electronically different healthcare centers through telemedicine. In the U.K, the Government has committed about USD $1.4 billion to implement ICTs in healthcare (Dwivedi, et al., 2002) and mobile healthcare is projected to be a 26 billion dollar industry by 2017 (Balandin et al.,

2014; Singh, 2014). A significant component of this funding is being used in developing a nationwide electronic platform (Balandin et al., 2014 Crompton, 2001). The large amount of money and resources committed to overhauling healthcare delivery with ICTs is largely responsible for the emergence of several telemedicine and e health platforms globally (Collms, 2001; Crompton, 2001).The primary goal of any telemedicine application is to transfer caregiver expertise from one location to another (Dwivedi, et al., 2002; Rao, 2001). For example, a local telemedicine program in our community is used to provide health consultation about orthopedics from a major health science's center to general practitioner in rural surrounding areas. Moreover, the World Health Organization has made Universal Health Care a priority with the goal of protecting people from being impoverished as a result of lack of or poor access to adequate health care. Thus, developments in ICTs is seen as a way to connect community based health services to more urban or global health initiatives (WHO, 2015).

Furthermore, Dwivedi et al (2002) reported that one of the most widely used applications of telemedicine is tele radiology - which include ICT use for Image acquisition, storage, display, processing and transfer from one geographical location to another location for diagnosis. With innovation in technologies, (telecommunications, multimedia and IT healthcare applications) telemedicine can play a significant role in transforming healthcare delivery. Countries like Singapore and Malaysia are good examples to the extent that individuals from economically advanced nations now seeks healthcare and elective surgeries from these countries and consider the services received to be equal or better than the ones they are used to receiving in their home countries. At the same time, countries like Malaysia already integrate telemedicine with the electronic health record concept by having a national telemedicine strategy already in place. As a result, Teleconsultations are becoming the norm rather than aberration in Malaysia. Also in Sweden, telemedicine is used as a method for reducing the length of hospital stays for children and adults (Dwivedi et al., 2002).

Another area where ICTs have offered valuable service to patients and health care teams is in managing multi-morbidity cases. Using ICTs has enabled integrated care to support patient self-management and collaborations among all caregivers in a manner that provides good and sustainable care (Noordman, van der Heide, Hopman, Schellevis, & Rijken, 2015; Rijken et al., 2013). As a result, ICTs *intervene* in the provision of care while improving the quality of care by making efficient use of resources (Goodwin et al., 2014; Boult et al., 2009; Nordman et al., 2015). Increasingly, integrated health care is being implemented globally. ICTs also allow for care pathways to be included in the type of care offered to the patient by multidisciplinary teams. A care pathway can cover aspects of a patient's care chain that are outside of hospitals including social worker, nurses, home care, general practitioners, pharmacist along with any other practitioner a patient might need (Brignole et al., 2006; Noordman et al., 2015; Pinder, Petchey, Shaw, & Carter, 2005; Stellato et al., 2015a, 2015b). Although most of the available studies on integrated care concern disease-specific care pathways (e.g. Brignole et al., 2006; Pinder et al., 2005; Stellato et al., 2015) these systems of care can be effective in other health related situations as well. Also, advances in technologies and innovations in health related technologies allow for better health care and monitoring in gerontology and the quality of life for homebound patients. This is especially true in cases where patients are connected to health equipment designed for monitoring heart rate, rhythm and blood pressure among other vital statistics (Anonymous, 1997; Dwivedi, et al., 2002; Stellato et al., 2015a). Equipment is usually installed in the homes of patients and is centrally monitored to the extent that those requiring emergency care or acute care can be treated by alerting emergency medical service professional or ambulatory care.

For example, Mrs. Rupp is a registered nurse in the US who makes house calls. Normally she could see about five or six patients a day with every home visit costing about $135. Using telemedicine Mrs. Rupp is able to see about 15 patients in four hours reducing the cost to about $36 for each televisit (teleconsultation) (Anonymous, 1997 cited in Dwivedi et al., 2002). This demonstrates how telemedicine can transform the healthcare delivery even at a low level. From a practitioner's perspective, telemedicine allows for the most efficient use of time, not to mention that it reduces cost for health care providers enabling them to care for more patients in the time allotted. Furthermore, patients report that the use of technology monitoring is very helpful and empowering. For instance one patient reports:

Taking my weight on a regular basis has always been difficult. I'm very lazy... Now, I get on the scale more easily in the morning and I regularly take my BP. Measurements are automatically sent to the platform, I don't have to do anything. Now I know that everybody knows and it's a good feeling. I could ask to be sent pill reminders but I have a very attentive wife and I don't think I need any further help, for the time being. I guess that being able to keep a watch on you makes it easier to actually do the right things for your life and health (Stellato et al., 2015a, p. 7).

Another study that assesses the use of telemedicine in palliative care found that Telemedicine allowed greater access to the healthcare system, reduced the need to employ emergency services, improved assessment/control of symptoms, and provided greater orientation and confidence in the care given by family members through early and proactive interventions (Hennemann-Krause, Lopes, Araújo, Petersen, & Nunes, 2015). Web conferencing in particular, proved to be a good adjuvant to home monitoring of symptoms, complementing in-person assistance (Hennermann-Krause, 2015).

Multidisciplinary teams through e-health or telemedicine offer important advantages in terms of helping to coordinate activities between different hospital departments, locations, and or agencies. This approach also offers practitioners the venue to discuss their diagnoses and recommendations with the rest of the team. More significant is the fact that the team can be interactive and provide an educational function for all practitioners and medical students in same or different area of specializations and disciplines (Robertsons, et al., 2010).

CHALLENGES FACING MULTIDISCIPLINARY HEALTHCARE TEAMS

Findings from early media space identified a number of the major issues affecting technology-mediated communication and interaction. These included: a range of novel communicative asymmetries introduced by audio-visual technologies (e.g. Heath and Luff 1992); the role played by the physical medium in which social activities occur and on how these activities are conducted, (e.g., Gaver 1992); and the embodied actions of participants (e.g. looking at the same thing at the same time), that need to be mutually available if people are to successfully coordinate their actions with others (e.g. Robertson 1997, 2000). However, there are challenges or problems that arise as individuals in multidisciplinary teams interact via ICTs. First is the issue of access to technology (Olaniran, 2007). For instance, when participants in remote communication situations do not have equal access to the same technology, interaction and communication may become challenging not to mention disjointed, fractured or impossible. Furthermore, not all technology access is created equal. One access location may be operating at the latest state of the art network connection and speed while another location may be operating at a lesser speed or have an unstable network connection. All these will affect the process and quality of interactions that may influence eventual participation (Olaniran, 2009a, 2009b).

The interdependencies among team members or participants in the interaction and the physical along with the social environments in which these interactions occur are important and have been alluded to in prior literature. For example, the role of physical space in the negotiation of ongoing relationships between people and the resources they use in collaboration is important in terms of accomplished or aspired goals (e.g. Dourish, 2006; Harrison &Tatar 2008; Ciolfi et al., 2008). Furthermore, as one discusses multidisciplinary teams in health care settings, it is important to realize that there are different concepts of place and their implications for technology design and development (Olaniran, 2007, 2009a; Robertson, et al., 2010).

Toni Robertson et al., (2001) found that the physical spaces, in which local MDTMs were held, influence how participants' interaction occurred and how this interaction was experienced by members located in different physical spaces connected via video. Olaniran (2009a) also found that the physical setting or space in which videoconferencing meeting occur influences how meeting attendees behaved or participated. In particular, the different social, organizational and technology aspects of local meetings had their own histories, processes, and practices that appeared meaningless during local meetings became salient during video conferencing. This necessitated an increase in the discussion of various actions and activities. Along with discussion, participants required additional explanation as to how and why these activities related to the basic function and aims of the MDTMs (e.g., namely the management of patient treatment). These explanations included the origins of activities, if, and in what ways, the variations were important, and how relevant practices would be addressed in the future (Robertsons, et al., 2010).

For example, in cancer MTDMs settings surgeons usually initiate each meeting with a list of patients to be discussed. Nurses coordinate with their respective surgeons and circulate this patient list to the relevant team members such as: radiologists and pathologists. Nurses also make sure that all appropriate images are ordered and available to all participants during these mediated meetings. Among other materials included for in MDTM meetings are clinical data showing patients' medical records, relevant medical history, summary of surgeries, current and past treatments, and risk factors. This information is also made available to practitioners for reference during the meeting. With all of this available information, other options such as, the suitability of patients for inclusion in clinical trial protocols or other experimental procedures can also be discussed. Robertsons et al. (2010) recorded that the presentation of radiology and pathology images 'sits in the middle' during a patient discussion. Also, the progression of, and references to images often structure both the initial presentation of each patient's condition and the discussion that ensues (Schmidt et al. 2007). Robertsons et al. (2010) concluded that there are two different kinds of images that may need to be transformed in some way so that they can be made publicly available for a group of people to examine conjointly. At the same time, there are reported *local* variations in how these images were transformed, which accounted for the most miscommunications within the video-mediated meetings (Luff et al 2003). Furthermore, data and presentation materials are subject to idiosyncratic differences as to the numbers of individuals that get to see them and how or whether they are used for teaching purposes. For instance, the size of the MTDM influences how the pictures and visual aid are presented so that they are clearly visible to participants. At the same time, a teaching hospital has additional obligations of preparing the materials in a manner in which junior, up and coming medical students can learn without encumbering additional cost to the hospital and the team (Robertsons, et al., 2010).

COMMUNICATION AND OTHER LOGISTICAL ISSUES

As communication scholars, there are clearly communication challenges that are of concern in medical record keeping and other standardization that ICTs bring to CSCW multidisciplinary healthcare teams (Scholl & Olaniran, 2013). Often transmitted data needs to be interpreted in a manner that gives a broad picture or an overview of a patient's care, which may not always be accurate. However, incidents such as these do not occur in isolation. The truth is that the nature of healthcare involves fuzzy, complicated work conducted by multiple individuals whose activities are unavoidably and intricately linked. This often includes scenarios within healthcare settings where attempts to complete a patient's medical record through the addition of brief details of complicated diagnostic information becomes detrimental to future interpretation by the patient's general practitioner. As a result, brief details added to a patient's medical record can be documented and presented to the GP in such a way that it drastically impacts how this information is utilized in future diagnosis and additional clinical practice (Heath and Luff, 1996). For instance, hospital physicians may be called upon to fill in gaps of a patient's medical record through the construction of a *discharge letter* sent to the patient's general practitioner. Often, these discharge notes or instructions are written by nurses (Stellato, 2015) which may simply contain a general summary of doctor's (surgeon's) instructions and hence remains subject to interpretation and unintentionally leading to error. There are times that this document reveals inaccuracies within record keeping that result from the error in translation or the misinterpretation of information (Scholl & Olaniran, 2013; Winthereik & Vikkelso, 2005). The resulting discharge letter is considered a poor document that only provides a polished and crude version of the course of events at the hospital or place of treatment. Therefore, when documents such as these are shared with MTDM teams, there is an increased risk of error and miscommunication.

POTENTIAL SOLUTIONS/IMPLICATIONS

No matter the nature or type of technology used by MDTMs, the ultimate goal should focus on the most effective way to coordinate care (van Servellen, 2009). Given the challenges alluded to above, practitioners and scholars must examine the nature of MDTMs and the ICTs they use in order to effectively collaborate across medical disciplines in an efficient manner. It is paramount that technology should not be implemented without reason or need. Technology is merely a tool and should be used only to assist MDTMs in making the best medical decisions. In other words, ICTs should be chosen carefully and more importantly, this chosen technology should fit the medical situation, not the other way around. From this standpoint, Short, Frischer, and Basford (2004) suggest using decision support systems in the area of medical informatics. The system provides physicians with advice on treatments while identifying potential risks. Specifically, doctors enter data on the patient and the system supports doctors by improving their diagnoses through provision of *previous experience* that a doctor might be lacking and consequently, reducing medical errors (see also, Scholl & Olaniran, 2013). Similarly, decision support systems can be used as a tool for transferring information in MTDMs, that is, transferring information among healthcare personnel and at different levels of care (Olve, Vimarlund, & Agerbo, 2006; Stellato et al., 2015a). Nonetheless, where they are appropriate, the costs and disadvantages of ICTs "could be lowered by improving coordination, because better-coordinated care among different health disciplines reduces fragmentation and diminishes redundancy" (Retchin, 2008, p. 932). Evidence indicates that when ICTs are properly implemented, they have *a positive* impact on behavior, as well as operational, process, and clinical outcomes especially when phased in (Banas, Erskine, Sun, &Retchin, 2011; Richardson et al., 2012; Scholl & Olaniran, 2013). For instance, Banas et al. (2011) suggested a three phase implementation just for adopting an electronic health record. The three phases consist of: a) preparatory phase which focused on training and technical application; b) adaptive period - designed to engage clinicians at their own pace, and c) practice transformation which focuses on optimization of the platform to incorporate changes after implementation.

Notwithstanding, MTDMs need to exceed mere digitization of health records. As such, increased coordination and the best application of ICTs can be achieved by applying Retchin's (2008) three factors of temporality, the urgency of care, and authority structure to address or better understand the challenges we previously discussed. To this end, producing the best health outcomes and maximizing the use of appropriate technology requires that a multidisciplinary team: 1) determine the nature of the care needed, 2) understand what levels of temporality, urgency of care, and authority structure they need to implement, and 3) determine the best formats and combinations of ICTs to accomplish their goals.

Some teams who solely work on chronic conditions (e.g., heart failure, diabetes, terminal illness) and primary care, which require more time to make and implement medical decisions may jeopardize patients when team members feel the need to schedule/conduct meetings in order to brief each other or discuss upcoming medical procedures beforehand (Kane, Groth, & Randall, 2011; Kane & Luz, 2006; Stellato et al., 2015a). However, because level of urgency is linked with authority structure (Retchin, 2008), matters that can be handled in a linear, one-step-at-a-time fashion that might also lend themselves to more opportunities in shared decision making (e.g., distributed authority structure), saving time in the long run. Thus, it is crucial that MDTMs plan ahead. For example, some ICTs can link remote team members to allow them to share leadership and much needed expertise in a timely manner.

At the same time, a low level of urgency would imply more flexibility in terms of time. This means that team member involvement would not be restricted to scheduling synchronous communication. Team members that are remotely located can use a wide range of ICTs to stay in touch and provide their input. For instance, Singh et al. (2010) report on the use of telehealth in a rural public health district in Georgia to provide non-urgent, primary care to geographically dispersed patients and physicians. As reported in their longitudinal study, the system allowed providers and technical support staff in and outside the district to collaborate and share in the leadership process (see also Balandin et al, 2014; Stellato, 2015a). Additionally, technology allows primary care providers to consult with specialists four hours away within flexible time frames that were convenient for all parties. These providers also had access to sophisticated equipment that allowed for the transfer of images and video to assist in consultations. Therefore, the flexibility of time within non-urgent cases helps in releasing members to communicate asynchronously or when not all participants can be available at the same time. In such scenarios, the use of other ICTs, such as pagers, IMs, smartphones and emails and other devices that support video and data transfer will do well (Scholl & Olaniran, 2013).

For more acute medical matters (e.g., aggressive treatment of late-stage cancer, emergency room or intensive care), MDTMs are best conducted concurrently, with more centralized leadership. As with non-urgent care, telehealth technologies are also ideal. However, key providers directly responsible for the provision of care must be readily available to take part in the synchronous communication that is a part of telemedicine. Therefore, members who have access to the more sophisticated technologies might have to take on more centralized, authoritarian roles in order to prevent any delays or inefficiencies that might occur in the provision of critical patient care. More portable devices should also be used to supplement the synchronous ICTs in order for team members to have the same access to crucial information and images (e.g., Stellato et al., 2015a). Such devices tend to be underutilized, but can influence clinician confidence (O'Neil-Pirozzi, Kendrick, Goldstein, & Glenn, 2004; Stellato et al., 2015a). Also crucial is that the team is supported by qualified personnel to anticipate and repair any breakdowns in the information flow (Nelson, Houston, Hoffman, & Bradham, 2011). Preplanning by both providers and technical staff is essential to ensure the efficiency of the ICT system.

Earlier, the issue of some MDTM members' unequal or limited access to ICTs was acknowledged. This inequality might be experienced when some members have contact with more synchronous forms of technology (e.g., teleconferencing facilities) while providers in rural areas are limited to email or phones that do not allow multiple users. This inequity in access to same ICTs or interoperability of ICTs is more exacerbated among geographically dispersed participants and cross-border interactions (Balandin et al., 2014; Olaniran, 2007, 2010). Consequently, temporality may be an issue because such limitations might reduce some health care teams to working sequentially rather than concurrently, thus, restricting them to non-urgent care cases. This includes cases such as caring for a patient recovering from a leg amputation with no complications. In such a case, there is no need for centralized leadership as one person can determine the level of care needed without delay. With matters that are more urgent, less sophisticated technology that supports a central authority structure might be ideal, such as messaging tools (e.g., email, text), that the team leader can use to disseminate large amounts of information to team members who are not charged with shared leadership roles.

The second challenge previously mentioned involves the unintended impacts of physical space on the group's communication dynamic and decision-making processes. It is well documented that the occupation of physical spaces significantly influences the communication that takes place within the health care team (Olaniran, 2009; Robertson et al., 2010). Retchin's (2008) framework can shed more light on when and why these technologies influence the team dynamic. With regard to temporality, however, the concurrent nature of some tele medical settings can draw increased attention to the organizational aspects of a meeting, such as who sits at the center of a table or who occupies the spot closest to the camera during a teleconference. Team members need to be made aware of these factors and attempt to draw more attention to the task and less on the contextual aspects of the group dynamic. In situations when the structure of authority needs to be more centralized, the physician or health professional in the leadership position has a unique opportunity to make the group mindful of the aspects that become more salient during electronic (rather than face-to-face) meetings. This task becomes increasingly important when the nature of the medical care is urgent (e.g., intensive care) and the task needs immediate attention. In instances when authority needs to be centralized and group members must meet electronically, or when it is most practical for one of the specialists on the team to lead the discussion, it might be more important for the specialist to occupy a portion of the physical space that draws more attention to her or him, which might not receive as much attention if the meeting were held face-to-face (Scholl & Olaniran, 2013).

The third challenge presented earlier was the potential to misinterpret medical information, which often results from the need to fill in the gaps left by missing data. It is reasonable to expect that urgent care situations requiring quick decisions might compel health care professionals to make hasty inferences that result from incomplete or inaccurate information. Such cases might require a more centralized— rather than shared—authority within the medical team. Key decision makers in these centralized roles might be positioned to expose team members to electronic medical records systems (Meredith, 2009; Scholl & Olaniran, 2013). Meredith (2009) found that access to a robust patient record system can lead to user satisfaction as well as benefits to clinical staff, such as fewer errors and greater access to patient information during crises. Given that urgency is related to authority structure, Retchin (2008) advises that high-urgency situations often require one or more professionals on the team to possess more authoritative power. Such a person also has the opportunity to decide which ICTs on which the group will rely to best convey medical information accurately and expediently; technologies that are well suited for sequential communication (e.g., email, digital image transfer, text messaging) might help achieve this goal. This overall strategy might help professionals avoid inaccuracies in interpretation or inappropriately fill in the missing gaps in data.

Regarding record accuracy, standardization might account for how medical practitioners distinguish areas of responsibilities or division of labor, thus accounting for decisions regarding how to structure authority within the MDTM. Consequently, it might be useful to document information in a way where specific practitioners and organizations document or prepare records or focus more on the specific places in an organization where coordination and integration efforts took place (Winthereik &Vikkelso, 2005). Because the information would be exchanged in a sequential manner, this might leave room for more shared leadership among team members who need and/or have access to those medical records. Winthereik and Vikkelso (2005) suggested that a particular place of coordination might include situations in which the secretary in the GP clinic has to review records (e.g., discharge letter) to prepare for patients who call the clinic to make appointments or ask questions about current and future care.

Furthermore, it is argued that understanding how a secretary acts as a bridge between two organizations is useful when designing a useful discharge letter than attempts to create a common standard that does the coordination by itself. However, one needs to weigh the additional cost or work that will be created in multiple organizations to safeguard against medical error or the increase in health care delivery cost altogether. What it all boils down to is the idea that ICTs by themselves, however useful, cannot meet the complex, multidimensional needs of patients (Pulignano, Del Sindaco, Di Lenarda, & Sinagra, 2006; Salerno, 2015; Scholl & Olaniran, 2013). Therefore as MTDMs work in care delivery, integrated ICT-supported care should be used in a way that addresses the subjective and quality of care in IT-supported health and social care interventions. As a result, ICTs should not replace personal and social interactions (Salerno, 2015; Stellato et al., 2015a, 2015b).

It is important to note that healthcare professionals will always find ways to work around categories that do not fit their methods and even per chance informally seek additional information as needed. However, it is also important to make certain that these incidents are not left to chance. In an attempt to integrate healthcare work using ICTs to create standardization, additional work is needed and required (Berg & Goorman, 1999; Berg, 2004). Berg argues for a 'law of medical information', that deals with problems of using the same information for clinical, research, and management purposes such that the more purposes information is used for, the more work is required to accurately translate the information taken into account the context from which it is produced or generated (Berg, 2004; Scholl & Olaniran, 2013; Winthereik, 2003; Winthereik & Vikkelso, 2005). Winthereik and Vikkelso (2005) contend that GPs already have a large amount of work in order to re-vitalize the discharge letter as a clinical tool; thus, further standardization of the discharge letter content may increase bureaucratic work, in addition, to lead to the production of clinically non useable data. This is because clinical tasks are often too complicated to be framed in limited codes which often lead to inaccurate reports. For instance, a fully standardized discharge letter is intended to be useful everywhere and ought to require little interpretation by its intended receiver. The truth is that GPs need to figure out exactly the nature of care at a treatment center to crack the code of text. In essence, this process requires that GPs, along with their own responsibilities, must also take on the duty that belongs to a hospital, act as a safety mechanism and check up on what was done at the hospital in order to verify that it was clinically and medically competent. Not only would this be very time consuming through added work, but it may even require knowledge and skills that the GP may not have.

FUTURE RESEARCH DIRECTIONS

A thorough understanding of the communication that takes place in MDTMs, as well as the presence and impact of ICTs on these teams' functioning, can help scholars and practitioners take the next steps to further these areas of research. First, we still know relatively little about the communication and experiences that take place in health care teams (Cioffi, Wilkes, Cummings, Warne, & Harrison, 2010; Scholl &Olaniran, 2013; Varpio, Schryer, & Lingard, 2009), despite what we already know about their positive effects on patient outcomes (Ellingson, 2002). We can gain more insight by capturing these teams in action. This would allow scholars to document and understand how they talk, exchange information and alter their messages to resolve conflict and reach consensus. In other words, it would answer the question as to what steps these teams take to engage in problem-solving. Through the technology MDTMs often use, the verbal and many nonverbal exchanges to convey their message. These exchanges can be audio and/or video recorded and transcribed for data analysis. The emergent transcripts can enable professionals and scholars to see which technologies have the greatest measured outcomes in a particular context. Using Retchin's (2008) conceptual framework, these differences in outcomes can be measured across different levels of temporality, urgency, and authority structure, as well as across different media forms.

ICT use that encourages shared authority has implications for role ambiguity that MDTM members experience. Retchin (2008) states that "the role definitions in a co-managed model of care can be surprisingly ambiguous, and expectations frequently differ" (p. 931) from what is expected. The added responsibilities adopted by non-physician professionals could likely lead to an increased workforce that could substitute for direct care normally provided by physicians. Given current trends, it would be advantageous to investigate how ICTs facilitate the shifts in responsibility and decision making. In particular, scholars might ask how role ambiguities could be exacerbated or improved along with the use of specific ICTs, as well as the types of communication exchanges that take place.

Future research might also address the way medical and allied health students receive training in group communication, computer-mediated communication, and the use of ICTs. Retchin (2008) again warns that, "our current educational curricula may be insufficient to prepare health professionals for roles in a health care team" (p. 931). Given this projection, medical educators can explore ways to increase the emphasis on computer-mediated communication and teamwork in medical and professional training. Particular emphasis can be placed on the role ICTs play in increasing group participation, giving more voice to non-physician team members, and increasing efficiency when exchanging data and medical records across the digital divide.

CONCLUSION

Multidisciplinary health care collaboration is inevitable given our aging population and the increased prevalence of chronic illnesses that require coordinated care. Multidisciplinary health care has been shown to have a positive impact on several health outcomes, despite the fact that we still know relatively little about what actually occurs within these groups. Many collaborative models have been used to describe and explain the nature of multidisciplinary health care teams. Retchin's (2008) conceptual framework in particular, illustrates how temporality, urgency of care, and structure of authority can help us understand the impact of ICTs on the group process, as well as assist multidisciplinary collaborators in meeting health care objectives. Information and communication technologies play an increasingly prominent role in patient care and how inter-professional teams coordinate their care. Despite their positive impacts, ICTs present some challenges: limited or unequal access, unintended effects of physical space on the group dynamic, the potential to misinterpret medical information, and the lack of a universal format for medical records. However, in light of the challenges that ICTs might bring to the multidisciplinary setting, a collaborative health care framework that considers temporality, urgency of care, and structure of authority can provide ways to overcome these challenges, as well as pave the way for future research.

REFERENCES

Balandin, S., Shabaev, A., & Stibe, S. (2014, October). Enhancing ICT-Based multidisciplinary collaboration in cross-border context: FRUCT Facilitatedkarelia ENPI project success stories. *Proceedings of the 2014 16th Conference on Open Innovations Association (FRUCT16)* (pp. 9-15). IEEE.

Balka, E., Bjorn, P., & Wagner, I. (2008).Steps toward a typology for health informatics. *Proceedings of the Conference on Computer Supported Cooperative Work*, San Diego, USA (pp. 515-524). New York: ACM Press. doi:10.1145/1460563.1460645

Banas, C. A., Erskine, A. R., Sun, S., & Retchin, S. M. (2011). Phased implementation of electronic health records through an office of clinical transformation. *Journal of the American Medical Informatics Association*, *18*(5), 721–725. doi:10.1136/amiajnl-2011-000165 PMID:21659444

Berg, M. (Ed.). (2004). *Health Information Management: Integrating Information in Health Care Work*. New York: Routledge.

Berg, M., & Goorman, E. (1999). The Contextual Nature of Medical Information. *International Journal of Medical Informatics*, *56*(1-3), 51–60. doi:10.1016/S1386-5056(99)00041-6 PMID:10659934

Big sister is watching you: telemedicine. (1997, January 11). *The Economist, 342*(7999), p. 27.

Brignole, M., Ungar, A., Bartoletti, A., Ponassi, I., Lagi, A., & Mussi, C. et al.. (2006). Standardized care-pathway vs usual management of syncope patients presenting as emergencies at general hospitals. *Europace*, *8*(8), 644–650. doi:10.1093/europace/eul071 PMID:16864618

Ciolfi, L., Fitzpatrick, G., & Bannon, L. (Eds.). (2008). Settings for collaboration: The role of place. *Computer Supported Cooperative Work*, *17*(2–3).

Collms, J. (2001, Jan, 9). So far and yet *so* near with telemedicine. *The Times, London (UK)* [IDD Edition], p. 2.

Crompton, S. (2001, June 5). Virtual hospital speeds recovery. *The Times, London (UK)*, p. 2.

Dourish, P. (2006). Re-space-ing place: "place" and "space" ten years on. *CSCW. Proceedings of Conference on Computer Supported Cooperative Work* (pp. 299–308). Banf, Canada. New York: ACM Press. doi:10.1145/1180875.1180921

Dwivedi, A., Bali, R., James, A., Naguib, R. N., & Johnston, D. (2002). Merger of knowledge Management and information technology in Healthcare: Opportunities and challenges. *Proceedings of the 2002 IEEE Canadian Conference on Electrical & Computer Engineering* (pp. 1194-1199). doi:10.1109/CCECE.2002.1013118

Ellingsen, G., & Monteiro, E. (2007). Seamless Integration: Standardisation across multiple local settings. *Computer Supported Cooperative Work*, *15*(5-6), 443–466. doi:10.1007/s10606-006-9033-0

Fitzpatrick, G., Kaplan, S., & Mansfield, T. (1996). Physical spaces, virtual places and social worlds: a study of work in the virtual. *Proceedings of the 1996 ACM conference on Computer supported cooperative work* Boston, Massachusetts, United States (pp. 334–343). doi:10.1145/240080.240322

Gärtner, J., & Wagner, I. (1996). Mapping acting and agendas: Political frameworks of systems design and participation. *Human-Computer Interaction*, *11*(3), 187–214. doi:10.1207/s15327051hci1103_1

Gaver, B. (1992). The affordances of media spaces for collaboration. *CSCW Proceedings of the Conference on Computer Supported Cooperative Work*, Toronto, Canada (pp. 17–24.). New York: ACM Press.

Hailey, D., Roine, R., & Ohinmaa, A. (2002). Systematic review of evidence for the benefits of telemedicine. *Journal of Telemedicine and Telecare*, *8*(Suppl. 1), 1–7. doi:10.1258/1357633021937604 PMID:12020415

Harrison, S., & Dourish, P. (1996). Re-place-ing space: The roles of place and space in collaborative systems. *Proceedings of the Conference on Computer Supported Cooperative Work*, Cambridge, MA (pp. 67–76). New York: ACM Press. doi:10.1145/240080.240193

Harrison, S., & Tatar, D. (2008). Places: People, events, loci—the relation of semantic frames in the construction of place. *Computer Supported Cooperative Work*, *17*(2–3), 97–133. doi:10.1007/s10606-007-9073-0

Heath, C., & Luff, P. (1992). Media space and communicative asymmetries: Preliminary observations of video-mediated interaction. *Human-Computer Interaction*, *7*(3), 315–346. doi:10.1207/s15327051hci0703_3

Heath, C., & Luff, P. (1996). Documents and professional practice: 'bad' organisational reasons for 'good' clinical records. *Proceedings of the 1996 ACM Conference on Computer Supported Cooperative Work,* Boston, USA (pp. 354–363). New York: ACM Press. doi:10.1145/240080.240342

Hennemann-Krause, L., Lopes, A. J., Araújo, J. A., Petersen, E. M., & Nunes, R. A. (2015). The assessment of telemedicine to support outpatient palliative care in advanced cancer. *Palliative & Supportive Care*, *13*(04), 1025–1030. doi:10.1017/S147895151400100X PMID:25159308

Johns, P. M. (1997). Integrating information systems and healthcare. *Logistics Information Management*, *10*(4), 140–145. doi:10.1108/09576059710187555

Kane, B., Groth, K., & Randall, D. (2011). Medical team meetings: Utilising technology to enhance communication, collaboration and decision-making. *Behaviour & Information Technology, 30*(4), 437–442. doi:10.1080/0144929X.2011.591576

Kane, B., & Luz, S. (2007). Multidisciplinary medical team meetings: An analysis of collaborative working with special attention to timing and teleconferencing. *Computer Supported Collaborative Work, 15*(5-6), 501–535. doi:10.1007/s10606-006-9035-y

Lefley, H. (1998). Training professionals for rehabilitation teams. In P. Corrigan & D. Giffort (Eds.), *Building teams and programs for effective psychiatric rehabilitation* (pp. 13–23). San Francisco: Jossey-Bass.

Luff, P., Heath, C., Kuzuoka, H., Hindmarsh, J., Yamazaki, K., & Oyama, S. (2003). Fractured ecologies: Creating environments for collaboration. *Human-Computer Interaction, 18*(1), 51–84. doi:10.1207/S15327051HCI1812_3

Nelson, L., Houston, T., Hoffman, J., & Bradham, T. S. (2011). Interdisciplinary collaboration in EDHI programs. *The Volta Review, 111*(2), 267–279.

Noordman, J., van der Heide, I., Hopman, P., Schellevis, F., & Rijken, M. (2015). Innovative health care approaches for patients with multi-morbidity in Europe. *Nivel.* Retrieved from http://www.nivel.nl/sites/default/files/bestanden/Rapport-CHRODIS.pdf

O'Neil-Pirozzi, T. M., Kendrick, H., Goldstein, R., & Glenn, M. (2004).Clinical influence on use of portable electronic memory devices in traumatic brain injury rehabilitation. *Brain Injury, 18*(2), 179–189. doi: PMID:14660229.10.1080/0269905031000149560

Olaniran, B. (2007a). Challenges to implementing e-learning and lesser developed countries. In A. L. Edmundson (Ed.), *Globalized e-learning cultural challenges* (pp. 18–34). Hershey, PA, USA: Idea Group, Inc. doi:10.4018/978-1-59904-301-2.ch002

Olaniran, B. A. (2007b). Culture and communication challenges in virtual workspaces. In K. St-Amant (Ed.), Linguistic and cultural online communication issues in the global age (pp. 79-92). PA: Information science reference (IGI Global). doi:10.4018/978-1-59904-213-8.ch006

Olaniran, B. A. (2009a). Organizational Communication: Assessment of Videoconferencing as a Medium for Meetings in the Workplace. *International Journal of Human Technology Interaction, 5*(2), 63–84. doi:10.4018/jthi.2009040104

Olaniran, B. A. (2009b). Discerning Culture in E-Learning and Knowledge Management in the Global Workplace. *Knowledge Management & E-Learning: An International Journal, 1*(3), 180-195.

Olaniran, B. A. (2010). Challenges Facing the Semantic Web and Social Software as Communication Technology Agents in E-learning Environments. *International Journal of Virtual and Personal Learning Environments, 1*(4), 18–30. doi:10.4018/jvple.2010100102

Olve, N., Vimarlund, V., & Agerbo, M. (2006). Elderly healthcare, collaboration and ICT - Enabling the benefits of an enabling technology. In *Vinnova Report 2006:05.* Swedish Governmental Agency for Innovation Systems, Stockholm, Sweden.

Pinder, R., Petchey, R., Shaw, S., & Carter, Y. (2005). What's in a care pathway? Towards a cultural cartography of the new NHS. *Sociology of Health & Illness, 27*(6), 759–779. doi:10.1111/j.1467-9566.2005.00473.x PMID:16283898

Pulignano, G., Del Sindaco, D., Di Lenarda, A., & Sinagra, G. (2006). The evolving care of the elderly with heart failure: From the 'high-tech' to the 'high-touch' approach. *The Journal of Cardiovascular Medicine, 7*(12), 841–846. doi:10.2459/01.JCM.0000253827.79816.05 PMID:17122668

Retchin, S. M. (2008). A conceptual framework for inter professional and co-managed care. *Academic Medicine, 83*(10), 929–933. doi:10.1097/ACM.0b013e3181850b4b PMID:18820522

Richardson, J. E., Abramson, E. L., Pfoh, E. R., & Kaushal, R.HITEC Investigators. (2012). Bridging Informatics and Implementation Science: Evaluating a Framework to Assess Electronic Health Record Implementations in Community Settings. Proceedings of the *AMIA Annual Symposium* (p. 770). PMID:23304351

Rijken, M., Struckmann, V., Dyakova, M., Melchiorre, M. G., Rissanen, S., & van Ginneken, E. (2013). ICARE4EU: Improving care for people with multiple chronic conditions in Europe. *Eurohealth, 19*(3), 29–31.

Robertson, T. (2000). Cooperative work, women and the working environments of technology design. *Australian Feminist Studies, 15*(32), 205–219. doi:10.1080/08164640050138716

Robertson, T. (2002). The public availability of actions and artefacts. *Computer Supported Cooperative Work, 11*(3-4), 299–316. doi:10.1023/A:1021214827446

Robertson, T., Li, J., O'Hara, K., & Hansen, S. (2010). Collaboration within different settings: A study of co-located and distributed multidisciplinary medical team meetings. *Computer Supported Cooperative Work, 19*(5), 483–513. doi:10.1007/s10606-010-9124-9

Salerno, D. (2015). Development of e-Health Services and Integrated/Coordinated Cares. *International Journal of Integrated Care, 15*(5).

Scholl, J. C., & Olaniran, B. A. (2013). ICT Use and Multidisciplinary Healthcare Teams. In M. Cruz-Cunha, I. Miranda, & P. Gonçalves (Eds.), *Handbook of Research on ICTs for Human-Centered Healthcare and Social Care Services* (pp. 627–645). Hershey, PA: Medical Information Science Reference; doi:10.4018/978-1-4666-3986-7.ch033

Short, D., Frischer, M., & Bashford, J. (2004). Barriers to the adoption of computerized decision support systems in general practice consultations: A qualitative study of GPs perspectives. *International Journal of Medical Informatics, 73*(4), 357–362. doi:10.1016/j.ijmedinf.2004.02.001 PMID:15135754

Singh, R., Mathiassen, L., Stachura, M. E., & Astapova, E. V. (2010). Sustainable rural telehealth innovation: A public health case study. *Health Services Research, 45*(4), 985–1004. doi:10.1111/j.1475-6773.2010.01116.x PMID:20459449

Singh, S. (2014).The 10 Social and Tech Trends That Could Shape the Next Decade. *Forbes*. Retrieved from http://www.forbes.com/sites/sarwantsingh/2014/05/12/the-top-10-mega-trends-of-the-decade

Stellato, K., Humar, F., Montesi, C., Radini, D., Antonione, R., Sinagra, G., & Di Lenarda, A. (2015). Integrated Outpatient Care in Advanced Heart Failure: The Beehive Person-Centered Model. *International Journal of Person Centered Medicine*, *4*, 23–30.

Stellato, K., Radini, D., Pellizzari, M., Pordenon, M., & Pletti, L. (2015a). New Frontiers of People-Centered Integrated Care for Complex Chronic Disease. *Journal of Palliative Care Medicine*, *5*(234), 2.

Thomas, E. J., Sexton, J. B., & Helmreich, R. L. (2003). Discrepant attitudes about teamwork among critical care nurses and physicians. *Critical Care Medicine*, *31*(3), 956–959. doi:10.1097/01. CCM.0000056183.89175.76 PMID:12627011

Van Servellen, G. M. (2009). *Communication skills for the health care professional: Concepts, practice, and evidence*. Jones & Bartlett Publishers.

Varpio, L., Schryer, C. F., & Lingard, L. (2009). Routine and adaptive expert strategies for resolving ICT mediated communication problems in the team setting. *Medical Education*, *43*(7), 680–687. doi:10.1111/j.1365-2923.2009.03395.x PMID:19573192

Voida, A., Voida, S., Greenberg, S., & Ai Hi, H. (2008).Asymmetry in media space. *Proceedings of the Conference on Computer Supported Cooperative Work* CSCW '08 (pp. 313–322). San Diego, USA, New York: ACM press.

Wallace, S. (1997). Health information in the new millennium and beyond the role of computers and the Internet. *Health Education*, *97*(3), 88–95. doi:10.1108/09654289710162488

Winthereik, B. (2003). ''We Fill in Our Working Understanding'': On Codes, Classifications and the Production of Accurate Data. *Methods of Information in Medicine*, *42*(4), 489–496. PMID:14534655

Winthereik, B. R., & Vikkelso, S. (2005). ICT and Integrated Care: Some Dilemmas of Standardising Inter-Organisational Communication. *Computer Supported Cooperative Work*, *14*, 43–67. doi:10.1007/s10606-004-6442-9

Technical Discussions: Consideration of the recommendations on strengthening community-based health-care services. (2015). World Health Organization.

Wright, K. B., Sparks, L., & O'Hair, H. D. (2008). *Health communication in the 21ˢᵗ century*. Malden, MA: Blackwell Publishing.

This research was previously published in the International Journal of Reliable and Quality E-Healthcare (IJRQEH), 5(1); edited by Anastasius Moumtzoglou, pages 18-31, copyright year 2016 by IGI Publishing (an imprint of IGI Global).

Chapter 33
CARMIE:
A Conversational Medication Assistant for Heart Failure

Joana Lobo
Fraunhofer Portugal AICOS, Portugal

Liliana Ferreira
Fraunhofer Portugal AICOS, Portugal

Aníbal JS Ferreira
University of Porto, Portugal

ABSTRACT

The incidence of chronic diseases is increasing and monitoring patients in a home environment is recommended. Noncompliance with prescribed medication regimens is a concern, especially among older people. Heart failure is a chronic disease that requires patients to follow strict medication plans permanently. With the objective of helping these patients managing information about their medicines and increasing adherence, the personal medication advisor CARMIE was developed as a conversational agent capable of interacting, in Portuguese, with users through spoken natural language. The system architecture is based on a language parser, a dialog manager, and a language generator, integrated with already existing tools for speech recognition and synthesis. All modules work together and interact with the user through an Android application, supporting users to manage information about their prescribed medicines. The authors also present a preliminary usability study and further considerations on CARMIE.

INTRODUCTION

As modern Medicine developed, the consumption of pharmacological drugs has raised exponentially (Sullivan, Behncke, & Purushotham, 2010). With the multiplicity of medication regimens, modern Pharmacology brought large amounts of information to be managed by patients and healthcare staff. At the same time, and in part due to the world population ageing, the number of patients suffering from chronic

DOI: 10.4018/978-1-5225-3926-1.ch033

illnesses is growing (Giles, 2004). Such diseases usually demand treatments with numerous pharmaco-logical prescriptions that require strict medication management. One of these diseases is heart failure (HF), presenting high prevalence, especially in the USA and Europe, and significant health expenditure due to frequent patient hospitalization and readmissions (Ziaeian & Fonarow, 2016). Typically, senior HF patients need around 13 different drugs per day, at home, of which a significant number are not prescribed (Ewen et al., 2015). With such complex medication regimens for HF, patients spend a lot of effort gathering the information required to successfully manage their disease, but still having trouble in keeping track of this information (Ferguson et al., 2010). Compliance is also an important outcome predictor among patients with chronic diseases like HF. In general, medication adherence is remarkably lower than self-reported adherence (Nieuwenhuis, Jaarsma, van Veldhuisen, & van der Wal, 2012). A study (Cabral & Silva, 2010) showed that the poor adherence to therapeutic prescriptions is a major problem of public health in Portugal, where the main reasons for nonadherence are the patient's fear of asking questions to their doctors, and the difficulty in listening to or understanding caregivers' explanations on how to deal with the prescribed regimen. As slight improvements in functional capacity are of the utmost importance to HF patients, prescribed treatments should be taken seriously. Existing HF home-monitoring programs have proved to be helpful with reduced readmissions and prolongation of survival (Stewart & Horowitz, 2002). However, due to the unaffordable costs and insufficient number of medical personnel, the required specialized healthcare staff cannot offer daily home-assistance. It was suggested by Ferguson et al. (2010) that the use of automated intelligence assistance to manage medication can foster patient survival. Therefore, there is a need for automated systems, for health communication and management, that can provide intelligence assistance to HF patients within a home health environment.

This work aims to encompass the next technological step towards a virtual personal medication advi-sor: a conversational system capable of interacting with users through natural language, mostly voice, to help them manage their condition and the prescribed medication regimens. A virtual medication advisor shares its guidelines with information therapy, which supports that providing specific evidence-based medical information to certain patients at the right time can help them making positive behavior changes and improving self-consciousness of healthcare (Mettler & Kemper, 2002). It is expected that the con-versational assistant described in this work can bring together the advantages of information therapy and mobile technologies, improving disease outcomes through a patient centered approach.

The smartphone-based assistant developed, named CARMIE, aims to deliver information and knowledge-based advice to help chronic diseases' patients managing complex prescription regimens. In-home medication monitoring is facilitated by providing personalized intelligence assistance on posol-ogy, interactions, indications, and adverse reactions. Another objective is to motivate the user through interactive dialogue and cues, trying to increase medication adherence. It is expected that, in result of using the proposed system, well-informed and home-monitored patients will be showing increased patient survival, as well as reduced re-hospitalization and mortality rates, in addition to allowing better responsiveness and distribution of work time among healthcare staff. Patients with chronic diseases will be able to live more independently with greater compliance, satisfaction, and understanding of their therapeutic regimens.

As an initial approach, CARMIE was developed in European Portuguese, opening an unexplored path on the integration of intelligence assistance in Portuguese healthcare. Furthermore, the scope of the conversational assistant developed is restricted to medication regimens for HF, due to its well-defined pharmacological practices, which greatly depend on self-care and self-management to lengthen patient survival (McMurray et al., 2012). One of the particularities of this project, lies in the fact that the pharmacological information needed by CARMIE is retrieved from an ontology, a knowledge representation model.

Herewith, this paper starts by presenting a background on conversational systems for healthcare. The remaining sections present the CARMIE system, from the design methodologies to its interactions and system architecture, as well as an evaluation and discussion of findings and overall performance.

BACKGROUND

Intelligent agents can offer an expansive framework for developing computerized systems that can independently collect and deliver information, as well as make comprehensive decisions (Hudson & Cohen, 2010). This makes these systems able to provide intelligence assistance to patients within a home care setting. In general, intelligent agents for healthcare support can serve the following purposes: reminders, communication, surveillance, education, and support (Hudson & Cohen, 2010). Especially suitable for health communication and support, conversational systems can be intelligent agents with the ability to deliver assistance using spoken natural language (NL), engaging in dialogue with the user. The main steps of a conversational system include understanding what the user says, planning an appropriate reaction, and articulating the response through generated natural language. For this, these agents usually follow a modular structure composed by modules for speech recognition, natural language understanding (NLU), dialogue management, natural language generation (NLG), resource communication, and speech synthesis (McTear, 2002). Such technologies require a high level of system architecture and complex coordination among its different components (Mellish & Evans, 2004).

Health informatics research has been addressing the needs of patient homecare and medication management with the development of several types of patient-centered technologies and design guidelines (Siek et al., 2011; Wilcox et al., 2012). In general, studies of technology for self-management of medication include web-based personal health applications (Siek et al., 2010), multi-compartment medication devices including pillboxes and medicine cabinets (Paterson, Kinnear, Bond, & McKinstry, 2016), medication schedule tracking applications (Walker, Elder, & Hayes, 2014), sensor-driven reminder systems (Kaushik, Intille, & Larson, 2008), mobile phone messaging (Jongh, Gurol-Urganci, Vodopivec-Jamsek, Car, & Atun, 2012), chatbots (Hawig, n.d.) and virtual intelligent assistants (Dahl et al., 2011). In this scenario, intelligent assistants are amongst the most complex but complete and multimodal systems.

Many of these technologies have shown positive outcomes on medication adherence and patient self-care (Anglada-Martinez et al., 2015; Vervloet et al., 2012). However, they present limitations that need to be further addressed by new assistive technologies. It was suggested that providing voice inputs is essential for delivering health information for medication management (Siek et al., 2011) and that multimodality of information is especially important for technological assistants for senior users (Dahl, Coin, Greene, & Mandelbaum, 2011). In addition, information should be tailored both in timing and in content (Vervloet et al., 2012). Siek et al (2011) also pointed the need for a freely available standard library of pictures and medication information to be easily integrated in medication management systems.

Conversational assistants started to be developed mainly for general-use applications, for other than health related purposes (Axelrod, 2000; Baptist, 2000; Cardoso, Flores, Langlois, & Neto, 2002). One of the first medical applications focusing on the development of conversational assistants' modules, namely NLG, was GALEN-IN-USE, an implementation of openGALEN resources for collaborative and multilingual representation of surgical procedure classifications (Wagner, Rogers, Baud, & Scherrer, 1999). Since then, most of the conversational assistants, using NLU and NLG, for healthcare were conceptual approaches or partial prototypes, such as Chester (Allen et al., 2006; Ferguson et al., 2010), CARDIAC (Galescu, Allen, Ferguson, Swift, & Quinn, 2009) or HOMEY/HomeNL (Giorgino et al., 2005; Rojas-Barahona, Quaglini, & Stefanelli, 2009). Chester was a prototype intelligent assistant for health communication, to engage daily with the user, using spoken or typed natural language, for collecting, analyzing, and delivering information about the patient's condition. With this system, Ferguson et al. (2010) demonstrated the feasibility of spoken language interfaces for managing patient health information. However, they also identify significant ethical, legal, social, and technical challenges. CARDIAC is another English NL dialogue system conducting spoken health monitoring interviews for chronic HF patients. Rather than providing medication assistance, it collects information about the current state of patient's health, from objective (weight) to subjective (pain, fatigue, exercise) conditions (Galescu et al., 2009). HomeNL was a proof-of-concept dialogue system for the management of patients with hypertension. The study discusses ergonomic aspects of the assistant, including dialog adaptation and refinement of language models. HomeNL was able to influence condition outcomes, with averaged blood pressure values decreasing in the dialog-system treatment group compared with a control group (Giorgino et al., 2005). In general, these past works showed that virtual assistants can be effective in improving healthcare. The major drawbacks of the presented prototypes were the lack of portability and insufficient knowledge base to answer to user's needs in real homecare settings.

Smartphones, one of the most widespread technologies nowadays, brought, with mHealth applications and portable connected health, a new potential to promote medication adherence and self-management of chronic diseases. Mobile conversational intelligent assistants started to appear. Dahl et al. (2011) presented Cassandra, an avatar-based personal assistant for senior users to help them manage daily life tasks, such as taking medication or shopping, using a smartphone interface. In 2013, NextIT Corporation, a company with a strong experience in conversational agents for business and military applications (Artstein, Gandhe, Gerten, Leuski, & Traum, 2009), presented Alme for Healthcare. This virtual assistant combines an intricate natural language model with the friendly interface of a virtual health assistant to drive interactive dialogues with patients on their channel of choice: using spoken conversation, typed entries or screen taps (NextIT, 2013). The landscape of commercial multimodal assistants is increasing. They are mainly comprised by multi-platform chatbot-based solutions, with text/touch/speech multilingual interaction and wide-range features for personal daily management: from medication reminders, to guidance through a treatment/exercise regimen, encouragement on keeping a wellness plan on-track, record and share health data or achievements, search for useful information, etc. (Hawig, n.d.). The new generation of mobile conversational systems has also started to deploy their conversational interfaces on other portable devices such as wearables and social robots (McTear, Callejas, & Griol, 2016).

DESIGN AND IMPLEMENTATION

CARMIE was designed together with an iterative patient-centered approach to personal healthcare. During the development process, the system aimed for simplicity, portability, and full applicability in home healthcare settings. Herewith, a portable and public platform, the Android mobile system, was used as the technological support for the assistant. Thus, CARMIE is a virtual agent within an Android application that listens to and speaks to users regarding HF care and pharmacological information.

A modular architecture, this is, a top-down design, was chosen for CARMIE. The system was developed in small autonomous modules, each performing different functions but altogether working as a single structure, allowing easier debugging and updating. As stated by Mellish and Evans (2004), having a modular structure is important for a conversational assistant, in which different tasks occur simultaneously and specific modules can be reused by other systems.

CARMIE is composed of three essential internal modules: the language parser, the dialog manager and the language generator. Additionally, they integrate with two external modules, respectively for speech recognition and speech synthesis. Each internal module needs its own resources to fetch the necessary data. A schematics overview of this structure and respective information flow can be seen on Figure 1.

The agent was designed for users who speak European Portuguese, so it can be used on a Portuguese Healthcare setting. Thus, the external speech modules selected had to support European Portuguese. Providing the best packages for this language, Google Voice[1] and iSpeech[2] technologies were chosen for recognition and synthesis, allowing the internal components to directly interact with the user.

As a conversational system, CARMIE is very dependent on linguistic resources like European Portuguese linguistic knowledge databases and domain specific lexicons. Linguateca (Costa, Santos, & Cardoso, 2008) is a resource center for computational processing of the Portuguese language providing useful materials for linguistic analysis. Some of these resources, namely a general domain Portuguese lexicon and dictionary (Costa et al., 2008), were adapted and integrated on the developed language parser and language generator.

The virtual assistant CARMIE was settled to provide information on posology, drug indications (common targets and uses for a certain pharmacological drug), and adverse reactions (side-effects and harms of the usage of a pharmacological drug under the recommended administration conditions). Subcategories of posology data include administration dosage, route, frequency, and drug name. All the required pharmacological information was retrieved from an OWL (web ontology language) based ontology created using the PharmInx (Pharmacological Information Extraction) system developed by Aguiar et al. (2012). PharmInx automatically extracts and models information from Portuguese medi-

Figure 1. Schematics showing the information flow among the different modules of CARMIE and its resources system architecture

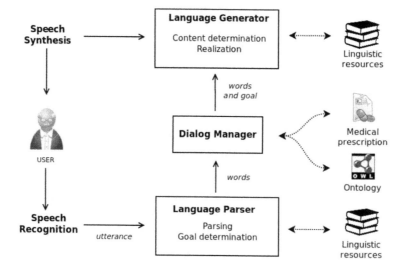

cal therapeutic records and leaflets. This tool was mainly developed to extract posology information using extensible knowledge models, structuring entities, and their respective relations extracted from pharmacological texts. PharmInx extracts this data from Portuguese free-form texts, with high precision when it comes to posology records. After extraction, the ontology is automatically populated by the information extracted. During CARMIE development, ontology design, and maintenance was handled by the Protégé framework, whereas a Jena application programming interface was used for ontology population. An organized and structured representation of pharmacological information was, thus, assembled in European Portuguese. The medication advisor used this knowledge representation model but restricted to HF pharmacology domain. The fact that CARMIE is based on ontology knowledge gives distinctive value to this conversational agent.

A personal medication assistant with access to user's medical prescriptions can deliver more reliable and tailored information to patients. To validate this, the current prototype of CARMIE was given access to simulated medical prescriptions, in the form of text files. Each prescription contains a list of prescribed medicines for that user, along with the respective posology. Future implementations will included a module to automatically receive and extract information from an authentic electronic medical prescription, allowing any physician to make his patients' prescriptions available to CARMIE.

Language Parser

The language parser, or NLU module, processes and segments what is perceived by the speech recognition module, using tokenization, phrase chunking, and part-of-speech (POS) tagging. In other words, this module breaks up the recognized text into meaningful elements (tokens), divides phrases and annotates, for each word in the sentence, its corresponding POS or its lexical category. The UIMA Hidden Markov Model tagger (Apache UIMA Development Community, 2011) was trained and adapted for Portuguese so it could be used by the language processing components. After tokenization and lexical classification, the parser identifies names and verbs on recognized sentences, in order to spot keywords, extract necessary information, and infer the intention of user's utterances. This parsing process relies on the linguistic resources, a Portuguese lexicon and dictionary. Processed information will then go to the dialog manager.

Dialog Manager

The dialog manager's (DM) purpose is goal analysis and information retrieval. When uttered words are tagged and keywords identified, the system attributes an intention to what the user said and, accordingly, delineates a goal for the response. A set of communicative goals were defined for CARMIE, such as, Existence, Information, List, Permission, and Reason. These goals are used for question classification. Understandable user utterances are not unlimited, and ideally follow a certain structure. It was settled that the main keywords that establish utterance's goal, and thus what the user requests from the system, are the first two words of the question - usually interrogative pronouns or verbs. This is enough to associate a goal to each of the possible main intentions behind user utterances. Also, system performance is simplified. For example, if the user wants to retrieve information on a specific pharmacological property, he should voice an appropriate question (e.g. "What is the frequency of Carvedilol?"). The system will associate that utterance with the communicative goal Information. Similarly, if the user asks if he has permission for taking a medicine (e.g. "Can I take Bisoprolol?"), CARMIE would identify the goal as Permission. Other types of utterances will trigger different goals.

After goal identification, the system selects the correspondent type of response. Depending on the goal, the DM tries to identify a known medicine name and a featured keyword (e.g. frequency, dose, reaction, etc.). Information is retrieved from the ontology and medical prescription, when necessary. The DM will look for medicine names on the ontology through specific SPARQL (SPARQL Protocol and RDF Query Language) queries and will check the user's prescription to know if the uttered medicine is prescribed. The DM can also suggest a similar medicine name if uttered medicines are invalid or not prescribed, by performing a Levenshtein Distance iterative routine (Hjelmqvist, 2012) to assess similarity between two strings: the name of the uttered medicine and of each prescribed medicine. The name on the prescription that has the closest similarity to the uttered medicine name is suggested to the user (e.g. "That medicine name does not exist. Do you mean <similar medicine name>?"). The user then confirms this judgment of the DM.

A highlight of CARMIE is its medical inquire. This feature is initiated when a user says that he does not feel well, or when the goal is set as Permission and the uttered medicine is not prescribed. For instance, if a user asks if he can take a certain medicine (e.g. "Can I take <medicine name>?"), the DM checks if that medicine name is present on his medical prescription. If yes, CARMIE gives a positive answer, as well as information about the prescribed frequency for that drug. If not prescribed, the system considers atypical the fact that the user asked if he could take a medicine that is not prescribed, since it is common for patients with chronic conditions to take nonprescription medication when they feel unwell (Mattila et al., 2013). Therefore, the DM identifies a secondary intention behind user's question and initiates a medical inquiry. The medical inquiry was designed especially for HF patients to assess if the user has symptoms that characterize deterioration of HF. Questions, such as, "Do you have swollen feet or legs?" or "Do you have shortness of breath?", are asked by CARMIE. The user must answer yes or no accordingly. By evaluating the positive answers and the risk of each symptom, CARMIE gives suitable advice to the user. Moreover, the DM generates a text file with the date, patient answers to the enquire, and an observation field. This medical report can be sent by email or text message to the healthcare staff registered as responsible for that patient.

Language Generator

Real-time NL generation is essential on dialogue frameworks. Moreover, NLG has to be psycho-linguistically realistic and stylistically suitable, while delivering the requested information in accordance with the right context. CARMIE's NLG module builds appropriate sentences to answer to the user according to the keywords and goal identified by the DM. The final objective is, not only to output informative text, but also to produce direct and suitable statements that can elucidate the user without causing any ambiguity. CARMIE favors short and simple sentences instead of fewer but longer and complex phrases. In addition, language generation in CARMIE is language and application-specific, using grammar rules and lexicons particular to the healthcare domain.

Hybrid language generation systems were identified as more successful and flexible (Galley, Fosler-Lussier, & Potamianos, 2001). When acceptable performance can be achieved without using complex linguist approaches, canned text and templates should be sufficient for realization (Reiter & Dale, 1997). More complex approaches should make use of meaning text theory and phrase- or feature-based methodologies. Therefore, CARMIE takes a hybrid and practical approach to NLG: simple and typical phrases are generated by canned-text and template-based approaches, whereas sentences requiring more interaction, initiative and complexity use a combination of phrase and feature-based methods.

Canned-text is implemented when fixed instructions or direct answers are required. For example, when an error occurs, a statement is randomly selected from a list of fixed sentences, such as, "I did not understand. Can you repeat please?". The template based approach is used for fixed sentences containing "gaps" for the information that can differ but always occupies the same place on the phrase. This is used, for instance, with greetings dependent on the time of the day or while listing the prescribed medicines: "Your doctor prescribed <number of medicines> medicines: <medicine name1> <medicine name2>…". Sentences generated using phrase and feature based methods are more complex and contain the answers with information from the ontology. Each sentence is specified according to a certain phrase pattern consisting of phrase elements such as verb, subject, object, noun modifier, post-modifier, and punctuation. Furthermore, generation is dictated by the characteristics of the desired sentence, according to a feature-based methodology. A unique set of qualifiers, such as negative/affirmative or singular/plural, allow the sentence to be effectively generated.

An Extensible Markup Language (XML) lexicon is used to get the appropriate word order, as well as conjugation in gender and number. This linguistic resource was specifically created for this module. The restricted lexicon allows the system to be lighter and faster, but with all the necessary data to generate NL within a personal medical advisor context. This lexicon contains a set of words that may be necessary for CARMIE's responses to the user, as well as the necessary information for every word that may be used. Each word element is characterized by several word features (category, number, gender, conjugations, etc.). The NLG module analyses this information and selects the suitable word for the phrase element that is being built, according to the XML lexicon and the keywords that were recognized.

User-Agent Interaction

The medical assistant CARMIE can start its engagement with the user by generating a simple greeting and then waiting for a user utterance. Due to the complexity of coherent and complete conversational systems, the range of possible user utterances will always be limited. Ideally, the user should be free to say whatever he wants, independently of the words or syntactic structure chosen. However, for now, the multilayered and automated nature of a medical assistant does not allow CARMIE to have such a wide flexibility. The user can interact with the system with somewhat restricted utterances, mostly in the form of questions and because this assistant is more focused in answering user's queries about information related to his medicines. Every uttered question will be interpreted by the system and an appropriate answer will be given, making use, if necessary, of the information retrieved from CARMIE's resources. For example, if a patient asks "What are the medicines that the doctor prescribed?", CARMIE will list the names of all the medicines on the prescription of that patient. When user utterances are invalid or misheard by the system, CARMIE replies with a random set phrase requesting the user to repeat or reformulate the question.

As a mixed-initiative assistant, the system can take the initiative by asking at a certain time of the dialog, for example, "How are you feeling today?" and wait for a response. Another example of CARMIE's initiative is the medical inquiry, producing and sending a medical report that allows healthcare staff to be updated with patient condition when he does not feel well, or has symptoms typical of HF worsening.

As the dialog proceeds, everything said by the user or by the system is shown on the smartphone's screen within a dialog list that can be scrolled up and down. Some screenshots of CARMIE user-system example interactions are shown in Figure 2.

Figure 2. Screenshots with examples of transcribed interaction with CARMIE Android application, featuring (a) Google Voice popup, (b) example of system initiative, (c) one step of the medical inquire, (d), (e) and (f) examples of dialogue. Original interfaces are presented in Portuguese language to the user.

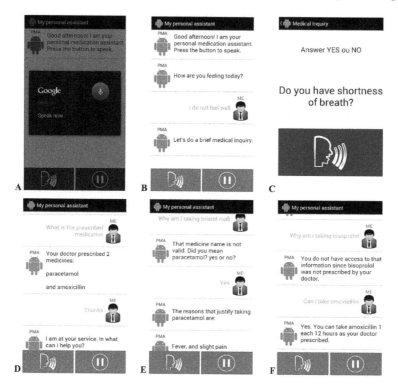

EVALUATION

There is still no consensual nor flawless method to evaluate a conversational system, especially regarding its NLU and NLG modules (Baptist, 2000). The difficulty of achieving a full formal evaluation of conversational assistants lies in their heavy dependence on the context where the dialog happens, as well as in the limited comparability of the results (Artstein, Gandhe, Gerten, Leuski, & Traum, 2009). Even so, a sufficient indicator of quality for these systems is the collective experience of its users (Baptist, 2000). Herewith, to validate the concept behind CARMIE, a semi-formal evaluation of the system was performed through a task-based usability test and questionnaire to assess system's feasibility, performance and drawbacks.

A usability assessment with senior HF patients would have been the best option for evaluating CARMIE. However, as the system is still in its early stages of development and as tests with these patients require special procedures, the performed usability study could not include these target users. The study was thus performed with 11 native Portuguese adults, between 22 and 30 years old, who were familiar with mHealth applications and worked regularly with senior patients.

For the usability test session, each participant was asked to simulate a senior HF patient and to complete two tasks using only CARMIE and a small support list. This list included the names of a set of medicines to be used during the session, as well as of a set of example utterances to interact with CARMIE. Before the experiment started, it was highlighted that one should never take a medicine that was not prescribed. The goal of the first task was understanding which medicine, from the simulated list of drugs previously presented, was prescribed to reduce fever. The participant had to use CARMIE to obtain this information, and, in case an appropriate drug was included in the list, the participant had to identify which. On the second task, the participant, still simulating an HF patient, was asked what should she do if she was feeling very tired and her legs were swollen. The minimum number of user questions to CARMIE to be able to complete the task was defined as two and three, respectively for task 1 and 2. After completing both tasks, participants could spend some time talking and freely using the system.

The objective of the test was to evaluate the system design, user task accomplishment, and user satisfaction. The study analyzed questions such as "Is spoken interaction useful and enjoyable?", "Does the flow of the application matches user expectations?", or "Is one able to retrieve the desired information?" For the described study, a Samsung Galaxy Nexus GT-I9250 with Android 4.0, and with the CARMIE application installed, was used. Each session was video recorded.

After the test, each participant was asked to evaluate the assistant by filling out a paper-based usability questionnaire. This questionnaire consisted of 16 statements that were evaluated by the participants using a 4-point Likert scale, from 1 (strongly agree) to 4 (strongly disagree). The questionnaire was based on the System Usability Scale (SUS) (Brooke, 1996), although some statements were adapted or added to directly address usability issues of HF senior patients. Each statement used was related to one of the following categories: usability, coherence, naturalness, quality of the information, or HF-directed usability. For example, the statement "I felt the dialogue with the system was natural." evaluated the naturalness of the system, while the statement "If I had to follow strict medication regimens, I think I would use this system frequently." evaluated HF-directed usability of the conversational assistant. The final SUS score (0 to 100) was calculated based on Brooke (1996), after normalization for 4-point scale used.

RESULTS

All the participants ended up completing the two assigned tasks - some of them faster and more easily than others. Each user made, on average, four questions to CARMIE before being able to complete each task. During the sessions, the most frequently uttered question was "Can I take <medicine name>?"

Questionnaire results are summarized in Table 1. Overall, system coherence, naturalness and quality of information scores were the most consistent among participants. Quality of information received the best average score. The final SUS score, calculated using the average scores for each question, was 88. This is equivalent to a 'very good' or 'B' rank score, showing that the users felt that the system was simple and useful.

On another hand, many participants commented that they felt that CARMIE was not very intuitive on the first try. Participants needed an initial time of interaction with the system before they got to fully understand how it worked and then it got easy to use. This was confirmed as most users completed task 2 faster than task 1. In addition, difficulties with the speech recognition of some keywords were observed for the majority of the participants, especially in what relates to medicines' names. Some participants suggested further adaptations necessary to make the application more accessible for senior patients. These and other identified drawbacks are discussed on the following sections.

Table 1. Average score (1 to 4) given by the participants grouped by category of questionnaire's statements, with the respective mean deviation

	Average Score	**Mean Deviation**
Usability	3	0.87
Coherence	4	0.63
Naturalness	3	0.68
Quality of Information	3	0.74
HF-directed Usability	3	0.80

DISCUSSION

Through the usability study performed, the virtual assistant CARMIE has proved to be capable of completing basic interaction tasks with users to address pharmacological and treatment information for HF daily care. In general, user engagement with CARMIE was successful. As proposed, the assistant generated phrases that were coherent, short, and easy to understand, being able to cope with user's requests. During the sessions, CARMIE's strengths were shown to be its simple interface, usefulness and direct way of acquiring tailored healthcare information.

The predominant verbal interaction and lack of visual interface indicators may explain why some participants felt that CARMIE was not very intuitive during the first task. It was concluded that some explanatory cues for first time users must be added to facilitate the initial interaction with the assistant.

Regarding the technological aspect, there was a successful integration of the developed NLU and NLG modules with external speech recognition and synthesis modules. Still, limitations were identified. As a preliminary conversational agent, CARMIE lacks in flexibility, mainly due to restricted phrasings and a fixed output vocabulary. The system should be able to understand and answer to a wider variety of user utterances. The Android implementation brought CARMIE closer to a mixed-initiative conversational system, but work is still needed to evolve this system initiative and increase, even more, user engagement. The complexity of CARMIE is not yet on a stage where stochastic models are compulsory for NLG. Even so, this could be one of the strategies towards improving system flexibility. In addition, a spell checker for the generated sentences seems to be necessary to recognize possible mistakes in users' queries, such as for the names of medicines.

A major limitation of this study is that it was not conducted with the final target age group. Questionnaire results regarding general usability of the system could differ for senior users, mainly because they would have less experience in interacting with mobile applications compared with younger participants. On CARMIE's case, it is possible that this gap will not be so evident, as the interaction is mainly verbal, not requiring much effective manipulation of the smartphone itself. Either way, this has still to be tested on further iterations of the study. For now, observations from the current study will allow refining the medication assistant.

A comparative analysis of CARMIE's results to the ones of previous studies cannot be performed since the few case studies done to assess usability of home-healthcare virtual assistants were done in a clinic context, featuring only individual system modules or different evaluation strategies (Ferguson et al., 2010; Galescu et al., 2009; Giorgino et al., 2005). An additional limitation is the fact that CARMIE is developed to be used in European Portuguese, a language still immature in what concerns natural language research, resources and tools, especially NLG and virtual intelligent assistants.

According to Chester's case study (Ferguson et al., 2010), and to what was seen through the usability test, patients are positive in general about intelligent systems for self-care. However, they are also very concerned about the privacy of their data. This is an important potential barrier to the acceptance of this type of personal health application and more efforts are necessary on this topic.

Challenges

It is important that CARMIE remains a medical information-provider rather than a decision-maker. This conversational system does not aim be a physician's replacement. According to Ferguson et al. (2010, p. S14), "Technology should be developed to complement and augment human decision-making." In addition, it is important to maintain a good granularity for the information delivered by the intelligent assistant. The type and amount of information that is appropriate to give may not be the same for every patient. For example, the long list of the adverse effects of prescribed medicines can pointlessly stress patients, especially as most of these events are very rare or irrelevant (Wilcox et al., 2012). Further personalization of the intelligent assistant could avoid unnecessary anxiety on the user (Krämer, Hoffmann, & Kopp, 2010). This can be done by adapting and selecting the information given to patients according to priorities or user social context. This can possibly prevent problems of excess of information and make the assistant more robust.

As discussed previously, healthcare ICT systems targeted for elderly users may face some barriers. Since older patients often do not have technical literacy or easy access to technology, the adherence to a computerized-assistant could be low. Senior patients may view the technology as intrusive and not suitable to their lifestyle, offering resistance to the introduction of new equipment or new habits. Even so, by studying human-computer interactions and redesigning the technology for this user group, it is possible to slowly change the way older people see ICT-based assistants. With this objective, some future directions for CARMIE are proposed.

Future Work

Before further experiments, the authors will focus on improving the conversational assistant. CARMIE can be better tailored to patient needs. The next step will be to broaden the type of pharmacological information delivered to the user, especially including listing and verification of possible medication interactions that may endanger user's health. Another improvement will be the incorporation of user's medical history and past medical records, complemented with a variety of patient basic information, such as name, age, sex, educational level, and physiological data (height, weight, blood pressure, etc.). The connection of CARMIE with a hospital Electronic Medical Record or even the patient's Electronic Health Record would be the best way to ensure the access to reliable, quality and updated information while ensuring security and privacy of the patient's health data. CARMIE can be set to use this information to adjust its dialogue and initiative.

Additional functionalities were suggested to make the agent more helpful, for example, the integration of CARMIE with visual information of pills and medicine boxes, as well as with a barcode reader. As some patients may not able to read, they may not recognize their pills nor know what is written on the medicine package or prescription. Previous research also supports the use of these visual or automated supports for helping elderly patients manage medication (Siek et al., 2011). In addition, incorporation with already existent medication reminders or alerts can also increase system helpfulness.

After these improvements, it will be important to conduct a study with senior HF patients on a homecare setting, with the objective of measuring the impact of conversational agents like CARMIE on patient daily self-care.

From a technical perspective, CARMIE's NL modules can be iteratively refined, especially by increasing the granularity of utterance interpretation and of the phrase elements that will be part of generated sentences. This will gradually result in a more complex and enhanced agent, smoothing some of system limitations, such as the lack of flexibility, initiative and naturalness. Other improvements can include the implementation of statistical or stochastic methodologies that will give to the system the ability to learn common user utterances or underlying intentions, the ability to build more complete approaches for NLG, or the ability of automated vocabulary growth. This increase in complexity can also be followed by additional intelligent modules to detect speaker identity, emotional state or degree of motivation.

CONCLUSION

Healthcare technologies are evolving towards interactive and personal health management intelligent assistants. These new technological solutions can lead to a pro-active attitude towards disease monitoring and management. The medication advisor CARMIE was successfully developed as an mHealth system, interacting in real-time through spoken natural language in European Portuguese, to deliver HF care information and help users manage their medication regimens. The strong points of the developed system were found to be its simplicity, quality of delivered information, user engagement, coherence, and its architecture aimed to enhance modularity. A uniqueness of CARMIE lies on the use of ontologies as the source of pharmacological information. In contrast with the high users' expectations for full-fledged conversational assistants, the current system lacks in flexibility and initiative. Future work will focus on improving system's granularity and complexity.

The system was envisioned within a patient-centered approach to personal healthcare, namely heart failure care, so that home-monitoring and treatment efficacy can be enhanced. This could contribute to reducing the burden and high costs related with HF readmissions and mortality rates. The specific evidence-based information given by CARMIE can help patients make positive behavior changes. Simplicity and interactivity of the system triggered user engagement with pharmacological information. User satisfaction with CARMIE can raise treatment compliance and self-consciousness of home healthcare, working together with physicians to modify disease outcomes.

REFERENCES

Aguiar, B. L., Mendes, E., & Ferreira, L. (2012). Information extraction from medication leaflets. *Paper presented at 1st PhD Students Conference in Electrical and Computer Engineering*, Porto.

Allen, J., Ferguson, G., Blaylock, N., Byron, D., Chambers, N., Dzikovska, M., & Swift, M. et al. (2006). Chester: Towards a personal medication advisor. *Journal of Biomedical Informatics*, *39*(5), 500–513. doi:10.1016/j.jbi.2006.02.004 PMID:16545620

Anglada-Martinez, H., Riu-Viladoms, G., Martin-Conde, M., Rovira-Illamola, M., Sotoca-Momblona, J. M., & Codina-Jane, C. (2015). Does mHealth increase adherence to medication? Results of a systematic review. *International Journal of Clinical Practice*, *69*(1), 9–32. doi:10.1111/ijcp.12582 PMID:25472682

Apache UIMA Development Community. (2011). *Tagger Annotator Documentation - version 2.3.1*. Retrieved from https://uima.apache.org/d/uima-addons-current/Tagger/hmmTaggerUsersGuide.html

Artstein, R., Gandhe, S., Gerten, J., Leuski, A., & Traum, D. (2009). Semi-formal evaluation of conversational characters. In *Languages: From Formal to Natural* (pp. 22–35). Heidelberg: Springer. doi:10.1007/978-3-642-01748-3_2

Axelrod, S. (2000). Natural language generation in the IBM Flight information system. *Proceedings of the 2000 ANLP/NAACL Workshop on Conversational Systems* (Vol. 3, pp. 21-26). Stroudsburg. doi:10.3115/1117562.1117567

Baptist, L. M. (2000). *Genesis II: a language generation module for conversational systems*. Unpublished Master dissertation, MIT, Department of Electronic Engineering, Cambridge.

Brooke, J. (1996). SUS - A quick and dirty usability scale. In P. W. Jordan, B. Thomas, B. A. Weerdmeester, & I. L. McClelland (Eds.), *Usability evaluation in industry* (pp. 189–194). London: Taylor and Francis.

Cabral, M. V., & Silva, P. A. (2010). Adherence to therapy in Portugal: attitude and behaviour of the Portuguese population towards medical prescription. University of Lisbon, Instituto de Ciências Sociais, Lisboa, Portugal.

Cardoso, P., Flores, L., Langlois, T., & Neto, J. (2002). Meteo: a telephone-based Portuguese conversation system in weather domain. *Proceedings of the 3rd International Conference on the Advances in Natural Language Processing*. Springer-Verlag Berlin Heidelberg. doi:10.1007/3-540-45433-0_26

Costa, L., Santos, D., & Cardoso, N. (Eds.). (2008). *Perspectivas sobre a Linguateca*. Aveiro, Portugal: Linguateca.

Dahl, D. A., Coin, E., Greene, M., & Mandelbaum, P. (2011). A conversational personal assistant for senior users. In D. Perez-Marin & I. Pascual-Nieto (Eds.), *Conversational Agents and Natural Language Interaction: Techniques and Effective Practices* (pp. 282–301). Hershey, PA: IGI Global. doi:10.4018/978-1-60960-617-6.ch012

Ewen, S., Baumgarten, T., Rettig-Ewen, V., Mahfoud, F., Griese-Mammen, N., Schulz, M., & Laufs, U. et al. (2015). Analyses of drugs stored at home by elderly patients with chronic heart failure. *Clinical Research in Cardiology; Official Journal of the German Cardiac Society, 104*(4), 320–327. doi:10.1007/s00392-014-0783-2 PMID:25373382

Ferguson, G., Quinn, J., Horwitz, C., Swift, M., Allen, J., & Galescu, L. (2010). Towards a personal health management assistant. *Journal of Biomedical Informatics, 43*(55S), S13–S16. doi:10.1016/j.jbi.2010.05.014 PMID:20937478

Galescu, L., Allen, J., Ferguson, G., Swift, M., & Quinn, J. (2009). Speech recognition in a dialog system for patient health monitoring. *Proceedings of the IEEE International Conference BIBM 2009: Workshop on NLP Approaches for Unmet Information Needs in Health Care*. Washington, DC: IEEE. doi:10.1109/BIBMW.2009.5332111

Galley, M., Fosler-Lussier, E., & Potamianos, A. (2001). Hybrid natural language generation for spoken dialogue systems. *Proceedings of the 7th European Conference on Speech Communication and Technology*. Springer-Verlag Berlin Heidelberg.

Giles, T. D. (2004). New perspectives in the prevention and treatment of chronic heart failure with reduced systolic function. *American Journal of Hypertension, 17*(5S), S249. doi:10.1016/j.amjhyper.2004.03.663

Giorgino, T., Azzin, I., Rognoni, C., Quaglini, S., Stefanell, M., Gretter, R., & Falavigna, D. (2005). Automated spoken dialogue system for hypertensive patient home management. *International Journal of Medical Informatics, 74*(2-4), 159–167. doi:10.1016/j.ijmedinf.2004.04.026 PMID:15694621

Hawig, D. (n. d.). Florence [Software]. Retrieved from https://florence.chat

Hjelmqvist, S. (2012). *Fast, memory efficient Levenshtein algorithm*. Retrieved from www.codeproject.com/Articles/13525/Fast-memory-efficient-Levenshtein-algorithm

Hudson, D. L., & Cohen, M. E. (2010). Intelligent agents in home healthcare. *Annals of telecommunications -. Annales des Télécommunications, 65*(9), 593–600. doi:10.1007/s12243-010-0170-6

Jongh, T. D., Gurol-Urganci, I., Vodopivec-Jamsek, V., Car, J., & Atun, R. (2012). Mobile phone messaging for facilitating self-management of long-term illnesses. *Cochrane Database of Systematic Reviews*, 12. PMID:23235644

Kaushik, P., Intille, S. S., & Larson, K. (2008). Observations from a case study on user adaptive reminders for medication adherence. *Paper presented at Second International Conference on Pervasive Computing Technologies for Healthcare*. doi:10.4108/ICST.PERVASIVEHEALTH2008.2545

Krämer, N. C., Hoffmann, L., & Kopp, S. (2010). Know Your Users! Empirical results for tailoring an agent's nonverbal behavior to different user groups. In J. Allbeck, N. Badler, T. Bickmore, C. Pelachaud, & A. Safonova (Eds.), *Intelligent Virtual Agents,* LNCS (Vol. 6356). Springer Berlin Heidelberg. doi:10.1007/978-3-642-15892-6_50

Mattila, M., Boehm, L., Burke, S., Kashyap, A., Holschbach, L., Miller, T., & Vardeny, O. (2013). Non-prescription Medication Use in Patients with Heart Failure: Assessment Methods, Utilization Patterns, and Discrepancies with Medical Records. *Journal of Cardiac Failure, 19*(12), 811–815. doi:10.1016/j.cardfail.2013.10.009 PMID:24184371

McMurray, J. J., Adamopoulos, S., Anker, S. D., Auricchio, A., Böhm, M., Dickstein, K., & Zeiher, A. et al. (2012). ESC Guidelines for the diagnosis and treatment of acute and chronic heart failure 2012: The Task Force for the Diagnosis and Treatment of Acute and Chronic Heart Failure 2012 of the European Society of Cardiology. *European Heart Journal, 33*(14), 1787–1847. doi:10.1093/eurheartj/ehs104 PMID:22611136

McTear, M., Callejas, Z., & Griol, D. (2016). *The Conversational Interface: Talking to Smart Devices.* Springer. doi:10.1007/978-3-319-32967-3

McTear, M. F. (2002). Spoken dialogue technology: Enabling the conversational user interface. *ACM Computing Surveys, 34*(1), 90–169. doi:10.1145/505282.505285

Mellish, C., & Evans, R. (2004). Implementation architectures for natural language generation. *Natural Language Engineering, 10*(3-4), 261–282. doi:10.1017/S1351324904003511

Mettler, M., & Kemper, D. W. (2002). Information therapy: Health education one person at a time. *Health Promotion Practice, 4*(3), 214–217. doi:10.1177/1524839903004003004 PMID:14610991

Next, I. T. Corporation. (2013). Alme [Software]. Retrieved from http://www.nextithealthcare.com/

Nieuwenhuis, M. M., Jaarsma, T., van Veldhuisen, D. J., & van der Wal, M. H. (2012). Self-reported versus true adherence in heart failure patients: A study using the Medication Event Monitoring System. *Netherlands Heart Journal; Monthly Journal of the Netherlands Society of Cardiology and the Netherlands Heart Foundation, 20*(7-8), 313–319. doi:10.1007/s12471-012-0283-9 PMID:22527915

Paterson, M., Kinnear, M., Bond, C., & McKinstry, B. (2016). A systematic review of electronic multi-compartment medication devices with reminder systems for improving adherence to self-administered medications. *International Journal of Pharmacy Practice,* n/a. doi:10.1111/ijpp.12242 PMID:26833669

Reiter, R., & Dale, R. (1997). Building Applied Natural Language Generation Systems. *Natural Language Engineering, 3*(1), 57–87. doi:10.1017/S1351324997001502

Rojas-Barahona, L. M., Quaglini, S., & Stefanelli, M. (2009). HomeNL: Homecare Assistance in Natural Language. An Intelligent Conversational Agent for Hypertensive Patients Management. *Proceedings of the 12th Conference on Artificial Intelligence in Medicine,* (pp. 245-249). Springer-Verlag. doi:10.1007/978-3-642-02976-9_35

Siek, K. A., Khan, D. U., Ross, S. E., Haverhals, L. M., Meyers, J., & Cali, S. R. (2011). Designing a personal health application for older adults to manage medications: A comprehensive case study. *Journal of Medical Systems*, *35*(5), 1099–1121. doi:10.1007/s10916-011-9719-9 PMID:21562730

Siek, K. A., Ross, S. E., Khan, D. U., Haverhals, L. M., Cali, S. R., & Meyers, J. (2010). Colorado Care Tablet: The design of an interoperable Personal Health Application to help older adults with multimorbidity manage their medications. *Journal of Biomedical Informatics*, *43*(5), S22–S26. doi:10.1016/j.jbi.2010.05.007 PMID:20937480

Stewart, S., & Horowitz, J. D. (2002). Home-based intervention in congestive heart failure: Long-term implications on readmission and survival. *Circulation*, *105*(24), 2861–2866. doi:10.1161/01.CIR.0000019067.99013.67 PMID:12070114

Sullivan, R., Behncke, I., & Purushotham, A. (2010). Why do we love medicines so much? *EMBO Reports*, *11*(8), 572–578. doi:10.1038/embor.2010.108 PMID:20634806

Vervloet, M., Linn, A. J., van Weert, J. C. M., de Bakker, D. H., Bouvy, M. L., & van Dijk, L. (2012). The effectiveness of interventions using electronic reminders to improve adherence to chronic medication: A systematic review of the literature. *Journal of the American Medical Informatics Association*, *19*(5), 696–704. doi:10.1136/amiajnl-2011-000748 PMID:22534082

Wagner, J. C., Rogers, J. E., Baud, R. H., & Scherrer, J. (1999). Natural Language Generation of Surgical Procedures. *International Journal of Medical Informatics*, *53*(2-3), 175–192. doi:10.1016/S1386-5056(98)00158-0 PMID:10193887

Walker, C. M., Elder, B. L., & Hayes, K. S. (2014). The Role of a Self-Directed Technology to Improve Medication Adherence in Heart Failure Patients. *The Journal for Nurse Practitioners*, *10*(10), 856–863. doi:10.1016/j.nurpra.2014.08.011

Wilcox, L., Feiner, S., Liu, A., Restaino, S., Collins, S., & Vawdrey, D. (2012). Designing Inpatient Technology to Meet the Medication Information Needs of Cardiology Patients. *Proceedings of the ACM SIGHIT International Health Informatics Symposium*. New York: ACM. doi:10.1145/2110363.2110466

Ziaeian, B., & Fonarow, G. C. (2016). Epidemiology and aetiology of heart failure. *Nature Reviews. Cardiology*, *13*(6), 368–378. doi:10.1038/nrcardio.2016.25 PMID:26935038

ENDNOTES

[1]   http://developer.android.com/reference/android/speech/package-summary.html
[2]   https://www.ispeech.org/developers/android

This research was previously published in the International Journal of E-Health and Medical Communications (IJEHMC), 8(4) edited by Joel J.P.C. Rodrigues, pages 21-37, copyright year 2017 by IGI Publishing (an imprint of IGI Global).

Chapter 34
A Collaborative M–Health Platform for Evidence–Based Self–Management and Detection of Chronic Multimorbidity Development and Progression

Kostas Giokas
National Technical University of Athens, Greece

Panagiotis Katrakazas
National Technical University of Athens, Greece

Dimitris Koutsouris
National Technical University of Athens, Greece

ABSTRACT

The ageing process of EU population has played a key role raising the prevalence of chronic disease, with more than 80% of people in the last age group (65-74) reported to be having three or more long-term Multimorbidity or Multiple Chronic Conditions (MCCs). The main problem is that currently, clinicians have limited guidance, as well as evidence of how to approach care decisions for such patients. As a consequence, the understanding of how to best take care of patients with multimorbidity conditions, may lead to improvements in Quality of Life (QoL), utilization of healthcare, safety, morbidity and mortality. The root of this problem is not narrowly confined to guidelines development and application, but is inherent throughout the translational path from the generation of evidence to the synthesis of the evidence upon which guidelines depend.

DOI: 10.4018/978-1-5225-3926-1.ch034

INTRODUCTION: OBJECTIVES OF PRESENT RESEARCH

The vision of the proposed research is to develop an *m-health ecosystem*, leading to an evidence-based self-management and detection of chronic *multimorbidity development and progression*, where clinical data will be periodically collected by an *engaged* and *empowered chronic patient* through an extensive on–intrusive use of market available and ad hoc made m-health apps that co-produce additional clinical data. The ecosystem above systematically *interoperates and integrates* into the Electronic Health Records available in the *private cloud environment* of local or national European healthcare organizations. This challenging approach is expected to highly contribute and increase the self-management attitude of the patient, as well as the research conducted on multimorbidity, by supporting clinicians and researchers to understand the clinical course of disease in detail and improve clinical outcomes. Three main layers of Scientific and Technological Objectives represent the load-bearing pillars of the proposed *m-health ecosystem* including *knowledge, applications and services* that will enable more effective and efficient:

1. **Health Promotion:** Improve self-management, patient management and patient-patient/patient-doctor collaboration:
   a. Promote self-management pathways for chronic elderly patients and increase the level of awareness of their health condition.
   b. Create and Test an m-health ecosystem enabled, personalized, patient – centric care model in different European healthcare systems leading up to a step forward in the cross-border harmonization.
   c. Increase the level of patient-patient and patient-doctor interaction by encouraging the patient to have a more active role in changing their behaviour by reaching healthcare goals.
2. **Public Health:** Combine the benefits of self-management with the need of increased research evidence on multimorbidity:
   a. Create additional insights to increase the level of knowledge in the estimation of the occurrence and distribution of multimorbidity.
   b. Contribute to and Support the development of consensus on self - management and care of multimorbidity, engaging it as a subject on expert panels focused on the care of older adults.
   c. Increase the daily evidence of the role of contextual and lifestyle-related factors in the development of multimorbidity.
   d. Aggregate and analyse the informative asset generated by the platform to enrich and better describe the natural history of multimorbidity both on a patient and community level.
3. **Standard, Business Models and Regulations:** Increase the patients and doctor confidence in technology as a foundation to create an holistic care process driven as a patient-centric healthcare system:
   a. Design *innovative care models* supported by an effective combination of disruptive technologies like *cloud, social, mobile* and *analytics*, which are developed in full respect of *patient privacy* and *safety*.
   b. Deploy a set of application and services contributing to the widespread of most relevant standards and protocols for interoperability of personal health systems (e.g. Continua Health Alliance, HL7, IHE, etc.) as well as IEEE based connectivity standards

c.   Contribute to the implementation of the results reached by the Working Party set up under Article 29 of Directive 95/46/EC, dealing with Data Protection Directive applied to the use of apps on smart devices.

BACKGROUND: THE CO-OCCURRENCE OF CHRONIC DISORDERS - MULTIMORBIDITY

The ageing process of EU population has played a key role raising the prevalence of chronic disease, with more than 80% of people in the last age group (65-74) reported having *three or more long-term conditions*. This condition is defined as *Multimorbidity or Multiple Chronic Condition (MCC)*. Multimorbidity is defined as the co-existence of two or more chronic conditions, where one is not necessarily more central than the others. Multimorbidity affects the quality of life, ability to work and employability, disability and mortality. The number of individuals with MCC is expected to increase dramatically in coming years (Anderson & Horvath, 2002). The term *multimorbidity*, captures multiple, potentially interacting, medical and psychiatric conditions, so it may be more appropriate and *more patient-centered* for the older population than considering it from the perspective of a single index condition, which is the traditional approach. The main problem is that currently clinicians have limited guidance or evidence as to how to approach care decisions for such patients (Boyd et al., 2005). As a consequence the *understanding of how to best care patients* with multimorbidity may lead to *improvements in quality of life (QOL), utilization of healthcare, safety, morbidity* and *mortality*. According to a recent study (Wallace & Salive, 2013) the suggestion for these *signs, symptoms, and syndrome*, is to be carefully and systematically addressed, since many never reach the level of a specific diagnosable "disease" with an ICD code; however, they can cause considerable suffering and require extensive health care. With rare exceptions, *nowadays clinical practice guidelines focus on the management of a single disease*, and do not address how to optimally integrate care for individuals whose multiple problems may make guideline-recommended management of any single disease impractical, irrelevant or even harmful. The root of this problem, however, is not narrowly confined to guidelines development and application, but is inherent throughout the translational path from the *generation of the evidence* to the synthesis of the evidence on which the aforementioned guidelines depend on. Recently, the emphasis has been placed on the role of "pragmatic clinical trials" to lead the care of real world populations. It is essential to note that without appropriate *standardized data management and analytic techniques* to account for heterogeneity of treatment effects, the results of such trials may be misleading about whether specific patients benefit more or less from therapies than the average patient. *The generation of evidence is related to the possibility of collecting and analysing data from daily routine care settings including the strong collaboration of the patient themselves that, if duly empowered to self-management, can maximize the synergies with the healthcare actors.* Multimorbidity deals with complex clinical manifestations of conditions, such as *signs* (visually observable patient abnormalities), *symptoms* (abnormal perceptions of illness that only patients can report, such as pain, itching, fatigue, depressive feelings), and *syndromes* (clusters of signs, symptoms, and other clinical phenomena that may or may not be indicative of a specific underlying disease).

MAIN FOCUS OF THE CHAPTER (STATE OF THE ART)

Issues, Controversies, Problems: Proposed Concept

Disease management is a *healthcare model* that could help physicians, patients and managed care organizations to improve outcomes and control costs through coordinated and proactive interventions.

To effectively implement this model, a trans-disciplinary approach is needed posing inevitable challenges for complex healthcare systems.

There are several core issues that disease management professionals deal with: *engaging patients* in their health management, *handling multiple* and *coexisting* chronic disease states, *supporting physician decision-making*, and *using data and decision making supporting technologies* to early identify and propose appropriate interventions. All of these aforementioned issues, if well implanted, need to lead to a more efficient utilization of resources and, eventually, cost savings.

Recently some Disease-Management Programmes (DMPs) have produced better results than in the past according to a study made by McKinsey (Brandt, Hartmann, & Hehner, 2010). The study analysed a wide range of DMPs from countries around the world to determine the characteristics that differentiate successful and unsuccessful programs. Five traits seemed to be the most important in ensuring that DMPs meet their goals: *program size, simplicity of design, a focus on patients' needs, the ability to collect data easily and analyse results* (Brandt et al., 2010), and the *presence of incentives* that encourage all stakeholders to comply with the program.

Out of the five characteristics that can help ensure that a disease-management program achieves its clinical and financial goals, the proposed research concept aims at contributing to:

- **Patient Focus:** The interventions they include apply to the vast majority of enrolled patients, as well as simple and straightforward to implement. In line with the Self-management technology support proposed in our research, the patients are given ongoing, disease-specific coaching and resources to access the most relevant information to maximize their ability to care for themselves.

- **Information Transparency:** Many early DMPs did not have good mechanisms to prove their effectiveness because they did not have systems in place to monitor what patients were doing and what results were being achieved. In some cases, there were no clearly defined measures to gauge the programs' success and no established methods for data collection (Brandt et al., 2010). Starting from these assumptions, the four factors connected in the disease management process envisaged to be supported by the proposed technology are listed below and inherited by the successful DMPs mentioned before. All the four factors will be taken into consideration in the absence of any one of them can reduce the likelihood of achieving an optimal outcome.

Factor 1: The monitoring must be timely conducted on a regular basis,

Factor 2: The monitoring must be comprehensive covering all necessary (disease and patient specific) vital signs and symptoms,

Factor 3: The data must be shared appropriately with the care team,

Factor 4: The data must be meaningful and actionable for the patient or the relatives in case of cognitive impairment or dementia present in the subject.

Involving patients actively in their care is critical for controlling disease management costs associated with monitoring and assessment. Encouraging and supporting patients to become more engaged in their healthcare will simultaneously encourage and support the goals of disease management (Intel Health, 2007). In this approach to healthcare, the more a patient becomes an equal partner in his or her care team, the more efficiently and effectively programs are likely to run.

The following set of proposed *enabling services* is expected to highly impact the routine care management of chronic patients by supporting clinicians and researchers to better understanding the underlying mechanisms of multimorbidity:

A Patient-Specific Content Management Suite (PS-CMS) available for healthcare operators in charge for the management of primary chronic condition, to "drag and drop" specific services and generate zero-code mobile apps to be "prescribed to the patient. These apps are needed to collect specific data from patients and complete the possible lack of information retrieved from the Data Management and Orchestration Service (DMOS). The list of services will include interoperability modules based on the widely used IEEE 11073 Health information protocol[1] to easily connect the set of point of care sensors (e.g. Continua Alliance[2]), as these are defined by the doctor and may also be needed to complement information related to the patient, to the mobile devices.

A set of personalized content management technologies and services based on intelligent tools and techniques, able to provide functionality for assessing relevance and reliability of web content. These will offer personalised, intelligent interventions (e.g. prompts, recommendations, remarks) to promote the self-engagement of patients. They will also compare and estimate how new, surprising and valuable different associations in the form of similarity and analogy may be in a particular context to increase the effectiveness of recommendations. Finally, they will offer personalised search and exploration for the users to focus on the aspects most relevant to their condition.

A Data Management and Orchestration Service (DMOS) founded on the hybrid cloud paradigm, able to manage the enormous variety of structured and unstructured data available for the same subject and collected from disparate data sources, e.g. the m-health ecosystem interacting with the EHRs/PHRs. The DMOS will act as a single point of truth to manage unstructured data (collected from m-health apps) available on a local level in the smartphone or public cloud (e.g. back end of the Health APP provider), as well as more structured data from private clouds of healthcare data sources (such as patient information managed and stored in local, regional or national private clouds where EHRs are accessible by the network of healthcare providers). Instead of duplicating mobile apps already existing in the market and generating highly relevant data such as BMI calculators, calories counter, diet and food tracker, insulin calculators, the DMOS will tie the data generated by a meaningful healthcare driven process aimed at transforming those data into valuable information. Issues related to *privacy, security and health information communication* related to safety and quality of data generated through mobile applications, will contribute to the progress in establishing regulations and definitions of standards, as expected by the European Commission's eHealth Action Plan 2012 – 2020.

A HL7 categorization system, included in the hybrid cloud-based DMOS environment, able to clean, normalize and translate data collected from mobile applications in HL7 format with the purpose of producing standardized and comparable data regardless the source of data generation (e.g. regardless if produced in a structured healthcare IT environment or in daily life environment such as home settings, and collected by mobile applications).

Detailed *analysis* and *predictive models* running in the *hybrid cloud analytics tools*, able to create *common clusters of primary chronic conditions* associated with *physiological parameters, lifestyle as well as social determinants and their interactions* to *early* recognise *signs, syndromes and symptoms leading to a possible* arise of secondary chronic diseases before multimorbidity.

The proposed model is addressing different type of healthcare actors interested in analysing and connecting clinical and patient information across varied settings and time periods to generate longitudinal and comprehensive views of patient care, identify unknown risk factors combination affecting the generation of multimorbidity, or aggregating data for epidemiological and public health use.

SOLUTIONS AND RECOMMENDATIONS: APPROACH AND METHODOLOGY

The proposed research will follow an iterative, collaborative and cooperative approach at a very early stage. From a technological development perspective, the design and development methodology will be focused on the core of the system, the patient. The methodology, called *Mixed Methodology* in literature (Daraghmi, Cullen, & Goh, 2008), will be based on a co-design principle including *Participatory Design* (Schuler & Namioka, 1993), *User Centred Design* (Noyes & Baber, 2012) to develop a usable interface and to develop a reliable and acceptable system by eliciting users participation in the design phase, integrated with *Rapid Application Development* (Beynon-Davies & Holmes, 1998; Guelfi & Savidis, 2006) for early deployment. This type of methodology includes *usability engineering* approaches to evaluate the new system by validating each development stage against old and emergent requirements. The implemented methodology will consist of three stages with each stage iteratively performed. It will also follow a new generation of Participatory Design based on three modules (Third Generation of Participatory Design, 3GPD (Pilemalm & Timpka, 2008)). The *first module* covers the pre-design stage when the project plan, schedules, and contacts with stakeholders are set up. The *second module* represents requirements analyses, design and prototyping stages. Finally, the *third module* is the post-design stage including full implementation and completion of requirements' specifications. The new generation of 3GPD is resource-effective, can be integrated with other methods such as rapid methods, and provides full documentation (Pilemalm & Timpka, 2008). From a Health Research perspective, the availability of *large databases in UNIPG (Università degli Studi di Perugia³) and ARC (Aging Research Center⁴)*, which are based on a national sample of 60+ old adults and include information on medical, social and psychological states (cross-sectional assessment) and events (follow-up assessments), allows the proposed research to carry out a retrospective study whose results will be implemented in the knowledge management system (DSS and predictive models), following these steps:

1. Development of a Health Index which can summarise the health status of older adults and trace the time-related changes: medical as well as functional aspects will be integrated. This index will characterise the subjects with multimorbidity and trace their progression to unfavourable health outcomes.
2. Validation of the index in other populations as a predictive tool for health changes from the complete absence of disease and functional impairment to the development of chronic multimorbidity and disability.
3. Identification of the biological and medical factors that lead to a higher risk of developing multimorbidity and consequent disability.
4. Identification of the social and environmental factors that can modulate the onset and progression of chronic multimorbidity.

Once the platform is developed and integrated, a *small-scale clinical trial* will be set-up in (possibly three) different and appropriate pilot sites, whose main objectives will be:

1. The development and validation of a Health Index to be used as a predictive tool for health changes,
2. The characterisation of the target users enrolled for the trial and risk stratification,
3. The design of personalised interventional program models for patients living in senior houses,
4. The monitoring of the *patients (half acting as a test group with apps and sensors; half as a control group without them)* living in their own homes, with particular attention to those with higher level of multimorbidity severity, and the regular updating of the model according to newly collected data,
5. The verification of the proposed system's effectiveness, stability and reliability as a tool to empower patients in self-management through validation and comparison tests,
6. The refinement of the developed solutions, applications and approaches on the basis of the research findings, and finally
7. The evaluation of clinical and non-clinical outcomes.

CLINICAL PROTOCOL

The clinical protocol included in the pilot study is devoted to the *validation* of the proposed methodology in young-old subjects (age 65-75 years) suffering from two or more of the following index diseases (hypertension, diabetes, monitoring, heart failure, arthritis, impairment in cognitive functions) and with a score <3 in all the 14 CIRS-G (Cumulative Illness Rating Scale-Geriatric) items.

The index of chronic diseases were chosen according to the epidemiological data on prevalence of chronic conditions in European's old age population (Busse, 2010), showing the most prevalent ones as considered in the study. We excluded cancer to have a more homogeneous population with a low risk of mortality during the study. The number of almost two or more chronic diseases to define multimorbidity was decided on the basis of the main epidemiological studies recently reviewed by Marengoni et al. (Alessandra Marengoni, Winblad, Karp, & Fratiglioni, 2008).

The CIRS scale was chosen because of its quite simple use, validation in geriatric population and guidelines for scoring. Briefly, the CIRS rates 14, conceptually valid, body systems (supporting content validity) on a five-point (pathophysiologic) severity scale. It has been slightly adapted to form the CIRS-G (CIRS-Geriatric), for which guidelines to enhance reliability have been formulated (Miller et al., 1992). The severity of each category ranges from 0 to 4 according to the following level of severity:

0. No Problem,
1. Current mild problem or past significant problem,
2. Moderate disability or morbidity / requires "first line" therapy,
3. Severe /constant significant disability / "uncontrollable" chronic problems,
4. Extremely Severe / immediate treatment required / end organ failure / severe impairment in function.

To have a study population with comorbidity not too severe to preclude the use of ICT technologies, we will include in the pilot study subjects with a score *<3 in all CIRS-G categories.*

PRINCIPLES OF PROPOSED SOLUTION

We believe that the combination of:

1. Appropriate *self-management* and *patient empowerment strategies* supported by
2. The extensive use of *knowledge management systems*, which provide data management and data analytics capabilities, and
3. *Mobile apps* for continuous, non-intrusive daily life patient monitoring information collection,

can be seen as an innovative type of clinical support system for the identification of multimorbidity related early signs and symptoms.

The proposed m-*health ecosystem* is built employing the "Hub and Spoke" paradigm at any level, from organizational to technological perspective. The model is named after a bicycle wheel, which has a strong central hub with a series of connecting spokes (see Figure 1). In the sense of a Hub and Spoke model applied to the healthcare system the patient, the carers and local communities are central to the model (the HUB). In the Hub, patients and carers are expected to be involved in decision-making about their care, whereas community members are also expected to be involved in planning services to meet their needs. In our proposed solution *the patient is the "focus" of the HUB* and, thanks to the creation

Figure 1. Hub and Spoke Model

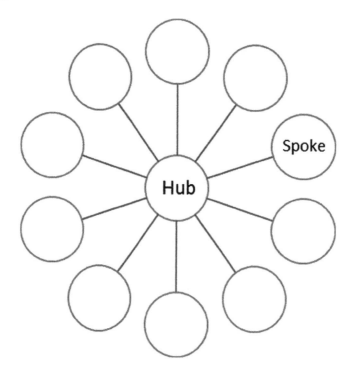

of the m-health based ecosystem around the patient, the objective is to contribute and move from the traditional *physician – centered model to a patient centred model.*

If the patient is the focus of the Hub, the Spokes are the different *levels of care and organisations* available in every European country, varying according to the national organizational models[5]. In a healthcare system, all the Spokes surrounding the Hub contribute to record and generate information relevant to the patient's care and manage it through informative infrastructures such as Electronic Medical Records (EMRs), Electronic Health Record (EHRs) and Personal Health Records (PHRs). *In the proposed research, we envision the access to accurate, relevant and comprehensive information that is essential to enable patients and carers to make informed decisions about healthcare treatment.* Based on the International Alliance of Patients' Organizations (IAPO) policy, one of the *Five Principles* needed to achieve a patient –cantered healthcare system in actually related to the *information.*, "Information must be presented in an appropriate format according to health literacy principles, considering the individual condition, language, age,, understanding, abilities and culture"(Groves, 2010).

This is the reason why, out of the three most widespread Health Record systems mentioned above, whose adoption varies considerably among various EU countries[6], the more relevant to be considered as complementary to the *proposed m-health ecosystem* are the Electronic Health Records (EHRs) and the Personalized Health Records (PHRs). This choice is due to the fact that, in contrast to Electronic Medical Records (EMRs) (Garrett & Seidman, 2011; Pawola, 2011), *EHRs* are built to go beyond standard clinical data collected in a provider's office and are inclusive of a *broader view of a patient's care.* EHRs obtain information from/to *all the authorized actors* involved in a patient's care. EHRs also share information with other health care providers, such as laboratories and specialists. EHRs follow patients – to the specialist, the hospital, the nursing home, or even across the country. The *PHRs* contain the same types of information as EHRs—diagnoses, (initial) set up and access, medications, immunizations, family medical histories, and provider contact information—but are designed to be managed by patients. Patients can use PHRs to maintain and manage their health information in a *private, secure, and confidential environment.* PHRs can include information from a variety of sources including clinicians, home monitoring devices, and patients themselves. (HealthIT.gov, 2015) Attaining *patient engagement* for *Self-Management* starts from an information based process where the patient can understand the importance of *self-tracking his/her chronic condition management routines* by the use of mobile devices and *generate additional information to be integrated with EHR and PHR informative systems.*

Self-tracking with a smart phone or tablet is the best option available nowadays. However, engagement does not end with tracking. In addition to simply following these routines, patients need to *understand the long-term requirements* of self-managing their health. For this purpose, clinicians connect to their patients via a patient-clinician-patient communications loop through "Facebook type" posts in the patient personalized app (Giokas, Iliopoulou, Makris, & Koutsouris, 2015; Giokas, Tsirmpas, Anastasiou, Costarides, & Koutsouris, 2015; Koutsouris et al., 2014). Clinicians can provide patient specific targeted information, which helps keeping health at the top of patients' minds. In our proposed solution, a dashboard called Patient-Specific Content Management Suite has been envisaged (see *proposed concept*). One important functional feature of the dashboard will be the possibility of setting up health engaging messages from the clinician, which will be dispatched according to the evolving patient's profile, as the last is tracked by the back end system level, which deals with progressive data insights and analysis. Feedback loops "work incredibly well to establish the awareness needed to change a person's mindset about health." (Kinsella, 2012) Nevertheless, patients often develop a malaise toward performing self-management routines and reporting findings. Psychologists call it "habituation: once people get used to something, they tend to get bored with it and move onto something else." (Cherry, n.d.) Hence, a challenge presented is as to how we keep people maximally engaged and responsive to their health condition and information regarding it. Since there is no one way to correct this digression, Dr. Kvedar (Founder and Director of the Centre for Connected Health in Boston) suggests developing *customized, contextual relevant and targeted information and goals for each patient* in order to maintain engagement or re-engage disconnected patients (Kinsella, 2012). Innovative Patient Portal 2.0, is expected to have the form of *integrated platforms* that provide, among other things, *"engaging and interactive content that is customized to (patients) based on age, gender, etc., social networking interactions that support patient-to-patient connections and mobile health applications"*. (Caressi, 2014) This innovation will involve changing not only the IT tools healthcare organizations leverage in engagement, but also the culture within *healthcare organizations to be more patient centric*. In addition to the *Self – Management and patient engagement* strategy to be implemented, *our proposed solution intends to approach multimorbidity from different perspectives* (*epidemiological, clinical and care science perspectives*) combined into a new and effective *m-health ecosystem* for professional use where *empowered patients actively contribute to the generation of the evidence* regarding clinical manifestations of conditions additional to the evidence recorded by formal and informal carers.

POSSIBILITY TO IMPLEMENT A PLATFORM FOR MULTIMORBIDITY

The proposed implementation of the platform modules will be based on the current knowledge on multimorbidity produced in the literature reviews ((Alessandra Marengoni et al., 2008; Meinow, 2008)), in which the operational definition of multimorbidity is reported.

Multimorbidity has been addressed from three perspectives, which have led to three major operational definitions:

1. **The number (commonly two or three) of concurrent longstanding diseases in the same individual:** This definition, which has been used mostly in epidemiological studies, includes both individuals who may live relatively unaffected by multimorbidity with the help of medications as well as those who face severe functional loss;
2. **The cumulative indices evaluating both number and severity of the concurrent diseases**: This definition is very suitable for clinical studies where the major aim is to identify persons who are at risk for negative health outcomes and who might benefit from specific interventions;
3. **The number of diseases, functional limitations and care utilisation:** In order to estimate the need for medical care and social assistance, health care studies take into account not only the cumulative effect of concurrent diseases, but also relevant factors such as symptoms, cognitive and physical dysfunctions, and psychosocial problems.

Given the complexity and heterogeneity of the health status of the elderly and the age-related pathologies, no single operational criterion will serve all research and clinical purposes effectively. "The common denominator of all the definitions is given by the concurrence of several chronic diseases whose severity can be graded or not with different methods" (*Handbook of Clinical Gender Medicine*, 2012). The above mentioned operational definitions will be the drivers for:

- The selection of the *target individual*, who is more suitable for the use of proposed ecosystem that will affect, in perspective,
- The *business model* stemming from this research,
- The selection of *parameters and the workflows* to be monitored by the ecosystem,
- The impacted *healthcare processes*, and finally
- The "spokes" impacted by the information collected through the ecosystem.

USE AND ADVANTAGES OF A HUB FOR MULTIMORBIDITY

The use of the m-health application for non-intrusive daily or periodical data collection is expected to provide a fundamental support for the monitoring of items and protocols that are used for the follow-up data collection, but this information concerns only the follow-up period in association with clinical information available in the EHRs/PHRs (Koutsouris et al., 2014). Traditionally, the follow-up monitoring protocol is based on informant interviews, clinical examinations, and testing by trained staff. The use of the proposed m-health tracking system is expected to ease the data collection process and help in increasing the amount of information (in the long term even replace) collected nowadays via patient-doctor interviews and self-administered questionnaires regarding social networking, leisure activities, nutritional assessment and health-related life quality assessment, info available in brief self-administered test or telephone-based test (performed by a trained nurse, psychologist or doctor) able to screen mild alterations in cognition; self-administered or nurse interview assessing demographic data, living arrangements, education, occupational history, current and past socioeconomic status, life habits, physical functioning, use of medical and social facilities, and formal and informal care received and provided. Many protocol items and clinical information can be collected by the engaged patient via the use of low cost or "prescribed apps", specifically addressing patient chronic conditions to be monitored or by exploiting a combination of apps already available in the app stores (see Figure 2).

All these apps can either be available for the patient's smartphone, because he/she decided to use it or can be "prescribed" by the clinician. Depending on the age and level of chronic condition, patients are persons who download health apps, buy wireless scales, buy activity trackers, collect and use that data to better improve their general health outcomes, or outcomes specific to the disease they have. Alternatively, apps can be prescribed by a clinician. According to a recent survey from health communications firm Digitas Health[7], almost 90% of chronic patients in the US would accept a mobile app prescription from their physician, as opposed to only 66% willing to accept a prescription for medication (Digitas Health, 2012). Intensive use of mobile apps lead patients to keep track of important health statistics, like blood pressure, weight and heart rate, progress during workouts, and might be of particular use when a

Figure 2. Examples of m-apps already available of health related data collection processes

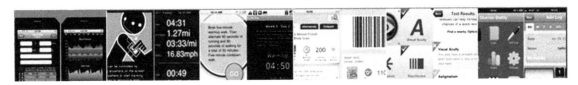

patient undergoes physical therapy; several eye tests can be performed on a smartphone to determine if a trip to the optician is needed; diabetes management applications that work on smart phones, act as a utility for diabetics to store a range of health statistics, etc. For this purpose, the proposed ecosystem is conceived to allow the clinician to manage a kind of "Patient-specific app prescription platform". The healthcare provider will be able to select from a specific dashboard, a set of apps to be prescribed to the specific patient with at least two options:

1.   Being able to select, in agreement with the patient, the apps already available in the market and prescribe it.
2.   Generating ad hoc apps trough "dragging and dropping" specific services and list of parameters needed specifically for that patient.

MAJOR CHALLENGES

Two are the major technological challenges to be addressed in order to offer those above two relevant options to the care provider.

The first challenge is to provide the opportunity to the doctor to *retrieve clinical related personal information* produced by the use of the apps available on the market. Technical, privacy and security issues will have to be addressed for this purpose. Although there are a subset of apps with impressive functionality (e.g. electrocardiogram (ECG) readers, blood pressure monitors, blood glucose monitors) it is clear that most of the healthcare apps available today are "only simple in design and do little more than provide information" (McNeill, 2015). This is stressed also in an assessment of multi-functionality: "although two-thirds of healthcare apps can display information, only half of these can also provide instructions, and only one-fifth could track or capture user entered data" (Aitken, 2013). We consider the personal data generated by the user/patient/citizen as his/her property and not app producer property. Starting from this assumption, in our proposed research we will deal with a new method of managing the personal data accessibility and management through a *privacy driven app data management architecture*.

The second challenge is for the platform to be able to offer the best and simplest user experience for the care provider. A *co-design approach* between *ICT partners, clinical partners* and *a selection of patients* (e.g. through focus groups), will be crucial to guarantee the best usability experience for the care provider and the patient. Health apps lack engagement because the people who design them are not usually part of the audience those applications are aimed at. This is usually addressed by the co-designing aspect. The care provider will be able to *generate ad hoc apps* by selecting not only the set of parameters to be manually entered by the patient themselves but also the set of design guidelines and industry standards of Continua Health Alliance[8] applied to the sensors and devices, APIs and related services to be included in the app, in case the patient and care provider agree about the need for an automated vital sign monitoring device. It is important to underline that the versatile possibility offered by the platform for data collection, manual or automated, can guarantee a better cost-effectiveness for the patient and his/her spending capacity without affecting the possibility of data collection during the patient's daily routine.

Last but not least, the area of disruptive *knowledge management* will be addressed by the proposed eco-system. Due to the high number of "spokes" surrounding the "hub", highly important variables considering the different EU healthcare models, as well as specific healthcare processes' variability, must be addressed in a flexible way by the proposed platform. Data and processes flow around the patient will have to be appropriately managed in order to involve both distributed systems and distributed healthcare operators, invoked at the right time and for the right amount of information needed. These challenges will be addressed by the so-called Knowledge Management System.

The knowledge management system will provide the "bridge" between the m-health ecosystem and the Electronic and Patient Health Records context. It is important to notice that *sharing* and *compiling* personal health data with multiple healthcare providers in a *patient-centric approach* is an additional and fundamental step that creates context and finally leads to improved patient adherence and engagement. The co-designing approach will be also exploited, to understand the patients' requirements in terms of attractive contents, needed to keep the "fidelity" of the patients with the described environment. A semantic search engine able to retrieve patient specific engaging contents is included in this research. Finally, the implementation and the business model expected to be created through the m-health ecosystem enabled by the proposed solution, will contribute in boosting the modernization of health services and the penetration of EHRs and PHRs at a European level. It is important to notice that EHRs and PHRs are part of all European national governments' intention to modernise and revitalise the health services. However, EHR adoption varies considerably in Europe. The Nordic countries have been using the technology for more than ten years, but adoption in the U.K., Germany, France and Spain is "on course". This will allow the release of a combined portal for professionals and patients, giving them *secure and smooth* access to health information.

FUTURE CHALLENGES: AMBITION

The Clinical Knowledge Perspective

Human health is a dynamic and multidimensional status, and this is especially evident in aging when health changes occur more frequently and at an increased rate. Studies on health in the elderly have mostly focused on defining a "dream scenario" of healthy aging rather than on constructing a practical definition based on objective and subjective measures of health. The health of a person can be defined from several perspectives: *absence or presence of diseases* (morbidity, often described in terms of medical diagnoses); *capability to perform daily activities* (physical and cognitive functioning including a range of alterations from simple impairment to disability); and *subjective perception of own health*. Until now most of the literature has taken into account only singular dimensions (Alessandra Marengoni et al., 2011). The relevance of disability rather than morbidity has already been reported by Marengoni et al. (A Marengoni, von Strauss, Rizzuto, Winblad, & Fratiglioni, 2009). In addition, physical function, as measured through tests of balance, walking speed, grip strength, and chair stands, at midlife or later, is a good predictor of survival (Cooper, Kuh, & Hardy, 2010). Decline in physical function after the age of 65 years old, is also a predictor of late-life disability (Hirsch, Buzková, Robbins, Patel, & Newman, 2012).

In our research, we intend to use a more holistic approach to health assessment, by using the model for health and health changes in older adulthood as described in Figure 3, where the diagonal line represents the time dimension starting at any age from a healthy status (no dysfunction and no morbidity) up to a terminal phase.

Figure 3. Health as a continuum process in aging

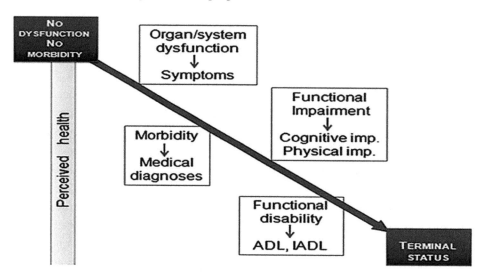

The primary objectives of this research are to address two research questions:

1.   How can we measure the health status of older adults in a more comprehensive way?
2.   What are the chains of events that culminate in the development of poor health in the elderly?

Specifically, we aim to:

- *Create a summary index* to define current health status based on physical and cognitive functionality, morbidity, and disability: *Aging Health Index (AHI)*. This summary score, combining many dimensions of health into a singular description, will allow comparison in and between populations, comparison between different time periods, and in the same individual at different phases of the adult life.
- *Describe the health status of older adults* using the AHI across different age groups and genders, and about self-reported general health status by the use of the m-health ecosystem.
- *Trace the chains of events leading to poor health*, as well as any functional dependence, using the AHI.
- *Relate the AHI to work capacity and engagement in society.*

THE M-HEALTH ENABLED SELF-MANAGEMENT APPROACH

The self-management model aims to empower the person to be a more active participant in their care. Support for people to self-manage may be available from local resources and services, community and voluntary groups, schools and national organisations. However, people may need help to access this support. Self-management support should be tailored to the needs of local communities, particularly the needs of individuals and communities who traditionally find it harder to engage with services. The internet is now a major source of health information where people who look at consumer-created web content, change their behaviour afterwards. In the Healthcare sector, patients look at such a resource to discuss their condition and medication and to see how others are coping.

The world of *e-patients* is developing in recent years, as well as the number of e-patients is rapidly growing (Rainie, 2012). In the running FP7 funded project Empower a survey made on patients with chronic diseases (diabetes type 2 patients), there is evidence of an increased need of sense-making in diabetes care. *Empowering patients can be powerful agents initiating a change in the way healthcare is delivered, and medicine is practiced.* E-Patients are empowered patients that use technology to obtain additional information and be prepared when they meet with their healthcare provider. E-Patients want to *share medical decisions* with their healthcare provider, *want to access their EHR,* request a *second opinion* when facing major decisions and *use digital technologies for accessing health information.* This is the new healthcare trend of "Medicine 2.0" (Van De Belt, Engelen, Berben, & Schoonhoven, 2010) where applications, services, and tools, in particular Web-based services for health care are used by consumers, caregivers, patients, health professionals, and biomedical researchers, through *Web 2.0 technologies* (e.g. web and m-Health apps) and *Web 3.0 technologies* (semantic web approaches) to enable and facilitate specifically:

1. Social networking,
2. Participation,
3. Apomediation,
4. Openness,
5. Collaboration,

within and between these user groups.

Where health care consumers independently decide about subsequent disclosure of health data represent a disruptive innovation that inverts the current approach to medical records in that they are created by and reside with patients who grant permission for their use to institutions, clinicians, researchers, public health agencies, and other users of medical information. (Mandl & Kohane, 2008)

The consequence of patient empowerment strategy also leads to a gravity shift away from health care providers as the sole custodians of medical data. This approach opens up a series of opportunities and risks that must be carefully managed from different dimensions (privacy, technology, clinical, psychological, organizational etc.), as the multidisciplinary based strategy we propose does. The medical professionals need to know how patients use online and mobile technologies and how they use it in their decision-making, to make them equal partners in the care system. Patients who use internet without strategy or the required skills and take all the search results they find to their doctors are referred as *Googlers or cybercondriacs*[9] while patients using the internet with strategy and asking the opinion of the medical professionals about the content they find online can be considered as *equal partners.* There are pieces of information available online, but it is an expert's responsibility and duty to find out what the patient should ignore.

In order to support the healthcare provider in this critical and time consuming task, the proposed research envisages the development of an ambitious *personalised content management search engine* that will be able to provide an *innovative and engaging experience for the patient,* namely the possibility to have access to his/her specific chronic disease in clinically-validated communities of discussion, videos and blogs widespread in the web, based on validation rules developed in the project. Starting from a patient profile categorization and chronic disease evolution, the personalized content management search engine should be able to learn about the evolution patterns and start searching for the more suitable profile-matched social media, as well as other attractive contents, with the final objective of involving the patient in becoming more empowered and collaborative with the doctor and other patients interested in sharing experiences. The expected ambition will be built on a wide architecture, which aims at orchestrating multiple complementary competencies in different areas such as:

- **Mobile Health experts and clinical experts**: To create an m-health ecosystem that implements the APP prescription and patient specific ad hoc composition as an enabling technological support to self-management.
- **Experts in interoperability, mobile health, privacy and security**: To aggregate structured and unstructured patient information (m-health data) in the knowledge base, respecting the privacy and security standards for health data treatment, and use this *new knowledge and data type* as the main informative channel among the patient and multiple healthcare providers.
- **Experts in knowledge management computer science approaches and researchers on multi-morbidity**: To exploit the knowledge base to create a clinically validated decision support system for multimorbidity evolution patterns detection and prediction.
- **Experts in knowledge management computer science approaches and clinical professionals**: To specialize in *self-management* by developing innovative patient engagement approaches and facilitating patient-patient and patient-doctor interactions.

EXPECTED IMPACTS (FUTURE RESEARCH DIRECTIONS)

As discussed in the previous section, we aim at developing an m-health solution that will engage the patients in control and preventive care actions, so as to help reducing comorbidities. The proposed research intends to meet the needs of practicing clinicians which struggle with the uncertainness of applying disease-specific guidelines to older adults with multiple conditions of diseases, by engaging patients in collecting more frequent information on the symptoms of their diseases and the related treatments (Fried, Tinetti, & Iannone, 2011). This new approach in caring comorbidities will imply secondary prevention and treatments of the pathologies. It will see to patients being more involved in the health care decision making process and allow General Practitioners (GP) and health care specialists to interact with the bases of innovative organizational models that could imply a more outcome oriented reimbursement schemas (Bjornland, Goh, Haanæs, Kainu, & Kennedy, 2012). The implementation of such a solution should help in overcoming several barriers in the diagnosis and treatment of comorbidities, including the lack of outcome data, the role of primary and secondary care, the patients' and families' expectations, the lack of specific health care organizational models that address the multi-morbidity issues and the lack of incentive schemas for the health care professionals more in line with their activities of prevention, diagnosis and treatments of multi-morbidity (A.T. Kearney, 2012; WHO, 2011).

CONCLUSION

In conclusion, the proposed research aims to achieve several goals, which are hereby presented:

Self-management of multimorbidity of the pilots' trials participants is expected to be improved, accompanied with an increase in self-determination in multimorbidity risk prevention and treatment, while using the proposed solution.

The proposed solution will allow an increased involvement in self-management of health status, prevention of risk behaviours and self-monitoring of health parameters with the use of m-health apps. Thus, it will lead to an improvement or maintenance of multimorbidity index, as the latter is measured by CIRS-G and an increase of QoL, as it is assessed by the SF-36 scale.

Self-efficacy regarding patients with multimorbidity is also expected to be increased, in contrast to the number and costs of visits into outpatient consultation, treatments and hospitalization/re-hospitalization at the emergency departments, which are expected to be reduced.

The introduction of *Innovative self-care management pathways for multimorbidity*, based on an effective combination of disruptive technologies like *cloud, social, mobile* and *analytics* developed in full respect of patient privacy and safety will lead to an increased efficacy of *multimorbidity predictive models* for single patients, as well as for the target population. The number of identified cause-effect relationships between health-related behavior produced by the proposed solution is expected to increase, and the health condition of patients with multimorbidity is expected to be improved.

Introducing a *new behavioral model*, which shows the efficacy of the platform functionalities in producing behavioral changes for patients with multimorbidity, as well as a *health ecosystem* that enables a personalised patient-centric care model which leads to an increased cross-border harmonization of health care practices, will lead to an *innovative and sustainable business model* for multimorbidity prevention and treatments, and an *innovative solution* for multimorbidity health policy preventive campaigns management.

REFERENCES

Aitken, M. (2013). *Patient Apps for Improved Healthcare: From Novelty to Mainstream*. Retrieved June 18, 2015, from http://www.imshealth.com/deployedfiles/imshealth/Global/Content/Corporate/IMS Health Institute/Reports/Patient_Apps/IIHI_Patient_Apps_Report.pdf

Anderson, G., & Horvath, J. (2002). *Chronic Conditions: Making the Case for Ongoing Care*. Retrieved June 18, 2015, from http://www.partnershipforsolutions.org/DMS/files/chronicbook2002.pdf

Beynon-Davies, P., & Holmes, S. (1998). Integrating rapid application development and participatory design. *IEE Proceedings. Software*, *145*(4), 105. doi:10.1049/ip-sen:19982196

Bjornland, D., Goh, E., Haanæs, K., Kainu, T., & Kennedy, S. (2012). *The Socio-Economic Impact of Mobile Health*. Retrieved June 20, 2015, from http://www.telenor.com/wp-content/uploads/2012/05/BCG-Telenor-Mobile-Health-Report-May-20121.pdf

Boyd, C. M., Darer, J., Boult, C., Fried, L. P., Boult, L., & Wu, A. W. (2005). Clinical practice guidelines and quality of care for older patients with multiple comorbid diseases: Implications for pay for performance. *Journal of the American Medical Association*, *294*(6), 716–724. doi:10.1001/jama.294.6.716 PMID:16091574

Brandt, S., Hartmann, J., & Hehner, S. (2010). *How to design a successful disease-management program*. Retrieved June 19, 2015, from http://www.mckinsey.com/insights/health_systems_and_services/how_to_design_a_successful_disease-management_program

Busse, R. (2010). *Tackling chronic disease in Europe: strategies, interventions and challenges*. World Health Organization, on behalf of the European Observatory on Health Systems and Policies.

Caressi, G. (2014). Will Healthcare Clear the Engagement Hurdle? *Forbes*. Retrieved June 18, 2015, from http://www.forbes.com/sites/gregcaressi/2014/02/19/will-healthcare-clear-the-engagement-hurdle/

Cherry, K. (n.d.). *What Is Habituation? Review Your Psychology Terms*. Retrieved June 18, 2015, from http://psychology.about.com/od/hindex/g/def_habituation.htm

Cooper, R., Kuh, D., & Hardy, R.Mortality Review Group. (2010). Objectively measured physical capability levels and mortality: Systematic review and meta-analysis. *BMJ (Clinical Research Ed.)*, *341*(1), c4467. doi:10.1136/bmj.c4467 PMID:20829298

Daraghmi, Y.-A., Cullen, R., & Goh, T. (2008). Mixed Methodology Design for Improving Usability of e-Health systems. In *Proceedings of Health Informatics New Zealand*. HINZ.

Digitas Health. (2012). *The m.Book 2012 Edition, The Healthcare Marketer's Guide to Going Mobile*. Digitas Health.

Fried, T. R., Tinetti, M. E., & Iannone, L. (2011). Primary care clinicians' experiences with treatment decision making for older persons with multiple conditions. *Archives of Internal Medicine*, *171*(1), 75–80. doi:10.1001/archinternmed.2010.318 PMID:20837819

Garrett, P., & Seidman, J. (2011). EMR vs EHR – What is the Difference? *Health IT Buzz*. Retrieved June 18, 2015, from http://www.healthit.gov/buzz-blog/electronic-health-and-medical-records/emr-vs-ehr-difference/

Giokas, K., Iliopoulou, D., Makris, Y., & Koutsouris, D. (2015). Integrated system for continuous monitoring of COPD. In Handbook of Research on Trends in the Diagnosis and Treatment of Chronic Conditions.

Giokas, K., Tsirmpas, C., Anastasiou, A., Costarides, V., & Koutsouris, D. (2015). Contemporary heart failure treatment based on improved knowledge and personalized care of comorbidities. In Handbook of Research on Trends in the Diagnosis and Treatment of Chronic Conditions.

Groves, J. (2010). International Alliance of Patients' Organizations perspectives on person-centered medicine. *International Journal of Integrated Care*, *10*(Suppl), e011. PMID:20228908

Guelfi, N., & Savidis, A. (Eds.). (2006). *Rapid Integration of Software Engineering Techniques* (Vol. 3943). Berlin, Heidelberg: Springer Berlin Heidelberg; doi:10.1007/11751113

Handbook of Clinical Gender Medicine. (2012). Karger Medical and Scientific Publishers.

Health I. T.gov. (2015). *What is the difference between a Personal Health Record, an Electronic Health Record, and an Electronic Medical Record?* Retrieved September 1, 2015, from http://healthit.gov/providers-professionals/faqs/what-are-differences-between-electronic-medical-records-electronic

Hirsch, C. H., Buzková, P., Robbins, J. A., Patel, K. V., & Newman, A. B. (2012). Predicting late-life disability and death by the rate of decline in physical performance measures. *Age and Ageing, 41*(2), 155–161. doi:10.1093/ageing/afr151 PMID:22156556

Intel Health. (2007). *Reconceiving Disease Management: A Technology Perspective*. Retrieved September 1, 2015, from http://www.intel.com/pressroom/kits/healthcare/DiseaseMgmt_whitepaper.pdf

A.T. Kearney. (2012). *Improving the evidence for mobile health*. Author.

Kinsella, A. (2012). *Engaging Patients: A Challenging New Frontier in Healthcare Delivery | Tim Rowan's Home Care Technology Blog*. Retrieved June 18, 2015, from http://www.homehealthnews.org/2013/02/engaging-patients-a-challenging-new-frontier-in-healthcare-delivery/

Koutsouris, D., Iliopoulou, D., Lazakidou, A., Fotiadis, D., Petridou, M., Giokas, K., & Vellidou, E. et al. (2014). The use of telephone monitoring for diabetic patients: Theory and practical implications. *Smart Homecare Technology and TeleHealth, 2*, 13. doi:10.2147/SHTT.S41242

Kuhlmann, E., Blank, R. H., Bourgeault, I. L., & Wendt, C. (2015). *The Palgrave International Handbook of Healthcare Policy and Governance* (E. Kuhlmann, R. H. Blank, I. L. Bourgeault, & C. Wendt, Eds.). Palgrave Macmillan. doi:10.1057/9781137384935

Mandl, K. D., & Kohane, I. S. (2008). Tectonic shifts in the health information economy. *The New England Journal of Medicine, 358*(16), 1732–1737. doi:10.1056/NEJMsb0800220 PMID:18420506

Marengoni, A., Angleman, S., Melis, R., Mangialasche, F., Karp, A., Garmen, A., & Fratiglioni, L. et al. (2011). Aging with multimorbidity: A systematic review of the literature. *Ageing Research Reviews, 10*(4), 430–439. doi:10.1016/j.arr.2011.03.003 PMID:21402176

Marengoni, A., von Strauss, E., Rizzuto, D., Winblad, B., & Fratiglioni, L. (2009). The impact of chronic multimorbidity and disability on functional decline and survival in elderly persons. A community-based, longitudinal study. *Journal of Internal Medicine, 265*(2), 288–295. doi:10.1111/j.1365-2796.2008.02017.x PMID:19192038

Marengoni, A., Winblad, B., Karp, A., & Fratiglioni, L. (2008). Prevalence of chronic diseases and multimorbidity among the elderly population in Sweden. *American Journal of Public Health, 98*(7), 1198–1200. doi:10.2105/AJPH.2007.121137 PMID:18511722

McNeill, D. (2015). *Using Person-Centered Health Analytics to Live Longer: Leveraging Engagement, Behavior Change, and Technology for a Healthy Life*. FT Press.

Meinow, B. (2008). *Capturing Health in the Elderly Population: Complex Health Problems, Mortality, and the Allocation of Home-help Services*. Stockholm: Stockholm University.

Miller, M. D., Paradis, C. F., Houck, P. R., Mazumdar, S., Stack, J. A., Rifai, A. H., & Reynolds, C. F. III et al.. (1992). Rating chronic medical illness burden in geropsychiatric practice and research: Application of the Cumulative Illness Rating Scale. *Psychiatry Research*, *41*(3), 237–248. doi:10.1016/0165-1781(92)90005-N PMID:1594710

Noyes, J., & Baber, C. (2012). *User-Centred Design of Systems*. Springer Science & Business Media.

Pawola, L. (2011). *The History of the Electronic Health Record - Health Topics*. Orlando, Florida: HIMSS.

Pilemalm, S., & Timpka, T. (2008). Third generation participatory design in health informatics--making user participation applicable to large-scale information system projects. *Journal of Biomedical Informatics*, *41*(2), 327–339. doi:10.1016/j.jbi.2007.09.004 PMID:17981514

Rainie, L. (2012). *The Rise of the e-Patient | Pew Research Center*. Retrieved June 20, 2015, from http://www.pewinternet.org/2012/01/12/the-rise-of-the-e-patient/

Schuler, D., & Namioka, A. (1993). *Participatory Design: Principles and Practices*. Hillsdale, NJ: L. Erlbaum Associates Inc.

Van De Belt, T. H., Engelen, L. J. L. P. G., Berben, S. A. A., & Schoonhoven, L. (2010). Definition of Health 2.0 and Medicine 2.0: A systematic review. *Journal of Medical Internet Research*, *12*(2), e18. doi:10.2196/jmir.1350 PMID:20542857

Wallace, R. B., & Salive, M. E. (2013). The dimensions of multiple chronic conditions: Where do we go from here? A commentary on the Special Issue of Preventing Chronic Disease. *Preventing Chronic Disease*, *10*, E59. doi:10.5888/pcd10.130104 PMID:23618539

WHO. (2011). *mHealth: New horizons for health through mobile technologies: second global survey on eHealth*. World Health Organization Report.

KEY TERMS AND DEFINITIONS

CIRS-G: A metric to calculate the number and severity of chronic illnesses in the structure of the comorbid state of patients focusing on geriatrics.

Clinical Protocol: A medical guideline (also called a clinical guideline, clinical protocol or clinical practice guideline) is a document with the aim of guiding decisions and criteria regarding diagnosis, management, and treatment in specific areas of healthcare.

Disease Management Programme: Aim to help people get on top of their chronic disease and maintain a good quality of life. One of the aims of DMPs is to improve medical treatment in the long term.

Empowerment: Is the granting of patients to take an active role in the decisions made about his or her own healthcare.

Interoperability: The ability of different information technology systems and software applications to communicate, exchange data, and use the information that has been exchanged.

mHealth: A term used for the practice of medicine and public health supported by mobile devices.

Multimorbidity: Co-occurrence of two or more chronic medical conditions in one person.

ENDNOTES

1 https://standards.ieee.org/findstds/standard/11073-10425-2014.html
2 http://www.continuaalliance.org
3 http://www.unipg.it/en/
4 http://ki-su-arc.se
5 See Chapter 16: Health Policy in the European Union (Kuhlmann, Blank, Bourgeault, & Wendt, 2015) for a detailed description of the different typologies of health care systems in EU Member States.
6 EU Project: www.eurorec.org/RD/
7 http://www.digitashealth.com
8 http://www.continuaalliance.org/
9 http://en.wikipedia.org/wiki/Cybercondria

This research was previously published in M-Health Innovations for Patient-Centered Care edited by Anastasius Moumtzoglou, pages 52-71, copyright year 2016 by Medical Information Science Reference (an imprint of IGI Global).

Chapter 35

Non–Traditional Data Mining Applications in Taiwan National Health Insurance (NHI) Databases:
A Hybrid Mining (HM) Case for the Framing of NHI Decisions

Joseph Tan
McMaster University, Canada

Fuchung Wang
National Health Insurance Administration, Taiwan

ABSTRACT

This study examines time-sensitive applications of data mining methods to facilitate claims review processing and provide policy information for insurance decision-making vis-à-vis the Taiwan National Health Insurance (NHI) databases. In order to obtain the best payment management, a hybrid mining (HM) approach, which has been grounded on the extant knowledge of data mining projects and health insurance domain knowledge, is proposed. Through the integration of data warehousing, online analytic processing, data mining techniques and traditional data analysis in the healthcare field, an easy-to-use decision support platform, which will assist in directing the health insurance decision-making process, is built. Drawing from lessons learned within a case study setting, results showed that not only is HM approach a reliable, powerful, and user-friendly platform for diversified payment decision support, but that it also has great relevance for the practice and acceptance of evidence-based medicine. Essentially, HM approach can provide a critical boost to health insurance decision support; hence, future researchers should develop and improve the approach combined with their own application systems.

DOI: 10.4018/978-1-5225-3926-1.ch035

1. INTRODUCTION

Fueled by the massive amount of mandated data to be manipulated routinely and automatically, the resulting information deluge faced by healthcare insurance systems characterized by a single payer (monopolistic) and/or a few payers (oligopolistic) has, in turn, caused traditional information retrieval methods and data analysis to perform inadequately. As a result, the new interdisciplinary field of data sciences, encompassing both classical statistical methods and modern machine learning tools to support efficient and effective processing and mining of information as well as the discovery of knowledge (and hidden patterns) from enormous databases (Han, Kamber, & Pei, 2012; Gupta, 2014) is now gradually being realized and implemented.

Meanwhile, the growth of health expenditures is the most challenging risk to healthcare systems worldwide. In 2014, for example, the US government spent 1.1 trillion for Medicare and Medicaid. By 2030, expenditures for these two programs are projected to consume 50% of federal budget. Cost and spending factors drive needs for change. Given that healthcare organizations are typically characterized as complex adaptive systems with multi-stakeholders (Tan et al., 2005), they are also known to be highly information dependent; therefore, knowledge intensive technology is vital to the survival of these complex organizations and systems. Using health data analytics and data mining techniques to make business decisions for increasingly complex adaptive healthcare organizations and systems can effectively influence cost, revenues, and operational efficiency while maintaining a high level of care.

To date, various data mining (DM) methods and application systems approaches have been promoted. Unlike the traditional statistical and online analytical processing (OLAP) tools, these newer techniques have integrated algorithmic and inductive approaches to facilitate advanced data analysis and decision support to yield business intelligence (Rupink, Kukar, & Krisper, 2007). Some researchers have explored the use of DM in the development of a decision support system (DSS) to manage healthcare services (Sliver et al., 2001) while others have provided the outcome of mining methods in the value of quality improvement (Lee et al., 2011). Owing to rapid advances in data sciences (and big data processing technology) on the one hand and an increasingly complex, competitive environment on the other, newly mined knowledge is becoming pervasively critical to aid decision making in today's rapidly changing healthcare environments and systems.

Hybrid mining (HM) approach (Chen & Cheng, 2012) underlies a novel design for uncovering knowledge embedded in complex data systems linking multiple stakeholders as exemplified by the National Health Insurance (NHI) databases in Taiwan. In Taiwan, the national health expenditures in 2012 totaled 6.6% of GDP, although this compared favorably with 16.2% in the same year for the US. More surprisingly, apart from higher expenditures, life expectancy of those residing in the US is still lower than Taiwan by at least 2 years.

Structurally, the Taiwan NHI has been mandated and set up as a monopolistic social insurance plan, a mandatory healthcare plan characterized by a centralized disbursement of funds with its administration cost budgeted at only 1% of total expenditures. It is financed primarily through direct government funding, employment premiums and user co-payments. Patients just need to present their health insurance cards when visiting with a care provider. The National Health Insurance Administration (NHIA) will reimburse payments to the providers (Figure 1).

In 2002, in light of the need to avoid ongoing losses and for cost containment, NHI moved to alter the payment system from a fee-for-service to a global budget, foreshadowing a kind of prospective payment system (PPS). Meanwhile, Taiwan had plans to reform its payment schema to include case payment,

Figure 1. The framework of Taiwan National Health Insurance (NHI)

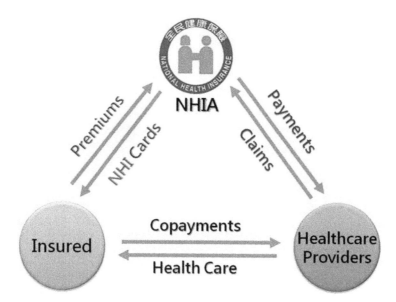

pay-for-performance and diagnostic related group (DRG) under the global budget (Cheng, 2009). As all claims are to be filed and processed electronically, the NHIA's automated IT-supported claims review system will check for the overall appropriateness of claims and also select a small percentage of these claims for individual professional review by clinical experts (Cheng, 2015).

Even so, it is important to clarify the underlying complex relations among embedded entities in the NHI databases in order to help decrease the nature of obstacles in the healthcare application. Accordingly, the goal of this paper is to showcase the HM approach based on the extant knowledge of DM projects and health insurance domain knowledge. Specifically, our research validates the approach by drawing on lessons learned in a case study setting aimed at facilitating evidence-based medicine to support multiple health insurance payment strategies. The rest of this paper is structured as follows. Section II overviews hybrid mining, emphasizing particular DM methods applicable to aid general decision and policy making within the healthcare insurance industry. Section III highlights the specific use of HM approach to aid health insurance claims processing and payment decisions. Section IV discusses lessons drawn from the case study demonstrating the results of using the HM approach as well as experiences of its use. The paper then concludes with insights into future work and research directions.

2. HYBRID MINING: AN OVERVIEW

Briefly, DM may be defined as the iterative process of analyzing data via either automatic or manual methods in order to discover implicit, but useful information and previously unknown patterns and relationships hidden in the data (a process often referred to as "knowledge discovery"). Today, many organizations are capitalizing on data analytics and DM methods to improve on product design in terms of consumer expectations and experiences and/or service marketing capabilities. In the case of insurance claims processing, as is with Taiwan NHI, the primary intent for mining the data would be to detect abnormal transactional patterns, and to predict future directions based on past experiences and current trends. In adapting to rapidly changing environments, new and rapidly expanding organizations are clearly in need of this technology.

As real-world problems tend to be highly nonlinear in nature, it is difficult, if not impossible, to develop a comprehensive model taking into account all of the independent variables impacting various organizational decisions using only conventional statistical approaches; instead, complex data analytics and new forms of DM approaches have been demonstrated to be more reliable and useful (Chen & Tsao, 2009). Meanwhile, the digital revolution has provided relatively inexpensive and available means to collect and store large amount of current and historic data. As databases grow in size, it will be increasingly more difficult to support all organizational activities, even routine decision making. HM will be an efficient alternative and has been proposed for processing and manipulating health insurance databases (Kuo, Lina, & Shihb, 2007). In an era of Big Data, accessing to a specific value in a huge data can be time consuming and require high power computing and processing. With growing accumulation of insurance data, HM for such big data can be a highly valued and efficient method (Ebadati & Tabrizi, 2016).

As traditional manual data analysis has its limitations, new methods for advanced data analysis and knowledge discovery have become indispensable, thereby promoting a new field of data sciences. These new approaches are based on algorithms integrating complex statistical tools, artificial intelligence, neural networks (NN), inductive rules, and predicate logic. In contrast to the traditional reactive DSS tools, these newer approaches will initiate analysis to create knowledge and predictive analysis, as the premise underlying DM is proactive. Broadly speaking, therefore, DM or data analytics may now be applied to solve specific and practical problems that have not even yet been identified by the user.

2.1. Hybrid Mining Approach

The promise of HM as the next generation of DM systems has already been discussed in the extant literature. The approach is based on a novel combination of existing approaches, as noted by a number of researchers (Chu & Tsai, 2007). This work is motivated by the obvious limitations of classical paradigms for DM that have been used in isolation. As each method carries its own advantages and shortcomings, mixing the use of different methods can be both complementary and desirable. Hybrid approach shows improved data analytic modeling accuracy and robustness (Kao, Zahara, & Kao, 2008). Research into the integration of different methods and case applications of HM technologies will continue to broaden our knowledge of this evolving field.

Applying clustering to refine the design of NNs is a concept that originated in the mid-1990s (Balakrishnan et al., 1996; West, 2000). Essentially, hybrid design architecture use NNs guided by clustering algorithms to generate more accurate classifiers. Following the success of the HM application, there has been increasing number of studies investigating HM approaches. Examples of tasks that can be facilitated by the use of HM include constructing the credit scoring models from a credit database and designing an effective credit-scoring model. West (2000), for example, investigated the credit scoring accuracy of five NN models, and reported that non-parametric and hybrid design architecture would be very useful in developing effective credit scoring models. He then concluded that hybrid architecture should be considered for credit scoring applicants.

Kuo and his colleagues (2002) developed a two-stage method by first allowing self-organizing map to determine the number of clusters and then, employing the K-means algorithm to classify samples into cluster. As well, Lee and his colleagues (2002) integrated the back-propagation NNs with traditional discriminant analysis approach to achieve greater accuracy and easier interpretation of mining results. Chen and Huang (2003) also presented a work involving two interesting credit analysis problems and resolved them by applying NNs and genetic algorithms techniques. Hsieh (2005) proposed a hybrid system based on clustering and NN techniques, leading to a hybrid architecture that generates more accurate classifiers. Lee and Chen (2005) proposed a two-stage hybrid modeling procedure with artificial NNs and multivariate adaptive regression while Huang and Wang (2006) combined genetic algorithms with support vector machine classifier. For many years to come, HM methods preserve the strengths and also maximize the applications. Ebadati and Tabrizi (2016) presented hybrid clustering to serve as an important unsupervised approach that finds a structure for big data. Altogether, results of past research showed that HM is a promising addition to the existing repertoire of DM methodology.

Today, HM approach is well developed not only technologically but also in applied studies. For example, there has been great progress achieved in the application of DM techniques focusing on credit scoring competition of the consumer credit market (West, 2000; Lee et al., 2002; Chen & Huang, 2003; Lee & Chen, 2005). Sadatrasoul and his colleagues (2013) investigated hybrid methods focus on credit scoring from 2000 to 2012 in four categories and found two of the frequently used combinations are "classification and classification" and "clustering and classification". These hybrid methods can identify and extract potentially good v. bad groupings of applicants; importantly, the researchers also argue strongly for the potential to knowledge transfer (KT) the use of similar forms of scoring models in other applications. Specifically, in the case of big data insurance claims processing, for example, it is purported that an equivalent scoring model can be efficiently used to resolve a practical problem of detecting patient visits with abusive utilization pattern based on intelligent profiling of the patient visit information extracted from insurance claims database(s).

2.2. Enhanced Health Care With Better Mining

The routine delivery of healthcare services generates massive streams of both structured and unstructured data in a mix of administrative and clinical domains about patients, hospital procedures, bed costs, other fees and claims processes. In this age of rapid knowledge diffusion and digital health transformation, and given that data, in and of themselves, represent strategic resources for healthcare institutions, the use of data analytics and DM in many areas of healthcare services delivery to track patient treatment effectiveness, improve healthcare procedures and management, enhance customer relationship management and detect frauds and abuses (Durairaj & Ranjani, 2013), is something that cannot be overly emphasized.

Today, many healthcare organizations are moving towards implementing DM technologies to help control costs and improve the efficacy of patient care. As clinicians and managers continue to find values in data analytics and new DM approaches through their respective power to unlock new patterns (Durairaj & Ranjani, 2013; Srinivasan & Pavya, 2016) in data, it has been argued that such a trend will lead to the potential improvements of organizational resource utilization and, ultimately, patient health and well being. Moreover, as these newly discovered patterns are oftentimes based upon evolving clinical practices, they can, in turn, be used to set new standards of evidence-based care and best practices.

Broadly speaking, health data analytics and DM offer community-based gains that improve healthcare forecasting, analyses, and visualization (Payton, 2003). Therefore, if healthcare decision makers can make clever use of health data analytics and DM techniques, new knowledge can be automatically generated on a timely basis. For example, a patient's length of stay (LOS) (Hachesu, 2013) is a major component in the costing of inpatient treatment. Based on the premise that it is possible to reduce costs through reduced inpatient LOS, the knowledge acquired will, in turn, lead automatically to a reduction of cost. Another example is applying HM in the medical prescription domain. Although the prescribing behaviors among health professionals for treating both acute and chronic diseases are diverse and difficult to predict, mining those data from a nationwide prescription database will be a great benefit to develop a smart medication recommendation model to reduce costs, eliminate potential drug abuses and improve patient safety and compliance (Syed-Abdul et al., 2014).

Applying HM techniques and other emerging approaches in data sciences appropriately and refining them into some repeatable steps for analyzing available data and uncovering business insights are critical for many reasons (Sliver et al., 2001). One such reason is that managers and clinical users often have to rerun these tools on the same or different data sets repeatedly in the same sequence over time so that they can measure and determine whether the actions they have taken will lead to the desired effect. Another reason is to be able to semi-automate the analysis to achieve greater process efficiencies. A third reason is that users can easily apply these tools to other institutions, and possibly, other industries. The last but not least, mining in healthcare using a hybrid approach or other emerging techniques in the data sciences might provide better result while comparing with more traditional, but limited statistical approaches.

Put together, a novel hybrid data mining approach for knowledge extraction and classification in health services and medical databases will benefit the coordination of health services delivery and healthcare management significantly. The approach might combine self-organizing map, K-means with NN-based classifier to clustering all data and fusing them through the use of serial and parallel fusion in conjunction with neural classifier (Hassan & Verma, 2007). Besides, association rule is also a popular method to be added into any HM approaches. Valuable knowledge can be discovered from the application of HM techniques in healthcare databases. These new applications can be naturally classified into three broad categories, including that of descriptive (or clinically diagnostic), predictive (or clinically prognostic) and prescriptive (or clinically therapeutic) modeling, in order to increase the quality and safety of care and decrease the medical expenditure.

3. FRAMING DECISIONS ON HEALTH INSURANCE PAYMENTS

With escalating healthcare costs over the past decades, timely analysis of healthcare information has become an issue of growing importance. Addressing the effectiveness of association rules and neural segmentation in analyzing and retrieving unknown behavioral patterns from huge datasets, the Australian Health Insurance Commission (HIC) had collected detailed claims information and established a homogeneous claim database through the administration of various programs. As the medical reimbursement process is time consuming, this specific case will show that health data analytics and advancing DM algorithms could be used successfully on large, real-time customer data, with reasonable execution time. Moreover, the applied HIC project had also demonstrated that the intelligent applications of these algorithms could result in quantifiable benefits for the interested and participating organizations, thereby helping to identify specific actions that have to be taken (Cabena et al., 1997). Moreover, efficient reimbursement process is not the only objective to help determine health insurance payments. There are many payment decisions that also need information system to support such as the framing of payment policy-related decisions.

3.1. Applying HM to Payment Information System (PIS)

Healthcare payment models can be segregated into several different types (or, forms). In many well-structured healthcare payment models, quality is a key component. However, there is no incentive to take any cost saving in fee-for-service, which is the most traditional form of healthcare payment models. Therefore, the insurance companies or government agencies usual need a payment information system (PIS) to deal with the huge claims to identify the errors, potential abuses and frauds. As noted in the aforementioned HIC project, HM approach could improve fee-for-service reimbursement process while undergoing a payment reform process involving, for example, the transition from fee-for-service to value-based systems. To achieve this goal, advancing health data analytics and DM algorithms should be used to predict health outcomes and to provide a framework for analyzing policy decision information using emerging and alternative developing models.

Chae and his colleagues (2001) demonstrated how decision tree algorithm and the association rules that provided an occurrence relationship among risk factors could be used in a policy analysis for hypertension management. While logistic regression provides insights into general risk factors for hypertension, it does not provide specific information on the segment characteristics of age or risk factors that may be useful for policy analysis. This kind of cases will be very useful payment information to help frame health insurance decision in pay-for-performance (P4P) or other value-based reimbursement environments, as healthcare providers are only compensated if they meet certain metrics for quality, safety and efficiency.

Another research explored the use of artificial NNs in the development of a DSS to manage healthcare non-clinical services. The advantage of using this system is that healthcare managers can provide their own risk assessment values such as point score system (or use of balanced scorecard) based on their own knowledge and corporate objectives (Rupink, Kukar, & Krisper, 2007). While developing and applying intelligent decision models that is based on a DM method, the project team members (and users) may also find that applying the DM to decision support through supporting structure and utility function development from pre-classified patient data may (and can) also lead to the discovery of hierarchical decision models and improved performance both in terms of classification accuracy and the discovery of meaningful concept hierarchies (Bohanec, Zupan, & Rajkovic, 2000).

Simply stated, administrative v. clinical decision as well as policymaking processes are ways of determining the best alternative path(s) or choice(s) to follow for the delivery of healthcare services. "Decision support" means using the methods and tools for supporting people (decision or policy makers) involved in the decision-making (or policymaking) process. DM and decision support approaches (including data analytics) are often complementary and supplementary. In this sense, both the information from retrospective data and existing medical knowledge are combined in data analytics and data mining to construct potentially useful and highly predictive medical decision model.

Claims-based databases or healthcare utilization databases are made of routinely collected records originally intended for management purposes. They are the main component of healthcare PIS for reimbursement of health insurance. In recent decades, some national data holders of administrative healthcare databases have started to recompile these databases and made these available for academic research purposes. One of the most well known administrative healthcare databases is National Health Insurance Research Database (NHIRD) in Taiwan. NHIRD studies were also published across multiple disciplines in a growing number of journals (Chen et al., 2010). However, most of them used traditional data analysis to describe or predict health outcomes and the relationships among studied variables; unfortunately, only a few applied DM methods for complex computation have emerged only in the last few years due to a limitation of knowledge in data sciences.

Meanwhile, inappropriate payments by insurance organizations or payers occur because of errors, potential abuses and frauds. The scale of this problem is large enough to make it a priority issue for many health systems worldwide. Joudaki and his colleagues (2015) recommended general steps to data mining of healthcare claims. Shin and his colleagues (2012) proposed the scoring model to detect outpatient clinics with abusive utilization patterns based on profiling information extracted from insurance claims database. Lin and Yeh (2012) take advantage of DM technology to design models and find out cases requiring for manual inspection so as to save time and manpower.

Put together, healthcare insurance programs rely not only on traditional data analysis methods but new knowledge discovery processes for analyzing the claims database to enhance the effectiveness and efficiency of PIS. However, traditional methods of detecting healthcare frauds and abuses are inefficient and time-consuming (Joudaki et al., 2015); moreover, they are inadequate to evaluate the different payment decisions in the diverse reimbursement system. HM approaches will ease the statistical and computing power needed to manipulate the massive data volume, variety, velocity and veracity in real claims-based settings. In such settings, the respective disease incidence rates may and can also be computed on a national basis given the availability and accessibility of national databases with long follow-up periods as characteristic of the design of a population-based, public-health oriented databases to help reduce any chance of selection bias.

3.2. A Framework for Payment Decision Support

Achieving a framework for health insurance payment decision support will serve to crystallize the role of HM-based systems in health insurance payment. Based on a review of the extant literature and to ensure that the design and implementation of support systems be available in practice, our research applied the design perspective to synthesize and propose such a fundamental framework. Two of the frequently used mining technologies, that is, clustering and association rule, can be combined within the HM approach to yield the most cost-effective payment decision from scoring model.

This framework, as depicted in Figure 2, was based on the extant knowledge of hybrid data mining and health insurance payment projects. The framework combined DM and decision support to be used as a template for quantifiable and/or subjective evaluation to be made by researchers and practitioners. Notably, the original method to process the health insurance payment decision follows the sequence of dotted lines as shown in Figure 2 for which the processing was automated with semiautomatic claims review checks applied to a selection of a small percentage of all claims being targeted for professional review by clinical experts. The framework integrated with HM would reduce the percentage and identify the precise claims to be set aside for professional review to improve the efficiency of payment decision in the review process. The results also provided feedback into the model scoring to improve the effectiveness. Next, we reviewed how such a framework is to be applied into payment decision so as to fit into the diverse reimbursement system and explained why it worked via the NHI case.

Figure 2. The framework for health insurance payment decision support

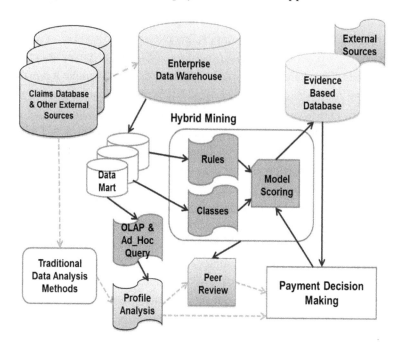

4. THE NHI CASE

Launched in 1995, the NHI system of Taiwan was established to provide healthcare insurance for all Taiwan residents. NHI is a compulsory program; to date, 99.9% of the population is enrolled, including nationals and foreign workers, even inmates since 2013 (Cheng, 2015). From the healthcare delivery side, about 93.5% of the providers have joined the program.

The NHI provides a uniform package for all insured, and the benefits are very comprehensive, covering a wide range of services even though Taiwan spends only 6% of its GDP on health care. Patients are free to choose providers and there is no significant waiting time to see a doctor. Meanwhile, medical expenditures are contained by the global budget payment system (Cheng, 2009; Cheng 2015). As a monopolistic system, the NHIA is the only agency authorized to administer the program and collects premiums from the insured, their employers, and the government based on an individual's monthly income. Owing to the fact that the NHI is a single payer, its administrative cost is relatively low. It is less than 1% of the NHI medical expenditures, which is small compared to relative spending of many Western countries. A key factor leading to the program's success is the adaptation of information system (IS) from its very inception (Cheng, 2009; Cheng 2015). With its modernized health IT/IS infrastructure and platform, it has been easier for Taiwan than it is for the US to enhance the cost effectiveness and the quality of health care being delivered (Reinhardt, 2008). This is because since 1996, not only is 99% of claims being processed electronically, but the smart-card program to connect multi-providers in health care has also been successfully implemented by 2004 in Taiwan. Given the state of health data digitization in Taiwan, the NHIA can almost track all ongoing transactions in real-time throughout the nation's healthcare system.

Figure 3 shows the primary NHI PIS structure. Notably, it differs from several other countries in that except for out-of-pocket expenses, patients need not pay directly when visiting with a care provider. Essentially, the respective care providers would initiate the claims to the NHIA for payment in the reimbursement process. This benefits the patient as it reduces their financial burden while the pressure of the cash flow from the side of the providers is increased. As the NHIA reimburses medical payments to care providers on a monthly basis, it is critical for the PIS to complete the entire claims processing within 60 days. Notwithstanding, the NHIA is established to support, on a long-term basis, the continuing success of the NHI program as defined by sustained high-quality medical services with comparatively low cost. The reimbursement system has been designed specifically to facilitate the efficiency and cost-effectiveness of the claims review process. Additionally, the complete system is subject to strict privacy and security controls through the NHI Virtual Private Network (VPN) that only NHI-contracted health services providers can access and use.

In 2015, the number of claims for outpatient treatment and medical orders totaled 43 million and 160 million per month respectively and the number of claims for outpatient was 300 thousand per month. As noted, these claims must be reimbursed within 2 months of the visit dates with the monthly provisional payment totaling NT$ 50 billion (approximately 1.6 billion US dollars). In order to manage such a massive utilization of medical resources while simultaneously assuring the care quality, the NHIA developed and implemented various review mechanisms to examine the appropriateness of submitted claims (National Health Insurance Administration, 2015) with the aim of completing all procedural reviews in a timely fashion. Aside from prospective and on-site reviews, retrospective review is the key mechanism used by the NHIA. With retrospective review, two approaches are adopted, namely, procedural review and professional review. The procedural review is fully automated, comprising auto-adjudication and profile analysis. In this process, the NHIA check the accuracy and completeness of claims data electronically; to

Figure 3. The NHI payment information system structure

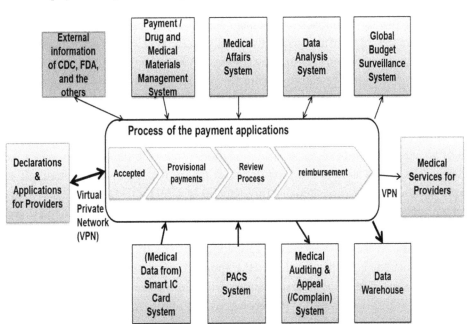

date, there are more than one thousand rules of auto-adjudication and hundreds of indicators for profile analysis that have been put in place by the NHIA.

For the professional review, about 3,000 physicians with various specialties have been contracted with the NHIA annually; briefly, these expert reviewers were entrusted to peer-review the rationality of medical procedures and services according to the claims data vis-à-vis the copy of original medical records available from the provider(s). Undoubtedly, the peer-review process can become expensive. How easy it is to realize the efficiency-effectiveness of the reimbursement process will depend largely on the balance of procedural review vis-à-vis the professional review. Some of the rules and indicators in the procedural review have been derived from more traditional statistical analysis and the feedback of professional review, while others have emerged from the scope of benefits dictated in the payment provision.

Following the procedural review, a selected subset of claims is being flagged down to undergo a professional review via two main approaches: (a) random sampling, and (b) ad hoc querying. For the random sampling, if some unnecessary treatments were found in the review, then the corresponding payment would be deducted not only in the reviewed claim but also in those associated claims as per the sampling rate to rollback costs of the total claim. While this approach could have impacted significantly on preventing abnormal claims, such cases, however, are difficult to capture with random sampling of the procedural review. For ad hoc querying initiated by the health records managers' experience in picking out some suspicious cases for the specific purpose of claims auditing, an advance analysis is often followed. In this case, the payment would be deducted upon auditing via the professional claim review process; still, a key challenge here is to intelligently model this decision process as a semi-automated process that can be incorporated and streamlined into the routine procedural review.

In 2014, the deny rate of primary review stands only at around 0.28%~2.66% and is likely to decrease over time. One reason for this anticipated decline is that, depending on the type of claims, a good portion of the procedural review was becoming increasingly difficult to identify the frauds and abuses with the more traditional rules and indicators no longer applicable. Another reason is that providers argued against the impact of having a rollback mechanism linked to the rate of deducted payments arising from the random sampling. Many Taiwanese rely heavily on the government-managed health insurance system to share a large part of their healthcare expenses. With growing demands on NHIA payments, however, the fraudulent and abusive claims of some healthcare services providers' behaviors have challenged the integrity of the system. To overcome these challenges, it was proposed that a HM framework be incorporated into the system.

As shown in the NHI case, the concept of clinical pathways to facilitate automatic and systematic construction of an adaptable and extensible detection model was eventually implemented for the NHIA claims processing. First, it was found to provide the critically needed system safeguard; second, past empirical experiments have demonstrated that this detection model is efficient and capable of identifying some fraudulent and abusive cases that were not detected via a manually constructed detection (Yang & Hwang, 2006); and finally, the model has also been evaluated objectively by a real dataset gathered from the NHI program. In the sub-sections to follow, we discuss in more details the various ways in which decision support has been provided via HM approaches for the different aspects of the NHIA claims processing system, including decision support for (a) the diverse reimbursement process; (b) quality improvement (QI) via the pay-for-performance (P4P) program; and (c) the implementation of the diagnostic related groupings (DRGs) program.

4.1. Diverse Reimbursement Process

The objective of the NHIA claims review under a global budget system has shifted gradually from the containment of medical expenditure to the assurance of medical care quality. The NHIA has developed a series of plans that are structured to improve the quality of care while keeping costs under control. These plans offer healthcare providers incentives to care for the patients' overall well being by reimbursing them based on clinical outcomes (National Health Insurance Administration, 2015). To assure and improve on the care quality, the NHIA has to maintain an ongoing, strong functioning profile analysis database with DM methods as well as a management model for case anomalies.

Soon following the establishment of the NHIA, the PIS was also implemented to review the delivery of medical services to prevent waste and safeguard care quality. Information technology (IT) is used in conducting both the procedural and professional review, but especially the procedural review, which relies on profile analysis based on specific medical criteria to conduct automated audits, and improve efficiencies and effectiveness of claim reviews. While the traditional DM were occasionally used, it was, however, difficult to implement such methodology into the reimbursement process. For example, the mining association rules for discovering relation between variables in NHIRD (Lin et al., 2013) have been popular and well researched, but there remained a lack of applicable standards for evaluating highly specialized medical services. Most of the extant traditional mining literature focused more on the technical methods and paid little attention to the practical implications of their findings for decision makers (Joudaki et al., 2015).

The decision support provided by the application of HM to facilitate claims review and payment processing can be more specialized and precise. HM can help the NHIA to extract useful information from millions of claims and identify or flagged out a smaller subset of the claims or claimants for further assessment. The healthcare quality indicators have also been identified and the DSS has also been designed to analyze and monitor trends of quality indicators with tutorial for QI activities embedded in the system. In addition, the NHIA can continue to entrust peer review to the medical associations to ascertain joint management with medical providers. Further, the NHIA is able to keep adding more quality indicators to monitor the performance of healthcare providers and to disclose all of these quality information to the public so as to reduce the asymmetry of medical information between healthcare providers and the general public.

According to the framework for health insurance payment decision support, a process DM workflow is shown in Figure 4, which aggregates the numerous monthly claims into a provider profile claims.

Using the past claims data of individual care provider the process could identify and classify the different grouping of providers. For example, the high fraud suspicious group would require more resources on the professional review. Meanwhile, the review results also provide a chance to verify and modify the credit-scoring model. Rather than retrospective claim reviews, the workflow is designed to segment the providers into different reimbursement processing level. This means essentially that better performing providers could have less of a percentage (level B) or none (level A) of their claims going into the professional review. Besides the other payment schemes such as case payment plans, family doctor plan, and the integration of care plans could be separated or embedded in the workflow to calculate their levels concurrently.

To fit in with the NHIA newest strategy, a HM approach was considered as a solution to resolve the aforementioned challenge of finding a way to semi-automate the abuse and fraud detection as a hybrid model that can be simulated into the routine procedural review and to increase the effectiveness of the

Figure 4. The hybrid mining based decision support workflow for reimbursement process

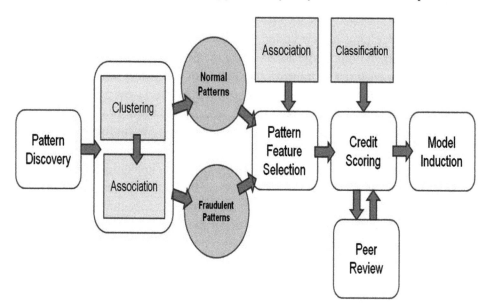

procedural review when using the mining techniques. In particular, the aim was to create a better application mimicking the real world. This case presents a HM approach in mimicking physicians' behavior for healthcare management. The design was based primarily on clustering and NN techniques. Effective segmentation of general practitioners' (GPs) practice patterns makes it easier to detect and investigate health fraud by recognizing and quantifying the features of claims and characteristics of providers.

Here, we used clustering techniques to preprocess the input data and used NNs to construct the scoring model. The clustering stage involved a classification process. A self-organizing map clustering algorithm was used to determine the number of clusters automatically as well as the starting points of each cluster. Then, the K-means clustering algorithm was used to generate clusters of samples belonging to new classes. In the NN stage, samples with new class labels were used in the design of the scoring model. Compared with the traditional mining approach on the basis of real physicians' behavior datasets, the proposed method demonstrates that the HM can be used to build an effective dynamic scoring model to develop a data-driven initiative to analyze and model the formal relations between GPs' practice patterns and health fraud. A sample of scoring result is provided in Table 1; we consolidated these ideas and implemented them into the reimbursement process with the decision support function.

NHIA officers who are responsible for the retrospective review process had further confirmed that the hybrid model was superior to the single mining method both in terms of perception and actual assessment outcomes. A hybrid model supporting the assessment of the provider performance needs to take into consideration also patients characteristics, provider characteristics, correlation between outcomes of patient within the same provider and the number of patients opting to be treated by the provider. These underlying factors motivate the centrality of HM analysis. Beyond this, the hybrid model applies DM techniques to support the key policymakers in Taiwan government in managing and building up the healthcare management knowledge from submitted claims information of healthcare providers. The scoring results also offered feedback to providers via the NHI VPN mentioned previously, and aided the providers to gain specific knowledge of their claims situation.

Table 1. A sample of scoring result

Credit scoring Cluster(3) 710 Physicians(16.4%) High variation in diseases High price per claim		
Fraud possible	Cluster(3-1) 16 belongs to Class A Providers	Cluster(3-2) 45 belongs to Class B providers
	Cluster(3-1) 420 belongs to Class A providers	Cluster(3-2) 229 belongs to Class B providers
Inappropriate possible	Cluster(3-1) 90 belongs to Class A Providers	Cluster(3-2) 125 belongs to Class B providers
	Cluster(3-1) 346 belongs to Class A providers	Cluster(3-2) 149 belongs to Class B providers

In summary, not only did the hybrid model proved to contribute new knowledge, but, as a result of applying the newly discovered knowledge in terms of changing physicians' behaviors, the desired outcome(s) serve as a good reference for the prevention of fraud and potential abuse in claims processing. Ultimately, this implies that such a model can serve as a key mechanism that would, over the long run, normalize most of the outliers, scaling them back to normal based on the repeated cycle of automated reviews and quality control built into the system. More generally, such a PIS may also now be deemed generally applicable to other monopolistic national healthcare systems.

4.2. QI via Pay-for-Performance (P4P) Program

Over the years, the NHIA had engaged in a number of QI initiatives. Among five of the pilot programs implemented in the late 2001, the pay-for-performance (P4P) program was relatively popular. Essentially, the program permitted voluntary participation by primary care physicians, hospitals, or clinics and other care facilities. To participate in the program, providers must adopt some quality assurance (QA) steps such as meeting the qualification or certification requirements, following the treatment guidelines and certain other protocols. Apart from sending in the claims data, these providers must also store their self-reported performance data electronically in a website that is linked directly to NHIA for easy access and review. The NHIA will then review the claims with other fee-for-services claims monthly and also complete processing of the claims reimbursement within 2 months. Adding to the self-reported performance data based on the outcome or process depending on how the program quality requirements have been satisfied, these reviews will then let the NHIA to determine within the following year on whether the claims "bonus" payments would also be reimbursed (or not).

An example of P4P is in diabetic care, which falls into a process-based payment category. Taiwan's monopolistic system is an ideal platform for P4P program as the system embodies an information infrastructure that yields comprehensive and up-to-date information on the actual care being delivered to the patients. Although some research has already applied DM techniques to detect fraudulent or abusive reporting by healthcare providers via their invoices for diabetic outpatient services, the goal of these reimbursement "bonus" plans, however, is to improve healthcare quality over the longer term.

Specifically, in the NHI case, we aggregated the diabetic care cases claims with self-reported performance data to make a classification. The diabetic data in this instance was those captured from the northern area of Taiwan with 6,274 diabetic patients. The diabetic registries and databases systematically collected patient information, while our analysis showcased a method of applying DM techniques, and some of the data issues, analysis problems, and results. The accumulated information could then be used both for proactive feedback to providers to improve the coverage rate and for incentive to encourage new providers to join the program.

Table 2 presents the optimal clustering result in our specific case, showing only the most critical variables with a total of five clusters that were found to be statistically significant.

Our next step was to join the historic claims data with the five clusters to identify the proper payment with multilevel analysis so as to differentiate between those claims that are patient level within a single provider and those claims that are characterized as among providers. Again, it was found that applying the HM approach here would help the NHIA to share precise information among invited providers to join the program as their patients' profiles is similar to those characterizing successful and high performing providers. Following the different payment analysis, the results and methods would subsequently yield

Table 2. Clustering result in diabetic patients

CLUSTER	Patients	Gender (F)	Family History	Tri glycerides	HbA1c	Pathological Changes of Foot	Standard Payment	Payment Range
A	1,899	100%	42%	180.76	8.529	84%	60	±10
B	964	1.04%	100%	188.9	8.271	71%	45	±6
C	1,337	0.67%	49%	198.41	8.65	100%	50	±6
D	1,280	76.88%	50%	188.66	8.61	87%	35	±3
E	794	55.09%	93%	246.75	9.642	0%	55	±6

a solution for the policymaking not only in diabetes management but also for other chronic diseases management.

The aforementioned example is very similar to the research that has applied DM method to classify consumers' behavior in choosing among Taiwan hospitals (Lee, Shih, & Chung, 2008). In this study, Lee et al. sorted the factors of consumers' behavior into four categories, taking into account patient risk adjustment, which will have a normative commitment by the providers. Then, they developed a back propagation NN classification model. They found that the applied model demonstrated the usefulness of 85.1% classification rate in sorting out consumers' styles. Hence, evidence exists to suggest that the NN model is useful in identifying emerging patterns of consumers' choices for Taiwan hospitals.

Conversely, instead of a NN model, a decision tree would be very simple to fit into a P4P program. For example, the NHIA had used the important variables in patients' profiles to identify which kind of providers will continue to join the family doctor program in order to earn the bonus payment, and which will quit; these representing the split between the decision on a decision tree. Additionally, today's capability on the visualization of results when decision support is to be combined with the complex rules can provide a convenient tool to the policymakers, especially having to decide on classification such as the diagnostic related groupings (DRGs), which is discussed next.

4.3. Implementing the DRG Policy

In contrast to the aforementioned cases, this section outlines how decision support can benefit the implementation of a DRG policy. Traditionally, past applications of the DM methodology have often been conducted with the analysis of one DRG by OLAP (Sliver et al., 2001) and to support the exploration of trajectories of care for healthcare providers. Jay and his colleague (2013), for example, developed a mining approach for grouping and analyzing trajectories of care using claim data for which patients were automatically grouped into 19 classes. The resulting profiles were clinically meaningful and economically relevant. In the case reported here, we will introduce an integrated method via HM approach to aid the DRG policymaking.

DRGs are divided into 25 major diagnostic categories (MDC) and relative weight (RW) is a value assigned to each DRG to reflect relative resource consumption for the group. The RW is used to calculate the total payment for the case. As part of expensive medical materials paid by patients will not be counted towards a DRG, some hospitals would like to abandon those claims. It will impact the RW calculation and the payment decision will have bias in the long term. An orthopedics DRG sample of HM approach combining automated methods and statistical knowledge is shown in Figure 5 and Table 3. Data mining is a core of the payment decision support process. HM approach can help the NHIA to extract useful information from thousands of claims and identify a smaller subset of the claims or claimants for further assessment.

5. CONCLUSION AND DISCUSSION

Overall, most of the identified literature focused more on the technical methods used in DM, and paid little attention to the practical implications of their findings for health managers and decision makers. Our research provides a good example of a study that provides managerial implications of their findings for dealing with healthcare fraud and other related abuses. However, an effective and efficient reimburse-

Figure 5. The claim of DRG for orthopedics

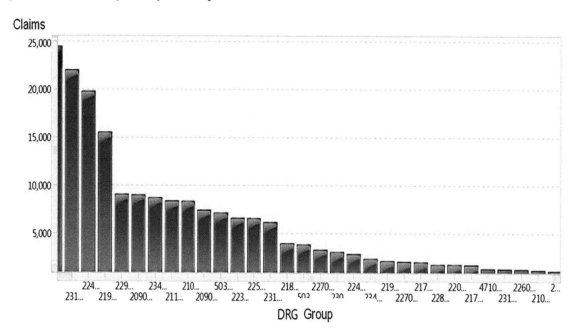

Table 3. Comparison between hybrid mining model and the hospital claims

Hospital	Claims	Model Consistent		Percentage of Low Consistent
		<50%	>50%	
A	41	9	32	22.0%
B	43	9	34	20.9%
C	129	18	111	14.0%
D	111	12	99	10.8%
E	123	18	105	14.6%
F	26	3	23	11.5%
G	16	5	11	31.3%
H	4	1	3	25.0%
I	17	2	15	11.8%
J	10	1	9	10.0%

ment process is not always a guaranty for the payment decision. Providers might modify or upcode the data to avoid having their submitted claims to go into the review process. On-site review is necessary to verify the provider behavior and has a better performance outcome than just including a DM approach. Therefore, to improve the uptake of HM methods, future studies should pay more attention to the policy implications. The rest of this section will concentrate on the general limitation and implications of our presented work.

5.1. Practice Implications

Altogether, our research supports the idea that HM-based system can serve as an efficient decision support in health insurance reimbursement decisions. The HM is both an efficient and cost effective approach in saving the cost of peer review and providing a flexible and an impromptu healthcare management mechanism. Furthermore, fraud detection is only one part of a bigger program of combating healthcare fraud, abuse and waste. Fraud detection should note the pitfalls that healthcare delivery policies such as fee-for-service can create that might increase the possibility of fraud and abuse. The integrated HM approach to facilitate health insurance payment decision should be covered by diversified decision support as shown in Figure 6.

Regardless if the insurance companies or government agencies would like to apply DM methods or not, macro payment such as global budget or fee schedules should have more mining applications as the decision making is a parallel process of examining large sets of different claims data to uncover hidden patterns, unknown correlations, trends, and other useful information. The traditional mining results can be accumulated and combined with the management strategy. However, it is a passive decision approach as it supports decision processes through new knowledge acquired without producing explicit decision suggestions or solutions. Conversely, the HM approach offers an easy-to-use tool, enabling business us-

Figure 6. Diversified payment decision support

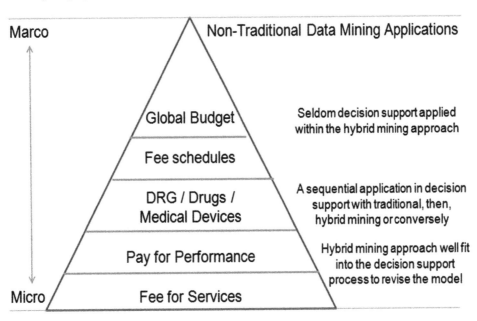

ers to exploit DM models with only having a relatively fundamental understanding of the DM concepts. It also helps them to interpret the models intelligently. Beginning in September 2014, a Central Intelligence System (CIS) was launched to further screen claimed costs. The system included HM approach to automatically target important items and picks out anomalies that are then listed for peer review or specially marked, and it also provides information on the anomalies, enhancing the efficiency of the reviews and payment decisions via an evidence-based learning paradigm this is shaped by the respective physician or patient's behavior being investigated.

Our research also found that most errors or problems of DM happened during the data cleaning and assessment stages, both of which are related to the domain issues. Learning of the healthcare data analysis process is a very time consuming process. It is definitely not only useful for the beginners but for the experts, as there are diverse emerging approaches and no one single approach is deemed to be the most appropriate at any one time. When an inappropriate method is used, it can also lead undesirably to data misinterpretation. Typically, the healthcare trial can be segmented into three parts, namely, the structure, process and outcome. Most of the DM projects ignored the difference among variables relating to the three parts, and simply combine them as a single whole. Oftentimes, the result will not be useful for the decision makers and policymakers. Besides, the validity of DM would also be put into question, such as in terms of the structure as mistakes are made in choosing variables among the three healthcare trial stages. The hybrid model is useful to help resolve a number of these noted challenges and/or application issues. However, it does require more time, additional learning, and/or cost, making it a difficult task to persuade those traditional data analysts who have typically relied on the cause-outcome paradigm to switch their methodological perspective.

In this era of big data, as data sources and technology advance, HM approach can be used to improve the odds that a certain treatment will result in a favorable outcome for diversified payment decision support. The goal of diversified payment decision support is to use high confidence approach that not only can benefit the cost effectiveness of resources allocation, but predict actionable interventions or treatments that will improve long-term health outcomes. The NHI case explores the HM approach combined with an application system (PIS) that policymakers can use to advance the science and art of claims processing and/or when the needs arise to develop payment policies in monopolistic healthcare system.

HM-based DSS is already here and its usage is growing rapidly. While applying mining methods to classify consumers' behavior in choosing hospitals, evidence has shown to suggest that the model is useful in identifying existing patterns among hospitals' consumers. What we need is conscious action, the real action that can deliver what has been envisioned for the society as a whole. Last but not least, social consensus on privacy and security is still very critical. The conflict between the sweeping power of technology to access and assemble personal information about privacy and security is an ever-growing concern.

5.2. Limitations and Future Research

Briefly, the content of our research comprises HM approach in the NHI. It does not go into detail on results obtained in each payment decision support. This paper includes an exploratory analysis of the main characteristics of the payment decision; however, additional aspects could have been included, but for the fact that detailed health information and statistics are subject to privacy and confidentiality rules. It is necessary to be very careful in the use and/or application of NHI-based data so as to avoid the bias and confounding issues. One potential problem of information bias, for example, is the possibility of "upcoding" a certain claim. Similarly, when data are not covering the entire patient medical records, there is also the potential of confounders in generating a decision based only on partial records. Models need to available to adjust continuously in order to improve the cost effectiveness and robustness of the statistical methods employed, even in a HM approach.

The presented case explained and demonstrated how a DM project may be improved through the use of the HM approach, which was composed of design, domain and assessment levels. Accordingly, the design process should synchronize with the other two components in order to ensure that it can be implemented in the real world. This work also showed that DM techniques can support the design of future IS for managing and building up the healthcare knowledge through the analysis of health insurance reimbursement data. The framework presented also illustrates how the hybrid model can help to turn data into knowledge. In Taiwan, the next generation PIS planning is underway and we are all looking forward to support the new "just-in-time" reimbursement process in a universal patient data environment. It is hoped that the results we obtained from using a HM approach will also encourage other users in applying the framework for future cases.

Extending the integration of different methods and the application of hybrid technologies will broaden our understanding on this emerging topic. In future case applications, other quality indicators can be analyzed to effectively support a hospital-wide continuous quality improvement activity and the DSS should be well integrated with the hospital order communication system to support concurrent review. It is anticipated that new applications of HM in healthcare data can be achieved for such areas as the hospital infection control, the ranking of hospitals, or the identifying of high-risk patients. In this sense, the hospital information management system will be developed within a knowledge management context in which users can share and use the knowledge mode effectively. The HM results can also be an effective means of understanding behavioral trend of each physician group, and as a tool for building evidence in effective credit scoring models. Finally, comorbidity is associated with deteriorating health outcomes, more complex clinical management, and increased healthcare costs. Future research should pay more attention on using HM and other emerging approaches to identify the value of health services planning and financing in such increasingly complex cases.

REFERENCES

Balakrishnan, P. V., Cooper, M. C., Jacob, V. S., & Lewis, P. A. (1996). Comparative performance of the FSCL neural net and k-means algorithm for market segmentation. *European Journal of Operational Research*, *93*(2), 346–357. doi:10.1016/0377-2217(96)00046-X

Bohanec, M., Zupan, B., & Rajkovic, V. (2000). Applications of qualitative multiattribute decision models in health care. *International Journal of Medical Informatics*, *58*, 191–205. doi:10.1016/S1386-5056(00)00087-3 PMID:10978921

Cabena, P. et al.. (1997). *Discovering Data Mining: From Concept to Implementation*. Prentice Hall.

Chae, Y. M., Ho, S. H., Cho, K. W., Lee, D. H., & Ji, S. H. (2001). Data mining approach to policy analysis in a health insurance domain. *International Journal of Medical Informatics*, *62*(2), 103–111. doi:10.1016/S1386-5056(01)00154-X PMID:11470613

Chen, M. C., & Huang, S. H. (2003). Credit scoring and rejected instances reassigning through evolutionary computation techniques. *Expert Systems with Applications, 24*(4), 433–441. doi:10.1016/S0957-4174(02)00191-4

Chen, T. C., & Tsao, H. L. (2009). Using a hybrid meta-evolutionary rule mining approach as a classification response model. *Expert Systems with Applications, 36*(2), 1999–2007. doi:10.1016/j.eswa.2007.12.050

Chen, Y., & Cheng, C. (2012). Identifying the medical practice after total hip arthroplasty using an integrated hybrid approach. *Computers in Biology and Medicine, 42*(8), 826–840. doi:10.1016/j.compbiomed.2012.06.006 PMID:22795228

Chen, Y., Yeh, H.-Y., Wu, J.-C., Haschler, I., Chen, T.-J., & Wetter, T. (2010). Taiwans national health insurance research database: Administrative health care database as study object. *Scientometrics, 86*(2), 365–380. doi:10.1007/s11192-010-0289-2

Cheng, T. (2009). Lessons from Taiwans universal national health insurance: A conversation with Taiwans health minister Ching-Chuan Yeh. *Health Affairs, 28*(4), 1035–1044. doi:10.1377/hlthaff.28.4.1035

Cheng, T. (2015). Reflections on the 20th anniversary of Taiwans single-payer national health insurance system. *Health Affairs, 34*(3), 502–510. doi:10.1377/hlthaff.2014.1332 PMID:25732502

Chu, B. H., Tsai, M. S., & Ho, C.-S. (2007). Toward a hybrid data mining model for customer retention. *Knowledge-Based Systems, 20*(8), 703–718. doi:10.1016/j.knosys.2006.10.003

Siami, M., & Hajimohammadi, Z. (2013). Credit scoring in banks and financial institutions via data mining techniques: A literature review. *Journal of AI and Data Mining, 1*(2), 119–129.

Durairaj, M., & Ranjani, V. (2013). Data mining applications in healthcare sector: A study. *International Journal of Scientific and Technology Research, 2*(10), 29–35.

Ebadati, E. O. M., & Tabrizi, M. M. (2016). A hybrid clustering technique to improve big data accessibility based on machine learning approaches. In *Information Systems Design and Intelligent Applications* (pp. 413-423).

Gupta, G. K. (2014). *Introduction to Data Mining with Case Studies*. PHI Learning Pvt. Ltd.

Hachesu, P., Ahmadi, M., Alizadeh, S., & Sadoughi, F. (2013). Use of data mining techniques to determine and predict length of stay of cardiac patients. *Healthcare Informatics Research, 19*(2), 121–129. doi:10.4258/hir.2013.19.2.121 PMID:23882417

Han, J., Kamber, H., & Pei, J. (2012). *Data Mining: Concepts and Techniques*. Morgan Kaufmann Publishers. doi:10.1007/978-1-4419-1428-6_3752

Hsieh, N. (2005). Hybrid mining approach in the design of credit scoring model. *Expert Systems with Applications, 28*(4), 655–665. doi:10.1016/j.eswa.2004.12.022

Huang, C., & Wang, C. (2006). A GA-based feature selection and parameters optimization for support vector machines. *Expert Systems with Applications, 31*(2), 231–240. doi:10.1016/j.eswa.2005.09.024

Jay, N., Nuemi, G., Gadreau, M., & Quantin, C. (2013). A data mining approach for grouping and analyzing trajectories of care using claim data: The example of breast cancer. *BMC Medical Informatics and Decision Making*, *13*(1), 130. doi:10.1186/1472-6947-13-130 PMID:24289668

Joudaki, H. et al.. (2015). Using data mining to detect health care fraud and abuse: A review of literature. *Global Journal of Health Science*, *7*(1), 194–202. PMID:25560347

Kao, Y. T., Zahara, E., & Kao, I. W. (2008). A hybridized approach to data clustering. *Expert Systems with Applications*, *34*(3), 1754–1762. doi:10.1016/j.eswa.2007.01.028

Kuo, R., Ho, L., & Hu, C. (2002). Integration of self-organizing feature map and k-means algorithm for market segmentation. *Computers & Operations Research*, *29*(11), 1475–1493. doi:10.1016/S0305-0548(01)00043-0

Kuo, R., Lina, S., & Shihb, C. (2007). Mining association rules through integration of clustering analysis and ant colony system for health insurance database in Taiwan. *Expert Systems with Applications*, *33*(3), 794–808. doi:10.1016/j.eswa.2006.08.035

Lee, T., & Chen, I. (2005). A two-stage hybrid credit scoring model using artificial neural networks and multivariate adaptive regression splines. *Expert Systems with Applications*, *28*(4), 743–752. doi:10.1016/j.eswa.2004.12.031

Lee, T., Chiu, C.-C., Lu, C.-J., & Chen, I.-F. (2002). Credit scoring using the hybrid neural discriminant technique. *Expert Systems with Applications*, *23*(3), 245–254. doi:10.1016/S0957-4174(02)00044-1

Lee, T., Liu, C.-Y., Kuo, Y.-H., Mills, M. E., Fong, J.-G., & Hung, C. (2011). Application of data mining to the identification of critical factors in patient falls using a web-based reporting system. *International Journal of Medical Informatics*, *80*(2), 141–150. doi:10.1016/j.ijmedinf.2010.10.009 PMID:21115393

Lee, W. I., Shih, B. Y., & Chung, Y. S. (2008). The exploration of consumers behavior in choosing hospital by the application of neural network. *Expert Systems with Applications*, *34*(2), 806–816. doi:10.1016/j.eswa.2006.10.020

Lin, K., & Yeh, C. (2012). Use of data mining techniques to detect medical fraud in health insurance. *International Journal of Engineering and Technology Innovation*, *2*(2), 126–137.

Lin, Y., Chen, Y., Hu, S., Chen, H., Chen, J., & Yang, S. (2013). Identifying core herbal treatments for urticarial using Taiwans nationwide prescription database. *Journal of Ethnopharmacology*, *148*(2), 556–562. doi:10.1016/j.jep.2013.04.052 PMID:23684721

National Health Insurance Administration. (2015). National Health Insurance Annual Report.

Payton, F. C. (2003). *Data Mining in Health Care Applications*. IGI Publishing. doi:10.4018/978-1-59140-051-6.ch015

Reinhardt, U. E. (2008). Humbled in Taiwan. *British Medical Journal*, *336*(7635), 72. doi:10.1136/bmj.39450.473380.0F PMID:18187722

Rupink, R., Kukar, M., & Krisper, M. (2007). Integrating data mining and decision support through data mining based decision support system. *Journal of Computer Information Systems*, (Spring), 89–104.

Shin, H., Park, H., Lee, J., & Jhee, W. C. (2012). A scoring model to detect abusive billing patterns in health insurance claims. *Expert Systems with Applications, 39*(8), 7441–7450. doi:10.1016/j.eswa.2012.01.105

Sliver, M., Sakata, T., Su, H.C., Herman, C., Dolins, S.B., & O'Shea, M.J. (2001). Data mining techniques in a healthcare data warehouse. *Journal of Healthcare Information Management, 15*(2), 155–164. PMID:11452577

Srinivasan, B., & Pavya, K. (2016). A study on data mining prediction techniques in healthcare sector. *International Research Journal of Engineering and Technology, 3*(3), 552–556.

Syed-Abdul, S., Nguyen, A., Huang, F., Jian, W.-S., Iqbal, U., Yang, V., & Li, Y.-C. et al. (2014). A smart medication recommendation model for the electronic prescription. *Computer Methods and Programs in Biomedicine, 117*(2), 218–224. doi:10.1016/j.cmpb.2014.06.019 PMID:25092226

Tan, J., Wen, H. J., & Awad, N. (2005). Health Care & Services Delivery Systems as Complex Adaptive Systems: Examining Chaos Theory in Action. *Communications of the ACM, 48*(5), 36–44. doi:10.1145/1060710.1060737

West, D. (2000). Neural network credit scoring models. *Computers & Operations Research, 27*(11-12), 1131–1152. doi:10.1016/S0305-0548(99)00149-5

Yang, W. S., & Hwang, S. Y. (2006). A process-mining framework for the detection of healthcare fraud and abuse. *Expert Systems with Applications, 31*(1), 56–68. doi:10.1016/j.eswa.2005.09.003

ZahidHassan S. & Verma., B. (2007). A hybrid data mining approach for knowledge extraction and classification in medical databases. *Proceeding of the Seventh International Conference on Intelligent Systems Design and Applications* (pp. 503-510).

This research was previously published in the International Journal of Healthcare Information Systems and Informatics (IJHISI), 12(4); edited by Joseph Tan, pages 31-51, copyright year 2017 by IGI Publishing (an imprint of IGI Global).

Chapter 36
Interoperability in Healthcare

Luciana Cardoso
Minho University, Portugal

Fernando Marins
Minho University, Portugal

César Quintas
Centro Hospitalar do Porto, Portugal

Filipe Portela
Minho University, Portugal

Manuel Santos
Minho University, Portugal

António Abelha
Minho University, Portugal

José Machado
Minho University, Portugal

ABSTRACT

With the advancement of technology, patient information has been being computerized in order to facilitate the work of healthcare professionals and improve the quality of healthcare delivery. However, there are many heterogeneous information systems that need to communicate, sharing information and making it available when and where it is needed. To respond to this requirement the Agency for Integration, Diffusion, and Archiving of medical information (AIDA) was created, a multi-agent and service-based platform that ensures interoperability among healthcare information systems. In order to improve the performance of the platform, beyond the SWOT analysis performed, a system to prevent failures that may occur in the platform database and also in machines where the agents are executed was created. The system has been implemented in the Centro Hospitalar do Porto (one of the major Portuguese hospitals), and it is now possible to define critical workload periods of AIDA, improving high availability and load balancing. This is explored in this chapter.

DOI: 10.4018/978-1-5225-3926-1.ch036

INTRODUCTION

In healthcare, information systems have been growing, and consequently the volume, complexity and criticism of data become more and more difficult to manage. However, despite these systems contribute increasing the quality of healthcare delivery, information sources are distributed, ubiquitous, heterogeneous, large and complex and the Health Information Systems (HIS) need to communicate in order to share information and to make it available at any place at any time. Data are stored in multiple independent structures. Therefore it emerges the need to create a global system that brings together all the islands of information shared between services. It is necessary to develop a solid and efficient process of integration and interoperation that must take into consideration scalability, flexibility, portability and security.

Several methodologies presently exist to implement interoperable information systems in healthcare; it results in several common communication architectures and mainstream standards such as Health Level 7 (HL7). However, several concerns regarding the distribution, fault tolerance, standards, communication and tightly bound systems still exist broadly throughout the healthcare area. The multi-agent paradigm has been an interesting technology in the area of *interoperability*; it addresses many of such limitations (Miranda et al., 2012; Miranda, Machado, Abelha, & Neves, 2013).

The homogeneity of clinical, medical and administrative systems is not possible due to financial and technical restrictions, as well as functional needs. The solution is to integrate, diffuse and archive this information under a dynamic framework, in order to share this knowledge with every information system that needs it. So *AIDA – Agency for Interoperation, diffusion and Archive of Medical Information* is presented. AIDA is an agency that supplies intelligent electronic workers called proactive agents, in charge of some tasks, such as communicating with the heterogeneous systems, sending and receiving information (e.g., medical or clinical reports, images, collections of data, prescriptions), managing and saving the information and answering to information requests (J Machado et al., 2010; Miranda, Duarte, Abelha, Machado, & Neves, 2010; Peixoto, Santos, Abelha, & Machado, 2012).

With the growing importance of HIS, databases became indispensable tools for day-to-day tasks in healthcare units. They store important and confidential information about patient's clinical status and about the other hospital services. Thus, they must be permanently available, reliable and at high performance. In many healthcare units, fault tolerant systems are used. They ensure the availability, reliability and disaster recovery of data. However, these mechanisms do not allow the prediction or prevention of faults. In this context, the necessity of developing a *fault forecasting* system emerges. It is necessary to monitor database performance to verify the normal workload and adapt a forecasting model used in medicine into the database context. Based on percentiles a scale to represent the severity of situations was created (Silva et al., 2012).

The AIDA was implemented at Centro Hospitalar do Porto (CHP), in Portugal, and was subjected to Strengths, Weaknesses, Opportunities, and Threats (SWOT) analysis in order to ascertain what can be change to improve the system. This analysis can reveal what are the great strengths of the system as well as its major pitfalls. In addition, the opportunities than can be taken as advantages are highlighted and the key threats to the system are alerted (Pereira, Salazar, Abelha, & Machado, 2013).

The main goal of this chapter is to explain the importance of interoperability in the context of the quality healthcare delivery. In the background section a brief introduction about interoperability and its importance in the healthcare environment. The *intelligent agents* in interoperability section present a promising technology for interoperability implementation, namely the multi-agent technology. Combining the issues mentioned in the previous sections, a solution, the AIDA platform, is presented. In its section its architecture as well as its database is described. In order to improve AIDA performance, in the following sections fault forecasting systems are presented either from a database or from machines, which execute AIDA agents. The database, machines and agents' workload are also presented and discussed in these sections. In the last section the strengths, weaknesses, opportunities and threats of AIDA are analysed.

BACKGROUND

HIS around the world are in rapid transition, moving from the traditional, paper-based practices to computerized processes and systems to ensure the delivery of health care and improve the quality of the services (Weber-Jahnke, Peyton, & Topaloglou, 2012). The healthcare domain, specifically HIS have been a very attractive domain for Computer Science researchers and it is facing a growing number of challenges. HIS are at the heart of all these challenges. They can provide a better coordination among medical professionals and facilities, thus reducing the number and incidence of medical errors. At the same time, they can reduce healthcare costs and may provide a means to improve the management of hospitals (Palazzo et al., 2013).

HIS provide a composed environment of complex information systems, heterogeneous, distributed and ubiquitous, speaking different languages, integrating medical equipment and customized by different entities, which in turn were set by different people aiming at different goals. Everyday new applications are developed to assist physicians in their work, but those systems are built in "silos" and they have a little impact on their environment constituting isolated information islands, that limit the flow of information, while lack the ability to interact and communicate with other systems (Miranda et al., 2012; Palazzo et al., 2013; Peixoto et al., 2012; Weber-Jahnke et al., 2012).

The possibility and the need of communication are one of the main characteristics of the human beings. Similarly the HIS need to communicate and cooperate in order to enhance their overall performance and usefulness, to improve HIS, quality of the diagnosis, but mainly, to improve the quality in patient treatment. Cooperation and exchange of data and information is indeed one of the most relevant features, is the essence for the optimisation of existing resources and the improvement of the decision making process through consolidation, verification and dissemination of information (Miranda et al., 2012).

The perception of integration and interoperation must be introduced into this environment. Integration aims to gather and acquire information of distinct systems in order to reinforce or strengthen them, while interoperation concentrates on the continuous communication and exchange of information across cooperative systems. Therefore, the concept of *interoperability* has been presented; there is no definition for this term, however it can be said that interoperability is the ability of independent systems to exchange meaningful information and initiate actions from each other, in order to operate together for mutual benefit (Miranda et al., 2010). The main goal of interoperability in healthcare is to connect applications and data can be shared and exchanged across the healthcare environment and distributed to medical staff or patients whenever and wherever they need it. Interoperability is no longer a technological option, it is a fundamental requirement for delivering effective care and ensuring the health and well-being of million of patients world-wide (Rogers, Peres, & Müller, 2010).

Motivation

In the last decades interoperability and the respective implications for the delivery of healthcare has been a topic of study, and in 2003 it was found that the level of interoperability between systems in most health institutions was extremely low (Carr & Moore, 2003).

However, since 1987 the *Health Level Seven International (HL7)* was founded. It is a non-profit organization, which the main goal is providing a comprehensive framework and related standards for the exchange, integration, sharing, and retrieval of electronic health information that supports clinical practice and the management, delivery and evaluation of health services. HL7 provides standards for interoperability with multiple objectives like the improvement of care delivery, the optimization of the daily workflow, the reduction of ambiguity and the improving of knowledge exchange between all stakeholders (HL7, 2012).

There has been an intensive effort to develop standards adapted and optimized towards improving healthcare delivery. These standards have been able to give a definite structure or shape to low level interoperability in healthcare, in a firmly established and modular manner. Among these patterns HL7 is considered the most adaptable one in healthcare interoperability. HL7 started as a mainly syntactic healthcare oriented communication protocol at the application layer, the seventh layer of the Open Systems Interconnect (OSI) communication model. The initial versions of the protocol defined the message structure by loosely connected healthcare applications, and by classifying the different types of messages involved in this environment with the aggregation of standardized segments. It was uniquely syntactic, and according to the general models of interoperation is one of the lowest levels of this process. In the current version, the HL7 is focused on semantic interoperability, including the appropriate use of exchanging information in the sense of the communicating application's behaviour. This model contains relations and metadata in an abstract level that may enable far higher levels of integration, namely semantic interoperability and validation of exchanged information, using the relational mapping of each artefact (Miranda et al., 2012, 2010).

Interoperability in Electronic Health Record

Nowadays information technologies in medicine and healthcare are experiencing a difficult situation in which each staff person uses in the daily work a set of independent technologies that involve huge sets of information. This independence may be the cause of difficulty in *interoperability* between information systems. The overload of information systems within a healthcare facility may lead to problems in accessing the total information needed.

HIS have gained great importance and have grown in quality and quantity. With this information overload, it is necessary to infer what information is relevant to be registered in the Electronic Health Record (EHR) and Decision Support Systems (DSS) must allow for reasoning with incomplete, ambiguous and uncertain knowledge (Peixoto et al., 2012). The EHR is a core application which covers horizontally the healthcare unit and makes possible a transverse analysis of medical records along the services, units or treated pathologies, bringing to the healthcare area new methodologies for problem solving, computational models, technologies and tools.

Due to the complexity of each HIS, the possibility of a global information system emerges as something complex and incomplete. However, the need to gather significant information to be shared with other services and to communicate all relevant data related to the patient and the executed procedures, is not only of high value to the institutions, but also to the patient. In order to aggregate and consolidate all significant information, a solid and efficient process of interoperation or integration must be developed. This process must take into consideration scalability, flexibility, portability and security when applied to EHR. The complexity and sensitivity of the exchanged information require more than technological efficiency and pragmatic exchange of information. The dissemination of incoherent information and its introduction into the EHR may cause more than inconsistent records, and they may give rise to a wrong diagnose. In order to avoid this moral and ethical drawback a thorough validation of the exchanged and integrated information must be performed. The development of top-level interoperability frameworks is henceforth of an intrinsic nature or indispensable quality of the healthcare environment. The multitude and intricacy of services that must be performed by the EHR and Group Decision Support Systems (GDSS) require such a framework or otherwise would be inefficiently intertwined with other essential solutions (Miranda et al., 2010).

INTELLIGENT AGENTS IN INTEROPERABILITY

There is a variety of methodologies and architectures through which it is possible to implement interoperability between HIS. These methodologies are based on common communication architectures and standards such as HL7. However, there are still some concerns about the distribution, fault tolerance, and communication standards. The multi-agent technology has stood out in the area of *interoperability*, including interoperability in healthcare, addressing the concerns mentioned above.

This technology is closely related to the basic concepts that define a distributed architecture. The agent-based computing has been vaunted for its ability to solve problems and/or as a new revolution in the development and analysis of software. The agent-based systems are not only a promising technology, it is becoming as a new way of thinking, a conceptual paradigm for analysing problems and develop systems in order to solve problems related to the complexity, distribution and interactivity. Although there is no accepted definition for agent, it can be said that agents are understood as computational artifacts that exhibit certain properties such as (Jose Machado, Abelha, Novais, Neves, & Neves, 2010):

- **Autonomy:** The ability to act without direct intervention from peers, more specifically humans;
- **Reactivity:** Capacity for integration into an environment, perceive through sensors and acting to certain stimuli;
- **Pro-Activity:** Ability to solve intelligent problems as planning their own activities in order to achieve their goals;
- **Social, Emotional and Moral Behaviour:** Ability to interact with other agents and even change their behaviour in response to this interaction. They can communicate through constructs and protocols of low or high level, as well as means of addressing and direct communication. They can cooperate to achieve a certain common goal, as well as their individual goals, i.e. they must have the ability to negotiate with other agents.

In view of the above-described property, agents can be defined as autonomous and problem-solving computational entities capable of effective operation in dynamic and open environments. They are often deployed in environments in which they interact, and maybe cooperate with other agents that have possibly conflicting goals (Luck, McBurney, & Preist, 2003).

Agent-based software should be robust, scalable and secure. To achieve this, the architectures must allow compliant agents to discover each other, communicate and offer a service to one another. These architectures go beyond the capabilities of the typical distributed object oriented programming techniques and tools (Contreras, Germán, Chi, & Sheremetov, 2004).

Multi-Agent Systems for Interoperability

Multi-agent systems (MAS) offer a new and often more appropriate way of development of complex systems, especially in open and dynamic environments. Some key features of the agent technology support these capabilities. The autonomy and pro-activeness features of an agent allow it to plan and perform tasks defined to accomplish the design objectives. The social abilities enable an agent to interact in MAS and cooperate or complete fulfilling its goals. The MAS can be considered as a rich and highly adaptable technology with a keen interest in the area of *interoperability* among HIS (Jose Machado et al., 2010).

To develop these systems specification standard methods are required, and it is believed that one of the characteristics for its high acceptability and recommendation is simplicity. In fact, the use of *intelligent agents* to simulate human decision-making in the medical field offers the potential for software suitable for the development and practical analysis and design methodologies that do not distinguish between agents and humans. These systems can provide skill and effectiveness to monitor the behaviour of its own officers, with a significant impact on the process of acquiring and validating knowledge, i.e. MAS is aware of the evolution process of intelligent systems and it is capable of accomplishing actions, which usually are performed by human beings, as replace elements or delegate tasks.

The MAS is able to manage the entire life cycle of the agent, the availability of the modules of the HIS as a whole, keeping all agents freely distributed. New agents with the same characteristics and objectives can be created through the MAS depending on the needs of the system in which they are inserted. The structure of these agents and the MAS can be developed according to the services they provide and the logical functionality of systems that interact with them.

The agents in a healthcare facility configure applications or utilities that collect information in the organization. Once collected, this information can be provided directly to other entities, e.g. a doctor or to a server, stored in a file or sent by e-mail to someone (J Machado et al., 2010).

HL7 Services in the Multi-Agent System

The *HL7* standard plays an essential role in the implementation of interoperability, in the development of exchange of medical information, the standardization of medical documents into eXtensible Markup Language (XML) structures and vocabulary specification for rugged use in messages and documents. Although health informatics standards like HL7 are completely distinct from agent communication standards, HL7 services can be also implemented under the agent paradigm.

These agents based on HL7 services can communicate with services that follow different paradigms and communicate with other agents that use both the HL7 as communication agents. Although the HL7 standard can be implemented using other architectures, agent-based solutions enjoy a wide *interoperability* capability, being able to be integrated with the specific behaviours. These behaviours may become more effective if they use the machine learning paradigm and other artificial intelligence (AI) techniques in order to adapt to the environment and be able to avoid errors and correct the flow of information and knowledge extraction within the institution.

As mentioned previously, the HL7 standard does not limit its use to any technology or architecture; however, it aims to use regular communications between health systems oriented. There are, obviously, architectures and technologies that have become the most used, but the ones that stand out are those that are present by default in the information systems of specific equipment to perform various diagnostic methods.

However, in the process of communication and exchange of information, we cannot only worry about information systems, although information exchange with the devices is increasingly important. These devices usually communicate through loosely associated standards, i.e. directly with the information system (e.g., Medical imaging Information System, Cardiology Information System) or proprietary systems that may or may not be consistent with other information systems. This type of equipment usually follows a client - server architecture in which the equipment is in most cases only a client. So, it is understandable that there is considerable difficulty in establishing a system of uniformly understanding and fully communicating with all services within a hospital. Even with the adoption of standards, specifically HL7, different flavourings usually require distinct handling of the messages and its events. To resolve this situation, the solution is to refer to the use of agents that enable creating specific behaviours or agents that adapt to any situation by keeping all coupled systems (Miranda et al., 2012).

THE AGENCY FOR INTEGRATION, DIFFUSION AND ARCHIVE OF MEDICAL INFORMATION (AIDA)

Medical informatics is an area supported by two basic sciences, the Computer Science and the Health Sciences, which contributes to the improvement of quality in the provision of health services as it aims to better management of information resources and health. As mentioned in the previous sections, the interaction and communication based on specific protocols are fundamental to the successful implementation, execution and / or management of any HIS. Actually the HIS have to be described as a wide variety of distributed and heterogeneous systems that speak different languages, integrate medical equipment, are customized by different companies, which in turn were developed by different people aimed at different goals. This leads us to consider the solution(s) for a particular problem, part of a process of integration of different information sources, using different protocols through an *Agency for Integration, Diffusion and Archive (AIDA)* medical information, bringing health care methodologies to solve problems in medical education, computational models, tools and technologies (Duarte et al., 2010).

AIDA is a platform developed to allow the dissemination and integration of information generated in a healthcare environment. This platform includes many different integration capabilities; primarily uses Service Oriented Architectures (SOA) and *Multi-Agent Systems* (MAS) to implement interoperability, in accordance with standards, comprising of all service providers within a health institution (Miranda et al., 2010).

This platform, designed to ensure *interoperability* between the HIS, and is characterized by electronic appliances providing intelligent workers, here understood as software agents, which have a pro-active behaviour and are responsible for tasks such as communication between different sub-systems, sending and receiving information (e.g., clinical or medical reports, images, data collections, prescriptions), management and economics of information and responding to requests, with the necessary resources to carry them out correctly and timely. The main objectives are, as the name implies, integrating, disseminating and archiving large data sets from various sources (i.e., departments, services, units, computers, medical equipment, etc.). However this platform also provides tools to implement and facilitate communication with humans through Web-based services, i.e., the construction of AIDA follows the acceptance of simplicity, common objectives and addressing responsibilities (Duarte et al., 2010; Peixoto et al., 2012).

AIDA Architecture

Figure 1 shows the architecture where one can observe that AIDA is the central element in a healthcare environment, which ensures interoperability and communication between the following systems:

- **The Electronic Medical Record (EHR):** A kind of repository of information on the study of the health of an individual subject of care, in a format that can be processed by computer, stored and transmitted from a secure and accessible by multiple authorized users;
- **The Administrative Information System (AIS):** Seeks to represent, manage and archive the administrative information during the episode. The episode is a collection of all the operations assigned to a patient from start to the end of the treatment;
- **The Medical Information System (MIS):** Seeks to represent, manage and archive clinical information during the episode;
- **The Nursing Information System (NIS):** Seeks to represent and manage archive information on nursing practices during the episode;
- **The Information Systems of all Departments and Services (DIS):** In particular Laboratories (Labs), *Radiology Information System* (RIS) and Medical Imaging (PACS - Picture Archive and Communication System), which handles images standard DICOM format.

Figure 1. AIDA architecture

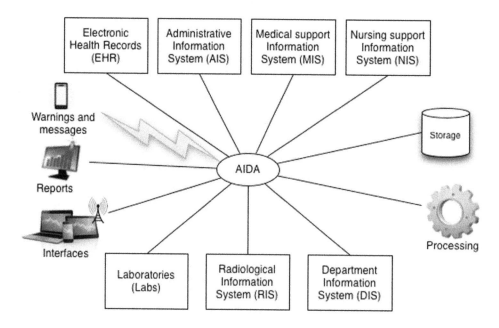

The presented architecture was expected to support medical applications and has the form of intelligent information processing Web systems. Its functional roles and information flowing among them are controlled with adjustable autonomy.

Health professionals gather information and its value is stored and distributed automatically to where it is needed. Every document created within a specialized service honouring certain rules, is kept closer to different departments. The coding tools and ordering are very useful for connecting different data to a particular problem, as the encoded data are very easy to access by AI based decision support systems. The built-in electronic sorting can be used not only for medical equipment or pharmacological prescriptions, but also for the acquisition of laboratory results and study images that are out of service at the origin. Furthermore, it can allow the centralization of exam display, thus allowing the results from different services sharing the same interface, improving the quality of service.

There are also different access permissions when dealing with medical data. Although they can only be viewed by authorized personnel, starting from any terminal within the health unit to even the laptop or PDA. Personal access must be flexible in order to allow professionals to access when needed. Medical information is so important in terms of privacy as well as in terms of significance. The messaging system allows creating, sending and receiving messages online. It can be very useful for the treatment of data, images or even to exchange files (Peixoto et al., 2012).

AIDA as a Multi-Agent System

Considering the previous sections it can be noted that the AIDA platform is a pure communication MAS, i.e., there is no external environment influence and the agents only communicate with each other via messages. However AIDA contains different types of agents:

- **The Proxy Agents (PAs):** Provide the bridges between users and the system in terms of questions that can be explained;, decisions may have to be taken and / or visualization of the results. The system interfaces are based on Web-related front-ends using Hypermedia pages that can be accessed through a standard Web browser;
- **The Decision Agents (DAs):** Provide mediation capacities, acting by accepting a task of PAs. They can break down tasks into sub-tasks, sending them to be processed by the CAs, later integrating the results (returned by CAs);
- **The Computing Agents (CAs):** Accept requests of DAs specific tasks, returning the results;
- **The Resource Agents (RAs):** Have all the knowledge needed to access a specific information resource;
- **The Interaction and Explanation Agents (IEAs):** Act on the basis of argumentative processes that are fed with data and / or knowledge from both the PA and the DAs. Note that the plans received by the DAs may be partial; in that mode, only after the completion of a task, a trace can be compiled and an application can be delivered to the APs and / or DAs (Jose Machado et al., 2010).

AIDA Database

Over the years, organizations have increased use of databases and today they are considered essential for everyday tasks (Godinho, 2011). Particularly in healthcare units, databases have a vital role, since they store very important information about the patients' clinical status, administrative information and other relevant information for the healthcare services. Therefore, it is crucial to ensure the availability, reliability, confidence and safety of databases. As a result, they must have the following characteristics (Bertino & Sandhu, 2005; Drake et al., 2005; A. Rodrigues, 2005):

- **Confidentiality:** The database must have mechanisms to prevent intruders, so that unauthorized persons cannot access and publicize the data stored (Bertino & Sandhu, 2005; Kim et al., 2010; A. Rodrigues, 2005);
- **Integrity:** The database must have mechanisms that prevent modification of data by unauthorized persons. Thus, it is possible to keep the information from the database incorruptible and inviolable (Bertino & Sandhu, 2005; Kim et al., 2010; A. Rodrigues, 2005);
- **Availability:** The databases must have mechanisms to access the required information in time. In addition, they should have mechanisms for fault prevention and tolerance, so that the system will thereby be able to continue operating despite the failure of any component not affecting the normal operation of the organization (Bertino & Sandhu, 2005; A. Rodrigues, 2005).

In healthcare units, it is important for databases to be available twenty-four hours a day, seven days per week, because the information is vital for solving the patients' problems and for hospital management. For this reason, it is essential to ensure the integrity and permanent availability of data even in the presence of faults (Godinho, 2011).

To achieve these goals, fault tolerance mechanisms based on the data or components redundancy are used. The main databases of CHP – including AIDA - are based on an Oracle Real Application Cluster (RAC) System. This mechanism is provided by Oracle for improving the availability and scalability of databases. A RAC system is composed by a shared database witch can be accessed through the server/computer that contains a database instance and an ASM (Automatic Storage Management) instance. In this way, it is possible access to the database across multiple servers (Ashdown & Kyte, 2011; Drake et al., 2005; Strohm, 2012).

In AIDA database, there is also another fault tolerance mechanism: a data guard solution. This mechanism consists in one or more standby databases (replicas of the original database), which should be in different places. In this way, when the master database is unavailable the replica can be used in read-only mode. It is essential that the master and the standby databases are synchronized and access is read-only during the recovering (Godinho, 2011). The Figure 2 presents the complete architecture of AIDA database with these two mechanisms.

DATABASE WORKLOAD AND FAULT FORECASTING IN THE AIDA DATABASE

The fault tolerant system adapted to AIDA database mentioned in the Section AIDA Database ensures the availability, reliability and disaster recovery of data. However, these mechanisms do not allow the prediction or prevention of faults. In this context, it emerges the necessity of developing a *fault forecasting* system. To achieve this goal it is essential to monitor database performance, verify the normal workload and then adapt a forecasting model to the database context.

Figure 2. AIDA Database Architecture with RAC and data guard solution systems

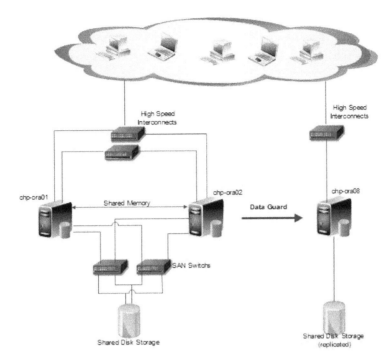

Monitoring Database Performance

The use of monitoring systems by organizations has been growing not only because they are useful to diagnose faults but also because they can help to ensure data security (Nair, 2008). Monitoring is not a simple process, and its complexity increases as it becomes necessary to monitor various components and systems with complex architectures. However, with the Oracle Systems it is possible to take advantage of several tools to help in this process. The performance views are one of these tools that enable to consult useful information for monitoring. The content of these views is refreshed periodically (Chan, 2008; Rich, 2013).

There are several statistics that can be used to characterize the behaviour of the database. According to the objective of preventing faults related to the resource limitation, some of them have been selected to monitor the following statistics (Chan, 2008; Godinho, 2011; Ramos, 2007):

- **DB Time:** Is the time elapsing between the instant of placing of the query by the user to the reception of all results, this time should be the lowest possible. In Oracle systems, this time is a sum of total time (including CPU time, IO time, Wait time) spent on all requests from users. Therefore it is a good indicator of the workload of the system. Typically, this time increases with the number of simultaneous users or applications, but it may also increase due to other system problems (Dias, Ramacher, Shaft, Venkataramani, & Wood, 2005; Godinho, 2011).

- **Numbers of Transactions:** Transactions are indivisible sequences of operations that perform some work on the database. A greater number of transactions can indicate more work. In Oracle databases, the number of transactions can be obtained by adding up the values of statistics "user commits" and "user rollbacks" since each transaction always ends with a "commit" command and any undo operation as a "rollback" command (Godinho, 2011; Schumacher, 2003; Shallahamer, 2007).

- **Number of Executions:** One transaction consists of set of operations in the database depending one the query. It is important to collect information about the number of operations because it may be the case that there are few transactions but many operations. In Oracle databases this information can be obtained by collecting, the "execute count" statistic (Shallahamer, 2007).

- **Calls Ratio (RC):** Ratio between recursive calls and total calls. A recursive call occurs when a user request needs one query SQL that needs another SQL query. The total of calls is the sum of recursive calls and user calls (when a user request can be resolved through a single SQL query). Ideally this ratio should be as low as possible, since the high number of recursive calls can indicate problems with the design of tables or an excessive amount of triggers running at the same time. This ratio can be calculated by the equation (Rich, 2013):

$$RC = \frac{recursive\,Calls}{\left(recursive\,Calls + user\,Calls\right)}$$

- **Number of Current Logons:** Each logon, i.e., session is associated with a piece of memory, so many simultaneous sessions can cause problems. Note that the number of logons does not represent the number of users because each user may have multiple sessions. In Oracle systems, the number of sessions can be obtained by statistic "logons current" (Chan, 2008).

- **Processor Utilization:** It is necessary to constantly monitor its utilization because it is one of the most important database components. Low values of processor utilization may indicate problems at the level of I/O. If the values are too high, it can compromise the functioning of the database. The percentage of utilization can be obtained thought a command of the operating system (Chan, 2008).

- **Memory Utilization:** The memory is a key component to the speed of the database systems. Depending on the data location the access speed changes. If the data is in memory, speed is greater. However, if the data is on disk, the access velocity is lower. This statistic is also accessible through the operating system commands (Schumacher, 2003).

- **Size of Redo File:** Represents the amount of redo entries (Kbytes). The redo files are used to store information about changes made to the database. An increase in the size of these files, indicates a higher number of operations and therefore a higher database load (Rich, 2013).

- **Buffer Cache Ratio (BC):** This ratio shows the percentage of data that is in memory cache, rather than in the disk. Normally, the BC is very high, so it is necessary to pay attention if BC decreases, this may indicate a lack of memory problems. BC can be calculated:

$$BC = \frac{\left(1 - physical\,Reads\right)}{\left(consistent\,Gets + block\,Gets\right) \times 100}$$

- **Amount of I/O Requests:** The I/O operations need a long time to process. A large number of these operations can indicate memory problems and frequent access to disc (Chan, 2008).
- **Amount of Redo Space Requests:** Indicates the lack of space to write in the buffer. Some delays may occur because it is necessary to write some data to disk to release memory. This can happen due to a poorly sized buffer, or excess entries generated simultaneously.
- **Volume of Network Traffic:** The network that interconnects all the components of the database. Therefore, the network is very important for database performance. If a volume of the network is increasing greatly, the database can be slow and compromise users' requests (Chan, 2008).

Modified Early Warning Score

In medicine, a model called the Modified Early Warning Score (MEWS), has been used for the prediction, in advance, of serious health problems. This model uses a decision table, like the Table 1, to evaluate the clinical status of the patient according to the monitoring of patients' vital signs. The set of these values represents the clinical status of the patient. (Albino & Jacinto, 2009; Gardner-Thorpe, Love, Wrightson, Walsh, & Keeling, 2006; Subbe, Kruger, Rutherford, & Gemmel, 2001).

Normally, if any of the parameters have a score equal to two, the patient must be in observation. In case, the sum of scores is equal to four, or an increase of two values, the patient requires urgent medical attention. In a more extreme situation, if a patient has a score higher than four, he is at risk of life (Devaney & Lead, 2011; Subbe et al., 2001).

Score Table

To evaluate the behaviour of the database it is essential to study its normal workload. So, after collecting the values of the statistics mentioned in the previous subsection during a month, it was possible to evaluate the state of the database based on percentiles and classifying the state through a decision table (Table 2). The statistics collected about the database (as mentioned in a previous section) are evaluated individually through the score table. Depending on the value of the deviation, abnormal situations are assigned granted scores such as in MEWS.

Table 1. MEWS scores

MEWS Score	3	2	1	0	1	2	3
Temperature (C)		< 35.0	35.1-36.0	36.1-38.0	38.1-38.5	> 38.6	
Heart rate (min⁻¹)		< 40	41-50	51-100	101-110	111-130	> 131
Systolic BP (mmHg)	< 70	71-80	81-100	101-199		> 200	
Respiratory rate (min⁻¹)		< 8		8-14	15-20	21-29	> 30
SPO$_2$	< 85	85-89	90-93	> 94			
Urine output (ml/kg/h)	Nil	< 0.5					
Neurological		New confusion		Alert	Reacting to voice	Reacting to pain	Unresponsive

Table 2. Database severity scores

SCORE	0	1	2	3
Value	< p75	p75-p80	p80-p90	> p90
Severity	Normal	Low Severity	Grave	Critical

According to the scores, two situations can happen: less serious situations wherein the sum of all parameters' score is equal or less than four and serious situations wherein the sum is more than four. The value four was elected because in MEWS the value four also means the limit between less and more serious situations. Furthermore, the system's administrators agreed that this should be the limit. They also agreed that this value may not be e permanent and could be changed. In the first situation a visual warning will be issued on the dashboard responsible for monitoring the system and in the second warnings will be sent (via email) to the database administrator, allowing him to take speedy action to prevent the occurrence of a fault in the database.

New limits are calculated at the end of each day, based on new measurements that are periodically collected.

AIDA Database Workload

The most critical period detected in the AIDA's *database workload* during a normal day in CHP was between 10:00 to 12:00. Three peaks were detected: DB time (6.9 seconds), percentage of processor utilization (32.63%) and number of sessions (941).

Verifying the following points it is possible to verify the average values of several statistics related to AIDA database:

- Transactions per second – 214;
- Percentage of processor utilization – 18;
- Percentage of the memory utilization – 98;
- DB time per second – 6;
- Number of sessions – 681;
- Number of I/O requests per second – 632;
- Number of operations per second – 742;
- Buffer cache ratio – 0.998;
- Number of redo size (KB/s) – 152;
- Recursive calls ratio – 0.14;
- Network traffic volume (bytes/s) – 686 135;
- Redo log space requests per second – 0.55.

It is possible to conclude that AIDA database has a high utilization. The average number of sessions is 681. Furthermore, one can observe that on average about 214 transactions per second are processed, resulting on about 742 operations per second in the database.

Figure 3 presents six graphs for the following metrics: number of sessions, percentage of memory, volume of network traffic, number of transactions, operations and requests for I/O per second. In all these

Figure 3. Extracting results from the monitor dashboard of AIDA

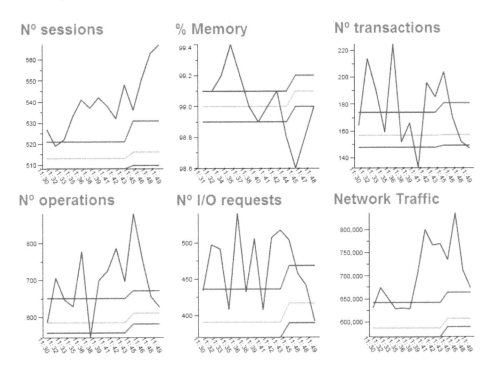

graphs there are four lines, the green corresponds to the 75th percentile, the yellow to the 80th percentile, the red to the 90th percentile and the blue is the value measured every minute. This excerpt was taken from one of the critical periods of the day, verifying that the blue line with some frequency exceeds the limits established by the percentiles indicating the presence of an abnormal situation.

If only considering the last measurement, it shows that the number of sessions and the volume of network traffic are above the 90th percentile, the number of operations per second is above the 80th percentile, and the number of requests for I / O operations is between percentile 75 and 80. The other metrics are in a normal situation, below the 75th percentile. In this case, the sum of the overall score would be 9, which would provide a warning email of abnormality. However, this situation does not cause database fault and for this reason it is necessary to update limits. Limits are updated at the end of the day taking account of all measured values that do not cause a fault, in this way the model improves its ability to represent reality.

It is important to note, that emails are sent only 15 to 15 minutes in order mean values be used to compare; thus avoiding the impact of small variations during the interval.

AGENTS WORKLOAD AND FORECASTING AND DETECTION OF FAULTS IN THE AIDA

Besides monitoring and preventing faults of the database, it is also important to monitor the behaviour of the agents individually as well as the computers they execute their tasks. It is also essential to monitor the agents and computers performance.

Monitoring Agents and Computer Performance

In order to collect information about the performance of the agents and computers the Windows Management Instrumentation (WMI) technology was used. WMI is the Microsoft approach for Web-Based Enterprise Management (WBEM), which is an industry initiative to develop a standard technology for accessing management. WMI uses the Common Information Model (CIM) standard to represent managed components such as systems, applications, networks, devices or even files. CIM is a standard, unified, object-oriented framework for describing physical and logical objects in a managed environment. To provide a common framework, CIM defines a series of objects taking into account a basic set of classes, classifications and associations. WMI objects can be accessed from scripts running either on a local machine or, security permitting, across a network. Besides that, it offers a powerful set of services including the retrieval of information and the event notification system. Furthermore, its utilization is easy because WMI uses a query-based language named Windows Query Language (WQL), which is a subset of the standard SQL (Structured Query Language) (Boshier, 2000; Costa & Silva, 2010; Lavy & Meggitt, 2001).

To characterize the agent performance, three metrics are collected (Microsoft, 2013a, 2013b):

- **Percent Processor Time:** Percentage of elapsed time that all of threads of the agent's process used the processor to execute instructions.
- **Working Set:** Maximum number, in megabytes, in the working set of the agent's process at any point in time. The working set is the set of memory pages touched recently by the threads in the process.
- **I/O Data Kbytes per Second:** Rate at which the agent's process is issuing read and write input/ output (I/O) operations. This property counts all I/O activity generated by the process, including file, network, and device I/O operations.

On the other hand, to analyse the computer performance, information about RAM memory and CPU and further about the disk free space is collected. These three metrics are collected in the available percentage of CPU, RAM memory and disk space. Being aware of these three parameters, it is possible to characterize the computer performance, as well as identify situations where the machine is at a crash state (Microsoft, 2013c, 2013d, 2013e) .

Agents and Computer Workload

During a month, the workload of the AIDA computers and agents was collected. As Figure 4 shows, among the five machines that execute AIDA agents, the hsa-aida08 computer is the one that consumes more CPU (an average of 14.09%) and the hsa-aida01 is the one that consumes more memory RAM (an average of 42,38%). On the other hand, hsa-aida01 is the one that consumes less CPU (an average of 5.5%), and hsa-aida08 and hsa-aida04 are the ones that consume less memory RAM (an average of 14.23% and 12.93%, respectively). It was also possible to confirm that the CPU's consumption was constant only varying from 5 to 10 percent in maximum. The consumption of RAM memory was very constant.

In Figure 5, the activity of the agent 101 during a day is presented. This agent is executed continuously in hsa-aida01. As it can be seen on the left side of Figure 5, the average of RAM memory consumption is constant and it rounds the 400-450 Mbytes. On the right side of Figure 5, it can be observed that the

Figure 4. Extracting results from the monitor dashboard of AIDA machines

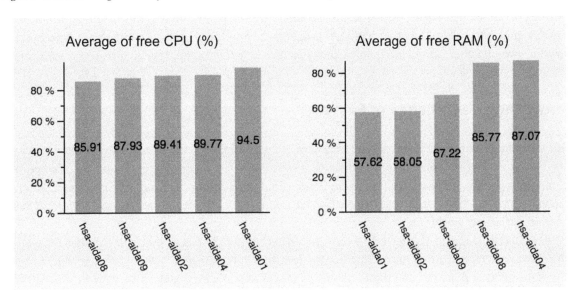

Figure 5. Extracting results from the monitor dashboard of AIDA agents. Activity of the agent 101 during a day (from 00:00 to 23:59) in hsa-aida01. Number of processes, average of CPU usage (%), RAM memory consumption (Mbytes) and I/O operations per second (Kbytes). On the right the number of processes and CPU consumption is highlighted.

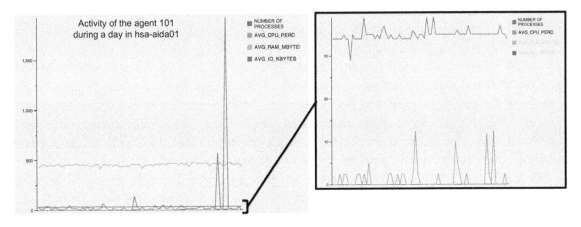

number of processes produced by agent 101 is about 35. These are the reasons for the high consumption of RAM in hsa-aida01. In Figure 5 it also can be observed that the average of CPU consumption badly exceeds the 10% and the I/O operations were constant during this day except for some operations at the end of the day.

The high number of agents that are executed in hsa-aida08 justifies the high consumption of CPU. In these machine agents that are responsible for archive transfer, billing, request processing and verifications are installed. Besides the number of agents, most of these are often executed, which also justifies the elevated use of CPU in hsa-aida08.

The hsa-aida04 is the machine that has more resources available as it can be seen in the Figure 5. So, it may be concluded that when a new agent is created, it should be installed in this machine. Monitoring AIDA machines, besides preventing faults of its agents, as it will be discussed in the next subsection, it allows the system administrators to manage the resources of AIDA computers in order to take advantage of them in the best way.

Forecasting and Detection of Faults

In this subsection two applications will be presented. One that prevents faults in AIDA computers (where agents are executed) and inherence prevents agent faults too. The other application quickly detects and informs the system administrator if an agent is not running. Both of these applications use a database independent from AIDA database, because if AIDA database is down the monitoring system of these applications are not interrupted.

When a fault occurs in an agent it is very important to quickly detect the fault in order to repair it in the shortest period of time, preventing bigger damages in the normal working flow of AIDA. Each agent registers its activity in a log file in the machine wherein it is executed, furthermore the errors that agents catch are registered in other log files, which contain only errors. Based on the time that agents take to refresh the log file with their newest activity, it is possible to characterize the normal activity of a specific agent, so it is possible to know how often an agent is executed. A minimum period of time (about two weeks) is useful to collect the intervals of time that characterize the agent activity. With a set of data collected about the intervals of time that an agent is executed and using a score table based on percentiles (similar with the score table presented in the previous section) it is possible to classify the state of agents activity, assigning a score such as it is done in MEWS.

Once the only variable used to calculate the score is the interval of time, the table for this situation has five states (from zero to four), moreover after doing tests the intervals between the percentiles 85, 90, 95 and 97.5 were assigned to this score table (instead of going from the percentile 75 until 90 such as the score table mentioned in the previous section). As for the model used on the database for *fault forecasting*, if the score obtained was less than four then a visual warning was issued on the monitoring dashboard, if the score was equal to four an email was sent to the system administrator in order to take speedy action to restore the normal working flow and prevent future damages. New limits are constantly calculated for each agent improving the application's efficacy. In relation to the errors recorded in the respective log file, the application detects when a new error appears and informs (by email) the administrator. To finish, this application is endowed with persistence in relation to the database state. If the database is down, all SQL statements are recorded in a file and the administrator is warned. When the database returns back to normal state, records are committed and the limits are refreshed. During the database down time, scores do not stop being calculated and abnormal situations are detected. However the limits are not refreshed and the limits used in the score table are the last ones.

The application related to the computer monitoring also uses a score table to identify critical situations. This application prevents faults in the AIDA machines and by inherence prevents agent faults too. Initially, there was an attempt to create a score table based on percentiles as the tables previously presented, but it did not succeed. The application sent several false positive warnings per day. The computer performance limits for a good operation is an issue that varies a lot. Those limits depend of the objectives that the system administrator wants for a specific machine. For example, the hsa-aida01 machine has agents that are running continuously and they are responsible for archiving transfers and provide Web services. This behaviour provokes, as it is possible to see in the previous section, a high consumption of RAM memory. In this case, the system administrator should increase the RAM limits in order to avoid being warned in regular situations. So, the score table was created with default fixed limits that also were discussed among the system administrators for the available percentage of CPU, memory and disk space and through a management page, the system administrator can change these limits for each metric either generally or specifically for one machine. The default score table for all computers, based on MEWS, are presented in Table 3.

Once again, if the sum of all parameter scores is more than four, serious situations are detected and a warning (email) is sent to the administrator. For example, if a machine has 12% of CPU available, 6% of RAM memory and 14% of disk's free space, the score is five, this situation is considered critical and the administrator will be informed to take preventive actions.

AIDA - SWOT ANALYSIS

Once the AIDA is a vital element of the normal operation of the HIS, it is very important to ensure that it offers the best functionalities and that users are satisfied. This analysis is intended to gather information about AIDA, in order to improve it. The *SWOT analysis* can reveal what are the great strengths of AIDA as well as its weaknesses. Furthermore, the opportunities are highlighted and the key threats to AIDA are alerted. The acronym SWOT means: strengths, weaknesses, opportunities and threats. Strengths represent the internal power that an organization owns to fight against the rivalry. Weaknesses represent aspects that reduce the quality of the product and/or of the service taking into account the customers opinion and/or competitive environment. Opportunities are defined as a set of conditions suitable for achieving certain objectives at the right moment, and threats are any inappropriate event or force in the external environment that causes damage to the organization's strategy. When this analysis is complete it is possible to use the strengths to develop new strategies; once weaknesses detected, these may be eliminated and some strategies may be reinforced; the opportunities should be explored; the threats should be countered. Strengths and weaknesses may be detected by an internal evaluation, on the other hand opportunities and threats by an external one. The organizational environment wherein the SWOT analysis is performed involves a huge number of elements and complex relationships of cause-and-effect, and is split in the internal and external environment. The first one can be controlled by the organization since it is very sensitive to the strategies implemented. There are internal factors such as management, culture at work, finance, research and development, staff, operational efficiency and capacity, technical frameworks and organizational structure. Nonetheless, external factors such as political, economic, cultural, social, technological and ambient, define the external environment, which is not controlled by the organization and acts homogeneously in all organizations included in the same market and the same

Table 3. Default scores table for fault forecasting in the AIDA computers

Scores	0	1	2	3
Available CPU (%)	> 50	50-25	25-10	< 10
Available RAM memory (%)	> 15	15-10	10-5	< 5
Disk's Free Space (%)	> 15	15-10	10-5	< 5

area. It may be concluded that opportunities and threats affect all organizations, however the probability of their impacts may be reduced by each organization (Dyson, 2004; Pereira et al., 2013).

In the following subsections the items of AIDA SWOT analysis in the CHP are presented.

AIDA Strengths

- Power management of change in the system;
- Ability to personalize objects like interface;
- High availability and full-time support;
- High accessibility;
- Security;
- Technologically modern system (R. Rodrigues et al., 2012; Santos, Portela, & Vilas-Boas, 2011) ;
- Ease of maintenance;
- Ease of use (Pereira et al., 2012);
- Credibility of the management team;
- Immediate access to detailed clinical information;
- Reports customized to meet the needs required;
- High computing power;
- Interoperability (Miranda et al., 2010);
- Ability to remotely access the system in a safe way;
- Failures prediction of databases (Silva et al., 2012);
- Fast detection of agents' abnormal activity;
- Failures prediction of machines wherein agents are executed.

AIDA Weaknesses

- System documentation non-existent;
- Graphical interface slightly confusing;
- Necessity of paper documentation in some services of the CHP;
- Insufficient education and training of health professionals;
- Computers are old and consequently slow.

Opportunities to AIDA

- Ability to integrate other applications;
- Ability to provide information via Internet;
- Ability to expand and sustain new services;
- Increasing importance of digital files;
- Government incentives;
- Extinction of paper use in the CHP;
- Modernization and organizational development;
- Projection of more efficient and usable interfaces;

- Developing better and more effective security protocols;
- Increasing expectation of citizens to obtain answers of clinical services faster and, at the same time, reliably;
- Use of mobile devices to access the system;
- Use of new technologies in order to enrich the system.

Threats to AIDA

- High degree of competition from other systems;
- Expansion of software companies for the health market;
- Competition/market pressure;
- Competition for scarce talented IT resources;
- Economic-financial crisis and subsequent financial constraints;
- Readiness to recover from disasters;
- Cyber attacks (hackers);
- System is based on Internet Explorer.

It may be concluded that AIDA in the CHP is a system of high relevance, endowed with many positive points such as interoperability, good usability, faults forecasting and high availability. On the other hand, a small number of weaknesses were detected such as the inexistent system documentation. This weakness is overcome by the full-time presence of technicians, who are always available to assist any healthcare professional.

The computerization of the entire clinical process in all services of the CHP is not an easy task. Nonetheless, all the efforts are being made for concretizing this main goal.

Relatively to interface, the Portuguese legislation forces the healthcare units to save all information about every patient, consequently when a professional accesses the clinical process of a specific patient, every clinical information about him has to be displayed, which can make the reading process a bit confusing.

The current Portuguese financial situation and the high cost of new technology acquisition made difficult replacing old computers. So it is very important to look at opportunities that may improve the AIDA. For example, the increasing importance of digital files creates a good opportunity to extinct the use of paper in the CHP. The other opportunities such as integrating new applications and services, improving security protocols and using mobile devices should be well exploited in order to fight against the competition.

The *SWOT analysis* shows few threats that the administration should realize. The biggest threat is the competition from other systems, despite the economic and financial crisis represents a big threat as well.

Security is an issue that the administrators should be always aware of, in spite of AIDA providing a high level of security. It is very important to ensure the security and confidentiality of its information and prevent cyber attacks. It is also very important to ensure the availability of the system. That means the system should have alternatives to disaster situations; if the system crashes, the CHP must not paralyze its activities.

CONCLUSION

This chapter demonstrates the importance and the impact that the interoperability causes in healthcare information systems. The usage of the HL7 standard embedded in a multi-agent system (endowed of autonomy, reactivity, pro-activity and social, emotional and moral behaviour) is fundamental to improve communication among heterogeneous systems, i.e., to achieve the interoperability among the healthcare information systems.

The intelligent and dynamic framework called AIDA is presented in this chapter. It constitutes a solution to accomplish the interoperability in healthcare units surpassing functional needs as well as financial and technical restrictions among clinical, medical and administrative systems.

The main core of AIDA platform is its database. The AIDA database must guarantee its confidentiality and integrity as well as its availability, which are ensured by fault tolerance mechanisms.

In order to prevent fault in AIDA database, a fault forecasting system based on MEWS model was adapted to the database context. Besides this system prevents database faults, it was possible to study the normal workload of AIDA database. In the Centro Hospitalar do Porto, a high utilization and workload of AIDA database (an average of 681 sessions, 214 transactions per second and 742 operations per second) was verified. It was also identified that the critical workload of AIDA is the period between 10:00 and 12:00.

A similar fault forecasting system for the computers wherein agents are executed was implemented. Detection of the faults system was also implemented. It enables detecting the agent fault in order to repair in the shortest period of time possible, preventing bigger damages in the normal working flow of AIDA. Furthermore, it was possible to study the computer and agents workload for the purpose of allowing the system administrators to manage the resources of AIDA machines and agents.

The SWOT analysis demonstrates that the system has a lot of strong points, as well as fewer weak ones. Through the identification of the system weaknesses, the system administrators can make up their minds. The evaluation proved to be a powerful tool, which has provided useful information to improve the quality of AIDA.

ACKNOWLEDGMENT

This work is funded by National Funds through the FCT - Fundação para a Ciência e a Tecnologia (Portuguese Foundation for Science and Technology) within project PEst-OE/EEI/UI0752/2014.

REFERENCES

Albino, A., & Jacinto, V. (2009). *Implementação da escala de alerta precoce - EWS*. Portimão.

Ashdown, L., & Kyte, T. (2011). *Oracle Database Concepts, 11g Release 2 (11.2)*. Oracle.

Bertino, E., & Sandhu, R. (2005). Database security - Concepts, approaches, and challenges. *IEEE Transactions on Dependable and Secure Computing*, 2(1), 2–19. doi:10.1109/TDSC.2005.9

Boshier, A. (2000). Windows Management Instrumentation: A Simple, Powerful Tool for Scripting Windows Management. *MSDN Magazine, 4.*

Carr, C. D., & Moore, S. M. (2003). IHE: A model for driving adoption of standards. *Computerized Medical Imaging and Graphics, 27*(2-3), 137–146. doi:10.1016/S0895-6111(02)00087-3 PMID:12620304

Chan, I. (2008). *Oracle Database Performance Tuning Guide, 10g Release 2 (10.2).* Oracle.

Contreras, M., Germán, E., Chi, M., & Sheremetov, L. (2004). Design and implementation of a FIPA compliant Agent Platform in.NET. *Journal of Object Technology, 3*(9), 5–28. doi:10.5381/jot.2004.3.9.a1

Costa, L., & Silva, F. (2010). Um Software de gerenciamento baseado no padrão WBEM-WMI. *Sistemas de Informação & Gestão de Tecnologia, 5.*

Devaney, G., & Lead, W. (2011). *Guideline for the use of the modified early warning score (MEWS).* Academic Press.

Dias, K., Ramacher, M., Shaft, U., Venkataramani, V., & Wood, G. (2005). Automatic performance diagnosis and tuning in Oracle. In *Proceedings of the 2005 CIDR Conf.* CIDR.

Drake, S., Hu, W., McInnis, D., Sköld, M., Srivastava, A., & Thalmann, L. ... Wolski, A. (2005). Architecture of Highly Available Databases. In M. Malek, M. Reitenspieß, & J. Kaiser (Eds.), Service Availability (Vol. 3335, pp. 1–16). Springer.

Duarte, J., Salazar, M., Quintas, C., Santos, M., Neves, J., Abelha, A., & Machado, J. (2010). Data Quality Evaluation of Electronic Health Records in the Hospital Admission Process. In *Proceedings of International Conference on Computer and Information Science*, (pp. 201–206). Academic Press.

Dyson, R. G. (2004). Strategic development and SWOT analysis at the University of Warwick. *European Journal of Operational Research, 152*(3), 631–640. doi:10.1016/S0377-2217(03)00062-6

Gardner-Thorpe, J., Love, N., Wrightson, J., Walsh, S., & Keeling, N. (2006). The value of Modified Early Warning Score (MEWS) in surgical in-patients: a prospective observational study. *Annals of the Royal College of Surgeons of England, 88*(6), 571–575. doi:10.1308/003588406X130615 PMID:17059720

Godinho, R. (2011). *Availability, Reliability and Scalability in Database Architecture.* Universidade do Minho.

HL7. (2012). *HL7 Website.* Retrieved from http://www.hl7.org/

Kim, S., Cho, N., Lee, Y., Kang, S.-H., Kim, T., Hwang, H., & Mun, D. (2010). Application of density-based outlier detection to database activity monitoring. *Information Systems Frontiers*, 1–11.

Lavy, M. M., & Meggitt, A. J. (2001). *Windows Management Instrumentation (WMI).* New Riders. Retrieved from http://www.google.pt/books?id=DD1jA3RgFEMC

Luck, M., McBurney, P., & Preist, C. (2003). *Agent technology: Enabling next generation computing (a roadmap for agent based computing).* AgentLink/University of Southampton.

Machado, J., Abelha, A., Novais, P., Neves, J., & Neves, J. (2010). Quality of service in healthcare units. *International Journal of Computer Aided Engineering and Technology*, 2(4), 436–449. doi:10.1504/IJCAET.2010.035396

Machado, J., Miranda, M., Gonçalves, P., Abelha, A., Neves, J., & Marques, J. A. (2010). *AIDATrace: Interoperation platform for active monitoring in healthcare environments*. Academic Press.

Microsoft. (2013a). *WMI Overview*. Retrieved August 16, 2013, from http://technet.microsoft.com/en-us/library/cc753534.aspx

Microsoft. (2013b). *Win32_PerfFormattedData_PerfProc_Process class*. Retrieved August 16, 2013, from http://msdn.microsoft.com/en-us/library/windows/desktop/aa394277(v=vs.85).aspx

Microsoft. (2013c). *Win32_PerfFormattedData_PerfOS_Processor class*. Retrieved August 16, 2013, from http://msdn.microsoft.com/en-us/library/windows/desktop/aa394271(v=vs.85).aspx

Microsoft. (2013d). *Win32_PerfFormattedData_PerfOS_Memory class*. Retrieved August 16, 2013, from http://msdn.microsoft.com/en-us/library/windows/desktop/aa394268(v=vs.85).aspx

Microsoft. (2013e). *Win32_PerfFormattedData_PerfDisk_LogicalDisk class*. Retrieved August 16, 2013, from http://msdn.microsoft.com/en-us/library/windows/desktop/aa394261(v=vs.85).aspx

Miranda, M., Duarte, J., Abelha, A., Machado, J., & Neves, J. (2010). Interoperability in healthcare. In *Proceedings of European Simulation and Modelling Conference*. ESM.

Miranda, M., Machado, J., Abelha, A., & Neves, J. (2013). In G. Fortino, C. Badica, M. Malgeri, & R. Unland (Eds.), *Healthcare Interoperability through a JADE Based Multi-Agent Platform* (Vol. 446, pp. 83–88). Intelligent Distributed Computing, VI: Springer. doi:10.1007/978-3-642-32524-3_11

Miranda, M., Salazar, M., Portela, F., Santos, M., Abelha, A., Neves, J., & Machado, J. (2012). Multi-agent Systems for HL7 Interoperability Services. In Procedia Technology (Vol. 5, pp. 725–733). Elsevier.

Nair, S. (2008). The Art of Database Monitoring. *Information Systems Control Journal*, (Ccm), 1–4.

Palazzo, L., Sernani, P., Claudi, A., Dolcini, G., Biancucci, G., & Dragoni, A. F. (2013). *A Multi-Agent Architecture for Health Information Systems*. Retrieved from http://netmed2013.dii.univpm.it/sites/netmed2013.dii.univpm.it/files/papers/paper5.pdf

Peixoto, H., Santos, M., Abelha, A., & Machado, J. (2012). Intelligence in Interoperability with AIDA. In *Proceedings of 20th International Symposium on Methodologies for Intelligent Systems* (LNCS), (Vol. 7661). Berlin: Springer.

Pereira, R., Duarte, J., Salazar, M., Santos, M., Abelha, A., & Machado, J. (2012). Usability of an Electronic Health Record. *IEEM, 5*.

Pereira, R., Salazar, M., Abelha, A., & Machado, J. (2013). SWOT Analysis of a Portuguese Electronic Health Record. In Collaborative, Trusted and Privacy-Aware e/m-Services (Vol. 399, pp. 169–177). Springer.

Ramos, L. (2007). *Performance Analysis of a Database Caching System In a Grid Environment*. FEUP.

Rich, B. (2013). *Oracle Database Reference, 11g Release 2 (11.2)*. Oracle.

Rodrigues, A. (2005). *Oracle 10g e 9i: Fundamentos Para Profissionais*. Lisboa: FCA.

Rodrigues, R., Gonçalves, P., Miranda, M., Portela, F., Santos, M., & Neves, J. ... Machado, J. (2012). Monitoring Intelligent System for the Intensive Care Unit using RFID and Multi-Agent Systems. In *Proceedings of IEEE International Conference on Industrial Engineering and Engineering Management (IEEM2012)*. IEEE.

Rogers, R., Peres, Y., & Müller, W. (2010). Living longer independently - A healthcare interoperability perspective. *E&I Elektrotechnik und Informationstechnik, 127*(7-8), 206–211. doi:10.1007/s00502-010-0748-8

Santos, M. F., Portela, F., & Vilas-Boas, M. (2011). *INTCARE: Multi-agent approach for real-time intelligent decision support in intensive medicine*. Academic Press.

Schumacher, R. (2003). *Oracle Performance Troubleshooting With Dictionary Internals SQL & Tuning Scripts*. Kittrell: Rampant TechPress.

Shallahamer, C. (2007). *Forecasting Oracle Performance*. Berkeley, CA: Apress.

Silva, P., Quintas, C., Duarte, J., Santos, M., Neves, J., Abelha, A., & Machado, J. (2012). Hospital database workload and fault forecasting. In *Step Towards Fault Forecasting in Hospital Information Systems*. Academic Press.

Strohm, R. (2012). *Oracle Real Application Clusters Administration and Deployment Guide, 11g Release 2 (11.2)*. Oracle.

Subbe, C. P., Kruger, M., Rutherford, P., & Gemmel, L. (2001). Validation of a Modified Early Warning Score in medical admissions. *QJM, 94*(10), 521–526. doi:10.1093/qjmed/94.10.521 PMID:11588210

Weber-Jahnke, J., Peyton, L., & Topaloglou, T. (2012). eHealth system interoperability. *Information Systems Frontiers, 14*(1), 1–3. doi:10.1007/s10796-011-9319-8

KEY TERMS AND DEFINITIONS

AIDA: Platform developed to ensure interoperability between healthcare information systems.

Database Workload: Database performance based on its main statistics.

Fault Forecasting: Prevention of failures through the monitoring of the performance of the object intended.

HL7: Standard for interoperability in healthcare.

Intelligent Agent: Autonomous programs that operate in an environment in order to achieve a goal.

Interoperability: Autonomous ability to interact and communicate.

Multi Agent System: System with multiple agents working together in order to achieve a global goal.

SWOT Analysis: Picking and discussion of strengths, weaknesses, opportunities and threats with the purpose of know better and improve a system.

This research was previously published in Cloud Computing Applications for Quality Health Care Delivery edited by Anastasius Moumtzoglou and Anastasia N. Kastania, pages 78-101, copyright year 2014 by Medical Information Science Reference (an imprint of IGI Global).

Chapter 37
Communication AssessmenT Checklist in Health:
Assessment and Comparison of Web-Based Health Resources

Juliana Genova
University of Ottawa, Canada

Jackie Bender
University of Toronto, Canada

ABSTRACT

There is no comprehensive and standardized tool for evaluating the communication quality of web resources for patients. The purpose of this study was to assess prostate cancer websites using the Communication AssessmenT Checklist in Health (CATCH) and to compare the results with those of the Consumer and Patient Health Information Section of the MLA (CAPHIS). CATCH is a theory-based tool consisting of 50 elements nested in 12 concepts. Two raters independently applied it to 35 HON certified websites containing information on prostate cancer treatment. The CATCH summary scores for these websites were then compared to the 2015 list of credible health websites published by CAPHIS. Websites contained a mean 24.1 (SD= 3.6) CATCH items. The concepts Language, Readability, Layout, Typography and Appearance were present in over 80% of sites. Content, Risk Communication, Usefulness, and Scientific Value were present in 50% or less. CATCH provided an overall score of the selected sites that was consistent with CAPHIS ratings. The prostate cancer websites evaluated in this study did not present treatment information in a useful, informative or credible way for patients. The communication quality of these resources could be improved with a clear strategic intent focused on decision-making, using CATCH as a guiding framework. CATCH is a tool that can be used independently or with other health resource evaluation tools to select the most trustworthy web resources for health information.

DOI: 10.4018/978-1-5225-3926-1.ch037

INTRODUCTION

Consumers in North America rely more and more on information gleaned from the Internet to inform their health-related decisions. The quality of this information may be a subject of concern, especially given the growing emphasis on shared decision-making between patient and health care professionals (Makoul & Clayman, 2006; Wong et al., 2000). Shared decision-making can improve the planning and carrying out of therapies (Brett et al., 2014; Brown, Brown, & Sharma, 2000), facilitate adaptation of new knowledge to specific patient communities (Brett et al., 2014; Collier, 2011; Fagerlin, Zikmund-Fisher, & Ubel; Frank, Basch, & Selby, 2014) and make information more accessible to patients by making it more user-friendly (Brett et al., 2014). There are a variety of tools to evaluate web resources, with a different scope, whose validity is not yet confirmed.

In order to make good health care decisions, people need to fully understand the risks and benefits of each treatment or therapy. Researchers have long stated that there is a gap between the evidence presented in the information, and the decisions people take, or between the creation of knowledge and its intended use (Bero et al., 1998; Dopson, Locock, Gabbay, Ferlie, & Fitzgerald, 2003; Lang, Wyer, & Haynes, 2007). If we consider knowledge translation as a two-step process, the first step would be filtering and distilling the evidence (Cohen et al., 2008; Grimshaw et al., 2006), while the second step would be the adoption or implementation of evidence. This second step is the most difficult to understand. Looking for an explanation, many researchers considered behaviour-change factors (Ajzen & Albarracen, 2007; Ajzen, Czasch, & Flood, 2009; S. Michie, Johnston, Abraham, & Walker, 2005; Susan Michie, van Stralen, & West, 2011). But the tipping point, between the presentation of the evidence, and its adoption, remains unexplained. The "packaging of information", warrants further attention as it may not adequately reflect the intended knowledge or effectively reach the intended audience.

In this study, we present a relatively new tool, the Communication AssessmenT Checklist in Health (CATCH). We use CATCH to evaluate the quality of health information on HON approved health websites intended for prostate cancer patients. We chose to focus on web resources for prostate cancer because it is the most common cancer in men (Collin et al., 2008), and it is also one of the most difficult cancers for patients to comprehend and formulate health decisions because of the variety of treatment options available (Clark, Wray, & Ashton, 2001; Stamey, McNeal, Yemoto, Sigal, & Johnstone, 1999). The results will allow us to draw a parallel between the websites with the highest overall CATCH score and the websites contained in the 2015 list of "Top health websites you can trust" published by CAPHIS.

INSTRUMENTS FOR HEALTH INFORMATION ASSESSMENT

Instruments Similar to CATCH

Numerous researchers have invested considerable effort in developing instruments that could streamline and filter health information, so that it becomes easier for the end-user to comprehend, evaluate and implement.

Some of those instruments take into consideration both the content and the form of the health message. The Guideline Implementability Appraisal tool (GLIA) (Shiffman, 2005) proposes a "Presentation and Formatting" dimension comprising two items. ADAPTE (T. A. Collaboration, 2009) highlights the importance of "Context of Use", " Strength of Evidence" and " Risks and Benefits". Other instruments focus on the scientific value of the evidence, its scope, purpose, clarity and presentation. These include the Appraisal of Guidelines for Research & Evaluation (AGREE) instruments (Brouwers, M. C. et al., 2010).

Another set of instruments analyzes the quality of information provided in health resources on the Internet. These include, LIDA (Borgmann et al., 2015; Soobrah & Clark, 2012) and DISCERN (Charnock, Shepperd, Needham, & Gann, 1999) which measure the accessibility, usability and reliability of the information. Still other validated instrument enable patients and providers to judge the quality of written consumer health information.The Information Comprehensiveness Tool (Warren, Footman, Tinelli, McKee, & Knai, 2014) assesses the comprehensiveness of health information, while a framework developed by Ferreira et al. (2013) evaluates its relevance.

The difference between all of these instruments and CATCH is the scope. CATCH takes into account all aspects of the health information, including the content and form, while the above-mentioned instruments focus either on the form or the content.

How CATCH Findings Coincide With Other Credible Sources

Numerous studies have assessed the quality of prostate cancer information on the Internet (Black & Penson, 2006; Pruthi, Belsante, Kurpad, Nielsen, & Wallen, 2011; Routh, Gong, Cannon, & Nelson, 2011) (Hellawell, Turner, Le Monnier, & Brewster, 2000). When systematically reviewed by Black and Penson in 2006, websites containing information on prostate cancer were found to be of sufficient quality to aid in decision-making but lacked currency, attribution, balance of evidence and comprehensiveness (Black & Penson, 2006). Prostate cancer websites have also been assessed for readability – the ease with which information is read and understood. Using Flesch Kindcaid Grade Level and Flesch Reading Ease Level tools, Ellmoottill et al. (Ellimoottil, Polcari, Kadlec, & Gupta, 2012) analyzed 62 eligible websites containing information on prostate cancer treatment options and only found 3 that were written below the recommended high school reading level (Ellimoottil et al., 2012). Concerning findings given that one third of the US population reads below a high school reading level (Ellimoottil et al., 2012). To our knowledge, the communication quality of prostate cancer websites has not been studied.

THE CATCH INSTRUMENT

CATCH (Table 1), whose development and preliminary validation is described in a prior publication (Genova et al., 2014) is based on Suitability Assessment Materials (SAM) (Doak et al., 1994), fundamental communication concepts from the theories of risk communication (Fischhoff, Brewer, & Downs, 2011), Tarde's theory of social values (Tarde, 1890; 1902), and concepts related to user-centered design (Neuhauser, 2011; Nielsen, 2004). The original CATCH is composed of 55 elements nested in 12 concepts ranging from appearance, form and content to fundamental communication concepts such as numeracy, objectivity, credibility, effectiveness, scientific value and usefulness. CATCH was initially applied to a set of printed education materials with proven effectiveness (Giguière, 2012) distributed to clinicians. This formative study demonstrated that CATCH has a good ability to discriminate between resources that are different, based on the quality of communication concepts, suggesting good construct validity (Genova et al., 2014).

Table 1. Concepts and elements for the Communication AssessmenT Checklist in Health (CATCH)

Concept	Element: Description
Appearance	
	1. Pictures, special fonts and colors
	2. Length: the material is no more than a page long.
Layout and typography	
	3. Clear layout: the text and graphics attract the reader's attention and create a visual path.
	4. Short to-the-point paragraphs: the resource uses short sentences of no more than 12 words, paragraphs of no more than 10 sentences with a single idea, and short and simple words.
	5. Subtitles: subtitles or subheadings are used to clearly group the information.
	6. Font size: the text is easy to read because the font size is not excessively small or large, at least 12 point, serif.
	7. Text clearly laid out and delimited by spaces: the text is well organized and easy to follow.
	8. Italics and capitals are used appropriately for references and subtitles or to enhance the layout.
Content	
	9. Purpose of the text is clearly stated in the title, illustration, or introduction.
	10. Limited scope: the scope of the resource is relevant to the stated purpose and is limited to defining the problem and the rationale, and providing a solution.
	11. Summary: the resource provides a summary or a review that reiterates and explains the central information.
	12. Information limited to key messages: the resource covers only a few key messages, ideally no more than three or four.
	13. Desired behaviors explained or modeled: best practices or recommended therapy procedures are clearly described.
Language and readability	
	14. Active voice: Sentences are written in the active voice whenever possible.
	15. Context given first: the situation is explained to the reader at the beginning of the message.
	16. Organizers (sometimes called "road signs") such as headers, captions, or transition words or statements briefly inform the reader of what is coming next.
Graphics	
	17. Graphics to facilitate understanding: the graphics are self-explanatory and facilitate understanding of the text.
	18. Relevance of graphics: graphics match and enhance the content; they should be simple in their meaning, without additional details that distract the reader. Moreover, they depict the recommended behavior.
	19. Captions: captions and/or legends are used for each figure, list, table, or other display supporting the text.
Risk communication	
	20. Risk clarity: the risk is clearly presented and defined. There is no ambiguity.
	21. Likelihood of the event: there is a greater than 50% likelihood that the event described in the message will happen.
	22. Risks presented in order of priority: risks are presented starting with the most important, to clarify all the issues at stake at each level of risk.
	23. Objective presentation of both harms and benefits: the resource provides complete information on harms and benefits. For example, reporting survival rates for 1 year is incomplete compared to 5 years.
	24. Standardized presentation of harms and benefits: for all the outcomes, harms are defined the same way and use the same variable as benefits.
	25. Absolute risk difference used

continued on following page

Table 1. Continued

Concept	Element: Description
	26. Consistent denominators and whole numbers: the resource uses the same denominators to present harms and benefits to ensure consistency, as well as whole numbers, which are easier to understand than fractions or decimals.
	27. Consistent time frames for harms and benefits: the resource expresses harms and benefits in the same temporal patterns.
	28. Clear difference between the risks at the baseline and the risks at follow-up: Risks at baseline and following treatment are clearly presented so that the reader can evaluate the degree of change between the two time periods.
	29. Use of positive and negative frames: the message highlights not only the harms, but also the benefits of the recommended action, and uses positive framing that is more productive than negative framing (e.g., survival versus mortality).
	30. Symbols (numbers, graphs, statistics, etc.): symbols are used to clearly convey the meaning of the probabilities presented.
Scientific value	
	31. Effectiveness of the recommendations: it is stated in the resources that adherence to the recommendations yields concrete and specific results.
	32. Robustness of the evidence: it is stated in the resource that the message is supported by sufficient, high quality data. It is convincing for professionals.
Emotional appeal	
	33. Communication of urgency: the message raises concerns that should be answered immediately to reduce the morbidity or mortality of patients.
	34. Timeliness and visibility of the topic: the resource addresses a topic covered by popular media because of a public debate, a scientific controversy, or because it features a celebrity with a disease.
	35. Vibrancy or intensity: a fast pace and the choice of words show that the author is invested in the subject or driven by the urgency to convey something. The resource, through its appearance and language, conveys a sense of urgency.
	36. Threat of the event: the message depicts a serious threat that cannot be ignored.
	37. Newness of the message: the document provides a new perspective or represents an innovation.
	38. Highlighting of danger: the message highlights a potential threat or danger relative to the topic presented.
Relevance	
	39. Consistency with experience, logic, and language of reader: the message's language, format, and structure correspond to the reader's level of education, language, and/or professional background.
	40. Cultural match: the resource is adapted to the culture of readers and takes into account their background, customs, beliefs, and expectations.
	41. Narrative included: contains personal testimonies or real life-examples to drive the message home.
Social value/Source credibility	
	42. Endorsement by renowned individuals or organizations: the document is "validated" by renowned clinicians, research scientists, professional organizations, or the government.
	43. Background of the author: the resource clearly states that its author has relevant experience.
	44. Disclaimer of conflict of interests: an official statement attests to the absence of any conflict of interest.
Social value/Usefulness for the patient	
	45. Time saving the resource states that the recommended behaviour saves time.
	46. Money saving: the resource states that the recommended behaviour helps save money.
	47. Non-threatening: the message does not highlight deficiencies or lack of training in the medical staff or the health system.
	48. Building of self-efficacy: the resource describes a technology or innovation that will give more self-confidence to the clinician and allow them to make an informed decision or trust his or her own judgment.
	49. Increased ease: the resource offers an easier and better way to do things.
	50. Better quality of life: the resource states that adherence to the targeted behaviour will facilitate healthcare processes and improve organization of the environment.

As a theory-based instrument, CATCH can, in our view, be applied to print or online content, using different media and targeting different audiences. To confirm this hypothesis, we assessed the usefulness of a modified version of CATCH specifically tailored for online health resources by using it to evaluate a set of web resources for prostate-cancer patients. The present study is a pilot designed to show how CATCH can be applied to online resources selected using the Health on the Net Code (HON code).

The HONcode

In the present study, we selected our sample of health information websites using the HON code search engine. The HON code is the oldest quality standard for health-related online information. To achieve the HON code seal of approval, websites must conform to a number of principles. HON code certified websites must have authoritative, reliable and accessible information, support patient-physician relation and confidentiality, and mention funding sources (Burkell, 2004).

It is hypothesized that the HON code guarantees, at least to some degree, the credibility of health information. Research suggests that the HONcode seems to be a reliable indicator of website quality. A recent study by Corcelles et al. evaluated online health information for patients with DISCERN and Journal of the American Medical Association (JAMA) benchmarks. The top 4% of the websites analyzed had the HONcode seal of approval. Similarly, a study by Kaicker, Dang and Mondal (Kaicker, Jatin, Dang, Wilfred, & Mondal, Tapas, 2013) concluded that sites that bore the HON code seal obtained higher DISCERN reconstruction content scores than those without this certification.

Recently, the Medical Library Association put together a list of pre-screened health websites called the Top 100 List of Health Websites You Can Trust (http://caphis.mlanet.org/consumer/index.html) to provide consumers and patients a resource to use in their daily practice. The criteria adopted to complete the list was developed by the Criteria for Assessing the Quality of Health Information on the Internet of the Health Summit Working Group, and included: credibility, sponsorship/authorship, content, audience, currency, disclosure, purpose, links, design, interactivity, and caveats. As these criteria seem to overlap to some extent with the elements we retained for CATCH, the second objective of this pilot study was to compare the rank order CATCH summary scores of the evaluated websites (Figure 3) to those endorsed by CAPHIS. As the previous study (Genova, Olson, & Bender, 2017) concerns health information for prostate-cancer, we will compare our results to those retained in CAPHIS' categories for Men's Health and Senior Health.

CATCH

The instrument was created based on a literature review of commonly accepted communication theories. First, we selected all the concepts that had some pertinence to evidence-based material and operationalized them so that they can be applied to the web resources. We used a mapping approach and applied them first to printed education materials Genova et al., 2014), then to web resources for prostate cancer patients (Genova et al., 2017) . This approach had twofold results. First, it validated the operationalized concepts and allowed us to organize them in CATCH. Second, it demonstrated the most frequent (not necessarily the most meaningful) and least frequent concepts used in the creation of health materials.

CATCH Concepts

CATCH uses several concepts from social sciences to evaluate the quality of the health information. We operationalized those concepts in elements, the rationale for which is described below.

The most important theory is risk communication, and one of its most important concepts is objectivity. We operationalized objectivity to first include numeracy. The reasons are simple: when risks and benefits have numerical expressions, they are easier to understand and use by people in distress when the ability to process information is decreased (Fagerlin, Zikmund-Fisher, & Ubel, 2011). Of course, numeric literacy plays a role: patients with higher numeric literacy rely more on abstract information (numbers, graphs etc), while patients with lower numeric literacy are more affected by emotion-based narratives (Salmon & Atkin, 2003), and whole numbers (e.g., 1 in 10,000) (Peters, 2012b; Sheridan et al., 2011).

We also operationalized objectivity to include: standard definitions, constant denominators, timeframes and clear prioritization of risks, costs and benefits. (Fischhoff, 2012; Fischhoff et al., 2011; Fischhoff, Watson, & Hope, 1984; Peters, 2012b). Another critical element of objectivity is the concept "less is more". Research shows that when patients are presented with less treatment choices, up to three, and when those choices are organized in order of importance, they make better decisions (Peters, Dieckmann, Dixon, Hibbard, & Mertz, 2007, Zikmund-Fisher, Windschitl, Exe, & Ubel, 2011).

Risk communication also has three important concepts: novelty, urgency and visibility of the danger, which usually appear together in health information (Genova et al., 2014). Novelty and urgency increase the perception of risk (Bandura, 2001), and have more impact on arguments (Ajzen, 1971) and opinion change (Murphy et al., 1998). There is a linear relationship between stronger fear-arousing conditions and greater message acceptance (Berkowitz & Cottingham, 1960; Sutton & Eiser, 1984). As Witte and Allen (2000) point out: "the stronger the fear aroused by a fear appeal, the more persuasive it is" (p. 601). Visibility, or use of celebrity names and hot topics (Genova et al., 2014) increase the impact of those elements.

Risk communication also has a subjective dimension that we operationalized as self-efficacy and effectiveness of the recommended response. A patient with high self-efficacy is more likely to perform the recommended action (Witte & Allen, 2000). Self-efficacy can be defined as a feeling of control over the material or social environment, or perceived behavioral control, self-esteem and self-confidence (S. Michie & Abraham, 2008; Woolf, Grol, Hutchinson, Eccles, & Grimshaw, 1999). Another important element is the effectiveness of the recommended response. If the response is perceived as leading to a quick, sure and efficient change, it may lead to behavior change (Witte & Allen, 2000; Witte, 2000; Ruiter & Kok, 2011).

Two more concepts can be seen as part of risk communication: narrative, and cultural match. A witness's account of his or her experiences through cancer will speak volumes to cancer patients. People relate to a message that is consistent with their experience, logic and language and they are more likely to adopt it. Patients tend to make sense of their environment through narrative, they think with stories (Morris, 2001). Similarly, cultural, racial, or sexual match, makes people feel as part of a group and allows them to more easily adhere to the information (Harter, Japp, & Beck, 2005) and ultimately, to adopt it.

Two more concepts can be seen as part of risk communication: positivity and conviction. Effective messages that highlight the positive outcomes (gain frames) have more impact than negative messages (Ruiter & Kok, 2011; Salmon & Atkin, 2003). As for the tone of the message, a vibrant, commanding or intense tone is appealing to patients and leads them to accept the information (Peters, 2012a).

Tarde's Theory of Social Value

Tarde based his theory on societal change on innovation and imitation, both triggered by value-credit (Tarde, 1902). Value-credit is composed of value-usefulness, value-beauty and value-truth. We operationalized this theory in the concepts of value-truth, as it relates to credibility of the source (Atkin, 1994), as endorsement by experts and disclaimer of interests. In CATCH, we operationalized value-usefulness as time-saving, money-saving (Brownson, Fielding, & Maylahn, 2009) and non-threatening for the patient. We operationalized value-beauty as "healthy environment" that promotes healing, or a treatment that avoids unnecessary surgical interventions or undesirable side effects.

Plain Language, Graphics and Content

CATCH also incorporates some elements of SAM (Doak et al., 1994) and notions related to the plain language, such as the active voice, use of short sentences, words which break the information into easier-to-process chunks (US Federal Plain Language Guidelines, 2010) and clean layout that facilitates reading (US Department of Health and Human Services, 2010) and creates a visual path (Doak, Doak, & Root, 1996) (Neuhauser, 2011). As for graphics, they should be culturally appropriate (Doak et al., 1996; Potomac & Doak, 2002), simple (Wright, 2001) and show only the behaviors to be encouraged (US Federal Plain Language Guidelines, 2010).

Application of CATCH to Web-Based Resources for Prostate Cancer Patients

A conceptual mapping approach was used to apply CATCH to the selected sample of web pages. Two raters (JB, JG) independently applied the 50 elements of the CATCH instrument to each web resource for prostate cancer patients.

Each web resource was rated along each CATCH element using a dichotomous scale indicating the presence/absence of the element. We wanted to find the presence or absence of each CATCH element and to compute the total occurrences. Once all the elements were computed, CATCH would give a comprehensive picture of the strategies used, their advantages and also disadvantages.

We used Excel and SPSS Version 21 to calculate the sum and sum percentage for each CATCH item and the total summary score for each web resource. We computed the scores for CATCH concepts by calculating the mean value of the items pertaining to each concept.

The raters compared their ratings and resolved any disagreements through discussion, which in some cases resulted in rewording of an element. Most disagreements among raters resulted from an unclear description of the elements or misunderstandings as to the degree of specificity required when coding for the presence or absence of an element.

RESULTS

Frequent Concepts

Table 1 displays all the concepts and elements of CARCH. Table 2 and Figure 1 show the most commonly addressed CATCH concepts. In order of frequency, they were Language and Readability, Layout

Table 2. Summary scores for CATCH concepts and elements (N=35)

CATCH Concepts and Items	Summary Score Sub-scale: X, SD (%) Item: n (%)
Appearance	28, 7.1 (80)
1. Pictures, special fonts and colours	33 (94)
2. Length: the material is no more than a page long.	23 (66)
Layout and Typography	31.3, 1.6 (86)
3. Clear layout	31 (89)
4. Short to-the-point paragraphs	30 (86)
5. Subtitles	33 (94)
6. Font size	29 (83)
7. Text clearly laid out and delimited by space	32 (91)
8. Italics and capitals	33 (94)
Content	19, 11.7, (54)
9. Purpose of the text	27 (77)
10. Limited scope	32 (91)
11. Summary	4 (11)
12. Information limited to key messages	10 (29)
13. Desired behaviours explained or modelled	22 (63)
Language and Readability	32.7, 2.1 (93)
14. Active voice	32 (91)
15. Context given first	35 (100)
16. Organizers	31 (89)
Graphics	13, 1.7 (37)
17. Graphics to facilitate understanding	14 (40)
18. Relevance of graphics.	14 (40)
19. Captions	11 (31)
Risk Communication	11.6, 12.2 (33)
20. Risk clarity	27 (77)
21. Likelihood of the event	33 (94)
22. Risks presented in order of priority	15 (43)
23. Objective presentation of both harms and benefits	7 (20)
24. Standardized presentation of harms and benefits	1 (3)
25. Absolute risk difference used	0 (0)
26. Consistent denominators and whole numbers	0 (0)
27. Consistent time frames for harms and benefits	0 (0)
28. Clear difference between the risks at baseline and the risks at follow-up	2 (6)
29. Use of positive and negative frames	20 (57)

continued on following page

Table 2. Continued

CATCH Concepts and Items	Summary Score Sub-scale: X, SD (%) Item: n (%)
30. Symbols (numbers, graphs, statistics, etc.)	0 (0)
Scientific Value	16, 7.1 (51)
31. Effectiveness of the recommendations	23 (66)
32. Robustness of the evidence	13 (37)
Emotional Appeal	19.2, 11.8 (55)
33. Communication of urgency	7 (20)
34. Timeliness and visibility of the topic	34 (97)
35. Vibrancy or intensity	7 (20)
36. Threat of the event	32 (91)
37. Newness of the message	15 (43)
38. Highlighting of danger	20 (57)
Relevance	12.7, 16.3 (36)
39. Consistency with experience, logic, and language of reader	31 (89)
40. Cultural match	7 (20)
41. Narrative included	0 (0)
Social Value/ Source Credibility	8.0, 8.0 (23)
42. Endorsement by renowned individuals or organizations	16 (46)
43. Background of the author	8 (23)
44. Disclaimer of conflict of interests	0 (0)
Social Value/Usefulness for the Patient	8.3, 11.8 (24)
45. Time saving	1 (3)
46. Money saving	2 (6)
47. Non-threatening	31 (89)
48. Building of self-efficacy	2 (6)
49. Increased ease	12 (34)
50. Better quality of life	2 (6)

and Typography, and Appearance. These elements were present in 80% to 93% of the web resources. As shown in Figure 2, the majority of the web resources evaluated contained fewer than 50% of the CATCH items. The mean CATCH summary score of the web resources was 24.1 (SD= 3.6). The scores ranged from 15 to 33, out of a possible 50.

Nearly all the web resources appropriately used italics and capitals, had clearly laid out text, subtitles and easy to read fonts. Although Appearance came in a close second, only 66% of the resources were the appropriate length for the web, about a screen long, and while many had graphics, most graphics were a simple stock image of the prostate gland. A handful of web resources contained embedded videos. In most cases, these were relevant to and facilitated understanding of the text.

Figure 1. CATCH element scores

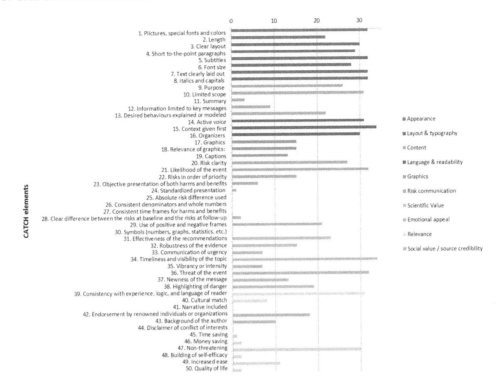

Poorly Represented Concepts

The concept Content was unequally distributed. Almost all of the resources had limited scope, clearly stated the context and were written in the active voice. But only 4 had summaries and 29% contained key messages or recommended a particular behavior or course of action. Web resources that did provide a recommendation, advised their readers to consult their physician.

Risk communication was poorly covered, beyond Risk Clarity and Likelihood of the Event, which were present in 94% and 77% of web resources respectively. Only 20% of resources contained a clear and objective presentation of the risks and benefits associated with each treatment option. Few web resources contained numeric presentation of the information, such as in a chart, graph or table, and none reported absolute risks or used consistent denominators or timeframes to describe the likelihood of harms and benefits. Positive and negative (gain and loss) frames, to invite patients to adopt a recommended behavior, were not used.

The Scientific Value of the web resources for prostate-cancer patients was also poorly addressed. Two thirds conveyed the effectiveness of the treatment options, but only 37% indicated that the message was supported by high-quality evidence. This finding goes hand-in-hand with the results for the concept Credibility. Less than 50% of the web resources reported that they were reviewed by a medical professional or organization, and only 23% reported the background of the author. We did not find any disclaimers of conflict of interests.

As for the concept, Emotional Appeal, only two elements were consistently covered: Threat of the Event, and Timeliness and Visibility. With regards to the concept Newness of the Message, less than

Figure 2. CATCH instrument score

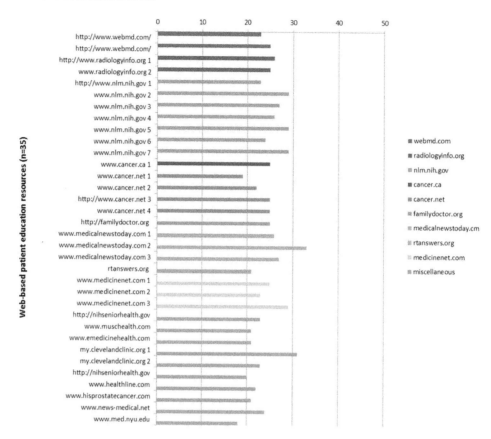

Figure 3. CATCH score according to websites

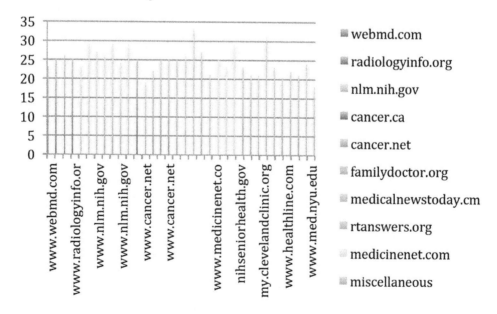

half of the web resources provided a new perspective or reported an innovation in prostate cancer treatment, and only about 20% of web resources conveyed the concepts Vibrancy or Intensity, or Urgency.

The concept Usefulness for the patient was also poorly addressed, ranging from 6 to 34%, with the exception of the element Non-Threatening which was evident in 89% of web resources.

Comparison to Other "Top Websites" Lists

There is another interesting result worth mentioning. As mentioned earlier, we conducted a search using the HON code search engine and the key words "prostate cancer treatment". We included the first five search results from each organization that pointed to different content, and selected the first 35 search results. The results from the HON code search engine also corresponded to the top ten web sites obtained using Google (we mention that because more than 75% of patients begin their search with one of these three search engines according to Pew Research Centre and visit only the top 10 websites listed in the results (Purcell, Brenner & Rainie, 2012). This finding suggests that the top websites produced by a search of the HON code website are also some of the most frequently visited sites on the web.

After applying CATCH to the different web resources, we gave a point for each element of CATCH present in the resources. This gave us the score of all the points obtained by the web-resource of the maximum 50 that could be obtained for each CATCH element resulting in an overall CATCH summary score for each web resources. It should be noted that our search was on web resources, not on websites, and it resulted in various web resources, sometimes from the same site. For those sites that yielded many hits in our search, we calculated the mean CATCH percentage score for all web resources retrieved from a particular site, resulting in a mean CATCH percentage for a given site.

As shown in Figure 3, our search retrieved seven resources from National Library of Medicine, National Institutes of Health, or NLM (https://www.nlm.nih.gov/), the mean CATCH score of which was 54%. We also have: two materials from the College of Radiology and the Radiological Society of North America (radiology.info) with a mean score of 51%; one resource from MedicineNet.com (medicinenet.com) with a score of 51%; two resources from WebMD (webmd.com) with a mean score of 48%; one from American Cancer Society (cancer.org) with a score of 50%; four resources from Cancer.net, the site with information approved by oncologists (cancer.net) with a mean score of 45%; and one from the American Academy of Family Physicians (familydoctor.org) with a score of 50% . The remainder of the web resources in our search yield have lower CATCH scores (as represented in Figure 3).

These results are consistent with those of published by CAPHIS (CAPHIS, 2015) in the categories relevant to our topic. In Men's Health section, one of the top five sites is the NLM (https://www.nlm.nih.gov/). This is also one of the best sites according to CATCH, with a median score of 54%. In the Senior Health section, NIH Senior's Health website (https://nihseniorhealth.gov/index.html), is the top listed site which according to CATCH, obtained 46%. Once again, it is a site of NLM.

DISCUSSION

In this section, we discuss the communication concepts exemplified on websites for prostate cancer patients. We will also highlight concepts and features that are missing or could be given more attention to improve the communication of the evidence in these web resources.

CATCH was used to assess the Appearance, Layout and Typography, Content, Language and Readability, Graphics, Communication of Risks, Emotional Appeal, Scientific Value, Relevance, Usefulness for the patient and Source Credibility of HON certified sites containing treatment information for prostate cancer patients.

In general, only the concepts of Appearance, Layout and Typography, and Language and Readability were well represented in the web resources on prostate cancer treatment options. This result can be explained by the fact that there are established user-centered standards and guidelines for the design of websites (Nielsen, 1999, 2004).

However, essential concepts were frequently missing. We found only 14 web resources that contained graphics, mostly similar stock images of the prostate gland. Pictures speak volumes, especially to an audience with lower literacy levels, like the general public (Ellimoottil et al., 2012). Similarly, Bender, Yue, To, Deacken, & Jadad (2013) found that a significant proportion of smartphone apps for cancer (at least 30%) used basic and repetitive images. Genova et al. (2014) also found poor use of graphics in printed education materials for clinicians; the pictures were only remotely connected to the content and overly complicated.

As far as the concept of Content is concerned, the most revealing finding is that there was no explicit statement of the purpose of the web resources for prostate cancer patients, except in the fact that the title of the page corresponded to the content. In that sense, these resources lacked a clear strategic intent. The purpose of the web resources for prostate cancer patients had to be inferred from the content and the organization of the materials. The purpose was not well defined and this ambiguity translated into poor communication of risks and incomplete information. If we suppose that patient education materials are supposed to inform and guide patient action, our evaluation shows these materials were not well-designed to achieve that purpose. In terms of guidance, only a few web resources took what might be called a minimalist approach to patient empowerment in that they recommended that patients ask their doctor about participation in a clinical trial.

This lack of strategic intent may in fact explain why many prostate cancer websites lack sufficient detail about treatment options (Ogah & Wassersug, 2013). It may also account for why risk factors were not presented objectively or consistently. We did not find any numerical representations of risks and advantages, such as charts, graphs, or numbers, aiming to facilitate decision-making and give them clear understanding of the situation. Timeframes, symbols and risk difference were not at all used. As for the organization of risks, most web resources did not present the side effects of prostate cancer treatments, the associated risks, and the eventual benefits. All of these factors are important for informed shared decision-making.

Also, the web resources did not use the strength of Emotional Appeal elements to encourage or empower patients. Positive frames were barely used and the tone was neutral, without patient narratives or a mention of cultural match.

The lack of strategic intent of the web resources evaluated is further illustrated by the low summary scores for the concepts Credibility and Scientific Value. The names, credentials and background of the authors or reviewers were rarely present, and none of the sites provided disclaimers of conflict of interests - results that are quite curious for medical websites. This finding is consistent with studies of the quality or credibility of information on prostate cancer websites, which has been reported to be lacking in currency, attribution, balance of evidence and disclosure (Black & Penson, 2006).

Web resources are not ends in and of themselves but rather a means to an end. Evaluating web resources entails assessing the fit between the content and the intended purpose. If a health information resource is designed with a clear strategy in mind - whether it is to inform, change perceptions or even attract visitors - it should be useful for that intended purpose. The prostate cancer websites in our sample did not score well in terms of Usefulness for patients - they did not adequately address the concerns that motivate patients to seek treatment information, such as quality of life (except for erectile dysfunction), reducing physical and emotional discomfort; saving time and money, or inconvenience. Warren et al (2014) found that many prostate cancer websites do not adequately address topics identified as important to patients, particularly related to treatment, recovery and quality of life issues. To improve the usefulness of websites containing information on prostate cancer treatment options, Rot, Ogah and Wassersug advise website developers to: (1) present all evidence-based treatment options, (2) regularly update and time stamp information (3) acknowledge that treatment recommendations may become out of date quickly, and (4) direct viewers to information on relevant, active clinical trials (2012).

Comparison of web resources with high CATCH summary scores to the websites published in the 2015 CAPHIS's trusted health website list, revealed many similar findings. The web resource with the highest CATCH summary score from our search was the NLM. The NLM was also one of the top-rated websites by CAPHIS. Of course, this could be attributed to our search strategy since we used the HON code search engine to identify websites, and the NLM is a HON certified website. However, these similar findings are also likely due to the similarity between the CATCH and CAPHIS rating criteria. According to the CAPHIS website, criteria for good quality health information resources include: credibility, sponsorship/authorship, content, audience, currency, disclosure, purpose, links, design, interactivity, and caveats.

The CAPHIS website evaluation criteria are similar to the CATCH elements in many ways. For example, CAPHIS concepts Credibility and Sponsorship/Authorship are related to CATCH elements 42, 43 and 44 and also 32, 33, 34, 35 and 37. The CAPHIS criteria of Content, is related to CATCH elements 9, 10, 11, 12 and 13. The CAPHIS concept of Currency is related to CATCH elements 21,32, 33, 34, 35 and 37. The CAPHIS concept of Disclosure is related to CATCH elements 20, and 22 to 30. The CAPHIS concept Purpose is related to CATCH elements 9 to 12, and Links, Design, and Caveats are clearly related to CATCH elements 1 to 32. The CAPHIS concept Audience is also present in CATCH in elements 39 to 41.

CATCH also contains two categories of communication concepts that are not captured by the CAPHIS criteria: Emotional Appeal (elements 33 to 38: Communication of Urgency, Timeliness and v=Visibility, Vibrancy or Intensity, Newness of the Message, Threat and Highlighting of Danger) and Usefulness for the Patient (elements 45 to 50: Time saving, Money saving, Non-threatening, Building of self-efficacy, Increased ease and Better quality of life).

Hence, CATCH provides a more comprehensive set of items to evaluate these shared concepts and a more comprehensive set of concepts as well. Therefore, we affirm that CATCH provides a more comprehensive and reliable indicator of the communication quality of a web resource.

Further studies are needed to formally assess the performance of the CATCH instrument as tool to evaluate the communication quality of web resources for prostate cancer, and for a broader spectrum of health topics.

CONCLUSION

CATCH is a theoretically based framework that can be used to evaluate the quality of various materials, whether they are patient or physician oriented, print or web-based.

The present study revealed that frequently consulted Websites for prostate cancer patients are not optimally designed to present health information in a way that is useful, informative and credible for patients. If the strategic intent is what guides content developers to create meaningful and valuable resources, with attention to detail, this was not the case here.

The fact that CATCH and CAPHIS yielded similar results, as far as the quality of websites is concerned, lends further support to the usefulness of CATCH as a reliable and comprehensive instrument that can be used alone or in conjunction with other instruments to improve communication with patients.

Communicating risks can be improved with more objective presentations of risks and benefits, numerical presentation of facts, and consistent timeframes. The purpose of the information on the websites must be clearer. The information should be credible and geared towards informed decision-making, not just gaining knowledge about diseases and treatments. The web resources did not offer any innovative approaches or new treatments, the potential negative side effects of treatments were downplayed, and the risks and benefits were organized just by the invasiveness of the treatment. If web resources are to change attitudes and behavior and more effectively support patients' active involvement in decisions related to their own care, communication elements such as vibrant and empathetic tone should become more common features of web-based patient resources.

REFERENCES

Aakhus, E., Granlund, I., Oxman, A., & Flottorp, S. (2015). Tailoring interventions to implement recommendations for the treatment of elderly patients with depression: a qualitative study. *International journal of mental health systems, 9*(1), 1-24.

Ajzen, I. (1971). Attitudinal vs. normative messages: An investigation of the differential effects of persuasive communications on behaviour. *Sociometry, 34*(2), 263–280. doi:10.2307/2786416

Ajzen, I., & Albarracín, D. (2007). *Predicting and changing behaviour: A reasoned action approach.* Lawrence Erlbaum Associates Publishers.

Ajzen, I., Czasch, C., & Flood, M. G. (2009). From Intentions to Behavior: Implementation Intention, Commitment, and Conscientiousness1. *Journal of Applied Social Psychology, 39*(6), 1356–1372. doi:10.1111/j.1559-1816.2009.00485.x

Atkin, C. (1994). Designing persuasive health messages: Effective dissemination of clinical health information (95-0015).

Bandura, A. (2001). Social cognitive theory: An agentic perspective. *Annual Review of Psychology, 52*(1), 1–26. doi:10.1146/annurev.psych.52.1.1 PMID:11148297

Bender, J., Yue, R., To, M., Deacken, L., & Jadad, A. (2013). A lot of action, but not in the right direction: Systematic review and content analysis of smartphone applications for the prevention, detection, and management of cancer. *Journal of Medical Internet Research, 15*(12), e287. doi:10.2196/jmir.2661 PMID:24366061

Berkowitz, L., & Cottingham, D. R. (1960). The interest value and relevance of fear arousing communications. *Journal of Abnormal and Social Psychology, 60*(1), 37–43. doi:10.1037/h0045247 PMID:13799520

Bero, L. A., Grilli, R., Grimshaw, J. M., Harvey, E., Oxman, A. D., & Thomson, M. A. (1998). Closing the gap between research and practice: An overview of systematic reviews of interventions to promote the implementation of research findings. *BMJ (Clinical Research Ed.), 317*(7156), 465–468. doi:10.1136/bmj.317.7156.465 PMID:9703533

Black, P., & Penson, D. (2006). Prostate cancer on the Internet—information or misinformation? *The Journal of Urology, 175*(5), 1836–1842. doi:10.1016/S0022-5347(05)00996-1 PMID:16600774

Borgmann, H., Wölm, J., Vallo, St., Mager, R., Huber, J., Breyer, J., & Tsaur, I. (2015). Prostate Cancer on the Web—Expedient Tool for Patients' Decision-Making? *Journal of Cancer Education, 32*(1), 135-140. PMID:26234650

Brett, J., Staniszewska, S., Mockford, C., Herron-Marx, S., Hughes, J. R., Tysall, C., & Suleman, R. (2014). Mapping the impact of patient and public involvement on health and social care research: A systematic review. *Health Expectations, 17*(5), 637–650. doi:10.1111/j.1369-7625.2012.00795.x PMID:22809132

Brouwers, M., Kho, M., Browman, G., Burgers, J., Cluzeau, F., Feder, G., & Zitzelsberger, L. et al. (2010). AGREE II: Advancing guideline development, reporting and evaluation in health care. *Canadian Medical Association Journal, 182*(18), E839–E842. doi:10.1503/cmaj.090449 PMID:20603348

Brown, G., Brown, M., & Sharma, S. (2000). Health care in the 21st century: Evidence-based medicine, patient preference-based quality, and cost effectiveness. *Quality Management in Health Care, 9*(1), 23–31. doi:10.1097/00019514-200009010-00004 PMID:11185879

Brownson, R. C., Fielding, J. E., & Maylahn, C. M. (2009). Evidence-based public health: A fundamental concept for public health practice. *Annual Review of Public Health, 30*(1), 175–201. doi:10.1146/annurev.publhealth.031308.100134 PMID:19296775

Burkell, J. (2004). Health information seals of approval: What do they signify? *Information Communication and Society, 7*(4), 491–509. doi:10.1080/1369118042000305610

Canadian Cancer Society. (1987). *Canadian cancer statistics.*

CAPHIS. (n. d.). Top. 100 List: Health Websites You Can Trust, the Consumer and Patient Health Information Section, Medical Library Association: Retrieved October 17 2008 from http://caphis.mlanet.org/consumer/index. html

Carter, N., & Miller, P., Murphy, Br., Payne, V., & Bryant-Lukosius, D. (2014). Healthcare providers' perspectives of the supportive care needs of men with advanced prostate Cancer. *Paper presented at the Oncology nursing forum*. doi:10.1188/14.ONF.421-430

Charnock, D., Shepperd, S., Needham, G., & Gann, R. (1999). DISCERN: An instrument for judging the quality of written consumer health information on treatment choices. *Journal of Epidemiology and Community Health*, *53*(2), 105–111. doi:10.1136/jech.53.2.105 PMID:10396471

Chua, H., Ho, S., Jasinska, A., Polk, Th., Welsh, R., Liberzon, I., & Strecher, V. (2011). Self-related neural response to tailored smoking-cessation messages predicts quitting. *Nature*, *20*(1), 1. PMID:21358641

Clark, J., Wray, N., & Ashton, C. (2001). Living with treatment decisions: Regrets and quality of life among men treated for metastatic prostate cancer. *Journal of Clinical Oncology*, *19*(1), 72–80. doi:10.1200/JCO.2001.19.1.72 PMID:11134197

Cohen, D. J., Crabtree, B. F., Etz, R. S., Balasubramanian, B. A., Donahue, K. E., Leviton, L. C., & Green, L. W. et al. (2008). Fidelity versus flexibility. *American Journal of Preventive Medicine*, *35*(5), 381–389. doi:10.1016/j.amepre.2008.08.005 PMID:18929985

Agree Collaboration. (2001). Appraisal of guidelines for research & evaluation (AGREE) instrument.

Collier, R. (2011). Federal government unveils patient-oriented research strategy. *Canadian Medical Association Journal*, *183*(13), E993–E994. doi:10.1503/cmaj.109-3978 PMID:21876023

Collin, S., Martin, R., Metcalfe, C., Gunnell, D., Albertsen, P. C., Neal, D., & Donovan, J. et al. (2008). Prostate-cancer mortality in the USA and UK in 1975–2004: An ecological study. *The Lancet Oncology*, *9*(5), 445–452. doi:10.1016/S1470-2045(08)70104-9 PMID:18424233

Davison, B., Szafron, M., Gutwin, C., & Visvanathan, K. (2014). Using a web-based decision support intervention to facilitate patient-physician communication at prostate cancer treatment discussions. *Canadian Oncology Nursing Journal/Revue canadienne de soins infirmiers en oncologie*, *24*(4), 241-247.

Giguere, A., Légaré, F., Grad, R., Pluye, P., Haynes, R. B., Cauchon, M., ... & Labrecque, M. (2012). Decision boxes for clinicians to support evidence-based practice and shared decision-making: The user experience. *Implementation Science; IS*, *7*(72). PMID:22862935

Doak, C. C., Doak, L. G., & Root, J. H. (1994). *Suitability assessment of materials*. Washington, DC: SAM.

Doak, C. C., Doak, L. G., & Root, J. H. (1996). Teaching patients with low literacy skills. *AJN The American Journal of Nursing*, *96*(12), 16M. doi:10.1097/00000446-199612000-00022

Dopson, S., Locock, L., Gabbay, J., Ferlie, E., & Fitzgerald, L. (2003). Evidence-based medicine and the implementation gap. *Health*, *7*(3), 311–330. doi:10.1177/1363459303007003004

Ellimoottil, Ch., Polcari, A., Kadlec, A., & Gupta, G. (2012). Readability of websites containing information about prostate cancer treatment options. *The Journal of Urology*, *188*(6), 2171–2176. doi:10.1016/j.juro.2012.07.105 PMID:23083852

Fagerlin, A., Zikmund-Fisher, B. J., & Ubel, P. A. (2011, October 05). Helping patients decide: Ten steps to better risk communication. *Journal of the National Cancer Institute, 103*(19), 1436–1443. doi:10.1093/jnci/djr318 PMID:21931068

Fagerlin, A., Zikmund-Fisher, B. J., & Ubel, P. A. (2011). Helping patients decide: Ten steps to better risk communication. *Journal of the National Cancer Institute, 103*(19), 1436–1443. doi:10.1093/jnci/djr318 PMID:21931068

Falk, E., O'Donnell, M., Tompson, St., Gonzales, R., Chin, S., Strecher, V., & An, L. (2014). *Neural systems associated with self-related processing predict population success of health messages.* Mass Commun Health.

Ferreira, D., Carreira, H., Silva, S., & Lunet, N. (2013). Assessment of the contents related to screening on Portuguese language websites providing information on breast and prostate cancer. *Cadernos de Saude Publica, 29*(11), 2163–2176. doi:10.1590/0102-311x00150312 PMID:24233032

Fischhoff, B. (2012). Duty to inform Communicating Risks and Benefits: An Evidence Based User's Guide.

Fischhoff, B., Brewer, N. T., & Downs, J. S. (2011). *Communicating risks and benefits: an evidence-based user's guide.* Food and Drug Administration.

Fischhoff, B., Watson, S. R., & Hope, C. (1984). Defining risk. *Policy Sciences, 17*(2), 123–139. doi:10.1007/BF00146924

Frank, L., Basch, E., & Selby, J. (2014). The PCORI Perspective on Patient-Centered Outcomes Research. *Journal of the American Medical Association, 312*(15), 1513–1514. doi:10.1001/jama.2014.11100 PMID:25167382

Genova, J., Nahon-Serfaty, I., Dansokho, S., Gagnon, M., Renaud, J., & Giguère, A. (2014). The Communication AssessmenT Checklist in Health (CATCH): A Tool for Assessing the Quality of Printed Educational Materials for Clinicians. *The Journal of Continuing Education in the Health Professions, 34*(4), 232–242. doi:10.1002/chp.21257 PMID:25530293

Genova, J., Olson, C. A., & Bender, J. (2017). Using the Communication AssessmenT Checklist in Health to Assess the Communication Quality of Web Based Resources for Prostate Cancer Transformative Healthcare Practice through Patient Engagement (pp. 163–191). Hershey, PA: IGI Global.

Grimshaw, J., Eccles, M., Thomas, R., MacLennan, G., Ramsay, C., Fraser, C., & Vale, L. (2006). Toward Evidence Based Quality Improvement. *Journal of General Internal Medicine, 21*(Suppl. 2), S14–S20. PMID:16637955

Guyatt, G., Oxman, A., Akl, E., Kunz, R., Vist, G., Brozek, J., & deBeer, H. et al. (2011). GRADE guidelines: 1. Introduction—GRADE evidence profiles and summary of findings tables. *Journal of Clinical Epidemiology, 64*(4), 383–394. doi:10.1016/j.jclinepi.2010.04.026 PMID:21195583

Guyatt, G., Oxman, A., Sultan, Sh., Brozek, J., Glasziou, P., Alonso-Coello, P., Jaeschke, R. (2012). GRADE guidelines 11—making an overall rating of confidence in effect estimates for a single outcome and for all outcomes. *Journal of clinical epidemiology.*

Harter, L. M., Japp, P. M., & Beck, C. S. (2005). *Narratives, health, and healing: Communication theory, research, and practice.* Lawrence Erlbaum.

Health On the Net Foundation. (n. d.). Retrieved 2014 from http://www.healthonnet.org/HONcode/Conduct.html

Hellawell, G., Turner, K., Le Monnier, K., & Brewster, S. (2000). Urology and the Internet: An evaluation of Internet use by urology patients and of information available on urological topics. *BJU International, 86*(3), 191–194. doi:10.1046/j.1464-410x.2000.00831.x PMID:10930912

Hoffman, A., Volk, R., Saarimaki, A., Stirling, C., Li, L., Härter, M., & Llewellyn-Thomas, H. et al. (2013). Delivering patient decision aids on the Internet: Definitions, theories, current evidence, and emerging research areas. *BMC Medical Informatics and Decision Making, 13*(Suppl. 2), S13. doi:10.1186/1472-6947-13-S2-S13 PMID:24625064

Jacobs, R., Lou, J., Ownby, R., & Caballero, J. (2014). A systematic review of eHealth interventions to improve health literacy. *Health Informatics Journal.* PMID:24916567

Kaicker, Jatin, Dang, Wilfred, & Mondal, Tapas. (2013). Assessing the Quality and Reliability of Health Information on ERCP Using the DISCERN Instrument. *Health Care: Current Reviews.*

Katz, E. (1999). Theorizing diffusion: Tarde and Sorokin revisited. *The Annals of the American Academy of Political and Social Science, 566*(1), 144–155. doi:10.1177/0002716299566001012

Klazinga, N. (2003). Development and validation of an international appraisal instrument for assessing the quality of clinical practice guidelines: The AGREE project [AGREE]. *Quality & Safety in Health Care, 12*(1), 18–23. doi:10.1136/qhc.12.1.18 PMID:12571340

Kobayashi, L., Wardle, J., & von Wagner, C. (2014). Limited health literacy is a barrier to colorectal cancer screening in England: Evidence from the English Longitudinal Study of Ageing. *Preventive Medicine, 61*, 100–105. doi:10.1016/j.ypmed.2013.11.012 PMID:24287122

Lang, E., Wyer, P., & Haynes, R. (2007). Knowledge translation: Closing the evidence-to-practice gap. *Annals of Emergency Medicine, 49*(3), 355–363. doi:10.1016/j.annemergmed.2006.08.022 PMID:17084943

Lazzarato, M. (2002). *Puissances de l'invention: la psychologie économique de Gabriel Tarde contre l'économie politique*: Les Empecheurs de penser en rond Paris.

Loblaw, D., Virgo, K., Nam, R., Somerfield, M., Ben-Josef, E., Mendelson, D., & Talcott, J. et al. (2007). Initial hormonal management of androgen-sensitive metastatic, recurrent, or progressive prostate cancer: 2007 update of an American Society of Clinical Oncology practice guideline. *Journal of Clinical Oncology, 25*(12), 1596–1605. doi:10.1200/JCO.2006.10.1949 PMID:17404365

Makoul, G., & Clayman, M. L. (2006). An integrative model of shared decision-making in medical encounters. *Patient Education and Counseling, 60*(3), 301–312. doi:10.1016/j.pec.2005.06.010 PMID:16051459

Michie, S., & Abraham, C. (2008). Advancing the science of behaviour change: A plea for scientific reporting. *Addiction (Abingdon, England), 103*(9), 1409–1410. doi:10.1111/j.1360-0443.2008.02291.x PMID:18783495

Michie, S., Johnston, M., Abraham, C., & Walker, A. (2005). Making psychological theory useful for implementing evidence based practice: A consensus approach. *Quality & Safety in Health Care, 14*(1), 26–33. doi:10.1136/qshc.2004.011155 PMID:15692000

Michie, S., van Stralen, M. M., & West, R. (2011). The behaviour change wheel: A new method for characterising and designing behaviour change interventions. *Implementation Science; IS, 6*(1), 42. doi:10.1186/1748-5908-6-42 PMID:21513547

Morris, D. B. (2001). Narrative, ethics, and pain: Thinking with stories. *Narrative, 9*(1), 55-77.

Murphy, M., Black, N., Lamping, D., McKee, C., Sanderson, C., Askham, J., & Marteau, T. (1998). Consensus development methods, and their use in clinical guideline development. *Health Technology Assessment (Winchester, England), 2*(3), i. PMID:9561895

Neuhauser, L. (2011). Readability, Comprehension and Usability. In B. B Fischhoff, N., & Downs, J. (Ed.), In Communicating Risks and Benefits: An Evidence-Based User's Guide. US Department of Health and Human Services Food and Drug Administration. Risk Communication Advisory Committee and consultants.

Nielsen, J. (1999). *Designing web usability: The practice of simplicity*. New Riders Publishing.

Nielsen, J. (2004). *Designing web usability*. Pearson Deutschland GmbH.

Norman, C. D., & Skinner, H. A. (2006a). eHEALS: The eHealth literacy scale. *Journal of Medical Internet Research, 8*(4), e27. doi:10.2196/jmir.8.4.e27 PMID:17213046

Norman, C. D., & Skinner, H. A. (2006b). eHealth literacy: Essential skills for consumer health in a networked world. *Journal of Medical Internet Research, 8*(2), e9. doi:10.2196/jmir.8.2.e9 PMID:16867972

Ogah, I., & Wassersug, R. (2013). How reliable are "reputable sources" for medical information on the Internet? The case of hormonal therapy to treat prostate cancer. *Paper presented at the Urologic Oncology: Seminars and Original Investigations.*

Oxman, A., & Group, GRADE Working. (2004). Grading quality of evidence and strength of recommendations. *BMJ (Clinical Research Ed.), 328*(19), 1490–1494. PMID:15205295

Peters, E. (2012a). Affect and emotion. Communicating Risks and Benefits: An Evidence Based User's Guide.

Peters, E. (2012b). Quantitative information. In B. B Fischhoff, N., & Downs, J. (Ed.), Communicating Risks and Benefits: An Evidence Based User's Guide: An Evidence Based User's Guide (pp. 53). US Department of Health and Human Services Food and Drug Administration. Risk Communication Advisory Committee and consultants.

Peters, E., Dieckmann, N., Dixon, A., Hibbard, J. H., & Mertz, C. K. (2007). Less is more in presenting quality information to consumers. *Medical Care Research and Review, 64*(2), 169–190. doi:10.1177/1 0775587070640020301 PMID:17406019

Potomac, M., & Doak, C. C. (2002). Pfizer Principles for Clear Health Communication.

Pruthi, R., Belsante, J., Kurpad, R., Nielsen, M., & Wallen, E. (2011). Robotic cystectomy and the Internet: Separating fact from fiction. *Paper presented at the Urologic Oncology: Seminars and Original Investigations.* doi:10.1016/j.urolonc.2009.04.010

Purcell, K., Brenner, J., & Rainie, L. (2012). Search engine use 2012.

Rot, I., Ogah, I., & Wassersug, R. (2012). The language of prostate cancer treatments and implications for informed decision-making by patients. *European Journal of Cancer Care, 21*(6), 766–775. doi:10.1111/j.1365-2354.2012.01359.x PMID:22574619

Routh, J., Gong, E., Cannon, G. M. Jr, & Nelson, C. P. (2011). Does a controversial topic affect the quality of urologic information on the Internet? *Urology, 78*(5), 1051–1056. doi:10.1016/j.urology.2011.06.050 PMID:21945281

Ruiter, R.A.C., & Kok, G. (2011). Planning to frighten people? Think again. *Writing health communication: An evidence-based guide for professionals.*

Salmon, C. T., & Atkin, C. (2003). Using media campaigns for health promotion. In Handbook of health communication (pp. 285-313).

Salonen, A., Ryhänen, A., & Leino-Kilpi, H. (2014). Educational benefits of Internet and computer-based programmes for prostate cancer patients: A systematic review. *Patient Education and Counseling, 94*(1), 10–19. doi:10.1016/j.pec.2013.08.022 PMID:24021418

Sheridan, St., Draeger, L., Pignone, M. P., Keyserling, T. C., Simpson, R. J., Rimer, B., & Gizlice, Z. et al. (2011). A randomized trial of an intervention to improve use and adherence to effective coronary heart disease prevention strategies. *BMC Health Services Research, 11*(1), 331. doi:10.1186/1472-6963-11-331 PMID:22141447

Shiffman, R., Dixon, J., Brandt, C., Essalhi, A., Hsiao, A., Michel, G., & O'Connell, R. (2005). The GuideLine Implementability Appraisal (GLIA): Development of an instrument to identify obstacles to guideline implementation. *BMC Medical Informatics and Decision Making, 5*(23). doi:10.1186/1472-6947-5-23 PMID:16048653

Smith, S. C., O'Conor, R., Curtis, L., Waite, K., Deary, I., Paasche-Orlow, M., & Wolf, M.S. (2015). Low health literacy predicts decline in physical function among older adults: findings from the LitCog cohort study. *Journal of epidemiology and community health.*

Soobrah, R., & Clark, S. K. (2012). Your patient information Website: How good is it? *Colorectal Disease, 14*(3), e90–e94. doi:10.1111/j.1463-1318.2011.02792.x PMID:21883807

Stamey, T. A., McNeal, J. E., Yemoto, C. M., Sigal, B. M., & Johnstone, I. M. (1999). Biological determinants of cancer progression in men with prostate cancer. *Journal of the American Medical Association, 281*(15), 1395–1400. doi:10.1001/jama.281.15.1395 PMID:10217055

Sullivan, Gail M. (2011). A primer on the validity of assessment instruments. *Journal of graduate medical education, 3*(2), 119-120.

Sutton, S. R., & Eiser, J. R. (1984). The effect of fear-arousing communications on cigarette smoking: An expectancy-value approach. *Journal of Behavioral Medicine, 7*(1), 13–33. doi:10.1007/BF00845345 PMID:6716470

Tarde, G. (1890). *Les lois de l'imitation*. Paris: Kimé éditeur.

Tarde, G. (1902). *Pstchologie économique. Tome second*. Paris.

Tarde, G. (1902). *Psychologie économique. Tome premier*. Paris.

Tennant, B., Stellefson, M., Dodd, V., Chaney, B., Chaney, D., Paige, S., & Alber, J. (2015). eHealth Literacy and Web 2.0 Health Information Seeking Behaviors Among Baby Boomers and Older Adults. *Journal of medical Internet research, 17*(3).

The ADAPTE Collaboration. (2009). *The ADAPTE Process: Resource Toolkit for Guideline Adaptation. Version 2.0*. Retrieved from http://www.adapte.org

US Department of Health and Human Services. (2010). *CfMMS*. Toolkit for Making Written Material Clear and Effective.

US Federal Plain Language Guidelines. (2010). User-Centered Design Basics). Retrieved from http://www.usability.gov/what-and-why/user-centered-design.html

Van der Vaart, R., van Deursen, A., Drossaert, C., Taal, E., van Dijk, J., & van de Laar, M. (2011). Does the eHealth Literacy Scale (eHEALS) measure what it intends to measure? Validation of a Dutch version of the eHEALS in two adult populations. *Journal of Medical Internet Research, 13*(4), e86. doi:10.2196/jmir.1840 PMID:22071338

Warren, E., Footman, K., Tinelli, M., McKee, M., & Knai, C. (2014). Do cancer-specific Websites meet patients information needs? *Patient Education and Counseling, 95*(1), 126–136. doi:10.1016/j.pec.2013.12.013 PMID:24447523

Witte, K., & Allen, M. (2000). A meta-analysis of fear appeals: Implications for effective public health campaigns. *Health Education & Behavior, 27*(5), 591–615. doi:10.1177/109019810002700506 PMID:11009129

Wong, F., Stewart, D., Dancey, J., Meana, M., McAndrews, M., Bunston, T., & Cheung, A. (2000). Men with prostate cancer: Influence of psychological factors on informational needs and decision-making. *Journal of Psychosomatic Research, 49*(1), 13–19. doi:10.1016/S0022-3999(99)00109-9 PMID:11053599

Woolf, St., Grol, R., Hutchinson, A., Eccles, M., & Grimshaw, J. (1999). Clinical guidelines: Potential benefits, limitations, and harms of clinical guidelines. *BMJ: British Medical Journal, 318*(7182), 527–530. doi:10.1136/bmj.318.7182.527 PMID:10024268

Wright, S. (2001). Contribution of a lecturer-practitioner in implementing evidence-based health care. *Clinical Effectiveness in Nursing, 5*(1), 30–34. doi:10.1054/cein.2000.0170 PMID:11761876

Zikmund-Fisher, B. J., Windschitl, P. D., Exe, N., & Ubel, P. A. (2011). 'I'll do what they did": Social norm information and cancer treatment decisions. *Patient Education and Counseling, 85*(2), 225–229. doi:10.1016/j.pec.2011.01.031 PMID:21367557

This research was previously published in the International Journal of User-Driven Healthcare (IJUDH), 6(2); edited by Ashok Kumar Biswas, pages 1-20, copyright year 2016 by IGI Publishing (an imprint of IGI Global).

Chapter 38
RFID–Enabled Healthcare

Amir Manzoor
Bahria University, Pakistan

ABSTRACT

RFID is a new technology that is quickly gaining ground in healthcare industry. RFID is being used in many areas of healthcare from asset tracking to patient care to access control. The objective of this article is to provide an extensive survey of existing literature to identify various applications of RFID in healthcare and ascertain how healthcare industry can gain long-term benefits of RFID technology. Findings indicate that RFID is being used in variety of healthcare applications. Findings indicate that effective use of RFID in healthcare requires various enablers, most important of which is the government support to use of RFID in healthcare. There also exist ethical/cultural issues related to RFID implementation that require close collaboration among RFID products manufactures and healthcare providers. This article also provides several recommendations for healthcare industry in order gain competitive advantage from the use of RFID technology.

INTRODUCTION

The healthcare industry is one of the largest sectors in many economies (Payton et al., 2011). Healthcare sector in USA created approximately 14.3 million jobs in 2008. This sector was expected to provide an additional 3.2 million jobs by 2018 (United-States-Department-of-Labor, 2010). At present, global healthcare sector is facing many challenges such as increasing operating costs, increasing number of medication errors, and ageing patient population. US healthcare expenses were expected to reach almost 20% of the GNP by 2017. That amounted to an increase of 15% in healthcare expenditure since 1963 (Middleton, 2009; Wurster et al., 2009). In Canada, healthcare expenses were expected to be almost 7.1% of the GNP by 2020, an increase of 1.1% since 2000 (Brimacombe et al., 2001). In Australia, healthcare expenses were estimated at 10% of the GNP (GS1-Australia, 2010). Each year, approximately 1.5 million Americans suffered from medication errors and these errors resulted in significant additional healthcare costs (National-Academy-of-Sciences, 2007). A study done in 2002 estimated that the population of people aged 85 and above in western countries would increase by 350% in 2020 (Wiener & Tilly, 2002). Another

DOI: 10.4018/978-1-5225-3926-1.ch038

study estimated that by 2050 the population of older Americans would increase by 135% (Newell, 2011). It is evident that there would be an increased pressure on healthcare expenditure, which will become more complicated given that, due to the economic crisis, several countries are facing critical challenges in providing healthcare services. Healthcare is a very different business due to various reasons. Patients are not typical consumers, they do not always make the decision as to when, and where they will seek which type of care and at what cost. Healthcare providers are not as autonomous as any other typical business could be. Various stakeholders, such as legislators, regulators, and payers often affect both clinical and business decisions of caregivers. For healthcare providers, efficiency is not merely good fiscal practice. It must be a critical component of their mission (Fosso Wamba, Anand, & Carter, 2013; Lefebvre, Castro, & Lefebvre, 2011a). Healthcare sector today provides strong institutional powers and policies for an effective use of information technology (IT). Healthcare sector considers adoption and effective use of IT a critical goal of modern healthcare system to enable better support service delivery (Menachemi & Brooks, 2006; Payton et al., 2011). IT offer many opportunities for healthcare transformation through business process reengineering. Effective use of IT could provide minimized data-entry errors, real-time access to patient data, improved clinical trials, streamlined processes, increased transparency, reduced administrative overhead, creation of new high-tech healthcare markets and jobs and improved overall healthcare management of individuals (PCAST, 2010; Burkhard et al., 2010). The estimated potential safety savings from adoption and use of interoperable electronic medical records systems in USA was approximately US$142–371 billion (Sherer, 2010). RFID technology is considered the next IT innovation expected to expand healthcare transformation (Fosso Wamba et al., 2008; Ngai et al., 2009a; 2009b; Oztekin et al., 2010a, 2010b; Fosso Wamba & Bgai, 2011). In order maximize efficiency and reduce waste, healthcare providers need to answer some tough questions such as what they have, where they have it, and where it needs to go. In order successfully track equipment and people, healthcare providers need a flexible and scalable system that provides automatic tracking with no dependency on clinical staff. One such system is RFID-bases system. All the capabilities enabled by RFID technology have the potential to facilitate new value creation in healthcare service innovation (Dominguez-Péry et al., 2011).

In short, RFID-enabled healthcare transformation projects could lead to tremendous benefits. These benefits include improved patient care, improved patient security, and safety, and improved organizational performance (Reyes et al., 2011). Use of RFID in healthcare can enable "new work practices to develop higher order capabilities for improving cost management, enhancing patient safety, and enabling regulatory compliance in hospital settings" (Lewis et al., 2009, p. 8). The high operational and strategic potential of the RFID technology is effective in the healthcare market. The value of the RFID market rose from about $ 5.63 billion in 2010 to almost $ 5.84 billion in 2011(Das & Harrop, 2011). The global market turnover for RFID readers and RFID tags alone was expected to reach $8.9 billion by 2015 (MarketResearch.com, 2011). In 2011, almost 150 million RFID tags were in use in the healthcare supply chain (Pleshek, 2011). The sale of RFID tags and systems was expected to reach almost $ 1.43 billion in 2019, an increase of 51% from 2009. Such an increase is due to the widespread of RFID-enabled healthcare applications, including the item-level tagging of drugs and various medical disposables, real-time locating systems for healthcare staff, patients and assets for improved efficiency and reduced losses, the compliance with safety requirements, and the availability of assets (Harrop et al., 2009). According to a latest study, the global RFID market was valued at US$ 1.9 billion in 2013 and is expected to grow at a CAGR of 13.9% from 2014 to 2040, to reach an estimated value of USD 5.3 billion in 2020. In 2014, North America held largest market share of nearly 51%. The various reasons contributing to this large market share included sophisticated healthcare infrastructure and increasing number of collaborations between medical device industry, regulatory authorities and nonprofit research organizations. It was expected that the increased research spending in the healthcare industry would further drive the RFID market in the years to come. With a CAGR of above 30%, Asia Pacific was one of the most important RFID market. Improved healthcare infrastructure and high economic growth in the countries of Asia Pacific regions were expected to boost the RFID market in the years to come. Furthermore, rising concern for patient safety and tracking of expensive medical devices, were among the key factors attributing to market growth in this region (Grand View Research, 2015).

The objective of this article is to provide an overview of RFID applications in healthcare. This overview would serve as a foundation for healthcare professionals with limited knowledge of information and communication technologies (ICT) to determine further directions of how RFID can be employed to solve their problems.

STAKEHOLDERS, THEIR ISSUES, AND RFID SOLUTIONS

Key stakeholders of healthcare sector can fall into following some major categories. The first category includes those involved in healthcare program operations e.g. Management, program staff, partners, and funding agencies. The second category includes those served or affected by the healthcare programs e.g. patients or clients, advocacy groups, community members, and elected officials. Third category includes those who are intended users of the evaluation findings e.g. persons in a position to make decisions about the program, such as partners, funding agencies, and the general public or taxpayers.

Stakeholders of healthcare industry face many issues today. In USA alone, more than 500 patients per day are killed sue to errors, accidents and infections in hospitals. This number does not include the mortality and suffering from millions of procedures that never needed to be done in the first place. At the same time, the employers and other purchasers paying for this care are losing "patience" with the slow pace of change in cleaning up the mess (Binder, 2013). Some key players of RFID market included SpaceCode Technologies, Terso Solutions Inc., Dolphin RFID, GAO RFID, Smartrac NV, Motorola, CAEN RFID, Zebra and Alien technology. Most of these players were constantly implementing innovative approaches in novel product development (Grand View Research, 2015).

Role of RFID in Healthcare

RFID uses radio waves to communicate between an RFID reader (also called RFID interrogator) and an electronic tag affixed to an object. RFID tags (active, passive, or semi-passive) are also called RFID chips or transponders. RFID tags can serve as a digital data store and each tag is encoded with a unique identifier that is tied to a database. Tags can be read using handheld or mobile readers, shelf or tabletop readers, or readers that can be installed at doorways. RFID readers communicate with the tags and retrieve the information to be sent to a host computer. This host computer acts as a RFID middleware and ensures communication between the RFID infrastructure and the different organizational systems (Asif & Mandviwalla, 2005). RFID operates without line-of-sight, provide dynamic item tracking to ensure patient safety, improved supply chain efficiency, improved overall safety, and operational efficiency. RFID systems greatly streamline inventory and asset tracking, virtually eliminating human error. Use of RFID systems provide detailed records of the movement of assets.

Issues and RFID Solutions

Following are some of the major issues faced by healthcare industry today and examples of various RFID solutions implemented by healthcare providers.

Asset Tracking and Management

Every hospital has high-value assets (such as wheel chairs, IV pumps, instruments, beds, etc.). If these devices move untraceable and we have no clear mechanism to determine their location, hospital staff can be unable to provide timely patient care. The turnover of these assets is essential for efficient operations of healthcare facility. While constant reporting on exact asset location is not required in all cases, but healthcare provider must be able to know the movement and have the ability to track where the asset goes. A wheel chair may cost around $150. However, it could cost $7,000 worth of clinical time per weak and up to 75% of maintenance time to search a wheel chair. To ensure effective performance of medical equipment regular, scheduled maintenance according to manufacturers' specifications is required. A typical hospital bed costs around $1200. Hospitals incur costs when no bed is available and patients spend extra time in an area that required heavy resources (such as ICU) (Motorola, 2013). According to another estimate, there is nearly $4,000 worth of hospital equipment per bed lost or stolen in the average hospital every year (RFID24-7.com, 2015). Most healthcare providers could make their operations better by increasing efficiency, especially in managing vast supplies of medical equipment. It is estimated that on average 15% of a typical hospital's mobile assets are lost or stolen during their useful life. That translates to an average cost of approximately $3,000 per item (Motorola, 2013). RFID is a highly adaptable technology that can be used to track and better manage critical healthcare assets and patients by enabling real-time identification, tracking, and tracing (Symonds et al., 2007; Bendavid et al., 2010; Fisher & Monahan, 2008). Based on particular needs, RFID-based solutions can include any mix of handheld, mobile, or fixed position readers and RFID tags can be used for virtually any type of item or for people. RFID-based systems can be implemented and be incrementally expanded. RFID tags are widely available, affordable, and inexpensive compared with Real Time Location System (RTLS) tags. RFID technology is a viable mean of checking, tracking, and tracing pharmaceutical products. RFID allows proper management of incident audit trails between the medical equipment and the healthcare staff (Booth et al., 2006). RFID readers doesn't require a line of sight to capture data and their range can be adjusted and modified to meet specific environmental needs and RFID tag types. Since RFID readers are capable of simultaneously capturing the data of multiple assets, the time required to take inventory can be reduced drastically. The RFID readers can be installed at strategic location where there is extensive movement of critical assets to detect and record inventory of such assets. This enables the healthcare provider quickly locate the assets based on their last known location. This quick asset location provides many benefits. These benefits include improved patient care and staff productivity, faster patient and room turnover, improved incremental revenue, tighter asset control, lower replacement costs, reduced patient care delays, reduced capital expenditure, speedy equipment requests, faster equipment delivery, enhanced equipment flow processes, and resource planning. Using data collected using RFID, healthcare providers can easily comply with requirements of the regulatory bodies.

Purdue Pharma L.P., a US-based pharmaceutical company, implemented individual item RFID tagging on its prescription pain relief medicine bottles to follow the products' movements throughout the supply chain (Burt 2005 and Havenstein 2005). Siemens and Isar River University Hospital, Munich,

Germany ran a project with RFID tagging of materials to test the use of active and passive RFID tags to track items used during surgery, and to track the surgical process itself to make sure item utilized during surgery are not inadvertently left behind inside a patient's body (Bacheldor, 2007f). The Royal Alexandra Hospital used a hospital-wide RFID asset tracking virtual asset library. The purpose of this library was to improve the use of assets, ensure the medical devices are available when needed, streamline routine scheduled maintenance, and reduce health and safety risks that could result if scheduled inspection plans are not met (Vilamovska et al., 2008; Britton, 2007). Southern Ohio Medical Center deployed a RFID-based asset tracking system to increase its efficiency of asset and equipment tracking. Medline Industries, a US distributor of medical supplies, marketed a RFID-based asset tracking system to detect any surgical asset left behind in patients after an operation. All surgical assets had RFID tags embedded. Hospital personnel passed a handheld wand containing an antenna connected to the RFID interrogator over the patient to pick up the RF signals of any tagged items left in the patient's body. (Sullivan, 2006). US-based Wayne Memorial Hospital deployed RFID technology for real-time asset location tracking and management. Hospital staff was able to keep track of the location and status of tagged assets (such as infusion pumps and wheel chairs) (Bacheldor 2007; RAND Corporation 2009). The UMass Memorial Medical Center (UMMC) in Massachusetts implemented RFID cabinets. These cabinets stored, tracked, and managed the utilization of high cost cardiac rhythm devices and supplies. UMMC was able to achieve approximately 38% reduction in inventory of selected high volume, high cost items (Collette and Johnson 2008). Ter Gooi Hospital employed Wi-Fi-based active RFID tags to track the location of infusion pumps and EKG machines (Wessel, 2007). Benefits from the application included better use of staff time, improved efficiency, and more timely care (Bacheldor, 2007h). Trondheim Hospital deployed an RFID-based uniform-tracking system. The system provided real-time inventory visibility of uniforms. With this system, Trondheim Hospital was able to reduce the space and labor costs with increased inventory accuracy. Texi, a Norway-based solution provider, developed an RFID system for the hospital inventory management where the RFID tags sewn into the garments were read by RFID readers. These RFID readers were installed in inventory closets and bins for soiled garments. The system provided 90% savings in space costs and resulted in an estimated (US$ 6 million) in space saving (O'Connor, 2007). Bon Secours Richmond Health System deployed a RFID enabled mobile asset management system to track and manage critical mobile medical equipment. This system was one of the largest RFID-based asset management system in USA (Vilamovska et al., 2008; Swedberg, 2008b; Harrop et al., 2008).

Inventory Management

Hospitals have massive inventories of consumables with diverse expiration dates. Because of this, many products are simply thrown away unused. Tagging consumables with RFID allows hospitals to not only eliminate manual inventory processes that waste time, but enjoy greater inventory accuracy and better utilize their consumables. Healthcare providers need to know when various consumables are nearing re-order status, with minimal staff monitoring. Inefficiency also affects inventory management and hospitals often face issues of misplaced, out of stock or expired medical supplies. This happens because no definitive system exists to monitor inventory changes. When there exist high usage levels and access by multiple users, monitoring stock level is often ignored. This absence of monitoring results in inaccurate inventories and unnecessary rush orders to meet patient needs. Many hospitals typically overstock IV because it is a commonly used medical supply often lost or misplaced. This overstocking typically costs hospitals $150,000 per year (Motorola, 2013). Hospitals may overstock other consumables as well such as dressings and instruments. This overstocking could result in tying up an average of 30% of hospital's capital (Motorola, 2013). Multiple RFID tags can be read at once to provide constant monitoring of inventory in a drug or supply cabinet. This way healthcare provider can better manage purchasing, reduce excessive inventories, and reduce delays in patient care. Fixed RFID readers, installed at supply room doors, are able to automatically and continuously record the asset location as it moves from one place to another. Handheld RFID readers provide on-the-spot reading of RFID tags and can be used to count inventory or locate a specific asset that could be misplaced in the supply room. RFID readers are capable of simultaneously capturing data of hundreds of assets. These readers can issue alerts when preset critical levels of inventory are reached. As such, use of RFID tags significantly reduces the time required for taking inventory of all assets in areas such as patient rooms, labs, procedure areas and stockrooms. Another benefit of the real-time, updated, and accurate inventory is to avoid out-of-stock situations for critical supplies needed for patients that would otherwise require rush orders at premium prices. With RFID reader and tagged supplies, items can be automatically dispensed and charged to the patients for proper billing, reduced lost and stolen supplies, reduced replacement costs, and increased revenue by eliminating non-charged consumables. Alerts can be issued to purchasers for expiring products to get timely re-orders. Drugs can be tagged with their national drug codes (NDCs), and LOT numbers. These numbers can be used to specify batch of the drug and drug expiration dates. When RFID is used to track medical inventory, software can issue warning against recalled or expired items. This way healthcare staff can remove compromised items and prioritize use of items that are expiring soon. Use of RFID tags with consumables can allow vendor-managed inventory where vendor would be responsible placing products in the hospital, and retains ownership of the given products until they are used. As such, hospitals can reduce their costs by paying only for this items that were used. In addition, hospitals need to spend less time managing and ordering products (RFID24-7.com, 2015).

DePuy Orthopedics, Inc., is a designer, manufacturer, and distributor of orthopedic devices and supplies. DePuy implemented RFID to track kits of critical operating room products shipped to sales agents and hospitals. Each kit and each part had an RFID tag attached. The system provided improved operational efficiency and labor productivity, time reduction in per-kit processing time and 99.99% read accuracy (ODIN 2008).

Time Management

Clinical time with patients is a critical resource for hospitals and many a times clinical staff spends too much time on non-patient care activities. Hospital nurses could spend an average of 20% of their time simply searching for portable medical equipment (Motorola, 2013). The ability to locate all hospital equipment in real-time has more benefits than just reducing asset loss. It also allows hospital staff to respond more quickly and accurately to emergencies.

Patient Tracking

Even with carefully designed plans of patient tracking, mistakes can happen. About 100 babies are switched at birth in U.S. hospitals every year (Motorola, 2013). Many patients need to walk around the facility as part of the recovery process. Many patients are vulnerable (such as people with mental disorders) and such hospitals need to restrict their movement. Practical solutions are required to balance patient freedom with patient safety. Errors in patient identification can lead to medication errors, delay in patient care, and lost valuable clinical time. One solution is RFID tagged wristbands. Patients wear these wristbands to enable positive patient identification (PPID). With positive patient identification, medication and treatment errors are reduced and patient movement can be recorded unobtrusively as they move around the facility. RFID readers are installed at key places to automatically record movement of patients and alerts can be issues to hospital staff in case vulnerable patients leave the designated areas.

Ospedale Treviglio-Caravaggio, an Italy-based hospital, implemented RFID to track admitted patients as they are admitted. Typically, when new patients arrived and admitted, the hospital followed a series of procedures for diagnosis or therapy. The patients were moved from one medical service area to another. This movement was difficult due to the dynamic nature of the system. For example, if x-ray procedure took long time, patients were taken for another procedure. Use of RFID allowed hospital administration to track the location of those patients or the procedures they had undergone (Swedberg, 2008a). Birmingham Heartlands Hospital used RFID-enabled wristbands to track patients and procedures, identify patients, and decrease incidents harmful to patients. (Bacheldor, 2007g). Xtag developed a RFID- based baby tagging system for safety and security. The system could also be used to track wandering patients in elder care facilities. The babies and elder patients wore an RFID bracelet with an embedded battery-powered RFID tag. The Xtag system offered one of the most secure protection system for the prevention of abduction attempts on the market in the world. The RFID tag was tamper proof and generated an alarm if the strap is cut, the tag is slipped of the ankle, the tag is removed underwater while bathing, or if the tag is disguised or damaged. RFID readers were designed to work with existing access control systems and picked up the signal and transmitted location data to the system (Maselli, 2003). ProSolutions, a Canadian firm specializing in RFID systems and integration, developed a RFID-based system (called BlueTag system) that protected newborn babies, Alzheimer's patients, and other individuals staying in hospital. The BlueTag system leveraged active ultrahigh-frequency (UHF) RFID tags embedded in bracelets and is used in 50 maternity wards in 10 countries around the world. (Bacheldor, 2008).

Healthcare IT Asset Management

Since typical IT equipment in healthcare environments is mobile, the inventory management can be time-consuming and misplaced or stolen equipment can increase costs because hospitals incur costs of hardware and staff costs of searching and re-deploying. There exist very stringent regulatory requirements related to security and control of financial and clinical records. The loss of medical equipment can also result in loss of data and consequently provide severe regulatory implications. Handheld RFID readers can provide a quick and efficient mean for hospital staff to track and manage inventory of equipment. Fixed RFID readers, installed at strategic and high-traffic locations can help keep track of important equipment (such as laptops and workstations on wheels (WOWs)) containing sensitive information.

RFID enable IT asset management provides faster service, improved security, accounting, and helps ensure and demonstrate compliance with HIPAA regulations regarding data security. With an up-to-date and accurate database of assets, hospitals can easily deploy the required upgrades and security updates on the assets. Any interruption in work (due to missing items or data) and time required to take inventory of assets can be effectively optimized.

File and Data Tracking

Healthcare regulatory requirements to safeguard patient records against loss or unauthorized access (e.g. by visitors, patients and other non-hospital personnel) are stringent and apply to both paper and digital records. There exist a variety of documents and data files that constitute patient records. These documents and data files may include charts, physician and pharmacy orders, and laboratory reports and imaging files. The dilemma here is that these documents must be circulated to be useful. RFID-based security solutions can be deployed to provide limited but secure clinical access on an as-needed basis to patient records while racking access. Handheld RFID readers can be used to locate a misfiled RFID-enabled files and folders minimizing the staff time needed to search for documents. Fixed RFID readers can track the movement of these files and folders around the facility. This feature could also help in forensic investigation. RFID technology is hard to counterfeit and provides greater security for sensitive financial and clinical patient-related information.

Huntsville Hospital used a RFID solution to verify a patient's identity and document the surgical process, from admission to discharge. Passive RFID tags were attached with patients. The objective of the system was to improve efficiency and communication that would directly improve surgical start times (Bacheldor, 2007e). The Emergency Health Centre (EHC) in Houston, Texas deployed a real-time RFID-based location tracking system to improve its patient care. On admission, patients wore RFID-enabled wristbands. These wristbands were tracked by RFID readers to record how much time patients spent to receive the needed medical care. Hospital staff received alerts from the system when beds and rooms were clean and ready for occupation. Emergency medical information service provider MedicAlert Foundation and California State University-Stanislaus (CSU) tested RFID-enabled medical cards to provide a more efficient method of collecting and forwarding patients' health-related data at the point of medical service (Swedberg 2007).

A number of RFID-related software applications were developed in Taiwan. Some of these applications focused on the use of radio frequency identification (RFID) technology to prevent spread of the severe acute respiratory syndrome (SARS) disease. These applications include computerized systems for monitoring the body temperature of healthcare personnel and patients in the hospital, track potential virus carriers and, when necessary, map their movements throughout hospitals and keeping track of people under quarantine in facilities separate from hospitals (Ioan, Turcu, Turcu, & Cerlinc, 2010).

Anti-Counterfeiting

Drug counterfeiting is an increasing global problem that results in patient's loss of money. Patients not only get inferior, non-economical products but also face significant health threats because these drugs contain dangerous substances. Pharmaceutical companies lose financially due to counterfeit drug trade and governments lose in terms of lost taxes and resources spent to combat counterfeiting. Worldwide counterfeit sales are increasing at about 13 percent annually, which is twice the rate of legitimate pharmaceuticals sales. Counterfeit sales were expected to reach $75 billion mark by 2010 (National Association of Boards of Pharmacy, 2009). RFID technology can help pharmaceutical companies, distributors, and hospitals to combat and deter drug counterfeiting. Counterfeit pharmaceutical products are a major threat to patient safety today. This is because these products may contain hazardous ingredients (Fuhrer &Guinard, 2006) and they may cause important financial losses to pharmaceutical firms (Dahiya, 2008).

According to some estimates, almost 10% of pharmaceutical products marketed worldwide in 2010 were counterfeit (Lefebvre et al., 2011b) and resulted in about US$ 75 billion in financial losses by the pharmaceutical industry (Dahiya, 2008). In this context, major US regulatory bodies (e.g., Food and Drug Administration) have issued adoption mandates. These mandates require pharmaceutical firms to adopt a unique identifier (or e-Pedigree) for the tracking and tracing of pharmaceutical products throughout the supply chain. These actions have caused a renewed interest in the adoption and use of RFID technology in healthcare sector. Some studies have even suggested that "RFID is an enabling technology that saves lives, prevents errors, saves costs and increases security. It removes tedious procedures and provides patients with more freedom and dignity" (IDTechEx, 2006, p-1). Hospital can work with pharmaceutical companies and pharmacies to tag and trace drugs across the supply chain. This way hospitals can assure the authenticity of their drugs. They can also use RFID to gain real-time data on parameters such as temperature and moisture levels, and configure their RFID systems to provide alerts in the case of conditions that could threaten medication quality (RFID24-7.com, 2015).

Patient Care

RFID technology offers an improved means of reducing errors in patient care, including adverse drug effects, allergies, patient–medication mismatches and medication dosage errors (Thuemmler et al., 2007; Tu et al., 2009; Aspden, Wolcott, Bootman, & Cronenwett, 2007). RFID technology can enable healthcare stakeholders to monitor all steps related to the patient blood collection and transfusion process, including the identification of blood bags at the collection point, the tracking and tracing of products from the collection point to the healthcare facility, and blood transfusion to a dedicated patient (Najera et al., 2011). Also, this technology makes it easier to manage patients with chronic conditions (Cresswell & Sheikh, 2008; Michael et al., 2008).

In healthcare facility operations, we see growing number of patients who are misidentified before, during or after medical treatment. These patient identification errors can result in improper medication of patients or entirely wrong treatment of patients. There could be inaccurate lab work and results reported for the wrong person, resulting in misdiagnoses related medication errors. Some hospitals are using RFID for correct patient identification and to prevent the above errors. By giving each patient an RFID-enabled bracelet encrypted with confidential medical history and treatment information, medical professionals are able to easily identify patients, access their records, easily see patterns, and update medical information (RFID24-7.com, 2015).

A hospital in Saarbrücken, Germany, used radio frequency technology to track bags of blood to record transfusions and ensure that patients get blood intended specifically for them. This RFID solution added significant security so the hospital can make sure the correct blood product is given to each patient (Wessel, 2006a). Italy's National Cancer Institute in Milan and Ospedale Maggiore hospital in Bologna used RFID technology to increase efficiency and safety in the management of the transfusion process. RFID tags were placed on blood bags and patient wristbands and staffs used handheld computers to register patients upon arrival, verify patient-blood group, and recognize patients and transfusion units at any time (Sini et al, 2008; Wessel, 2006c). Amsterdam Medical Centre used RFID to track and trace medical equipment, monitor the movements of patients and staff, and track and trace blood products. The goal of using RFID was to optimize schedules so more patients could be treated. A RFID-based system was deployed by St Vincent's Hospital, Alabama to provide patient-tracking and real-time clinical information. The system resulted in improved quality of patient care and increased revenues (Bacheldor, 2007b; Gambon, 2006). A concept developed by New Jersey orthopaedic surgeon Lee Berger, the noninvasive Ortho-Tag uses radio-frequency identification (RFID) technology designed at University of Pittsburgh to give physicians easy access to information about implants and patients often at the end of a long paper trail (Swedberg, 2008c). Arthur Koblasz developed a body-worn RFID tag. The body-worn RFID tags may include an upper body RFID tag located in a wrist band and a lower body RFID tag located in a sock worn by the monitored person. The RFID instrumentation located in the premises may include one or more antennas located in the floor, door, bed frame, and mattress. The systems may also activate response actions upon detecting specified movements, such as sending an alert message to a patient monitoring system, activating an alarm, activating a camera, and/or playing a recorded message to the person. The purpose was to prevent or detect specific types of movements of the person, such as falls from which the person has not recovered (Koblasz, 2007). The International Medical Centre of Japan implemented a Point of Act System (POAS) to provide real-time input at the point of action. POAS. POAS collected, managed and used consumption data at the point of care (e.g. hospital bed). POAS (Akyama, 2007).

Medication Error Reduction / Medication Compliance

According to National Coordinating Council for Medication Error Reporting and Prevention, a medication error is any preventable event that may cause or lead to inappropriate medication use or patient harm while the medication is in the control of the health care professional, patient, or consumer. Such events may be related to professional practice, health care products, procedures, and systems, including prescribing, order communication, product labeling, packaging, and nomenclature, compounding, dispensing, distribution, administration, education, monitoring, and use. Misidentification of drugs can have very serious consequences. One example is accidental administration of a non-prescribed lethal drug dose on a patient that resulted in paralysis. The reason for this incidence was the similar packaging of the drug. RFID can play an important role in reducing these errors. Drugs with RFID tags, can identify drugs so that healthcare staff do not have to rely on packaging to identify drugs. By scanning a drug's tag, all drug-related information can be accessed and verified. The misidentification of blood types is also a danger in health centers because blood transfusions of the incorrect type of blood can result in death. Blood containers with RFID tags can be scanned to verify the type being used is correct. The misidentification of other substances in use in the hospital can be similarly prevented with RFID as well (RFID24-7.com, 2015).

Germany's Jena University Hospital, the largest hospital in the German Federal State of Thuringia, used passive RFID tags to track medication in real-time from the hospital's pharmacy to intensive care and individual patients. Patients wore an RFID bracelet used for digital matching of medication to the individual patient. Handheld scanners read these bracelets and nurses gained instant access to detailed patient information displayed on a screen. The aim of using RFID was to reduce medication errors and improve workflow (Wessel, 2006b, 2007). Jacobi Medical Center in New York used handheld computers match the RFID tags on patients' wrists with bar-coded information on packets of medication to minimize medication errors and provide patients only the medication that has been prescribed to him or her. This system saved nurses time and allowed the nurse more time for direct patient care (Crounse, 2005). Medixine is a Finnish company that specializes in disease management. Medixine developed a system using RFID and mobile phones to make sure Alzheimer's patients take their medication (Collins,

2004a). A European trial, sponsored by Novartis and conducted by ECCT, an Eindhoven-based provider of medical consumer electronic devices, used battery-powered RFID tags embedded within medication blister packs. The trail showed that monitoring patients' compliance with medication prescriptions can help them comply with their medication schedule—thereby improving the benefits of taking the drug (Collins, 2006). A groups of pharmaceutical companies including Merck and Novartis used RFID tags, along with a range of bar code technologies, on individual items to detect dispensing errors and counterfeit drugs before they reached patients (Collins, 2004b). St. Clair Hospital, Pittsburgh, implemented a bar code software system to eliminate medication-dispensing errors (Swedberg, 2005).

Workflow Improvement

Memorial Medical Center in Long Beach, California implemented a RFID-based people/asset tracking system to improve the operations of its emergency department (Cross, 2006). The new system provided extensive data about emergency department use and patients trends and played key role in the quality improvement initiatives led by the hospital to reduce patients waiting time. This system also provided increased patient safety, better use of staff time, and increased facility capacity (Vilamovska et al., 2008).

US-based Providence Health Center implemented a RFID-based real-time locating system to track patients, staff, and equipment. The objective of the system was to improve its patient and operational processes and tracking of medical devices. RF signals emitted from active RF tags attached with patients/staff/equipment were received by RFID readers. These readers were typically mounted on the walls (Bacheldor, 2007d). Using a grant from Robert Wood Johnson Foundation, Shelby County Regional Medical Center in Memphis, Tennessee deployed a RFID-based patient tracking system to better manage its overcrowded emergency department. As a result, the typical patient stay time in trauma unit increased from 25% to 80% (Gearon, 2005).

Improved Staff Utilization

Healthcare staff spend so much of their time searching for equipment and consumables. More than one third of staff spends at least one hour per shift searching for equipment. This is a waste of valuable medical staff. Use of RFID can make hospital operations more efficient and cost-effective. The staff can spend more time with patients to assess their health problems, provide guidance and support, and perform post-operational monitoring. In this way, the staff provides higher quality healthcare for their patients (RFID24-7.com, 2015).

Improved Access Control

Use of RFID technology in healthcare can restrict access to equipment, medication, or information. This way the security of healthcare facility is improved. This access restriction can be applied to different areas such as pharmaceutical supply rooms and patient records. This can be achieved by using RFID badges programmed with the proper entry codes. With such access control, healthcare facilities can prevent the theft of supplies and drugs. Hospitals can also prevent trespassing into secure, confidential records by unauthorized persons (RFID24-7.com, 2015).

Temperature Sensing

Storage of various consumables of healthcare facilities (such as pharmaceuticals, tissues, organs, vaccines etc.) requires proper temperatures and humidity levels. This temperature and humidity controls is crucial to healthcare facility operations. Improper storage of a single material can put lives at risk and can result in significant financial and reputation losses. Given the importance of proper storage of consumables, many hospitals continue to rely on time consuming and error-prone manual documentation. RFID-enabled sensors can be placed inside the refrigerators containing consumables. These sensors can transmit radio signals to readers that include environmental data. Using an integrated software, hospital staff can be alerted when the temperature or humidity exceeds the defined threshold levels (RFID24-7.com, 2015).

COSTS OF HEALTHCARE RFID IMPLEMENTATION

The cost of the RFID technology (tags, readers, middleware, consulting, process design, troubleshooting, training, etc.) will impact return on investment (ROI) and value of RFID implementation. Direct RFID costs include the costs of RFID tags, RFID infrastructure, and RFID middleware. These direct costs are one key barrier to widespread adoption of healthcare RFID. According to Page (2007), the cost of RFID infrastructure can run from $200,000 to $600,000 or more for a facility-wide RFID tracking system in a medium-sized hospital. Davis (2004) reports that the costs for an RFID system can run from $20,000 to over $1 million depending on the size of the area where the technology is deployed and the application. According to Harrop et al., (2008), the prices of RFID tags will fall substantially in the near future. We can also make similar assumptions about prices of RFID infrastructure and middleware. One way to reduced RFID costs is by substituting RFID-designated reader networks with an existing Wi-Fi network (at the cost of worse granularity and network overload), or by using handheld devices at all times (leading to loss of user-friendliness).

ISSUES OF HEALTHCARE RFID IMPLEMENTATION

There exist many important barriers to wider-scale RFID implementation in healthcare (Ting, Kwok, Tsang, & Lee, 2011; Lefebvre, Castro, & Lefebvre, 2011a; Fosso Wamba, Anand, & Carter, 2013; Middleton, 2009; Buyurgan, Landry, & Philippe, 2013; Garfinkel & Rosenberg, 2006; Wamba, 2012; Ting, Kwok, Tsang, & Lee, 2011; Cheng & Chai, 2012; Yao, Chu, & Li, 2010).

Privacy, Security, Data Integrity and Legal Issues

Healthcare RFID implementation raise many issues pertaining to the protection of the privacy, security, integrity, legal issues, and ownership of the data collected through RFID applications. Within and across healthcare sectors, these issues are not addressed either fully or consistently. Benefits of using RFID in healthcare can be achieved when patients feel confident about security and privacy of the data being transmitted, security of technology, and the related policies (Sotto, 2008). According to Sotto (2008), there can be four categories of privacy concerns with respect to the use healthcare RFID. These concerns include the inappropriate collection of health information through RFID technology, the intentional misuse, or unauthorized disclosure of the data by an authorized data holder, the intentional interception of the transmitted/stored in RFID applications information and its subsequent misuse by unauthorized parties, and the unauthorized alteration of the data kept by an RFID application. To resolve the first issue, patients can be allowed to opt out of RFID systems, and by not using RFID chip to store any medical data on the RFID chip. Such data should instead be stored in a secure server in compliance with the Health Insurance Portability and Accountability Act (HIPAA) (Hagland, 2005). Encryption and authentication techniques can be used to address third issue. Halamka et al. (2006) suggests that RFID chips should serve exclusively for identification, and not authentication or access control.

RFID tags are susceptible to many of the same data security concerns associated with any wireless device. Without the manufacturer adding security options, standard RFID technologies are not yet suitable for secure proximity identification in health care applications as they can be subject to skimming, eavesdropping, and relay attacks. An attacker can beat the system by simply relaying the communication between the legitimate reader and token over a greater distance than intended. Passive tags in particular are considered to be *promiscuous* (automatically yielding their data to any device that queries the tag. This characteristic of tags raise concerns about skimming, interception, interference, hacking, cloning, and fraud, with potentially profound implications for privacy. While a variety of security defenses exist, such as shielding, tag encryption, reader authentication, role-based access control, and the addition of passwords, these solutions can raise complexity and costs. If RFID tags contain personal information, which could include health information, or data linked to personally identifiable individuals, without the proper security or integrity mechanisms in place, privacy interests become engaged. Personal health information is among the most sensitive types of information. As such, it requires stronger justifications for its collection, use and disclosure, rigorous protections against theft, loss and unauthorized use and disclosure, strong security around retention, transfer, and disposal, and stronger, more accountable governance mechanisms (Cavoukian, 2008).

The Unique Device Identifier (UDI) program was created by the U.S. Food & Drug Administration (FDA) to uniquely identify devices in the healthcare supply chain. Medical device manufacturers assign UDI numbers for every version of model of their devices. UDI numbers can be encoded into RFID tags and must also appear in human-readable form. UDI is a standardized numbering system and does not include any RFID specifications. The UDI requirements were developed to improve patient safety. UDI-complied RFID tags can be used to accurately track medical devices, boost the efficiency and effectiveness of device recalls, and simultaneously improve healthcare business processes and supply chain operations. The UDI rollout is in phases with labeling requirements going into effect for some devices in 2014. The program will be expanded to encompass more medical devices each year through 2020.

Technical Issues

There exist many technical issues related to RFID implementation. Some of these issues include the reliability and interoperability of RFID technologies, non-interference of RFID technology with other clinical information systems, and lack of RFID industry standards and best practices. This lack of standardization can also cause interoperability issues for RFID solutions offered by various providers. Practice of non-complying their RFID solutions with current medical regulations (HIPAA) is another barrier to RFID implementation (Fisher & Monahan, 2008). Vendors also do not normally tailor systems to specific healthcare provider needs and that could lead to maladaptation of technology. According to Fisher and Monahan (2008), limited standards also limit interoperability between RFID and existing systems in hospital. To solve these issues, European Union (EU) in 2007 adopted formally an ultra-wideband (UWB) frequency range for RFID healthcare application use in EU member countries. A significant implication of this decision was that RFID solution providers using UWB will need to alter their solutions to meet several new frequency limitations.

Operational / Managerial Issues

There exist a large number of operational/managerial issues related to healthcare RFID implementation. These issues include lack of guaranteed return on investment (ROI), lack of standardization in the risk calculations for identical RFID applications, difficulties in choosing the optimal mix of RFID technologies, lack of RFID best practices, implementation costs, implementation uncertainties, integration of the RFID systems into the existing IT systems, uncertain maintenance costs, and the limited availability of integrated RFID solutions. ROI of RFID implementation may not be guaranteed due to wide variability of RFID technologies and of settings within which they are deployed. Implementation costs and uncertainties are also due to the relatively little experience with healthcare RFID implementation (Anand & Wamba, 2013; Buyurgan, Landry, & Philippe, 2013). Lack of RFID best practices is because RFID technology is still relatively a young technology. Some other challenges to RFID implementation include building RFID infrastructure and bundling applications within hospital (Hagland, 2005). According to Dempsey (2005), hospitals also need to understand that there exist different types of RFID and each type has a different place in healthcare. Dempsey (2005) further suggests that RFID implementation can result in various organizational challenges and change in organizational processes.

Cultural and Ethical Issues

These issues include concerns about the surveillance potential of RFID, lack of understanding of the privacy and security threats associated with healthcare RFID, ethical, cultural, and social perceptions about RFID and its functions, and lack of potential patient acceptance due to the factors listed above (Wurster, Lichtenstein, & Hogeboom, 2008). According to Fisher and Monahan (2008), a closer examination is required of the social and organizational factors that contribute to the success or failure of RFID systems. The results of this examination should be intertwined in the preparatory work for RFID deployment. Expanding capability of interoperable RFID technology is increasing fear of potential privacy threats (Fisher and Monahan 2008). RFID implementation in healthcare has received much attention from those in healthcare community concerned about patient privacy. Boulard (2005) and O'Connor (2005) argues that true threats of RFID implementation related to personal data security and privacy have largely been misunderstood. These misunderstandings have resulted in many anti-RFID movements (Albrecht, 2007) and lobbying initiatives concerned with fear of surveillance threats (Boulard, 2005).

This lack of understanding of the real threats and benefits of healthcare RFID implementation can have severe implications for realization of true potential of RFID in improving the safety and quality of healthcare. This issue could become more serious if widespread awareness of RFID among consumers is not developed in near future. By 2009, only 18% Europeans were aware of RFID (Slettemeås, 2009). This implies that these issues can be harder to overcome among older populations. The acceptance of RFID by these older populations is key for the success of any healthcare RFID solution. National and global legislation, that addresses the privacy and legal issues, can help achieve this acceptance.

PRACTICAL/MANAGERIAL IMPLICATIONS AND RECOMMENDATIONS

Knowing the current state of operation is half the battle in improving it. Real-time information, collected, stored, and analyzed, provides the foundation from which healthcare professionals can glean the sort of business intelligence that can optimize workflow, improve utilization of valuable resources, and improve patient care and their outcomes. Data from RFID sensors provides capabilities to trigger event notifications, provide situational awareness regarding participant status in a workflow, track and manage assets, and even track and contain disease outbreaks. RFID data from multiple systems can be integrated and streamed in real-time into multiple clinical and administrative databases, and Big Data analysis tools can then be applied to dig deeper meaning from the relationships between seemingly disparate data types.

Healthcare providers can benefit from every extra minute saved. RFID tags worn on healthcare professionals ID badges and RFID tags on various assets create a perspective of action and location over time. This gives healthcare providers an objective look at how they're moving their assets/personnel through the hospital and how much time healthcare personals are actually spending with patients versus walking around trying to find needed information and equipment. Adjustments to design or process as a result of this knowledge may help staff feel less pressured as they move through their day, leaving them more capacity to focus on care and minimizing mistakes.

When compared to similar Automatic Identification and Data Capture (AIDC) technologies (e.g., bar-coding), RFID technology presents a vast range of advantages including: a unique item/product level identification, no need for line of sight, multiple tags reading, more data storage capability and data read/write capabilities (Asif & Mandviwalla, 2005). However, the high implementation costs of the technology remains a major inhibitor for its widespread adoption and use, as well as the substantial gap between the technology implementation costs and the RFID-enabled benefits (Bensel et al., 2008). Furthermore, the lack of common standard and the low operational performance level of RFID in a harsh environment continue to hamper its adoption.

There are many ways in which RFID solutions provide a justifiable return on investment, including productivity gains from automated workflow, better staffing-to-demand ratio, lower instances of HAIs, reduced staffing turnover and better protection against damages due to improved risk management. One of the most impactful areas may be increasing Medicare reimbursements for care based on patient survey results. This serves as a major incentive for hospitals to do all they can to ensure patients are not only objectively well cared for, but that they are aware of the quality of their care, feel positively about their experience and report as such. RFID tracking and monitoring provides an unbiased baseline by which providers can measure their performance and make timely improvements, and also serves as evidence of the quality of care provided. It is a transparent model that proves to patients that providers take their perceptions seriously, and aim to excel. It is also a reminder that they must be authentic in their reporting of the care they received. The practical balance of providing quality care efficiently has real impacts on the success of a healthcare organization, but so too does the patient perception of the quality of care.

Legacy information systems may need to be modified to accommodate the RFID system, technology, and information. Depending on the operating environment, the intended purposes, the technology contemplated, and the deployment method being considered, RFID technologies may not deliver sufficient accuracy or performance results to be suitable for mission-critical applications and uses. RFID systems are information systems that automatically capture, transmit and process identifiable information. Informational privacy involves the right of individuals to exercise control over the collection, use, retention and disclosure of personally identifiable information by others. RFID systems inherently poses privacy issues (Garfinkel & Rosenberg, 2006) and warrant a holistic systems approach to privacy. RFID tags contain unique identifiers. RFID tag data can be read at a distance, without line-of-sight even without consent of the individual who may be carrying the tag. This has compelling implications for informed consent. RFID information systems can also capture time and location data, upon which item histories and profiles can be constructed, making accountability for data use critical. Healthcare providers need to know what data is collected, how and for what purposes, where it is stored, how it is used, with whom it is shared or potentially disclosed, under what conditions, and so forth. There are inherent tensions between the, at times, competing interests of organizations and individuals over the disposition of the personal health information, especially over the undisclosed or unauthorized revelation of facts about individuals and the negative effects they may experience as a consequence. RFID information technologies can exacerbate a power imbalance between the individual and the collecting organization (Cavoukian, 2008).

The two major negative implications of RFID systems in healthcare organizations are the privacy of patient health information (PHI) and system implementation. The RFID-enabled medical products can be susceptible to privacy and accessibility issues. RFID tags can be secured by using passwords and access codes but it can be costly. The major concern of healthcare industry is how to minimize the cost of ensuring patient privacy at the highest level. In addition, the costs of implementing, operating, and maintaining RFID systems can be significant. RFID system can be extremely complex to deploy and for a healthcare organization to realize the positive impact of these systems we need investment of significant resources toward the implementation and maintenance of the system (Coustasse, Cunningham, Deslich, Willson, & Meadows, 2015).

Literature identifies many enablers for healthcare RFID implementation (Payton, Pare, Le Rouge, & Reddy, 2011; Cao, Baker, Wetherbe, & Gu, 2012; Wamba, 2012; Mehrjerdi, 2010; Wilkerson & McDonald Jr, 2007; Motorola, 2013; Newell, 2011; Ajami & Carter, 2013; Yao, Chu, & Li, 2010). The primary enabler for the use of RFID in healthcare delivery is the improvement in the quality of care. This quality of care is associated with implementation and capabilities of RFID. The improvement in the quality of care can be in terms of process control and capacity to support modern medicine practices, reduction of harmful incidents, improved resource use, delivery of safe, fast and unambiguous identification, and the creation of an operationally integrated hospital information system. Some short-term advantages of healthcare RFID include distant patient management (at home), biometric data collection, and telemetry and intelligent outpatient care. Given the increasing number of older people in many parts of the world including Europe, these benefits can be promising. RFID is also more efficient as compared to alternative solutions.

Use of RFID allows healthcare providers, analysts and researchers to identify a clear business case for specific RFID solutions that meet their needs best. For example, documentary evidence exists that shows good ROI of RFID inventory and asset management applications. Similarly, evidence shows clear benefit of installing real-time location systems for staff, patients and assets within healthcare facilities (Brimacombe, Antunes, & McIntyre, 2001). According to Murphy (2006), real-time RFID systems can provide clinical timesaving of up to two days a week. There are other uses of RFID (such as RFID-supported haemovigilance systems) that help provide positive, correct, patient-procedure and patient medication. All of these lead to improved patient care and bring direct (monetary) and indirect (e.g. reduced liability and additional treatment costs) benefits for healthcare providers. The falling RFID tag prices and vendor initiative for creating interoperable, cost-effective solutions are some other reasons that provide strong case for RFID adoption.

Healthcare is a complex system and as such the key to success of RFID implementation is the process of implementation. One reason for this is that the healthcare RFID is a relatively young and still developing technology. In its current state, RFID lacks established best practices and involve multiple technology that differ significantly in their functionality and purpose. Staged implementation is often recommended in case of RFID implementation. A staged implementation involves a well-planned and successful pilot, understanding of various RFID implementation-related issues (such as costs, types of tags, system operation, mix of technologies to be used, understanding of business processes, stakeholders analysis, support from top management, vendor selection, and staff training) (Murphy, 2006).

RFID is technically superior to alternative technologies and provide many significant benefits such as real-time data availability, ability to store more data, security of data using encryption, and user-friendliness.

Governments are involved at both national and international level to support healthcare RFID implementation. Governments provide various incentives (such as promulgation of explicit patient safety standards for healthcare RFID applications, the adoption of quality standards in national healthcare systems, and financial incentives for healthcare RFID adoption by healthcare providers (Motorola, 2013).

In the world of healthcare, "the more you know, the better." RFID applications, partnered with data evaluation technology, are a powerful tool in establishing a standard of applied awareness. Hospitals can derive a competitive advantage from this awareness that can dramatically change the way healthcare is deployed and managed to optimize hospital operations and patient outcomes. Use of RFID in healthcare can potentially change the delivery of health services in the years to come. One growing concern is the increasing costs of healthcare. Utilization of RFID technology may be a way to control healthcare expenditures.

FUTURE RESEARCH DIRECTIONS

There is plethora of opportunities for future research in this area. Prior research on IT-enabled firm performance suggests that the role and articulation of 'the underlying mechanisms' through which IT capabilities improve firm performance remain unclear" (Mithas et al.,2011, p-238). How the management of these new RFID-enabled healthcare capabilities should be realized to enhance healthcare performance? This area needs further research.

(Fosso Wamba& Chatfield, 2009) found that business value creation and realization from RFID projects was dependent on many contingency factors such as strong leadership, second-order organizational learning, resources commitment, and organizational transformation. Whether these factors are still relevant and the degree to which they still exist in healthcare sector today is a question that needs further research. This question is important given the fact that the context of the healthcare sector today provides high level of complexity (LeRouge et al., 2007). Another area that needs further investigation is technological, organizational and environmental factors that may have an impact on the adoption and use of RFID-enabled healthcare applications by applying current dominant IS adoption theories (Fichman, 2000). Much more research still needs to be done to evaluate whether the implementation of RFID technology in transfusion medicine is a feasible option for use in healthcare organizations' supply chains.

One of the key challenges of the healthcare sector is the difficulty of measuring the exact healthcare delivery costs to each patient, which allows a comparison of the costs with the outcomes (Kaplan & Porter, 2011). In this context, an area that needs future investigation is the assessment the business value of RFID-enabled item level tagging to evaluate its impact on the healthcare outcome and costs. Furthermore, to understand the influence of different healthcare stakeholders on their peers, it would be interesting to examine the business value from the co-adoption of RFID technology and other healthcare ISs (e.g., ERP, electronic medical records (EMR) systems etc.). Prior studies on IT adoption (Riggins & Mukhopadhyay, 1994) show a positive correlation between the level of business process reengineering and the use of and value gained from Its (Fosso Wamba & Chatfield, 2009). Therefore, additional research is needed to empirically investigate how to reengineer healthcare-related processes (patient, asset and staff) to achieve higher levels of business value from RFID-enabled healthcare projects.

Future research should also look at better strategies to incorporate RFID into healthcare processes and operations. Future studies need for example to identify the scope of the RFID-enabled healthcare project, then assess the potential impact of the technology in terms of incremental and/or process transformation. This assessment should also include the cascade effect that can be created by applying RFID at certain parts of the organization and/or operations. Developing a holistic performance measurement and management system to assess the value generated by RFID-enabled healthcare operations should be also included into future research.

It is proven that use of RFID technology can benefit healthcare industry in several areas. However, more research is needed on the governance and standardization of RFID utilization. Another research that could benefit healthcare industry is the research on health information technology and big data management in relation to RFID technology. Future research can also be done on connectivity and interoperability of RFID systems with hospitals' and providers' health information systems. Such research will be very important for continued implementation of RFID systems in the healthcare industry (Coustasse, Cunningham, Deslich, Willson, & Meadows, 2015).

CONCLUSION

This article presented a comprehensive overview of RFID technology adoption in the healthcare Industry including RFID applications and issues in the healthcare. More specifically, the chapter provided several examples of real-world RFID applications in the healthcare sector to illustrate emerging trends, and how various factors are influencing benefits creation from RFID technology in the healthcare sector.

This article also posits that the realization of the full business benefits from RFID-enabled healthcare applications will depend on many enablers namely better healthcare delivery, clear business case for certain RFID applications, smart implementation, technological superiority of RFID applications, and government incentives/support. The article also highlighted several avenues for future research on healthcare RFID. It can be said that there is a need for more healthcare RFID research. Also, given the sensitive nature of medical information, there is a need for more research on data management, security and privacy issues.

This article contributes to our understanding of RFID implementation in healthcare sector and its contribution to the efficiency of healthcare sector. The article also indicates that the policy makers should be aware of the opportunity to use RFID in healthcare and their policies and strategies should be formulated accordingly. Furthermore, effective use of RFID require various enablers, most important of which is the government support to use of RFID in healthcare. Furthermore, the ethical/cultural issues related to RFID implementation require close collaboration among RFID products manufactures and healthcare providers.

REFERENCES

About the issue. (2009). National Association of Boards of Pharmacy (NABP). Retrieved from http://www.dangerouspill.com/about_the_issue.html

Ajami, S., & Carter, M. W. (2013). The advantages and disadvantages of Radio Frequency Identification (RFID) in Health-care Centers; approach in Emergency Room (ER). *Pakistan Journal of Medical Sciences, 29*(1(Suppl)Suppl.), 443–448. doi:10.12669/pjms.291(Suppl).3552

Anand, A., & Wamba, S. F. (2013). Business value of RFID-enabled healthcare transformation projects. *Business Process Management Journal, 19*(1), 111–145. doi:10.1108/14637151311294895

Asif, Z., & Mandviwalla, M. (2005). Integrating the supply chain with RFID: A technical and business analysis. *Communications of the Association for Information Systems, 15*, 393–427.

Aspden, P., Wolcott, J., Bootman, J. L., & Cronenwett, L. R. (2007). *Preventing medication errors.* National Academies Press Washington.

Bacheldor, B. (2006, May 8). Report Sees Sharp Rise in Pharma RFID. *RFID Journal.*

Bacheldor, B. (2007a, October 29). Denver Health Adopting a Hospital-Wide RTLS System. *RFID Journal.*

Bacheldor, B. (2007b, October 9). Health Facility Uses RTLS to Provide 'Concierge' Care. *RFID Journal.*

Bacheldor, B. (2007c, April 23). Pharma RFID Adoption Still Slow. *RFID Journal.*

Bacheldor, B. (2007f, April 24). Siemens Launches RFID Pilot to Track Surgical Sponges, Procedures. *RFID Journal.*

Bacheldor, B. (2007g, April 10). Tags Track Surgical Patients at Birmingham Heartlands Hospital. *RFID Journal.*

Bacheldor, B. (2007h, December 12). Tergooi Hospital Uses RFID to Boost Efficiency. *RFID Journal.*

Bacheldor, B. (2008, February 13). BlueTag Patient-Tracking Comes to North America. *RFID Journal.*

Bendavid, Y., Boeck, H., & Philippe, R. (2010). Redesigning the replenishment process of medical supplies in hospitals with RFID. *Business Process Management Journal, 16*(6), 991–1013. doi:10.1108/14637151011093035

Bensel, P., & Gunther, O. et al.. (2008). Cost–benefit sharing in cross-company RFID applications: A case study approach. *Proceedings of the 29th International Conference on Information Systems (ICIS),* Paris, France (pp. 1–17).

Booth, P., Frisch, P. H., ... (2006). Application of RFID in an integrated healthcare environment. In Conference proceedings: *Annual international conference of the IEEE Engineering in Medicine and Biology Society. IEEE Engineering in Medicine and Biology Society* (pp. 117–119). doi:10.1109/IEMBS.2006.259389

Boulard, G. (2005). RFID: Promise or Peril? It may be easier than ever to track information, but it is causing concerns over privacy and civil liberties. *State Legislatures Magazine, 31*(10), 22–24. PMID:16397978

Brimacombe, G. G., Antunes, P., & McIntyre, J. (2001). *The future cost of health care in Canada, 2000 to 2020: balancing affordability and sustainability.* Conference Board of Canada.

Britton, J. (2007). An investigation into the feasibility of locating portable medical devices using radio frequency identification devices and technology. *Journal of Medical Engineering & Technology, 31*(6), 450–458. doi:10.1080/03091900701292141 PMID:17994419

Burkhard, R. J., & Schooley, B. et al.. (2010). Information systems and healthcare XXXVII: When your employer provides your personal health record—Exploring employee perceptions of an employer-sponsored PHR system. *Communications of the Association for Information Systems, 27*, 323–338.

Buyurgan, N., Landry, S., & Philippe, R. (2013). RFID Adoption in Healthcare and ROI Analysis. In *The Value of RFID* (pp. 81–96). Springer. doi:10.1007/978-1-4471-4345-1_7

Cao, Q., Baker, J., Wetherbe, J. C., & Gu, V. C. (2012). Organizational Adoption of Innovation: Identifying Factors that Influence RFID Adoption in the Healthcare Industry. In ECIS (p. 94).

Cavoukian, A. (2008, January). RFID and Privacy-Guidance for Health-Care Providers. Information and Privacy Commissioner of Ontario. Retrieved from http://www.longwoods.com/articles/images/rfid-healthcare.pdf

Cheng, C.-Y., & Chai, J.-W. (2012). Deployment of RFID in healthcare facilities—experimental design in MRI department. *Journal of Medical Systems, 36*(6), 3423–3433. doi:10.1007/s10916-011-9796-9 PMID:22072278

Collins, J. (2004a, November 16). Purdue Pharma Tags OxyContin. *RFID Journal.*

Collins, J. (2004b, November 19). Six U.K. Drug makers Pilot RFID. *RFID Journal.*

Collins, J. (2006, June 20). Novartis Trial Shows RFID Can Boost Patient Compliance. *RFID Journal.*

Coustasse, A., Cunningham, B., Deslich, S., Willson, E., & Meadows, P. (2015, June). Benefits and Barriers of Implementation and Utilization of Radio-Frequency Identification (RFID) Systems in Transfusion Medicine. *Perspectives.* Retrieved from http://perspectives.ahima.org/benefits-and-barriers-of-implementation-and-utilization-of-radio-frequency-identification-rfid-systems-in-transfusion-medicine/

Cresswell, K. M., & Sheikh, A. (2008). Information technology—Based approaches to reducing repeat drug exposure in patients with known drug allergies. *The Journal of Allergy and Clinical Immunology, 121*(5), 1112–1117.e1117. doi:10.1016/j.jaci.2007.12.1180 PMID:18313132

Cross, M. A. (2006). Keeping the ER on track. *Health Data Management, 14*(9), 68–69. PMID:17009590

Crounse, B. (2005). RFID: Increasing patient safety, reducing healthcare costs. *Microsoft.* Retrieved from http://www.microsoft.com/industry/healthcare/providers/businessvalue/housecalls/rfid.mspx

Dahiya, S. (2008). Counterfeit medicines: The global hazard. *Latest Reviews, 6*(4), 1–4.

Das, R., & Harrop, P. (2011). RFID Forecasts, Players and Opportunities 2011–2021.IDTechEx.

Davis, S. (2004). Tagging along. RFID helps hospitals track assets and people. *Health Facilities Management, 17*(12), 20–24. PMID:15637841

Dempsey, M. (2005). Weaving through the hopes and hype surrounding RFID. *Biomedical Instrumentation & Technology*, 2005(Suppl.), 19–22. PMID:16134535

Dominguez-Péry, C., & Ageron, B. et al.. (2011). A service science framework to enhance value creation in service innovation projects: An RFID case study. *International Journal of Production Economics*.

Fichman, R. G. (2000). The diffusion and assimilation of information technology innovations. In R. Zmud (Ed.), Framing the domains of IT management: Projecting the future through the past (pp. 105-128). Cincinnati, OH: Pinnaflex Educational Resources, Incorporated.

Fisher, J. A., & Monahan, T. (2008). Tracking the social dimensions of RFID systems in hospitals. *International Journal of Medical Informatics*, *77*(3), 176–183. doi:10.1016/j.ijmedinf.2007.04.010 PMID:17544841

Fosso Wamba, S., Anand, A., & Carter, L. (2013). A literature review of RFID-enabled healthcare applications and issues. *International Journal of Information Management*, *33*(5), 875–891. doi:10.1016/j.ijinfomgt.2013.07.005

Fosso Wamba, S., & Chatfield, A. T. (2009). A contingency model for creating value from RFID supply chain network projects in logistics and manufacturing environments. *European Journal of Information Systems*, *18*(6), 615–636. doi:10.1057/ejis.2009.44

Fosso Wamba, S., Lefebvre, L. A., Bendavid, Y., & Lefebvre, É. (2008). Exploring the impact of RFID technology and the EPC network on mobile B 2B ecommerce: A case study in the retail industry. *International Journal of Production Economics*, *112*(2), 614–629. doi:10.1016/j.ijpe.2007.05.010

Fosso Wamba, S., & Ngai, E. W. T. (2011). Unveiling the potential of RFID-enabled intelligent patient management: Results of a Delphi study. *Proceedings of the 44th Hawaii international conference on systems science*, Koloa, Kauai, Hawaii, USA.

Fuhrer, P., & Guinard, D. (2006). Building a smart hospital using RFID technologies. *Proceedings of the European conference on eHealth*, Fribourg, Switzerland (pp. 131–142).

Healthcare industry. (2010). GS1-Australia.

Gambon, J. (2006). RFID Frees Up Patient Beds. *RFID Journal*. (August 28)

Garfinkel, S., & Rosenberg, B. (2006). *RFID: Applications, security, and privacy*. Pearson Education India.

Gearon, Christopher. (2005) Technology. Behind the hype. *Hospitals & Health Networks*. 79(6), 22-24.

RFID in Healthcare Market Size Industry Report, 2022. (2015, November). *Grand View Research*. Retrieved from http://www.grandviewresearch.com/industry-analysis/rfid-in-healthcare-market

Hagland, M. (2005, February). Radianse in the News, Nine Tech Trends: Bar Coding and RFID. Retrieved from http://www.radianse.com/news-hci-feb2005-barcoding.html

Halamka, J., Juels, A., Stubblefield, A., & Westhues, J. (2006). The security implications of VeriChip cloning. *Journal of the American Medical Informatics Association*, *13*(6), 601–607. doi:10.1197/jamia.M2143 PMID:16929037

Harrop, P., Das R., et al. (2009). RFID for Healthcare and Pharmaceuticals 2009–2019. *IDTechEx*.

Harrop, P. & Crotch-Harvey, Trevor. (2008). RFID for Healthcare and Pharmaceuticals 2008-2018, IDTechEx. Retrieved from http://www.idtechex.com/research/reports/rfid_for_healthcare_and_pharmaceuticals_2008_2018_000146.asp

Healthcare: Career guide to industries. (2010). U.S. Department of Labor.

Rapid adoption of RFID in healthcare. (2006). *IDTechEx*.

Ioan, T., Turcu, C., Turcu, C., & Cerlinc, M. (2010). RFID-based Information System for Patients and Medical Staff Identification and Tracking. In C. Turcu (Ed.), Sustainable Radio Frequency Identification Solutions. *InTech*. Retrieved from http://www.intechopen.com/books/sustainable-radio-frequency-identification-solutions/rfid-based-information-system-for-patients-and-medical-staff-identification-and-tracking

Kaplan, R. S., & Porter, M. E. (2011). How to solve the cost crisis in health care. *Harvard Business Review*, 89(9), 46–64. PMID:21939127

Lefebvre, É., Castro, L., & Lefebvre, L. A. (2011a). Assessing the prevailing implementation issues of RFID in healthcare: A five-phase implementation model. *Int. J. Electron. Comput. Comm. Tech*, 5(2), 110–117.

Lefebvre, E., & Romero, A. et al.. (2011b). Technological strategies to deal with counterfeit medicines: The European and North-American perspectives. *International Journal of Education and Information Technologies*, 5(3), 275–284.

LeRouge, C., Mantzana, V., & Wilson, E. V. (2007). Healthcare information systems research, revelations and visions. *European Journal of Information Systems*, 16(6), 669–671. doi:10.1057/palgrave.ejis.3000712

Lewis, M. O., Sankaranarayanan, B., ... (2009). RFID-enabled process capabilities and its impacts on healthcare process performance: A multi-level analysis. Proceedings of ECIS 2009, Verona, Italy.

MarketResearch.com. (2011, Jnauary). RFID Readers and Tags – A Global Market Overview. Retrieved from http://industry-experts.com/verticals/other-reports/rfid-readers-and-tags-a-global-market-overview

Maselli, J. (2003, May 27). Xtag Unveils Infant Security System, *RFID Journal*.

Mehrjerdi, Y. Z. (2010). RFID-enabled healthcare systems: Risk-benefit analysis. *International Journal of Pharmaceutical and Healthcare Marketing*, 4(3), 282–300. doi:10.1108/17506121011076192

Menachemi, N., & Brooks, R. G. (2006). EHR and other IT adoption among physicians: Results of a large-scale state wide analysis. *Journal of Healthcare Information Management*, 20(3), 79–87. PMID:16903665

Michael, M. G., Fusco, S. J., & Michael, K. (2008). A research note on ethics in the emerging age of überveillance. *Computer Communications*, 31(6), 1192–1199. doi:10.1016/j.comcom.2008.01.023

Middleton, B. (2009). Re-engineering US health care with healthcare information technology-promises and peril.

Mithas, S., Ramasubbu, N., & Sambamurthy, V. (2011). How information management capability influences firm performance. *Management Information Systems Quarterly, 35*(1), 237–256.

Murphy, D. (2006). Is RFID right for your organization? Understand your process before implementing a solution. *Materials Management in Health Care, 15*(6), 28–33. PMID:16859241

Najera, P., Lopez, J., & Roman, R. (2011). Real-time location and inpatient care systems based on passive RFID. *Journal of Network and Computer Applications, 34*(3), 980–989. doi:10.1016/j.jnca.2010.04.011

Preventing medication errors: Quality chasm series. (2007). *National-Academy-of-Sciences*.

Newell, S. (2011). Special section on healthcare information systems. *The Journal of Strategic Information Systems, 20*(2), 158–160. doi:10.1016/j.jsis.2011.05.002

Ngai, E. W., Poon, J. K., Suk, F. F. C., & Ng, C. C. (2009a). Design of an RFID-based healthcare management system using an information system design theory. *Information Systems Frontiers, 11*(4), 405–417. doi:10.1007/s10796-009-9154-3

Ngai, E. W. T., Moon, K. K. L., Riggins, F. J., & Yi, C. Y. (2008). RFID research: An academic literature review (1995–2005) and future research directions. *International Journal of Production Economics, 112*(2), 510–520. doi:10.1016/j.ijpe.2007.05.004

Ngai, E. W. T., Xiu, L., & Chau, D. C. K. (2009b). Application of data mining techniques in customer relationship management: A literature review and classification. *Expert Systems with Applications, 36*(2, Part 2), 2592–2602. doi:10.1016/j.eswa.2008.02.021

O'Connor, M.C. (2005, February 17). Surveys Reveal Dubious Consumers. *RFID Journal*.

O'Connor, M.C. (2007, February 6). RFID Tidies Up Distribution of Hospital Scrubs. *RFID Journal*.

Oztekin, A., Mahdavi, F., Erande, K., Kong, Z. J., Swim, L. K., & Bukkapatnam, S. T. S. (2010a). Criticality index analysis based optimal RFID reader placement models for asset tracking. *International Journal of Production Research, 48*(9), 2679–2698. doi:10.1080/00207540903565006

Oztekin, A., Pajouh, F. M., Delen, D., & Swim, L. K. (2010b). An RFID network design methodology for asset tracking in healthcare. *Decision Support Systems, 49*(1), 100–109. doi:10.1016/j.dss.2010.01.007

Page, L. (2007). Testing gives way to implementation. Hospitals tune in to RFID. *Materials Management in Health Care, 16*(5), 18–20. PMID:17552344

Payton, F. C., Pare, G., Le Rouge, C. M., & Reddy, M. (2011). Health care IT: Process, people, patients and interdisciplinary considerations. *Journal of the Association for Information Systems, 12*(2), 3.

PCAST. (2010). *Report to the President realizing the full potential of the health information technology to improve healthcare for Americans: The path forward. President's Council of Advisors on Science and Technology (PCAST)*. Executive Office of the President.

Pleshek, J. (2011). RFID will see double-digit growth in the healthcare market. *Wtnnews.com*. Retrieved from http://wtnnews.com/articles/8824/

Reyes, P.M., Li, S., et al. (2011). Accessing antecedents and outcomes of RFID implementation in health care. *International Journal of Production Economics*.

RFID solutions for healthcare reducing costs and improving operational efficiency. (2013). *Motorola*. Retrieved from http://www.motorolasolutions.com/web/Business/Solutions/Industry%20Solutions/RFID%20 Solutions/RFID_in_Healthcare/_documents/_staticfiles/Application_Brief_RFID_in_Healthcare.pdf

Riggins, F. J., & Mukhopadhyay, T. (1994). Interdependent benefits from interorganizational systems: Opportunities for business partner reengineering. *Journal of Management Information Systems*, *11*(2), 37–57. doi:10.1080/07421222.1994.11518039

Sherer, S. (2010). Information systems and healthcare: An institutional theory perspective on physician adoption of electronic health records. *Communications of the Association for Information Systems*, *27*(7), 127–140.

Sini, E., Locatelli, P., & Restifo, N. (2008). Making the clinical process safe and efficient using RFID in healthcare. *European Journal of ePractice, 2*.

Slettemeås, D. (2009). RFID—the "Next Step" in Consumer–Product Relations or Orwellian Nightmare? *Challenges for Research and Policy*, *32*(3), 219–244. doi:10.1007/s10603-009-9103-z

Sullivan, L. (2006). *Medline Markets RFID System for Surgical Sponges*. RFID Journal.

Swedberg, C. (2005, September 12). Pittsburgh Hospital Pilots Hybrid System. *RFID Journal*.

Swedberg, C. (2007, February 16). MedicAlert Aims to RFID-Enable Medical Records. *RFID Journal*.

Swedberg, C. (2008a, January 3). Medical Center Set to Grow With RFID. *RFID Journal*.

Swedberg, C. (2008b, March 18). Surgeon Designs System to Monitor Orthopedic Implants and Promote Healing. *RFID Journal*.

Symonds, J., & Parry, D. et al.. (2007). An RFID-based system for assisted living: Challenges and solutions. *The Journal on Information Technology in Healthcare*, *5*(6), 387–398. PMID:17901606

Ten reasons why hospitals deploy RFID. (2015, September 3). *RFID24-7.com*. Retrieved from http://www.rfid24-7.com/white-paper/ten-reasons-why-hospitals-deploy-rfid/

Thuemmler, C., Buchanan, W., & Kumar, V. (2007). Setting safety standards by designing a low budget and compatible patient identification system based on passive RFID technology. *International Journal of Healthcare Technology and Management*, *8*(5), 571–583. doi:10.1504/IJHTM.2007.013524

Ting, S. L., Kwok, S. K., Tsang, A. H., & Lee, W. B. (2011). Critical elements and lessons learnt from the implementation of an RFID-enabled healthcare management system in a medical organization. *Journal of Medical Systems*, *35*(4), 657–669. doi:10.1007/s10916-009-9403-5 PMID:20703523

Tu, Y.-J., Zhou, W., & Piramuthu, S. (2009). Identifying RFID-embedded objects in pervasive healthcare applications. *Decision Support Systems*, *46*(2), 586–593. doi:10.1016/j.dss.2008.10.001

Vilamovska, A. M., Hatziandreu, E., Schindler, R., Oranje, C., Vries, H., & Krapels, J. (2008, July). Study on the requirements and options for RFID application in healthcare. *European Union*. Retrieved from http://ec.europa.eu/information_society/activities/health/docs/studies/200807-rfid-ehealth.pdf

Wessel, R. (2006a, February 27). German Clinic Uses RFID to Track Blood. *RFID Journal*.

Wessel, R. (2006b, June 9). German Hospital Expects RFID to Eradicate Drug Errors. *RFID Journal*.

Wessel, R. (2006c, September 26). RFID-enabled Locks Secure Bags of Blood. *RFID Journal*.

Wessel, R. (2007, June 1). Jena University Hospital Prescribes RFID to Reduce Medication Errors. *RFID Journal*.

Wiener, J. M., & Tilly, J. (2002). Population ageing in the United States of America: Implications for public programmes. *International Journal of Epidemiology*, *31*(4), 776–781. doi:10.1093/ije/31.4.776 PMID:12177018

Wilkerson, J. L., & McDonald Jr, C. L. (2007). RFID in Healthcare. *The Journal of Organizational Leadership & Business Texas A & M University Tex Ark Ana*.

Wurster, C., & Lichtenstein, B. P. et al.. (2009). Strategic, political, and cultural aspects of IT implementation: Improving the efficacy of an IT system in a large hospital. *Journal of Healthcare Management*, *54*(3), 191. PMID:19554799

Wurster, C. J., Lichtenstein, B. B., & Hogeboom, T. (2008). Strategic, political, and cultural aspects of IT implementation: improving the efficacy of an IT system in a large hospital. *Journal of Healthcare management/American College of Healthcare Executives, 54*(3), 191–206.

Yao, W., Chu, C.-H., & Li, Z. (2010). The use of RFID in healthcare: Benefits and barriers. *Proceedings of the 2010 IEEE International Conference on RFID-Technology and Applications (RFID-TA)* (pp. 128–134). IEEE.

This research was previously published in the International Journal of Information Communication Technologies and Human Development (IJICTHD), 8(2); edited by Hakikur Rahman, pages 26-46, copyright year 2016 by IGI Publishing (an imprint of IGI Global).

Chapter 39

Study of Real–Time Cardiac Monitoring System:
A Comprehensive Survey

Uma Arun
Center for Medical Electronics and Computing, M.S. Ramaiah Institute of Technology, India

Natarajan Sriraam
Center for Medical Electronics and Computing, M.S. Ramaiah Institute of Technology, India

ABSTRACT

Today's healthcare technology provides promising solutions to cater to the needs of patients. The development of wearable physiological monitoring system has reached home-centric patients by ensuring faster healthcare services. The primary advantage of this system is activation of alarms to alert the specialist in a nearby hospital to attend to any sort of emergency. Specifically, cardiac-related problems need special attention when a 24-hour Holter monitors ECG signals and identifies the level of abnormalities under various circumstances. Although several brands of Holters exist in market, there is a huge demand for digitized Holter recorders. These recorders can simultaneously analyse cardiac signals in real time mode and store the data and reuse them for next 24 hours. As home-centric based wearable cardiac monitoring system gains much attention recently, there is a need to design and develop a cardiac monitoring system by establishing a trade-off between the required clinical diagnostic quality and cost. This research study highlights a comprehensive survey of various cardiac monitoring systems under wire, wireless and wearable modes. This provides an insight into the need of the hour in bringing a cost-effective wearable system. The study provides an insight of the technological aspects of the existing cardiac monitoring system and suggests a viable design suitable for developing countries.

INTRODUCTION

Due to quality of lifestyle today, there is a huge increase in percentage of young age group (say 18 to 30 years) prone to chronic cardiac-related diseases. Electro cardiogram (ECG), which reflects the continuous cardiac activities, plays an important role in providing the required clinical diagnostic information

DOI: 10.4018/978-1-5225-3926-1.ch039

for the cardiology community. In the last two decades, Holter recorders have been used to monitor continuous cardiac episodes for 24-48 hours (Erik et al., (2015)). Their dynamic non-invasive monitors store the recordings and are validated later by a cardiologist for arrhythmias detection. Attempts have been made to design digital Holter recorders to overcome certain limitations. Due to the severity level of chronic cardiac-related disorder, there is a huge demand to recognize the related episodes in a real-time mode and to raise an alarm for the patient to consult a specialist immediately. On the other hand, these episodes can be transmitted in a real-time mode through cloud server and the specialist in a nearby hospital can direct the patient based on the severity level. Taking this trait into account, wearable physiological monitoring system has gained much attention in the recent years. Systems that make use these technologies are being introduced in market then and there.

Although wearable technology which is closely associated with home-centric based health care delivery gained popularity, its huge cost restricts its affordability to resource-constrained population. This research study provides an insight into real-time cardiac monitoring system, a comprehensive survey on various systems and signal processing techniques reported in the literature. The salient features and limitations of cardiac monitoring systems are also compared. Finally, a real-time cardiac monitoring system is proposed to overcome all these limitations.

CARDIAC MONITORING SYSTEM

Recent developments in the miniaturization aspect of sensors has created a huge impact on the wearable physiological monitoring related studies. Such sensing device ensures portability with less power consumption as well as effective energy utilization. The primary advantage of such systems are continuous monitoring of the signals in real-time by clinicians in a monitoring station along with activation of alarms during critical conditions.

In general physiological sensors, such as ECG, demand large energy due to high sampling rate and resolution and also impose limitations due to reduced user wearability. Holter systems are available for patients with cardiovascular diseases to record their cardio activities as demonstrated by Laze et al (1997). In 2001, there has been a notion of telemedicine using mobile phone by NegoslavDaja et al and with power efficient algorithms for Paroxysmal Atrial Fibrillation as proposed by Schreier et al. (2002). Gouaux et al. (2002) proposed a smaller and feasible device for telemedicine. However, it was still insufficient due to lack of processing of raw ECG signals in their devices.

Wireless sensing technology in the recent past decade can enables the healthcare delivery in a better manner and helps in monitoring of patients who are at risk. Although these sensor nodes offer potential low-power operation, the need to limit battery volume to enable a compact package and the need for supporting energy-intensive sensing systems require an energy management method (Winston et al., 2008). This must optimize the operation of sensors and other components further to meet measurement demands while minimizing energy. Energy usage of sensor nodes may be reduced by activating and deactivating sensors according to real-time measurement demand. For better brevity, Table 1 emphasize the various cardiac monitoring system reported in the literature .The report comprises of engineering principles, sensors used, design factor, signal processing and communication modalities adopted and advantage/limitations of each technique.

Table 1 shows a brief report of related literature.

Table 1. Brief study on literature: Cardiac monitoring system

Sl. No.	Title of Ref. Paper and Author	ECG Sensors	Amplification	Detailed Processor Information	Signal Processing	Transmission	Advantages
1	Real time ECG telemonitoring system design with mobile phone platform-(Cheng wen, et al., 2006)	Holter recording. Lead II ECG signal by prejelledelectrodes. ECG acquisition used in store and forward mode and real time mode	Instrumen-tation Amp with a gain of 1000.	Dual core processor (OMAP-5910).It integrates a DSP with an ARM.	HPF to reduce base line wander followed by IA and II order Bessel LPF to remove noise and movement artefacts.	ECG with information provided by GPS module in to an MMS message send it to the server through GSM/ GPRS module.	The communi-cation cost was reduced as this method transmitted only abnormal cases of ECG after real time acquisition and classification.
2	A wireless wearable ECG sensor for long term applications-(Ebrahim et al., 2012)	Wearable ECG sensor of wireless type-Thin capacitive electrode integrated with T shirt.	Instrumen-tation Amplifier LMC6001	Low power Microcon-trollerwith low operating voltage	IA followed by LPF, HPF, Notch filter of 60Hzand 10bit ADC.	ANT Protocol operates at2.4GHz and distance up to 30m.	Small size, Low weight and good quality of the measured signal. Sensor is good for long term monitoring.
3	Wearable physiological monitoring system using 2.4 GHz RF Transceiver-(Chihhuwang et al., 2007)	Wired type with ECG electrodes based in belt and 3axis Accelerometer (ADXL320) for movement.	ECG amplifier was incorporated in Physio-logical detector.	Microcon-troller MSP430 process and the data was stored in ring buffer.	ECG data and accelerometer data were converted into digital by ADC and fed into Microcon-troller	The output from microcon-troller goes to RF transceiver at 2.4GHz with FSK modulation.	Portable, wire-less and physiological monitoring system.
4	A computer based Wireless system for online acquisition, monitoring and digital processing of ECG waveforms-(Dipali Bansal et al., 2009)	Non-invasive disposable Ag-Ag Cl electrodes from RA, LA, RL after applying gel.	Cascaded amplifiers were used.Two stages of buffer amplifier, Unity gain amplifier followed by dc restoration amplifier with overall gain of 500.	Wireless FM transceiver	Matlab & Labview	FM wireless transmission	The ECG signal is transmitted in wireless FM so accurate measurement of cardiac output and cost effective.
5	MEMS wear biomonitoring system for remote vital signs monitoring - (Francis Tay et al., 2009).	ECG sensor integrated with SPO2 and temp sensor as a wearable T shirt in MEMS wear biomoni-toring	No separate amplifiers	Microcontrol-ler MSP430 (TI FG439)	The ECG signal was converted by ADC12 in the MCU with sampling frequency of 512Hz,Using two sym FIR LPF and HPF filtering is done	From MCU to patients PDA through Bluetooth. From here to doctors PDA through GSM network	All physiological signs will be immediately transmitted to patients PDA phone through bluetooth and to doctors PDA through GSM.
6	Toward a low cost and single chip holter: (Honding et al., 2011).	Wearable single chip ECG sensor using SoC holter with 1to 4 leads for 24 to 72 hours.	Preamplifica-tion was done by 3 stages to provide a gain of 500.	Nanocon-troller was used instead of MCU to provide low power based on 8 bit RISC processor.	AfterAfter amplification filtering by BPF and ADC of 12bit with sampling frequency of 1KHz.	With RS232 interface to Bluetooth/ Zigbee medium from the nanocon-troller.	With Single chip wearable Holter, large number of high risk population can be prevented from sudden death. Using a nanocontroller it was possible to reduce the energy consumption of Soc holter.
7	Real-Time ECG Transmission Via Internet for Nonclinical Applications-(Alfredo et al., 2001)	-----	Using Instrumen-tation Amp	PIC Microcon-troller	Instrumentation Amplifier & Analog to Digital Converter	Internet	
8	Smart Vest: Wearable multi parameter remote physiological monitoring system - (Pandian et al.,2008)	A number of tiny Wireless sensors placed on the human body to create body area network.		Sensors connected with washable shirt	Wearable	Remote	

continued on following page

Table 1. Continued

Sl. No.	Title of Ref. Paper and Author	ECG Sensors	Amplification	Detailed Processor Information	Signal Processing	Transmission	Advantages
9	Electrocardiogram (EKG) Data Acquisition and wireless transmission- (Patrick O Bobbie et al.)	Direct contact type electrodes	Instrumen-tation Amplifer using AD624	Microcon-troller	Low pass filter and notch filters were used after instrumentation amplifer.	Bluetooth and RF circuits. Transmission to PC and setup box.	Heart Patients with home based monitoring and useful in hospital without compromising patient mobility due to wires.
10	Wireless Sensor Networks for Monitoring Physiological Signals of Multiple Patients (Reza S. et al., 2011)	ECG sensor connected to amplifier	ECG amplifier and Noise cancellation using INA2322	Micro-controller MSP430F2274, CC2500 and wireless access point network connected to router and then through internet it reaches hospital.	In built Instrumentation amplifier with several opamps used for high pass feedback filtering and low pass filtering.	CC2500 and wireless access point network connected to router and then through internet it reaches hospital. The transmission from patient to access point through Texas InstrumentsSimpliciTI wireless communica-tion protocol.	This method was not using any Personal computer with the patient.
11	A Reliable Transmission Protocol for ZigBee-Based Wireless Patient Monitoring (Shyr-Kuen Chen et al., 2012)	ECG sensor was combined with accelerometer.	No amplifiers	Not much signal processing	3axis accelerometers were used for fall detection	Zigbee network	A reliable routing protocol for ZigBee-based wireless patient monitoring was used. It selects the closest data sink, therefore fast rerouting. A broken path was recovered in a short latency, and the reliability of the transmitted vital signs were assured.
12	Clinical Assessment of Wireless ECG Transmission in Real-Time Cardiac Telemonitoring (Alesanco et al., 2010)	The ECG signals were taken from MIT-BIH Arrhythmia database	No amplifiers	ECG signals were encoded before transmission.	There was no signal processing	The wireless Channel was used for the ECG transmission.	A real time ECG transmission protocol was used
13	A Mobile Care System With Alert Mechanism (Ren-Guey Lee et al., 2007)		Physiological parameter extraction device.	All physiological signals such as ECG, Spo2, -Blood pressure and pulse.	There was no signal processing	Mobile communication using Bluetooth	
14	Multi-Functional Device for Cardiologic Telemedicine and Diagnostic Holter (A Belardinelli et al., 2008)	No separate sensors.	TH16 was configured to acquire and store up to 20 standard ECG recordings or a 3 channels 24 hours holter monitoring.	No separate amplifiers.	TH16 was equipped with a six keys keyboard and a 240x320 display. It check the correctness of the electrode positions, review the acquired data and manage the internal ECGs archive, allowed the patient to insert notes during the holter monitoring, driving the patient or the doctor during the transmission of the ECGs to the server (A Belardinelli et al., 2008)	Communication between the TH16 and the server was digital and performed via either a PSTN or a GSM modem.	TH16 was a powerful and easy to use device, well tolerated by patients. The intermediary role of the family doctor between patient and specialist represent the best solution in order to optimize the procedures and refine the diagnosis (A Belardinelli et al., 2008)

RELATED LITERATURE

Cheng wen et al. (2008) have designed an ECG telemonitoring system based on a mobile phone platform. The signals were identified by the patient wearing Holter unit and abnormal heartbeats were transmitted in real-time system using GPRS or MMS. The Holter information through GPRS was then used to locate the patient in emergency. Real-time ECG classification algorithm was executed by a dual-core processor to identify abnormal beats with classification accuracy in the order 98%.

Ebrahim et al.,(2008) have showed that sensing vital signs using wireless medical sensors was promising compared to conventional, in-hospital healthcare systems. Due to high impedance between ECG signal source and the sensor, the signal quality was not as good as the signal coming from wet ECG systems.

ChihHu Wan et al., (2008) have proposed a wearable physiological monitoring system using low power RF transceiver. This system processes signals from patients and raises alarm to the central nursing station. In the detecting device, an ECG module is used to acquire the patient's ECG and a three axis accelerometer reflects his activity. An ADC-based microcontroller converts analog signal into digital data and transfers to RF transreceiver CC2500.The transreceiver provides wireless data communication for 2.4GHz signal.

Bansal et al., (2009) have suggested a cardiac monitoring system that comprise of an analog system and a FM transceiver pair interfaced through the audio port of a computer. The real-time acquired data was viewed and filtered using MATLAB software. The designed ECG system captured bio-signals faithfully in real-time wireless mode with minimum noise and had universal connectivity. The main drawback was their susceptibility to noise, lack of universal connectivity and off-line processing.

Francis Tay et al., (2009) have suggested a remote vital signs monitoring system that integrated wireless body area network and personal digital assistant phone technology. Four different physiological signs like ECG, SPo2, blood pressure and temperature were derived from ECG sensor and temperature sensor. All physiological signs and critical indices were transmitted to a patient's phone through bluetooth and further to a doctor's phone through global communication technology. The system offered a high standard of healthcare with cost reduction. The limitations were system performance and information security during transmission.

Hao ding et al., (2011) have designed an integrated single chip (SoC) wearable Holter, which recorded 1~4 leads ECG. This single chip SoC-Holter was relied on adequation algorithm architecture. To minimize energy consumption, CMOS technology (0.35μm) was used. The SoC-Holter had the following functions: signal conditioner, preamplifier, amplifier, filter, analog-to-digital converter, and nano-controller. The low-pass filter was composed of current division, degeneration and common-mode feedback circuits. Hence, an integrated, low cost, and user-friendly single chip Holter was feasible and a large number of high-risk populations were monitored. This SoC-Holter consumed less than 10 mW when the device was operating.

Pandian et al., (2008) have designed a wearable monitoring system using a washable shirt. It was with an array of sensors connected to a processing unit with firmware for monitoring physiological signal continuously. The wearable physiological system was called as smart vest. It consisted of sensors integrated with monitoring physiological parameters, wearable data acquisition, processing hardware and remote monitoring system. The wearable data acquisition system was designed using a microcontroller and interfaced with wireless communication and GPS modules. The monitored signals were ECG, PPG, temperature, pressure and heart rate. The drawbacks were limited availability of energy on network nodes. The maximum energy was consumed for communication capabilities. Hence, energy-conserving communication protocols were used. The bandwidth was limited and it was shared by all the nodes. Wireless sensor network suffered from the problem of node failure, noise interference from external sources as physiological signals were low in amplitude and frequency. Hence, reliable and efficient communication was needed.

Patrick O Bobbie et al., (2008) have suggested a platform of an EKG sensor capable of transmitting EKG signals to a PC or setup box. The signals were sampled at 250 samples at 12-bit resolution and transmitted wireless to remote monitoring system. The working of sensor was demonstrated using 802.11b. The device acquires EKG signal data prolific, is easy to obtain and effective. The development of functions that checks EKG waveform for abnormalities and alerts a doctor or a patient should be improved.

Reza S. Dilmaghani et al., (2011) have designed home centric based health monitoring using wireless sensor network where the remote node was connected to the local nearby hospital where as the host node was attached to the patient. The entire system were comprised of ECG sensors, MSP430 microcontrollers, a CC2500 low-power wireless radio and a network protocol called SimpliciTI protocol. The limitations were the need of additional access pointsto cover wider area and loss of data packets due to wireless environment.

Shyr-Kuen Chen et al., (2012) have designed a reliable routing protocol for ZigBee-based wireless patient monitoring. For a mobile sensor node, the new scheme selected the closest data sink as the destination in a WMN. Therefore, the latency of route query and the number of control messages was reduced simultaneously. The new protocol had the capability of fast rerouting. Therefore, a broken path was recovered with a short latency and reliability of the transmitted vital signs was assured. They implemented a ZigBee-based prototype of fall monitoring system based on the new routing protocol. In the system, a triaxial accelerometer and an ECG sensor to achieve real-time fall detection and physiological monitoring were integrated. When a fall event was detected, the closest router node to the sensor node was calculated. In addition, 4-s ECG signals were transmitted to the healthcare professional for notifying the patient status. The system was combined with the next generation WAN, such as LTE or WiMAX, to achieve pervasive healthcare. Through the integration with WiMAX, it improved the feasibility of wireless patient monitoring systems.

Alesanco et al. (2009) have suggested a study of wide-area wireless ECG transmission for real-time cardiac telemonitoring taking into account both technical and clinical aspects. The proposed technique had the facility of real-time monitoring by considering both channel parameters and tolerance of cardiologists to the effects of interruptions introduced during transmission. By using extensive wireless simulated scenarios, the compressed ECG signal was monitored on reception. A new protocol [reliable ECG transmission protocol (RETP)] was used to perform retransmissions of erroneous packets.

Hypertension and arrhythmia were chronic diseases which can be effectively prevented and controlled only if the physiological parameters of the patient are constantly monitored, along with the full support of health education and professional medicalcare. Ren-Guey Lee et al (2007) have suggested a role-based intelligent mobile care system with alert mechanism in chronic care environment. The system included patients, physicians, nurses and healthcare providers. Each of the persons uses a mobile phone to communicate with the server setup in the care center. For commercial mobile phones with Bluetooth communication capability, they have developed physiological signal recognition algorithms. This was implemented and built in the mobilephone without affecting its original communication functions. It was thus possible to integrate several front-end mobile care devices with Bluetooth communication capability to extract various physiological parameters of a patient [such as blood pressure, pulse, saturation of haemoglobin (SpO2) and (ECG)]. Thus, the physiological signal extraction devices only have to deal extraction and wireless transmission. Since they do not have to do signal processing, their form factor was further reduced to reach the goal of micro miniaturization and power saving. An alert management mechanism was included in back-end healthcare center to initiate various strategies for automatic emergency alerts. Within the time intervals in system setting, according to the medical history of a specific patient, the prototype system informed various healthcare providers in sequence to provide healthcare service.

A Belardinelli et al (2008)have suggested a more versatile, easy to use device that shortens the diagnosis time, avoids the patient to move to a healthcare center .The device was well tolerated by patients and the work flow allures the practitioners for the combination of its simplicity and effectiveness in reducing the time to reach the diagnosis, although a remarkable number of cardiac traces were not good enough to formulate a diagnosis, mainly due to contact loss in the patient's electrical circuit. All the causes of bad electrical connections were investigated and corrective measures were taken to improve the number of good quality signals.

DISCUSSION

From the literature table (Table 1) and the brief note on the existing real time cardiac monitoring system, it can be inferred that the design perspective of cardiac monitoring system varies from adopting a simple gel based electrodes to wireless dry electrodes. Attempts have been made to solve the power consumption, energy fixation, communication protocols, real time processor design, sensor selection and amplifier design. For wired and wireless scenario, accessibility to home centric healthcare delivery was not addressed efficiently. Most of the study restricts on the sample size, integration of the units was not addressed appropriately. Though wearable modes were reported, the effectiveness of the system in the context of patient's adaptability/comfortability was not addressed. For under developing countries, it is necessary that the healthcare delivery reach rural community by overcoming the constraints such as device cost, hazle free consultation. Screening procedure need to be introduced in such a scenario to take necessary steps to prohibit chronic cardiac related disorders. Hence the primary focus in terms of designing wearable real time cardiac monitoring system should rely on the wearable sensors with a system on chip(Soc) node where the entire preprocessing, feature extraction, classification of arrhythmias stages are configured with appropriate power drive to make the system to monitor the activities in a real time mode.

It can be inferred from the recent studies, most of the real time processor has the facility of configuring into Soc mode. For example, NI myRio processor, Cypress PSoc processor and Ardino processor can be adopted to configure the all possible operations into a single chip. On the other hand, several FGPA modalities are providing promising results for physiological monitoring applications which can program the entire operation into a single chip.

Attempts have not been made so far to make use of the local electronic components available in the market in the under developing countries. Several lab based projects have been developed by the biomedical engineering student community, where there are potentials to convert such attempts into appropriate level.

The following are the challenges while designing the real time cardiac monitoring system:

- The designed ECG system should record the rhythms continuously by rejecting artifacts and other external environmental noise etc., and the storage capability should enhance the facility of recordings more than 24 hours;
- The real time processor should ensure the precision, storage, power consumption capabilities compared to the existing system;

- Apart from establishing appropriate communication protocols, the processor shall be integrated into the Internet of Things (IOT) modules to ensure the real time access of recordings by the specialist at a remote place with a cloud computing server at the host end;
- The system should have the facility of converting raw data into digitized samples suitable for signal processing. Such a procedure is essential to develop automated detection of arrhythmias and generate an alert alarm signal to the patient or to the clinical specialist to take appropriate action to save the life of the patient.

REFERENCES

Aleksandrowicz, A., & Leonhardt, S. (2007). Wireless and Non-Contact ECG Measurement System -The Aachen Smart Chair. *Acta Polytechnica Czech Tech. Univ.*, *47*(4–5), 68–71.

Alesanco, A., & Garcıa, J. (2010). Clinical Assessment of Wireless ECG Transmission in Real-Time Cardiac Telemonitoring. *IEEE Transactions on Information Technology in Biomedicine*, *14*(5), 1144–1152. doi:10.1109/TITB.2010.2047650 PMID:20378476

Bai, J., & Lin, J. (1999). A pacemaker working status telemonitoring algorithm. *IEEE Transactions on Information Technology in Biomedicine*, *3*(3), 197–204. doi:10.1109/4233.788581 PMID:10719483

Bansal, D., Kahn, M., & Salhan, A.K. (2009). A computer based Wireless system for online acquisition, monitoring and digital processing of ECG waveforms. *Computers in biology and medicine*, *39*(4), 361-367. doi:10.1016/j.compbiomed.2009.01.013

Belardinelli, A., Muratori, L., Corazza, I., Magnalardo, M., Marangoni, F., & Zannoli, R. (2008). Multi-Functional Device for Cardiologic Telemedicine and Diagnostic Holter. *Computers in Cardiology*, *35*, 985–987.

Bobbie, P.O., Arif, C.Z., Chaudhari, H., & Pujari, S. (n. d.). *Electrocardiogram (EKG) Data Acquisition and Wireless Transmission*. Southern Polytechnic State University, Marietta, GA, USA.

Carson, E., Cramp, D.G., Morgan, A., & Roudsari, A.V. (1998). Clinical decision support, systems methodology, and telemedicine: Their role in the management of chronic disease. *IEEE Trans. Inform. Technol. Biomed.*, *2*(2), 80–88.

Chen, S.-K., Kao, T., Chan, C.-T., Huang, C.-N., Chiang, C.-Y., Lai, C.-Y., & Wang, P.-C. et al. (2012). A Reliable Transmission Protocol for ZigBee-Based Wireless Patient Monitoring. *IEEE Transactions on Information Technology in Biomedicine*, *16*(1), 6-16. PMID:21997287

Cheng Wen, Ming-Feng Yeh, Kuang-chiung, & Ren-Guey Lee. (2008). Real time ECG telemonitoring system design with mobile phone platform. *Measurement*, *41*(4), 463-470. doi:10.1016/j.measurement.2006.12.006

Chihhuwang, Ching-Cheng, Chen Tien, Chien Yu Chen. (2007). Wearable physiological monitoring system using 2.4GHz RF Transceiver. *Chung Hua Journal of Science and Engineering*, *5*(4), 59–62.

Coosemans, J., Hermans, B., & Puers, R. (2006). Integrating wireless ECG monitoring in textiles. *Sensors and Actuators. A, Physical, 130–131*, 48–53. doi:10.1016/j.sna.2005.10.052

Corbishley, P., & Rodríguez-Villegas, E. (2008). Breathing detection: Towards a miniaturized, wearable, battery-operated monitoring system. *IEEE Trmed. Eng., 55*(1), 196–204. doi:10.1109/TBME.2007.910679 PMID:18232362

Dilmaghani, R. S., Bobarshad, H., Ghavami, M., Choobkar, S., & Wolfe, C. (2011). Wireless Sensor Networks for Monitoring Physiological Signals of Multiple Patients. IEEE Transactions on Biomedical Circuits and Systems, 5(4).

Ding, H., Hou, K.M., Lecoq, L., Zhou, H., Sun, H., …, Murat, N. (2011). Toward a low cost and single chip holter: SoC-Holter. Journal of networks, 6(2), 181-189.

Fuhrhop, S., Lamparth, S., & Heuer, S. (2009). A Textile Integrated Long-Term ECG Monitor with Capacitively Coupled electrodes. *Proc. of the IEEE BioCAS* (pp. 21–24). doi:10.1109/BIOCAS.2009.5372095

Fung, E., Järvelin, M.-R., Doshi, R. N., Shinbane, J. S., Carlson, S. K., Grazette, L. P., & Peters, N. S. et al. (2015). Electrocardiographic patch devices and contemporary wireless cardiac monitoring. *Frontiers in Physics, 6*, 149. doi:10.3389/fphys.2015.00149 PMID:26074823

Gao, T., Pesto, C., Selavo, L., Chen, Y., & Ko, J. G. (2008) Wireless medical sensor networks in emergency response: Implementation and pilot results. *Proc. of the IEEE Conf. Technologies for Homeland Security* (pp. 187–192).

Gargiulo, G., Bifulco, P., Casarelli, M., Romano, M., Calvo, R.A., Jin, C., & van Schaik, A. (2010). An Ultra-High Input Impedance ECG Amplifier for Long-Term Monitoring of Athletes. *Med. Dev., 3*, pp. 1–9.

Gouaux. F, Simon-Chanutemps, L., Fayn, J., Adami, S., Arzi, M., …, Rubel, P. (2002). Ambient Intelligence and Pervasive Systems for the Monitoring of Citizens at Cardiac Risk: New Solutions. *Computers in Cardiology*, 2002, 289–292. doi:org/10.1155/2008/459185

Gunnarson, E., & Gundersen, T. (2005). A wearable ECG recording system for continuous arrhythmia monitoring in a wireless tele-home-care situation. *Proc. of the 18th IEEE Symp. on Computer-Based Medical Systems* (pp. 407–412).

Hernández, A.I., Mora, F., Villegas, G., Passariello, G., & Carra, G. (2001). Real-Time ECG Transmission Via Internet for Nonclinical Applications. *IEEE Transactions on information technology in biomedicine, 5*(3), 253.

Horsch, A., & Balbach, T. (1999). Telemedicine information systems. *IEEE Transactions on Information Technology in Biomedicine, 3*(3), 166–175. doi:10.1109/4233.788578 PMID:10719480

Hutten, H., Schreier, G., Kastner, P., & Schaldach, M. (1997). Cardiac tele monitoring by integrating pacemaker telemetry within worldwide data communication systems. *Proc. of the XIX Annual IEEE EMBS Conf.*, Chicago, IL, USA (pp. 974–976).

Jun, D., & Hong-Hai, Z. (2004). Mobile ECG detector through GPRS/internet. *Proc. of the 17th IEEE Symp. Computer-Based Medical System* (pp. 485–489).

Khoor, S., Nieberl, J., Fugedi, K., & Kail, E. (2003). Internet-based GPRS long-term ECG monitoring and non-linear heart-rate analysis for cardiovascular telemedicine management. *Computers in Cardiology* (pp. 209–212).

Laze, G. A. et al.. (1997). Usefulness of the addition of heart rate variability to Holter monitoring in predicting in-hospital cardiac events in patients with unstable angina pectoris. *The American Journal of Cardiology*.

Lee, R.-G., Chen, K.-C., Hsiao, C.-C., & Tseng, C.-L. (2007). A Mobile Care System with Alert Mechanism. *IEEE Transactions on Information Technology in Biomedicine*, *11*(5), 507–517. doi:10.1109/TITB.2006.888701 PMID:17912967

Lim, Y. G., Kim, K. K., & Park, K. S. (2006). ECG Measurement on a Chair without Conductive Contact. *IEEE Transactions on Bio-Medical Engineering*, *53*(5), 956–959. doi:10.1109/TBME.2006.872823 PMID:16686418

Lim, Y. G., Kim, K. K., & Park, K. S. (2007). ECG Recording on A Bed During Sleep Without Direct Skin-Contact. *IEEE Transactions on Bio-Medical Engineering*, *54*(4), 718–725. doi:10.1109/TBME.2006.889194 PMID:17405379

Margarit, M., Meyer, R. G., & Deen, M. J.Joo Leong Tham. (1999). A Low-Noise, Low Power VCO with Automatic Amplitude Control for Wireless Applications. *IEEE Journal of Solid-State Circuits*, *34*(6), 761–771. doi:10.1109/4.766810

Ng, K. A., & Chan, P. K. (2005). CMOS analog front-end IC for portable EEG/ECG monitoring applications. *IEEE Transactions on Circuits and Systems. I, Regular Papers*, *52*(11), 2335–2347. doi:10.1109/TCSI.2005.854141

Orlov, O. I., Drozdov, D. V., Doarn, C. R., & Merrell, R. C. (2001). Wireless ECG monitoring by telephone. *Telemedicine Journal and e-Health*, *7*(1), 33–38. doi:10.1089/153056201300093877 PMID:11321707

Ouwerkerk, M., Pasveer, F., & Langereis, G. (2008). Unobtrusive Sensing of Psychophysiological Parameters. In J.H.D.M. Westerink, M. Ouwekerk, T.J.M. Overbeek, W.F. Pasveer, B. de Ruyter (Eds.), Probing Experience (pp.163–193). Springer.

Pandian, M., & Safeer, K. (2008). Smart Vest: Wearable multiparameter remote physiological monitoring system. *Medical Engineering & Physics*, *30*(4), 99466–99477. doi:10.1016/j.medengphy.2007.05.014 PMID:17869159

Park, C. et al.. (2006). An Ultra-Wearable, Wireless, Low Power ECG Monitoring System. *Proc. of IEEE BioCAS*, 29, pp. 241–44 doi:10.1109/BIOCAS.2006.4600353

Park, S., Park, J., Ryu, S., Jeong, T., Lee, H., & Yim, C. (1998). Real-time monitoring of patients on remote sites. *Proc. XX Annual IEEE EMBS Conf., Hong Kong* (pp. 1321–1325).

Pavlopoulos, S., Kyriacou, E., Berler, A., Dembeyiotis, S., & Koutsouris, D. (1998). A novel emergency telemedicine system based on wireless communication technology—AMBULANCE. *IEEE Transactions on Information Technology in Biomedicine*, *2*(4), 261–267. doi:10.1109/4233.737581 PMID:10719536

Prance, R. J., Debray, A., Clark, T. D., Prance, H., Nock, M., Harland, C. J., & Clippingdale, A. J. (2000). An Ultra-Low-Noise Electrical-Potential Probe for Human-Body Scanning. *Measurement Science & Technology*, *11*(3), 291–297. doi:10.1088/0957-0233/11/3/318

Rocha, V., Seromenho, R., Correia, J., Mascioletti, A., Picano, A., & Gonçalves, G. (2008, May). Wearable computing for patients with coronary diseases. *Proc. of the IEEE Int. Conf. Automation, Quality Testing, Robotics* (Vol. 3, pp. 37–42). doi: 10.1007/s10916-015-0272-9

Spinelli, E. M., Martinez, N. H., & Mayosky, M. A. (1999). A Transconductance Driven-Right-Leg Circuit. *IEEE Transactions on Bio-Medical Engineering*, *46*(12), 1466–1470. doi:10.1109/10.804574 PMID:10612904

Tay, F., Guo, X., Xu, L., Nyan, M. N., & Yap, K. L. (2009). MEMS wear biomonitoring system for remote vital signsmonitoring. *Journal of the Franklin Institute*, *346*(6), 531–542. doi:10.1016/j.jfranklin.2009.02.003

Ueno.A*et al.* (2007). Capacitive Sensing of Electrocardiographic Potential through Cloth from the Dorsal Surface of the Body in a Supine Position: A Preliminary Study. *IEEE Trans. Biomed. Eng.*, 54(4), 759–766.

Virone, G., Noury, N., & Demongeot, J. (2002). A system for automatic measurement of circadian activity deviations in telemedicine. *IEEE Transactions on Bio-Medical Engineering*, *49*(12), 1463–1469. doi:10.1109/TBME.2002.805452 PMID:12542242

Wu, W. H., Batalin, M. A., Au, L. K., Bui, A. A. T., & Kaiser, W. J. (2008). Context-aware Sensing of Physiological Signals. *Artificial Intelligence in Medicine*, *42*(2). doi:10.1016/j.artmed.2007.12.002 PMID:18207716

Yama, Y.A., Ueno, A., & Uchikawa, Y. (2007). Development of a Wireless Capacitive Sensor for Ambulatory ECG Monitoring over Clothes. *Proc. 29th Ann. Int'l. Conf. IEEE EMBS* (pp. 5727–5730).

Zhang, F., & Lian, Y. (2009). QRS detection based on multi-scale mathematical morphology for wearable ECG device in body area networks. *IEEE Trans. Biomed. Circuits Syst.*, *3*(4), 220–228. doi:10.1109/TBCAS.2009.2020093 PMID:23853243

This research was previously published in the International Journal of Biomedical and Clinical Engineering (IJBCE), 5(1); edited by Natarajan Sriraam, pages 53-63, copyright year 2016 by IGI Publishing (an imprint of IGI Global).

Chapter 40
An ANT Analysis of Healthcare Services for the Nomadic Patients of Namibia

Tiko Iyamu
Namibia University of Science and Technology, Namibia

Suama Hamunyela
Namibia University of Science and Technology, Namibia

ABSTRACT

Patients seek attention and treatments to various types of diseases and symptoms. Diseases infection and symptoms are often not predictive. Normally, there is a spread and movement of people across the geographical locations, of both the rural and urban communities, in countries including Namibia. As such, healthcare could be needed at any location, and at any time. There is significant mobility of individuals and groups within a country. Unfortunately, the healthcare services are not always as mobile at the level and speed that individuals and groups does in Namibia. Hence, there is need for the mobility of healthcare services at both primary and secondary healthcare levels, particularly in the developing countries, such as Namibia. The population of Namibia is scantly spread among its towns and cities. The major towns and cities are situated, in the average of 175km far apart from each other, in the country's 825,418km square landscape. The spread necessitates movements of individuals and groups, particularly the old, poor, and nomadic people. Unfortunately, healthcare records in the country are not centralised and virtualised, making accessibility into patients' records difficult or impossible, from any location. As a result, healthcare service delivering is challenged. This study therefore explored and examined the possibility of mobility of healthcare services to those who live in the country. The study employed the qualitative research method, within which data was gathered from primary healthcare service providers, using open-ended questionnaires. The Moments of Translation from the perspective of actor-network theory (ANT) was used as a lens in the analysis of the data, to examine and understand the power and factors, which influences mobility of healthcare service in Namibia. Categorisation of Patients, Response Time, Understanding the Actors, Actors' participatory to service delivery, and Actors' Alliance were found to be the influencing factors in the provision of mobility of healthcare services.

DOI: 10.4018/978-1-5225-3926-1.ch040

INTRODUCTION

The movement and spread of the population in developing countries is argued to impact healthcare service provision (Rygh & Hjortdahl, 2007). To ensure effective healthcare services provision, states and healthcare organisations are engaged in transforming the industry. According to Sander Granlien and Hertzum (2012), to improve the quality and efficiency of healthcare many hospitals are involved in extensive efforts to substitute electronic patient records for paper records. Another effort that has been made by some organisations is the integration of health information systems to improve quality of healthcare service.

Also, the shift from curative to planning and preventing of disease outbreaks and control has significantly necessitated the need for healthcare data management, efficient service delivery, healthcare information flows between health practitioners and patients, as well as information sharing between healthcare levels of operandi (Chaulagai et al., 2005). The mission of curative, preventing and disease control can only be made possible if the information of the whole population based is made available to policy makers, healthcare profession, administrators, donors and all healthcare organisations.

However, different categories of patients exist in the healthcare sector and the needs for healthcare services are diverse. There is the nomadic patient. This inflates the need to investigate different dimensions of healthcare service provisions processes in a country. In Chang's (2011) argument, there is a scenario where the patient may visit a different healthcare organisation, either because the patient is dissatisfied with the treatment of his or her previous visit or the patient moves to a different location. Distinctively in this case is the mobility of healthcare services in Namibia.

Mobility in this paper refers to the state of easy accessibility of health services from any geographical location. The essentiality of mobility of healthcare is centred on factors such as portability, transferability and availability of healthcare information including real-time interaction between healthcare providers and the needing (Fardoun & Oadah, 2012). In healthcare, mobility is typically associated with mobile healthcare systems and applications, the use of health public kiosk, cellular phone devices, and other portable computing devices (Cisco, 2007), this paper argues that mobility can also be classified by the availability of healthcare services at different levels of healthcare operandi.

Mobility of healthcare services could be translated by various human actors (patients and healthcare workers), based on the different moments. Translation is a key tenet of actor-network theory (Latour, 1991). In actor-network theory (ANT), translation is influenced by interest of the actors (Iyamu, 2013). Translation takes place between the object and the actors it encounters as the initial program or script is altered through interaction.

ANT is popular for its ability to provide a rich and dynamic way of bringing together the socio-technical and non-technical aspects of the organization (Wickramasinghe et al., 2011). In ANT, society and organisations are a formation of different agents, and the agents interact to form heterogeneous networks (Law, 1992; Tatnall & Gilding, 1999; Cresswell et al., 2010). Networks define, describe and provide substance to agents. ANT then, deeply question and provide retorts to the existence of strong and weak (thus power) networks.

The Namibian healthcare levels of operandi cover both rural and urban areas following the thirteen political and administrative regional demarcations of the country. As a developing country, majority of Namibians still resides in rural areas. There is a significance movement of people between urban and rural areas.

The remainder of the paper in divided into five main sections. The first and second sections cover the literature review and research methodology, respectively. The third section presents the data analysis, which the findings. Based on the findings, the implications for the mobility of healthcare services in Namibia context are discussed in the fourth section. Finally, a conclusion is drawn.

The research was guided by two main questions: (i) What are the factors which influence the mobility of healthcare services in Namibia? (ii) What are the roles of human and non-human actors in the mobility of the mobility of healthcare services?

HEALTHCARE SERVICE

The healthcare sector in many countries consists of a large contingence of institutions and organisations, ranging from centres, small and medium to large and technologically advanced hospitals (Braa et al., 2007). The institutions are classified differently in many countries. In Namibia for example, the healthcare centres are classified according to geographical areas, namely, community (constituency) and district level, regional level and national level (Hamunyela & Iyamu, 2013). The levels of categories cover both rural and urban geographical locations. As in many developing countries, in Namibia, 58% of the population resides in rural areas while the remaining percentage resides in urban areas (NPC, 2012).

Due to the essentiality of healthcare, different studies have been conducted in pursuit to establish and describe health services to different healthcare seekers. Rygh and Hjortdahl (2007) examined how mobile health could be used as an innovative solution, to providing healthcare services to patients who reside in remote locations. The later stated that locality influences healthcare service delivery, therefore Mobile healthcare services are essential. This is affirmed by Faudoun and Oadah (2012) stating that, Mobile health greatly benefits patients who reside in remote areas.

Due to the geographical spread of citizens, mobile healthcare is highly essential, however, challenges do exist. According to Rygh and Hjortdahls (2007), healthcare providers in rural areas face numerous challenges in providing coherent and integrated services as compared to those in urban areas, which results from lack of mobile healthcare facilities. Also, the approaches that are often used by primary healthcare service providers in the rural areas are primitive and obsolete (MoHSS, 2007). This also could be attributed to the fact the recipients of the services do question or protest the act by the service providers.

Faudoun and Oadah (2012) emphasised that mobility means the use of mobile technologies to access healthcare service, from different places, at the same time; different places, at the different times; different time, different places; and same time, same place. Mobile of healthcare services includes electronic records, shared and accessed via mobile devices among healthcare providers and receivers. It is assumed that, with the mobile health technologies, healthcare problems, such as inadequacy of doctors and poor clinical examination as a result of insufficient skilled workers and scarcity of centre are eradicated (Narang, 2011). Since available healthcare providers can now remotely interact with patients and conduct analysis remotely. According to Istepanian et al. (2004), M-health offers a variety of benefits, such as timely access, monitoring patients remotely, and improved quality of patients care, to healthcare organisation, providers and patients.

The need for accessibility and quality of health information particularly in developing countries such as Namibia necessitates refection and attention. Thus, there is need for investigation on the mobility of services to improve delivering of healthcare. It has been empirically unveiled, it is important to have healthcare services at the communities' disposal, and at any location, as opposed to the difficulty of accessibility due to distances. The investigation to ensure achieving this objective was carried through a study. The methodology that was applied in the study is explained next.

METHODOLOGY

The case study research approach and the qualitative interpretive research method were employed. The case study approach was selected mainly because of its focus on real-life situation. According to Yin (2003), a case study can be described as the investigation of a contemporary phenomenon within a real-life context. The Namibian Ministry of Health and Social Services (MoHSS) was used as the case, in the study. In addition the MoHSS, the general populace were allowed to participate in the study.

Questionnaires and interviews were used, from the perspective of qualitative method. This was to allow the participants to share their subjective view of how they provide and receive healthcare services in the country. Hovorka and Lee (2010) argued that the qualitative method recognises and focuses on the subjective meaning which the participants bring to the context of the study. Upon completion of the questionnaire, follow up telephonic interviews were conducted to establish deeper understanding of the formation of networks and build of alliances. The two techniques are well established forms of data collection in social science studies.

The participants in the study were identified. A total of 23 people participated in the study. The participants included nurses (6), doctors (4), and patients (8) and non-patients (5), across the country. As at the time of the study, each of the participants had been in service, in their profession for at least five years. This was to ensure the quality of data obtained from them, in terms of the services that they render to nomadic patients of the country.

The data analysis was carried out, using the moments of translation from the perspective of actor-network theory (ANT). ANT was selected mainly because it allows us to examine the process of change, and the interaction that take place between technical and non-technical actors. Without the use of ANT, it would have been difficult or impossible to understand and exhume the processes and actors' influences in the mobility of healthcare services in Namibia. Translation occurs when actors start to define roles, distribute and redistribute roles and power, describe a scenario to form alliances of technical and non-technical. Translation stage involves a process of change, which occur via four major moments. The ANT translation stage involves a process of change, which occur via four major moments: problematization, interessement, enrolment and mobilization. This occurs when actors start to define roles, distribute and redistribute roles and power, describe a scenario to form alliances of technical and non-technical.

The Moments of Translation elements can be summarised as follows: (i) Problematization is the stage which reveals what necessitate the network formation. Uden & Francis (2011) elaborated that during problematisation, actors establish themselves as an obligatory passage point (OPP) between them and the network for indispensability. (ii) Interessement: at this stage, actors consciously or unconsciously reveal their individual or groups' interest on the item that has been problematized by the focal actor. (iii) Enrolment: process begins with a primary agent imposing their will on others for actions to be executed.; this act requires yielding from different actants. (iv) Mobilization: an enrolled actor speaks on behalf of the network, and tries to an interest to persuade others to partake in the activities of the network.

Namibian Ministry of Health and Social Services (MoHSS): The Case Studied

As it is in many countries, the Ministry of Health and Social Services (MoHSS) of Namibia coordinates and oversee the activities of the medical and health sectors in the country. The MoHSS is mandated to provide an integrated, affordable, accessible, quality health and social welfare services, which is responsive to the needs of the Namibian population (MoHSS, 2012). The population seek services from the available healthcare facilities which are located at different levels of operandi in the Namibia (Hamunyela & Iyamu, 2013). Processes and activities of the MoHSS are mostly performed manually (paper-based) or through health information systems (HIS). This can be a huge setback for the services which the MoHSS provides to the communities in the country such as distribution of the HIV treatment and immunisation against contiguous decease's outbreaks. Worse, the manual approach significantly delays centralisation of processes and activities (Hamunyela & Iyamu, 2013). This indeed is dangerous to patient needs, particularly those who are of intensive and chronic nature and nomadic patients.

In addition, there is mobility of individuals and groups within a country. Hence, there is need for the inclination of centralizing healthcare services at both primary and secondary healthcare levels in developing and developed countries. In Namibia, the geographical spread of the population, the widely held image of the healthiness of people in rural area, different groups with needs for healthcare (the old, the poor, nomadic people est.) necessitates the mobility of healthcare services.

DATA ANALYSIS

As mention earlier in the methodology section, the analysis of the data was done, using the lens of actor-network theory. The components of ANT that were followed in the analysis include Actor-Network, and Moments of Translation. In each of the sections of the analysis, the findings are presented and discussed.

Patients are attended to when seeking for health services at the centre, where a discussion (Translation) between the patient and the healthcare takes place. It is procedural to bring along a medical passport (a form of identity which issued by healthcare service providers) when seeking for health services and routine for the healthcare provider to note in the health passport the diagnosis taken and prescriptions. Interactions between healthcare and patients can be classified as part of a durable network that exists to offer services. It is a durable network because a fixt health centre exists and there are actants stationed at each centre.

Currently there are no records readily available when attending to in transit patients except for the health pass port and the medication labels which might not be available at times or lost. For example HIV patients who have been under the care of private doctors and wish to move to state hospitals might not be attended to or attended to after a long time due to communication break down between public and private centres. One of the common challenges encountered by the healthcare providers was a repetition of treatment course which were not effective. There were no records to show that the same treatment or test was carried out, and that it was not effective. One way to overcome these issues is implementation of an Electronic Patient Monitoring System (EPMS) and Electronic Dispensary Tool (EDT) linked to all health facilities providing HIV care for patients to be helped without relying on hard copies only.

Actor-Network

The human actors in the healthcare sector includes healthcare needing people, healthcare professionals (Doctors and Nurses), and the government MoHSS. The non-human actors consist of processes, ICT artefacts and other medical tools. As at the time of this study, different networks existed, some of them were in the categories of nurses' professionals, urban patients, rural patients, and tribal patients.

The actors had different interest. Each of the actors made a difference, either as a receiver or provider of healthcare service. The difference was based on the impact that the actors had on each other. For example, the knowledge a professional acquired in the course of providing health service to a patient.

Currently, there exist different networks to which actors belong. The enrolment of actors in the different networks was influenced by their interests. As gathered from the participants in the study, the primary interest of the general actors were, to receive service from the practitioners, and to render service to the patients. These interests were however, influenced and manifested by other factors and interests, which included spoken language, culture, and accessibility.

Moments of Translation

The moments which consist of four stages, namely problematisation, interessement, enrolment and mobilisation was employed in the analysis primarily to examine and understand the interactions which happen amongst the actors. This was to further understand the suitability, and transformation of the current *status quo* to era of mobility of service within the healthcare environment.

Problemetisation

The activities of the healthcare sector were initiated, problematised through two primary channels, patient and the government. The patients problematise an activity through illnesses, which were often varied. While the other focal actor, the government does same, problematise its healthcare related activities through the Minister of the Ministry of Health and Social Services (MoHSS).

The patients or their representatives (guardian) report incidents of illness, including vehicle accident involving human at the nearest healthcare centre. The incidents were recorded by the front-office professional, who normally were the Nurses. The Nurses escalate the incidents to the appropriate or respective specialist for further and detailed attention. Another criterion that was used for the referral of patients was language, to enable communication and precise understanding between actors (patient and specialist). The Nurses does so, record and escalate incidents based on the power bestowed on them by the authority of the organisation, which comes from their qualification to practice.

The government problematises all initiatives relating healthcare in the country through the Minister of health. The Minister further problematises the initiatives to heads of units and departments of agencies and organisation within the health sector, through workshops and strategic meetings. Unfortunately, the initiatives are not fit for the districts and rural communities, where they are considered needed most e.g. Unavailability of medical reports 'breaks' the continuity of HIV care between health districts.

Healthcare service providers are stationed at different locations of operands. The spread of the operands are far apart, of about 150kms in average. The travelling and nomadic people are therefore forced to seek healthcare service from the nearest location of medical operand.

There is a national policy which is intended to address the challenges of patients who are "on-transits" within the country. The policy defines "on-transit" as a maximum duration of three months stay from original or residence location. The implication is that, a patient who exceed that period may be denied the privilege which the on-transit healthcare service offers. Also, on-transit patient require a letter or medical passports in other to receive medical attention. The requirement is be able to access medical history, which includes previous diagnoses, treatments, and consultations. Unfortunately, some healthcare service providers are adamant on the requirement before service. The challenge is that many people inevitably lose or damage their medical passport. Some people do not always have the passport with them as the medical incidents are not always predictive. Even though the health passport is replaceable, the process is not real-time. As such, it delays treatment to the patient, worst, if the incident is severe.

Interessemment

As earlier revealed in the analysis, the actors had different interests. The actors were categorised into two main groups, healthcare service recipients and providers, which consist of patients and professionals, respectively. The interests of these groups were diverse, even though the primary goal was healthcare services.

The interest of the healthcare recipients were influenced by factors such as locations, type of health related service that was required, and the affordability of services. Proximity was a hindrance to many of the people who lived in the rural areas of the country. The healthcare facilities were far apart from each other. As a result, there were few options to those who need services such as Human Immunodeficiency Virus (HIV) patients, who needed to get their Antiretroviral (ARV) medications from healthcare centre. Due to the fewness of the facilities, the common ones were "General Practitioners". This made it difficult or impossible to access specialists and certain services.

The MoHSS for instance, interest concern its public mandate and social responsibility visible in different directorates and divisions that formed up the MoHSS. The MoHSS also has directorates and division managers in different roles that oversee the execution of duties (e.g. delivery of services), managing healthcare centres, recruit healthcare providers, procurement of necessary medications and other equipment's. These individuals set themselves up as the focal actors and as such, making rues for obligatory passage point.

The healthcare providers' interests were of professional progress, income, status and job descriptions. Healthcare providers in service benefited differently during the course of their duties, depending on the location and the responsibilities that they were assigned. Some of the benefits included flexibility and shifts working hours, housing subsidy, and free medical aid. Also, exposure to different health related cases which in long term can be attributed to experience gained.

ICT artefacts were used differently in the healthcare organisations to support the delivery of services, such as diagnostics and documentation of individual and group records. The use of ICT artefacts were also based on the interest of the users. The interests were informed by their technical skill and know-how of the technologies, and what they needed them for. Another factor was whether the technologies were supported for use in the environment that they were deployed. This played a critical factor in individual and group interest to make use of available technologies for healthcare services in Namibia. As a result, many of the professional anchor their interests on paper-based processes, which they were more comfortable with in delivering services. Paper technology is crucial to nomadic patients thus; it is required for them to forward the healthcare passport to receive the necessary services.

Enrolment to the Network

This process begins with a primary agent (in this case the MoHSS management) imposing their will on others in attempt to achieve for common goal. This was mainly because of the significant of participation of all key stakeholders, which determines the success of failure of healthcare initiatives in Namibia. However, participation was always a challenge, as a result, definition of roles and responsibilities were seen as critical.

The ministry defines the regulations, roles and responsibilities to healthcare providers, and standards of service deliveries at public healthcare centres. This process centred on negotiation and alignment of actants' interests within the different networks. The process was challenging in that it was always lengthy and difficult, and so many conflicts arose. The challenges were manifestation of the different cultural background, interests' focuses, as well as recording keeping. For example, some patients had relocated, and others had lost their health passport, and they needed medical attention. In such cases provision was made to create a new health passport for them through negotiation.

Even though health services were considered essential and critical, some patients would not enrol or reluctantly enrolled in the health related programs. This challenge was prevalence in the rural parts of the country. Many of the communities' members cited the same reason for their lack of participation in the health programs. Some of the reasons included accessibility, literacy, and affordability. For example, some of the participants in this study claimed that many needing healthcare are not literate enough to understand the messages which were used as medium of communication to them. Inscription occurs in this case in the sense that the primary interest of the MoHSS at different healthcare centres was to provide efficient services to all patients including the nomadic patients. Interest of all actants has been aligned and now there is a need to maintain the network. This results into a durable or not durable network.

Existence of conscious and unconscious networks of people, and their enrolments which were created overtime and space across the country signifies that there is need for durability and mobility of healthcare services. Thus, patients communicate their healthcare complains to healthcare providers, provide the healthcare passport if in possession, healthcare providers carry out the diagnosis process and offer prescriptions, again healthcare providers communicates the different cases encountered at reporting intervals to supervisors which in return reports to management (regional, district or national). Or though healthcare providers have power in durability of the network, MoHSS management have the most power to ensure the existence and the growth of the network.

Mobilisation

Due to the essentiality of health services in the country, it was vital for some actors from both MoHSS and the community to mobilise the healthcare service providers and recipients towards a common goal. During mobilisation, some actors were assigned the role of new initiators by becoming delegates or spokesperson for the focal actor (Iyamu &Tatnull, 2011). In this case, hospital matrons, and supervisors at different healthcare centres tried to mobilise healthcare providers to actively participate in the network (carry out their duties). This resulted to a stability of the process of delivering healthcare services in some areas, particularly in the urban areas.

As a result of the stability through adequate services, more patients became spokespersons to different healthcare centres. The self-appointed spokespersons encouraged others with the same or different health issue to seek healthcare services from designated locations of their preference. Also, the altitude and tribal inclination were the others factors which influenced mobilisation and of patients. For example, some patients recommended others to visit or seek assistance from health centres where majority of the health professional were on their tribal origin and spoke the same language as them.

FINDINGS AND DISCUSSION

This section presents the findings from the analysis of the data. They include Categorisation of Patients, Response Time, Understanding the Actors, Actors' participatory to service delivery, and Actors' Alliance.

Categorization of Patients

Categorization of patients was found to be significant, due to the different healthcare services they require, and how the services could be provided and by whom. The categorisation is divided into grouping and indexing:

1. **Grouping:** The actors require groupings, in terms of networks. The different networks, formed in accordance to categories, such as health related challenge, gender, spoken language, and resident location. This will help in terms of referral of patients, to specialist.
2. **Index Key:** Indexing of patients' record is critical. This is to enable searches, in the different categories, such as spoken language, tribal origin, current location, and illness type. This will help improve response time.

Some of the patients could only enrol in the network where there preferred language was used as the medium of communication. Even though interpreters were readily available, they preferred to express themselves than the use of translation. Enrolment into a network by many patients in some parts of the country was influenced by their culture. According to some of the participants, their tradition does not allowed them to be treated by professional of opposite sex.

Response Time

Following the process of problematization, from the moment of translation, we found *Response Time* to be crucial in delivering healthcare service to patients. This is even more critical because of the distances the patients have to travel to get the services. Response time is further viewed from two perspectives of significance, in the mobility of healthcare services in Namibia. The factors include the impact of bureaucracy and lack of access to real-time medical data:

1. **Bureaucracy:** The process of initiating medical attention is too bureaucratic for incidents which are health related. It is worst if the incident is severe, or become live-threatening. The situation can be more challenging in rural areas, and where there is no next of kin to provide relevant information about the patient.
2. **Real-Time Data:** There is lack of real-time data of patients' record. This makes it difficult for healthcare providers to provide relevant and instance services to patients, or to know of *previous diagnosis and prescriptions.*

Our interpretation of the findings indicates that the impact of bureaucracy and lack of access to real-time medical data requires cloud computing solution, as shown in Figure 1.

Cloud Computing (See Figure 1), depict the use of cloud computing solution to store, and access patients' data for health services in Namibia. Armbrust et al (2010:1) referred to cloud computing as *both the applications delivered as services over the Internet and the hardware and systems software in the data centers that provide those services.* This allows personnel or specialists to store and access patients' data from Private and Public hospital, including clinics, using different devices, such as laptop, mobile phones, and desktop. The architecture (See Figure1), using the cloud solution, enables all healthcare medical personnel in the country to have access to real-time data for their services.

The overall problem is the provision of healthcare services to the nomadic patients of the country. The MoHSS aim to provide effective services to all patients regardless of their dwelling status are currently a challenge, as many of the patients are given too much responsibility in addition to their individual illness. In response to the need for a more effective health services, highly qualified and skilled workforce is enrolled in this activities. Furthermore, procedures to deliver or receive healthcare services are enforced (e.g. only registered nurses can attend to patients or patients should carry their healthcare passport in case looking for healthcare services). This in turn leads to the consideration of suitable healthcare provision, healthcare received and medical history for patients. For healthcare service innovation by the MoHSS, the problematisation proposed by the instigators is that to improve healthcare services to all patients including the nomadic patients, there must be service innovations that enable the desired outcomes. This is seen as an OPP by the MoHSS to remain a competent healthcare service provider in the country. In the case of the patients, they need to be certain that they will receive adequate services at any time anywhere.

Understanding the Actors

In our examination of the empirical data, using the interessment tenet of the Moments of Translation, we found Understanding of the Actors to be significantly useful. In that, only through understanding of the involving actors mobility of healthcare services can be influenced. Understanding of the actors was shared from the perspective of awareness and technology know-how:

Figure 1. Patients data in the cloud

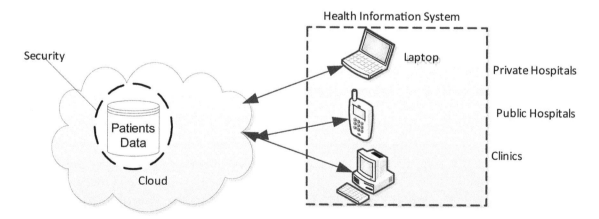

1. Awareness – the actants (healthcare providers and patients) took part in the healthcare services, including in the ways in which the services were provided and received, were based on their levels of awareness. For example some health professionals were became health professionals for personal benefits; and some patients' preference for healthcare services centres were influenced by factors, such as their knowledge of the type of services provided by the centres, the types of their illness, and knowledge of proximity to the centres.
2. Technology know-how - healthcare providers made use of the technologies that they were familiar and comfortable with. For example, some professional could hardly use computer systems to record or access patients' data. However, different technological tools are applicable in diagnosis and other services provision

As already established, the lack of awareness and technology know-how has detrimental implication on the mobility of healthcare services. Thus, a mobile kiosk provides a redress. The use of mobile kiosk will help to reduce or eradicate factors, such as proximity, as it changes location. Also, it could assist patients to garner more information that are offered and available in the different centres, as the patients visit the kiosk in their locations.

As shown in Figure 2, the mobile kiosk is intended to continually, move from one location to another. The kiosk is expected to move within cells (geographical location covered by base station), so it could access, and be accessed by hospitals and clinics, at any location, using any mobile device. According to Haeberlen et al (2004), mobiles devices include microwave ovens, Bluetooth devices, and cordless phones. However, personnel from the hospitals and clinics need to be able to make of mobile devices in order to access the mobile kiosk.

Figure 2. Mobile kiosk

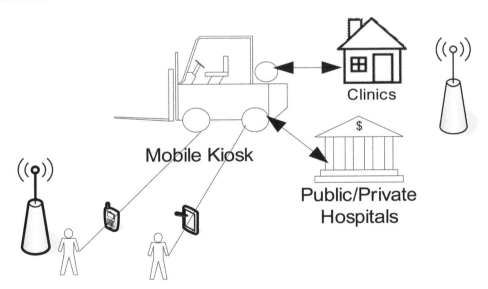

Actors' Participatory to Service Delivery

The analysis revealed that actors' participatory, drawing from the connection and relationship between human actors and interactive systems, is essential to the mobility of healthcare services in the Namibian context. The connection and relationship between the actors is enacted by different tools and devices, to enable and encourage participation in the MoHSS initiatives on health programs, across the country. The components of the participatory factor, connectivity of the actors and interactive system:

1. Connectivity of actors – connectivity will foster actors' enrolment in the mobility of healthcare services. As shown in Figure 2, users (healthcare service providers and patients) need to have application on their devices, which will enable them to easily access the mobile kiosks. The application should be symmetrical, in that it is user friendly to both literate and illiterate actors in their needs to access the kiosks. The application will enable users to easily access the kiosks, from any location including at impromptu times.

2. Interactive system – the interactive system establishes a step-by-step conversation, with the caller. The system is intended to scrutinize calls from the communities, thereby narrow the request or inquiring towards a specific need of the caller. This is purposely for efficiency and effectiveness of the mobile kiosks, in response to the community needs.

Actors' Alliance

The actors formed formal and informal alliances. The alliances were significantly helpful in understanding the challenges factors in the quest to provide healthcare services to the various communities in the country. The alliances were seen as forms of collaboration and political affiliation:

1. Collaboration –mobility of healthcare services require collaboration between community members and healthcare providers. The collaboration could be driven by an agent, but it is the responsibility of all that are involved in the mobility of healthcare services. The collaboration could happen at different levels, such as community members, health professional, and the government (MoHSS).

2. Political affiliation – the mobility of healthcare services in Namibia is endangered by tribal preference for services. This manifests from political affiliation of individuals and groups. Political inclination has potentials of influencing mobilisation of actors, to participate in the mobility of healthcare service in their communities. Political inclination is critical as some actors are heterogeneous in the networks, as shown in Figure 3.

Social Networking – the social networking approach will help to bring all actors together, in fostering the mobility of healthcare services in Namibia. According to Dwyer et al. (2007), ssocial networking is a type of virtual community that has grown tremendously in popularity over the past few years. Social networking has no boundaries, in terms of spoken language, and tribal origin. It brings people of common interest together in the same network.

Another important factor of social networking is that, an actor can be heterogeneous in that the actor can belong to more than one network, as shown on Figure 3. In this instance, the actor is able to influence and connect the networks to each other. This help to eradicate or silence tribal or political inclination which has potential to hamper the common goal, of the mobility of healthcare services.

Figure 3. Collaboration

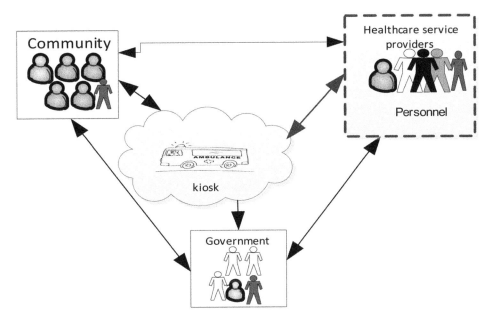

MOBILITY OF HEALTHCARE SERVICES IN NAMIBIA

People, technology and procedures are the actors in the process of healthcare service delivery. ANT's translation process that was followed in this study defines the formation of networks, which helped to identify the groupings and how they were created. The process starts with the main actor who defines the roles through problemitisation of the issue or item. This was done by localization of the issue, so as to foster relationship, and get more and regional actors to be interested, and partake in the initiative.

Although the employment of technical actants can be viewed as the consequences of the action of all actants to an extent, the ministry of health in this case has power to hire healthcare providers and extend the provision of services to all health service level of operation. This signifies authority to define procedures of service delivery e.g. change the national policy of the in transit patients or implement an Electronic Patient Management System (EPMS) at health centers. By so doing, associations of technical and non-technical actants are strengthen.

Moreover, the mobility of healthcare services is enabled and constrained within network such as community by the actions of actors, which often based on individual or group knowledge. Mobilisation is necessary to educate and inform actants about the services. Patients need to know about their rights to health services at any location and the importance of a health passport.

A health passport, referral letter or medication container was issued to patients by medical personnel at different locations or health centres across the country. Thus, the patients present whenever they needed health related treatment anywhere in the country. Challenge of presenting the above is that they are vulnerable to loss or results to unclear information on the passport or letter. The consequence of such loss and unclear information make services complex and complicated to both healthcare service providers and the patients. Hence it is critical to enforce electronic systems, which allow access to patients' health related records from anywhere across the country, and on real-time.

CONCLUSION

This paper presents a critical analysis of the role and account of actors in the mobility of healthcare services in Namibia. The analysis is of vital important to the Namibia, and other countries which has similar setup and challenges, in that it unveiled issues that the State government and many healthcare professional are not aware of, take for granted.

In the past, and continuous (before this study), the state Government as in many developing countries continue to invest and focus on technical issues, which often become "white elephants" due to lack of usefulness. This study revealed fundamental and primary issues, which makes technology useful and ease of use in the mobility of healthcare services across Namibia.

The paper emphasises on the importance of relationships between the actors (health professional and patients), and as well the significance of networks in the mobility of healthcare services at different health operandis. As at the time of the study, patients in transit were handled in accordance to the national health policy as promulgated by the MoHSS. The study revealed how healthcare service providers, through the use of spoken language and tribal origin, enable, and at the same time, constrain the services that they are supposed to render to the patients for better healthcare. These factors were often conscious, and sometimes unconsciously exhibited by the actors. However, little or nothing was known of the impact, the service providers of healthcare in Namibia.

REFERENCES

Armbrust, M. et al. (2010). A view of cloud computing. *Communications of the ACM, 53*(4), 50–58. doi:10.1145/1721654.1721672

Braa, J., Hanseth, O., Heywood, A., Mohammed, W., & Shawn, B. (2007). developing information systems in developing country: The flexible standards strategy. *MIS Quartely, 31*, 1–22.

Chang, P. (2011). Modeling the management of electronic health records in healthcare information systems. In *Proceedings of the 2011 International Conference on Cyber-Enabled Distributed Computing and Knowledge Discovery.*

Chaulagai, C. N., Moyo, C. M., Koot, J., & Moyo, H. B. (2005). *Design and implementation of a health management in Malawi: issues inovation and results* (pp. 2–10). Oxford University Press.

Cisco. (2007). *Mobility solution for healthcare: voice, text, images and information, delivered to the point of care.* Retrieved from http://www.cisco.com/web/strategy/docs/healthcare/07cs1084-Mob-ForHC_062708.pdf

Creswell, K., Worth, A., & Sheikh, A. (2010). Actor-network theory and its role in understanding the implementation of information technology developments in healthcare. *BMC Medical Informatics and Decision Making*, 10–67. PMID:20178586

Dwyer, C., Hiltz, S., & Passerini, K. (2007, August 9-12). Trust and privacy concern within social networking sites: A comparison of Facebook and MySpace. In the *Proceedings of the Thirteenth Americas Conference on Information Systems*, Keystone, CO.

Haeberlen, A. (2004). Practical robust localization over large-scale 802.11 wireless networks. In *Proceedings of the 10th Annual International Conference on Mobile Computing and Networking*.

Hamunyela, S., & Iyamu, T. (2013). Readness assessment model for the deployment of health information systems in the Namibian MoH. International Federation for Information Processing. In *Proceedings of the 12th Internation Conference on Social Implications of Computer in Developing Countries*, Jamaica.

Hovorka, D. S., & Lee, A. S. (2010). Reframing interpretivism and positivism as understanding and explanation: Consequences for information systems research. In *Proceedings of the International Conference on Information Systems* (Paper 188).

Istepanian, R. J. (2004). Guest editorial introduction to the specialon m-health: Beyond seamless mobility and global wireless health-care connectivity. *IEEE Transactions on Information Technology in Biomedicine*, 405–414. doi:10.1109/TITB.2004.840019 PMID:15615031

Iyamu, T. (2010). Theoretical analysis of the implementation of enterprise architecture. *International Journal of Actor-Network Theory and Technological Innovation*, 2(3), 27–38. doi:10.4018/jantti.2010070102

Iyamu, T., & Tatnull, A. (2011). *The impact of netwrork of actors on the infomation technology. Actor-Network Theory and Technology Innovation: Advancements and New Concepts Journal*. Hershey, PA: IGI Global.

Law, J. (1992). *Notes on the theory of the Actor-network: Ordering, strategy and heterogeneity*. Retrieved from http://comp.lancs.ac.uk/sociology/soc054jl.html

MoHSS. (2012). *Integrated healthcare delivery the challenge and implementations*. Retrieved from http://www.healthnet.org.na/documents.html

Namibia, M. (2007). *Community-based healtcare policy*. MoHSS.

Narang, J. K. (211). Quality of healthcare services in rural India: The user perspective. *VIKALPA*, 51-60.

NPC. (2012). *Namibia 2011 population and housing census*. Retrieved from www.npc.gov.na

Rygh, E. M., & Hjortdahl, P. H. (2007). Continuous and integrated health care services in rural areas. A literature study. *The International Electronic Journal of Rural and Remote Health Research. Education Practice and Policy*, 7(766), 1–10.

Sander Granlien, M., & Hertzum, M. (2012). Confirmatory factor analysis of service quality dimensions within mobile telephony industry in Ghana. *The Electronic Journal Information Systems Evaluation*, 15(2), 197–227.

Sinha, R. K. (2010). Impact of health information technology in public health. *Sri Lanka Journal of Bio-Medical Informatics*, 1(4), 223–236. doi:10.4038/sljbmi.v1i4.2239

Tutnall, A., & Burgess, S. (2002). Using actor-network to research the implementation of a B-B portal for regional SME in Melbourne. In *Proceedings of the 15th Bled Electronic Commerce Conference*.

Uden, L., & Francis, J. (2011). *Service innovation using actor-network theory. Actor-network theory and technology innovation: Advancements and new concepts journal, Advancements and new concepts journal.* Hershey, PA: IGI Global.

Wickramasinghe, N., Bali, R., & Goldberg, S. (2011). *Using S'ANT for facilitating superior understanding of key factors in the design of a chronic disease self-management model. Actor-network theory and technology innovation: advancements and new concepts journal, Advancements and new concepts journal.* Hershey, PA: IGI Global.

Yin, R. K. (2003). *Case study research design and methods* (3rd ed.). Sage Publications.

This research was previously published in the International Journal of Actor-Network Theory and Technological Innovation (IJANTTI), 6(1); edited by Ivan Tchalakov, pages 54-67, copyright year 2014 by IGI Publishing (an imprint of IGI Global).

Chapter 41
Activities and Evaluations for Technology-Based Upper Extremity Rehabilitation

Michelle Annett
University of Toronto, Canada & Autodesk Research, Canada

Fraser Anderson
Autodesk Research, Canada

Walter F. Bischof
University of British Columbia, Canada

ABSTRACT

Recent advances in projection and sensing have resulted in an increased adoption of virtual reality, video games, and interactive interfaces to improve patient compliance with rehabilitation programs. In this chapter, we describe the application of multi-touch tabletop surfaces to physical and occupational rehabilitation programs that are focused on the upper extremities. First, we detail the participatory design processes undertaken with local physical and occupational therapists to design and integrate a 'patient-friendly' multi-touch tabletop system in their workplace. We then explore the design considerations that informed the development of a suite of sixteen multi-touch interactive activities. The design considerations highlighted the need for customization and flexibility in the software, as well as the importance of supporting a variety of activity types. We then detail the laboratory-based methods that were used to evaluate the efficacy of the activity interventions as well as our deployment of the system in a local rehabilitation hospital. Our evaluation, which employed both qualitative and quantitative components (i.e., the Intrinsic Motivation Inventory, semi-structured interviews, kinetics and kinematics recorded from motion trackers and an electromyogram recorder), determined that it is the design of activities, rather than the utilization of technology itself, that impacts the success of technology-assisted rehabilitation. The chapter concludes with a discussion of the implications of our system and its deployment.

DOI: 10.4018/978-1-5225-3926-1.ch041

1. INTRODUCTION

More than 10% of Canadians are afflicted with impairments that influence their ability to perform everyday activities (CANSIM, 2009). These disabilities stem from a variety of causes, including aging, disease, stroke, trauma, or congenital health issues. Most commonly, patients have decreased motor functionality, memory problems, and an inability to focus on, or attend to, stimuli, leaving many unable to live independently or perform daily activities such as cooking, eating, or dressing. In traditional rehabilitation programs, occupational and physical therapists work closely with patients to perform exercises to regain or maintain physical (e.g., range of motion, coordination, balance, muscle strength, and muscle endurance) and cognitive (e.g., attention, short-term memory, visual-spatial abilities, and problem-solving skills) function to improve the patient's quality of life.

Current upper extremity rehabilitation activities, such as drawing images on paper, tracing letters in the air, or reaching for imaginary targets, require patients to perform repetitive movements that focus on increasing range of motion, coordination, muscle strength, and muscle endurance.

Most traditional motor and cognitive rehabilitation activities are monotonous and unexciting, providing sub-optimal patient engagement and immersion. It is very common for these activities to cause patients to exert only moderate amounts of effort or neglect them completely. In addition, therapists are limited in how they can manipulate the activities with respect to intensity and difficulty, and the subjective nature of patient performance makes the monitoring and evaluation of patient progress very difficult.

A new area of Human-Computer Interaction, *technology-assisted rehabilitation*, has begun to focus on the role that technology can play in improving patient abilities. It has been widely recognized that patient motivation and patient compliance with rehabilitation exercises are critical problems in physical therapy programs (Chang et al., 2011; Flynn & Lange, 2010; Gupta & O'Malley, 2006; Mumford et al., 2008; Rizzo & Kim, 2005; Saposnik et al., 2010). One approach to encourage compliance and increase motivation has been to use video games, as it is believed that patients can become as highly engaged with their therapy exercises as video game enthusiasts are with their games (Rizzo & Kim, 2005). For this reason, various technologies such as the Microsoft Kinect (Chang et al., 2011; Delbressine et al., 2012), PlayStation EyeToy (Rand et al., 2008), and Nintendo Wii (Saposnik et al., 2010) have become pervasive in therapy programs (Flynn and Lange, 2010). Preliminary research into integrating gaming, virtual reality, and haptics into rehabilitation programs has illustrated that technology-assisted rehabilitation can decrease the length of a patient's rehabilitation program, increase a patient's range of motion, muscle strength, and coordination, and provide rehabilitation opportunities in out-patient or rural settings (Gupta & O'Malley, 2006; Mumford et al., 2008).

Over the last decade, interactive surfaces and multi-touch tabletops have become very popular, partially due to their decreased cost. Interactive tabletops have several advantages (Hutchins et al., 1985) that make them excellent candidates for the rehabilitation process. By their very nature, multi-touch tabletops support natural and direct interaction (Wigdor and Wixon, 2011), that is, the user touches and manipulates an object or target directly instead of using a proxy device such as a mouse, keyboard, or joystick for interaction. As patients with cognitive disabilities often have trouble creating a mapping between a proxy object and target, this direct interaction provides an important advantage. Interactive tabletops also provide a large interaction space, which is to exercise gross motor function and encourage lateral upper-body movement (Annett et al., 2009; Mumford et al., 2008). Such interaction is not possible on small hand-held devices or tablets. Multi-touch tabletops have the potential to greatly enhance patient motivation and compliance with rehabilitation activities as they are highly interactive and immersive, and they support natural methods of user interaction. As immersive tasks can help to reduce the amount of pain or discomfort that patients experience (Berger-Vachon, 2006), we believe that the integration of multi-touch tabletops into the rehabilitation process can provide many benefits for both patients and therapists. Lastly, the sheer size and construction of tabletops allow them to support a patient's upper-body weight during an activity, thus allowing those with poor balance or muscular endurance to participate and benefit from activities as well.

In close collaboration with occupational therapists from the Glenrose Rehabilitation Hospital in Edmonton, Alberta, Canada, we have developed an interactive, multi-touch tabletop and a suite of upper extremity, motor-based applications. Our open-source system, *Ammi Interactive Rehabilitation Touch*, or AIR Touch (Figure 1), aims to provide therapists with an easy-to-use tool that can 1) be customized to meet a patient's abilities and needs, 2) increase patient motivation and engagement, and 3) record a variety of objective measurements.

2. RELATED WORK

The development of applications for multi-touch tabletops has steadily increased in the last decade due to the novelty, potential, and ease of construction and development of tabletop technologies. Multi-touch tabletops have been used for applications as diverse as remote interface control (Seifried et al., 2009), collaboration on navel ships (Domova et al. 2013), music composition (Jorda et al., 2007), children with autism (Bauminger-Zviely et al., 2013), and to explore genomic data (Shaer et al., 2010).

It has, however, only been in recent years that multi-touch tabletops have been used for rehabilitation. Mumford et al. (2008) describe an interactive surface that can be used to assess and treat traumatic brain injury. Mumford et al.'s system provides only coarse measures of patient progress, the implemented

Figure 1. The Air Touch System, (a) Version 1 and (b) Version 2

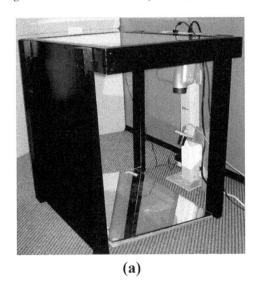
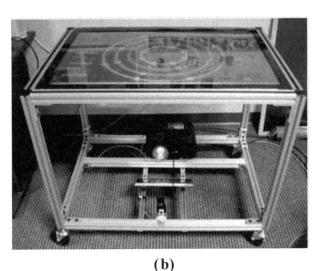

(a) **(b)**

activities do not appear to be intrinsically motivating, and the use of tangible objects prevents patients with poor fine-motor skills from using the system. Facal et al. (2009) describe a multi-touch surface that can be used to develop cognitive skills in the elderly, as did Augstein, M. et al. (2013, 2014), Dunne et al. (2010), Gamberini et al., (2009), Jacobs et al. (2013), Jung et al., (2013), and Kwon et al. (2013). As with Mumford et al.'s system, these systems do not support therapist interaction and do not appear to be overly engaging or motivating, nor do they have a breadth of activities suitable for a range of participant interests and abilities. In a slightly different vein, Hancock and colleagues sought to replicate sand-tray therapy, a type of therapy that allows children to use tangible objects to tell stories and talk about their emotions (2010). While Hancock et al.'s digital implementation did made use of digital 3D models and encouraged fine and gross motor movements, the focus of their work was not to improve upon these functions.

Work by Khademi and colleagues sought to compare the benefits of direct versus indirect interaction for stroke-rehabilitation (2014). Using objects, participants played a simplified version of the Fruit-Ninja game and found that direct interaction lead to higher player scores and higher scores on the Fugl-Meyer Assessment and Box and Block tests. Although this work demonstrated that direct-tangible interaction is preferable to indirect, the present exploration focuses exclusively on non-tangible interaction, to ensure that our system could be utilized by those who have decreased fine-motor skills and cannot grasp objects.

Apted et al. (2006) and Al Mahmud et al. (2008) have developed design guidelines for tabletop-based applications for the elderly. Some of their suggestions include maximizing the size of interface elements, reducing the number of interface elements, and utilizing familiar metaphors and common knowledge to increase user learnability and understanding. As motor skills, vision, and cognitive abilities are reduced in both, elderly and rehabilitation populations, we feel that these same guidelines should be applied to multi-touch tabletop activities.

While many existing works have advocated the use of engaging activities to encourage rehabilitation adherence, few have thoroughly considered the importance of activity design. In this work, we examine how activity design can affect the success of rehabilitation programs, examine evaluation techniques for technology-based rehabilitation activities, and provide design guidelines for developers of such technologies.

3. SYSTEM GOALS AND ITERATIVE DESIGN PROCESS

To better inform and situate the utilization of multi-touch tabletops within rehabilitation settings, we underwent a multi-stage, user-centric iterative design process with occupational and physical therapists from a local rehabilitation hospital in Edmonton, Alberta, Canada (i.e., the Glenrose Rehabilitation Hospital). The Glenrose Rehabilitation Hospital is the largest tertiary rehabilitation institution in Canada, with 220 clinical researchers, a school program for 300 children, 250 inpatient beds, and 30,000 outpatients a year, including both children, adults, and the elderly. The large diverse in-, out-, and day- patient population at the hospital provided a unique opportunity to immerse ourselves within a real-world clinical setting and provided first-hand contact with everyone involved in the rehabilitation process, from patients and caregivers to therapists and hospital administrators.

To better understand the needs of therapists and clients, we conducted a variety of large focus-groups with therapists and hospital administrators, organized one-on-one interviews with practicing therapists and administrators (before and after the installation of our prototype system), and shadowed a number of therapists and clients throughout the course of our iterative design process. It was through these events that rich information about the rehabilitation process and the current state of the art of rehabilitative activities and technologies was attained.

3.1. Goals

Given the variation in age and level of motor dysfunction in our target population, we learned that there is no single activity or exercise that can be used for every individual. Some patients have near-normal functioning, while others cannot move their fingers or wrists and rely exclusively on gross motor movements. In collaboration with our occupational therapist colleagues, four guiding objectives were developed to situate our research and development:

- **Objective 1:** *Engage patients and ensure that activities are easy to learn*
  - If activities are not intrinsically motivating or immersive, patients will not exert much effort.
  - When patients are immersed in an activity, they are less affected by their pain and thus may perform an activity longer.
  - Activities should build upon known metaphors and existing knowledge to maximize a patient's comfort level, especially for those with cognitive deficits.
- **Objective 2:** *Ensure that activities are repeatable and that meaningful performance measures can be recorded*
  - Objective performance measures can help to quantify a patient's progress.
  - Having repeatable activities ensures that the measures are meaningful and can be compared to past performance.
  - Informing patients about their performance can motivate them and may speed their recovery.
- **Objective 3:** *Leverage therapist expertise and their knowledge of a patient*
  - No system can or should replace the expert judgment and abilities of a therapist.
  - Therapists should be able to adjust the difficulty and type of activities to match a patient abilities, goals, and outcomes.
- **Objective 4:** *Decrease the setup and customization time so that the totality of a rehabilitation session can be spent on actual rehabilitation exercises*
  - Currently, too much time is wasted setting up and configuring equipment or activities to match the needs of the patient.
  - Ensure that any changes or modifications that need to be made can be done so without needing to restart an activity, log into the computer, etc.

3.2. System Design

The AIR Touch (Figure 1) is a cross-platform, multi-touch system that combines open-source software with a readily available multi-touch surface. Our multi-touch tabletop screen (90 cm x 55 cm) was designed and manufactured by NOR_/D[1] and was composed of layers of acrylic and diffuse materials. It uses the principle of Frustrated Total Internal Reflection to detect touch events (Han, 2005). The system uses a short-throw projector and mirror to rear-project digital content onto the acrylic screen.

All touch events are captured by a Point Grey Firefly MV infrared camera and processed using the open source, openFrameworks software library. The openFrameworks software library allows one to modify the touch sensitivity of the tabletop. As the target population has different levels of motor dysfunction, it was imperative that therapists were able to modify the amount of pressure required to generate touch events on the tabletop.

After a touch event is detected, it is relayed to our Apache Flex-based activities. Flex is an open-source extensible framework that combines ActionScript with an XML-derivative. Flex also has a large library of visually appealing user interface objects and animations that can be combined to create highly interactive, easy to use activities and interfaces for therapists and patients. To ensure that therapists would be able to customize activities as needed, all of the activity interfaces were designed such that parameters could easily be changed 'on the fly' with little to no effort on the part of the therapist (e.g., on-screen buttons, sliders, menus, colour pickers, etc. controlled the changing of colours, width of strokes, size and location of targets, etc.).

3.3. Feedback

The first version of the tabletop was rapidly constructed using plywood and lumber to quickly experiment with the form factor and gather feedback. Testing with the initial hardware configuration proved invaluable as it allowed therapists to quickly experiment with the potential of the technology. The feedback they provided was crucial in shaping later iterations of the hardware platform.

Some of the initial feedback we received regarded the physical configuration of the table. Several therapists requested the ability to adjust the height and angle of the interactive surface to support various patients (Figure 2). Portability was also a concern, as the initial prototype was heavy and not easily moved. Sanitary concerns were also raised, as the porous wood surface was not able to be sufficiently cleaned and disinfected for hospital use. Lastly, the aesthetics of a black, wooden table was a concern, especially as the table was meant to be a 'technological innovation' in the therapy process. Many therapists stated that it was important for patients to use technology and equipment that was commonplace for their able-bodied counterparts. The black table's appearance did not reflect the capabilities of the system and further created a divide between those with and without dysfunctions.

Taking this feedback into consideration, a second version of the interactive table was fabricated. This version was made out of extruded aluminium and plastic, allowing it to be easily sanitized and provide a more refined aesthetic. The table was mounted on lockable caster wheels with the computer, projector, and all the necessary hardware mounted to the frame. This allowed the table to easily be moved from room-to-room as necessary. The extruded aluminium also had an added benefit of making the tabletop appear similar to a large iPad, and thus removed some of the stigma regarding the use of old, out-dated equipment that had initially been reported.

As part of the feedback process, we determined that it was important to temper expectations and make therapists and patients aware of what was feasible and possible. For example, although we consulted with industrial designers and mechanical engineers to develop methods to adjust the height and angle of the table automatically, it was too difficult and expensive to implement many of the designs. Given the weight of the components, the rigidity and stability that the tabletop needed to have, and the calibration that was required to align the images from the projector with the touch events detected by the cameras, we opted to maintain the second version of the tabletop throughout the remainder of our iterative design process.

Figure 2. The Air Touch System in use by therapists and clients at the Glenrose Rehabilitation Hospital

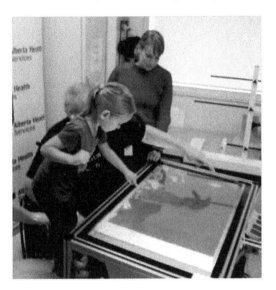
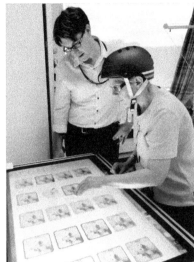

4. REHABILITATION-FOCUSED ACTIVITY DESIGN

Guided by the design objectives identified above, as well as Apted et al. (2006) and Al Mahmud et al.'s (2008) guidelines, we developed a suite of sixteen rehabilitation activities. Some activities were designed to replicate real-world activities (e.g., Finger Painting, Match Me, Touch Tessellation, Nomis Says) whereas others were novel and targeted specific motions and movements (e.g., Touch-A-Tap, Therapist Do-It-Yourself, Pop Those Balloons!). In addition, some were focused on harnessing creative expression and flow (Csikszentmihalyi, 1997; e.g., Photo Scrapbooking, Finger Painting), whereas others employed simple gamification elements (Deterding et al., 2011; e.g., Drumhab, Pop Those Balloons!, Touch Mazes).

Across all activities, we strove to ensure that any customizations or personalization that were possible would best represent the current and future needs of the client.

4.1. Activities

Herein, we describe each of the activities that were designed, detailing the rehabilitation goals that each targets and the activity-specific measures that can be recorded.

4.1.1. Finger Painting

Finger Painting is a multi-touch adaptation of traditional finger painting (Figure 3a). Patients are encouraged to use their hands and fingers as paint brushes. They are able to select various colors to paint with and are given the freedom to draw whatever they choose. The activity natural encourages fine and gross motor movements and artistic expression, while also camouflaging rehabilitation goals within a creative endeavour. As the activity is relatively unrestricted, it can be used leveraged by therapists as a 'blank canvas' for their own activities. For instance, therapists might ask patients to draw increasingly larger circles to encourage greater range of motion. During interaction with the activity, logs are recorded with the colors chosen, the length of paths drawn, and the resulting drawings are also saved (see Figure 3).

4.1.2. Paint-By-Number

Similar to Finger Painting, the Paint-By-Number activity also encourages the patient to use their hands as a paintbrush, but this time, to fill in a numbered outline (Figure 3b). The patient can touch one of the numbered paint buckets located on the screen to change the colour of their 'paintbrush'. This activity can be used to improve fine motor skills and to encourage gross motor movements such as flexion and elevation.

This activity can be customized by changing the image that is displayed, the location and size of the image, and the number of colours that are used. AIR Touch determines the accuracy of a patient's painting (i.e., if the painting was within the lines), if the correct colours were used, the number of paint strokes the patient made, the number of paint bucket selections that occurred, and the proportion of the image that was painted.

4.1.3. Touch Tracing

The Touch Tracing activity closely mimics an existing rehabilitation activity in which a therapist draws a pattern on a whiteboard and then asks the patient to trace overtop the pattern (Figure 3c). In the table-top adaptation, therapists can draw a pattern on the surface and then ask the patient to trace overtop of

Figure 3. Examples of the various stroke-based multi-touch activities that were implemented. (a) Finger Painting, (b) Paint-By-Number, (c) Touch Tracing, (d) Touch Mazes, and (e) Track Trace

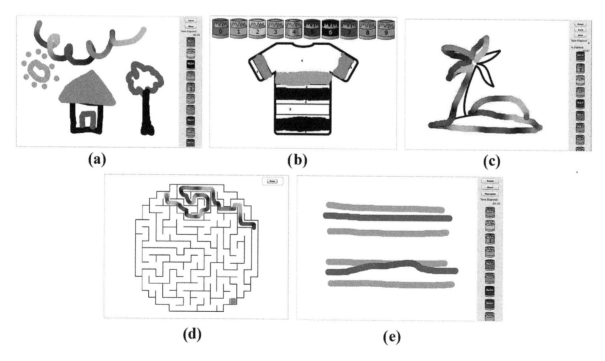

it. Alternatively, the therapist can load image files for tracing (e.g., complex patterns, letters, words, or outlines of emotionally salient images such as faces or animals). Both the therapist and patient can choose from a variety of different paint colours to make the activity more salient and meaningful.

Similar to the Paint-By-Number activity, therapists can change the size and location of the tracing pattern or image. This flexibility permits therapists to target both fine and gross motor skills. While this activity is performed, a number of measurements are recorded, including the accuracy of tracing (using a root-mean squared error formula), the average tracing speed, the percent of the pattern that was successfully traced, and the number of paint strokes the patient made.

4.1.4. Touch Mazes

Touch Mazes are based on traditional pen-and-paper mazes found in many children's books. During the activity, the patient traces their finger along the screen from the start point of the maze (indicated by a green square), through to the exit (indicated by a red square; Figure 3d). Similar to the Finger Painting and Touch Tracing Paint-By-Number activities, the colour of the paint strokes can be changed to increase activity enjoyment. A variety of maze complexities are available. Simpler mazes have larger tracks and are less cognitively challenging, whereas higher complexity mazes have narrower trackers and require more forethought. This allows for a wide range of patients to use the activity. As patients regain function, they can progress through different difficulty levels. This activity records the number of errors (i.e., maze wall crossovers), the average stroke speed, and the number of completed mazes.

4.1.5. Track Trace

The Track Trace application (Figure 3e) allows therapists to draw a set of tracks for patients to practice drawing through. Each track is defined by two therapist-drawn strokes, and the patient must then draw a line between them. This task is similar to the steering tasks commonly found within human-computer interaction (Accot and Zhai, 1999). This allows the therapist to control the length of the defined track, as well as the width, allowing precision control over fine motor difficulty (track width), as well as challenging the patient's range of motion (path length). Therapists can also make the track complex, with curves and corners, to add more of a cognitive challenge. The color of the tracks and the patient's paint color can also be changed to add more dynamism to the activity. Measures recorded during Track Trace include time-on-task, accuracy (total root mean squared error distance from track center), number of errors (track crossovers), as well as the paths themselves.

4.1.6. Touch-A-Tap

The Touch-A-Tap activity is a digital implementation of the Dynavision[2] systems that are common in rehabilitation institutions. With Touch-A-Tap, an array of targets is displayed on the screen, with only one 'activated' for the patient to touch at a given time (Figure 4a). After the patient touches the activated target, it deactivates, the next one activates, they touch it to deactivate it, and so on. Unlike the traditional Dynavision system, therapists can control a wide assortment of parameters, including the layout of targets (e.g., radial, rectilinear, random), the target size and spacing, and specific spatial areas to emphasize with the activation patterns. Both the colour of the targets and the activation color can be customized. These parameters give the therapist fine-grained control over the content of the activity and can help tailor the activity to a variety of patient needs. During performance, the activity logs the reaction times (per target), the target positions and layout, the touch error (using a root mean-squared error metric), and the total number of correct and incorrect selections.

4.1.7. Therapist Do-It-Yourself

This activity is analogous to an existing rehabilitation activity that requires therapists place targets in different spatial locations on a table so that a patient can reach out and touch them. In our table-based implementation of this activity, the therapist can touch the tabletop to define target locations. The defined targets are then presented to the patient in random or sequential order. Once the patient has touched a target, it 'flies away' and the next target in the sequence is presented.

For patients with asymmetric dysfunctions or with regions of neglect, this activity provides therapists with a tool to target their disability directly (Figure 4b). As a patient performs this activity, the target

Figure 4. Examples of the various targeting-based multi-touch activities that were implemented (a) Touch-A-Tap, (b) Therapist Do-It-yourself, (c) BeatGen, and (d) Drumhab

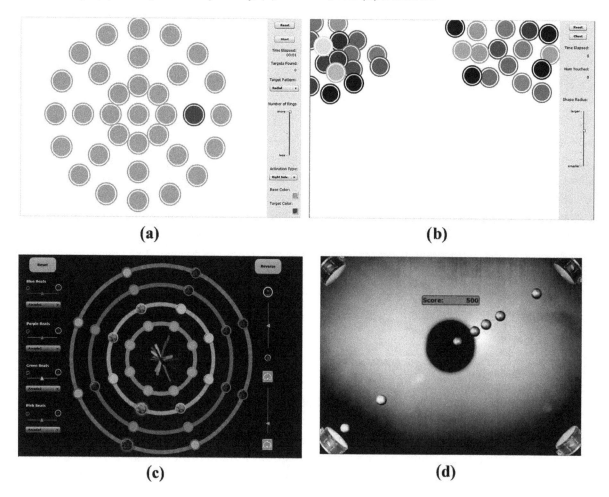

(a)

(b)

(c)

(d)

touch accuracy (as measured using the root mean squared error formula), the time between correct target selections, and the number of non-target touches are recorded.

4.1.8. BeatGen

The BeatGen activity is a music generation activity that allows patients to create audio loops through a simple, touch-based interface (Figure 4c). By touching various nodes, patients can add or remove audio samples from the loop. They are also able to configure the samples used, the volume of each sample, as well as the master volume and tempo. As the patient uses the activity, the loop is continually played in real-time, allowing for instantaneous feedback of their effects. This activity is especially appealing to younger patients, as it allows them to create electronic music in an analogous way to DJs. The application supports a wide range of motion, from the gross motor movement needed to touch the nodes on the far side of the table, to the more fine-grained motion of the slider. This allows the application to be used with a more diverse population. As the patient uses the activity, the time on task is recorded, along with the number and distribution of touch events, the parameters that were changed, and the resulting audio file.

4.1.9. Drumhab

We created a music-centric tabletop activity inspired by the popular Rock Band and Guitar Hero video games. In this activity, there are 'beats' that radiate from a centre orb and move towards four drums located in the corners of the tabletop (Figure 4d). The beats are synchronized to music and as each beat reaches its target drum, patient must use their hands as drumsticks to 'hit' the target drum to score points. If the drum is hit at the correct time, the beat 'explodes'.

A therapist can change the difficulty of Drumhab by choosing to display more or fewer beats on the screen, changing the speed of the beats, and selecting which drums are targets. As the drums are located in the corners of the tabletop, this activity promotes an increased range of motion. The speed at which the beats move can help to develop a patient's reflexes. As a patient performs this activity, a number of measures are recorded: the final score, the number of beats touched, the total number of beats that were presented, the number of false hits, and the beat touch accuracy (as defined by the root-mean squared error formula).

4.1.10. Nomis Says

Nomis Says is a virtual implementation of the classic Simon™ game. In Nomis Says, a therapist can modify the number of coloured quadrants that appear, change the size and location of each coloured quadrant, or change the number of times a patient can try to repeat a light-up sequence if they have made an error. Multiple patients, or a patient and caregiver, can take turns repeating the light-up sequences, or players can be responsible for one or two quadrants and touch them at the appropriate time (Figure 5a). Nomis Says provides many cognitive and motor challenges to patients (e.g., sequencing, divided attention, immediate recall, gross motor skills, and dexterity). Similar to other activities, Nomis Says records the length of each correctly reproduced sequence, the touch quadrant error (using the the root-mean squared error formula) and the number of false touch events.

Figure 5. Examples of the various game-based and creative multi-touch activities that were implemented. (a) Nomis Says, (b) Match Me, (c) Pop Those Balloons!, (d) Touch Tessellation, (e) Foggy Windows, (f) Photo Scrapbooking, (g) Third Party Applications (e.g., Google Earth)

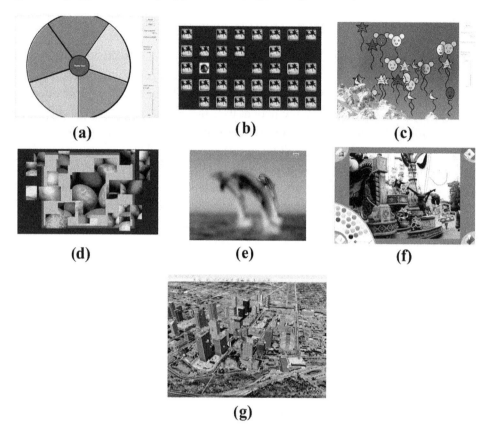

4.1.11. Match Me

Match Me is a digital implementation of the popular Concentration tile game that presents patients with an array of face-up or face-down touch tile pairs that need to be matched. This activity challenges gross motor movements, can increase sustained attention, and aims to improve visual neglect. To increase patient compliance and social interaction, family photos can appear on the tiles. A therapist can also choose to modify the number of touch tile pairs that are presented or change the location, pattern, or card background of the tiles. The Match Me activity supports both cooperation and competition: a patient can work with a partner to find matching touch tiles or complete against another player to find the most touch tile pairs (Figure 5b).

4.1.12. Pop Those Balloons

In Pop Those Balloons (Figure 5c), the patient is presented with a landscape that has floating balloons and is encouraged to think of their hands as stick pins. Using their stick pins, they must pop as many balloons as possible. Once a balloon has been popped, it 'fades out', disappears, and a popping sound is played. At this time, the patient's score increases, providing immediate positive feedback.

This activity aims to enhance hand-eye coordination as well as dexterity. Therapists can tailor this activity to meet the needs of a particular patient by modifying the number of balloons that appear, changing the speed at which the balloons float from bottom to top, or modifying the area of the screen to which the balloons float. While the patient is performing this activity, a number of metrics are gathered: the time between balloon pops, the number of popped balloons, the total number of balloons that appeared, and the balloon touch accuracy (using a root-mean squared error measurement).

4.1.13. Touch Tessellation

In Touch Tessellation, patients are presented with a number of tile-like puzzle pieces and must touch and drag each piece to complete the puzzle (Figure 5d). Touch Tessellation can test planning, decrease visual neglect, increase spatial relation skills, and challenge fine and gross motor skills. To customize the activity, a therapist can specify the size and number of puzzle pieces or modify the starting location of the puzzle pieces (e.g., to encourage patients to converse or perform gross motor movements). Patient photographs can be used and meaningful sounds can be played to encourage social dialog and emotional immersion. The activity records the number of puzzle pieces touched and drug, the number of joined pieces, and the patient's accuracy in touching each piece (using a root-mean squared error measurement).

4.1.14. Foggy Windows

In Foggy Windows, a patient is presented with a 'foggy window'. Patients must use their fingers or hands to 'defog the window' and reveal the hidden picture underneath. Foggy Windows can help patients exercise their gross motor skills and challenge figure-ground discrimination. To maintain patient engagement and compliance, therapists can modify the amount of fog that each window contains, the location of each window on the tabletop, or the size and type of the hidden object that is displayed (i.e., patient photographs, emails, or documents such as news stories can all be hidden). Foggy Windows can be used cooperatively, i.e., patients work with a partner to clean a window, or competitively, i.e., a patient and his or her partner have their own 'foggy window' and compete to clean them the fastest (Figure 5e). With Foggy Windows, it is possible to record the percent of the image that was defogged, the speed of each defogging stroke, and the areas where defogging occurred the most or least.

4.1.15. Photo Scrapbooking

In the Photo Scrapbooking activity, patients are encouraged to work cooperatively with a partner to modify personal pictures and make a scrapbook page. Patients can flip through a collection of their personal photographs to decide which one to modify and add to the scrapbook. In Photo Scrapbooking, patients can crop pictures, add stickers, paint, annotate, or alter picture attributes such as brightness or contrast (Figure 5f). Once a picture has been modified, it can be added to a scrapbook page, which can be saved, printed, or emailed to others. Photo Scrapbooking is an ideal collaborative activity because photographs naturally encourage emotional reactions and storytelling, and activate long-term memory. The editing of photos also challenges patients to exercise their fine and gross motor skills. This activity records the number and type of tools that were utilized, the length and duration of strokes (if one 'painted' on their image), the length and duration of touch events (if stickers were added), and the resulting images that were created.

4.1.16. Third Party Application Support

We have added a keyboard and mouse emulation extension to the AIR Touch system to support the use of third party applications. Interaction with Google Earth, for example, encourages patients to use their hands or fingers to navigate to places they have travelled to before or walk around their old neighbourhood (Figure 5g). Third party support also allows patients to play games with their family members, such as chess or checkers, browse the internet, or send emails using a virtual keyboard. This support allows patients to continue to stay connected to the outside world and practice skills that could be valuable once they finish their rehabilitation program. Given the variety of applications that can be used, this application only records the basic touch information (e.g., touch up, down, move, time between touch events, etc.).

4.2. Feedback

As mentioned, during our iterative design and implementation cycle, we consulted with a number of practicing occupational therapists. Discussions with these experts produced a number of guidelines that have influenced the design of our rehabilitation-centric activities and should be beneficial for others working in the area (Figure 6).

4.2.1. Communication

Encouraging communication during multi-user activities allows the trust between a patient and therapist to increase. It can also encourage patients to share their feelings and difficulties with their caregivers, and if using activities collaboratively, create bonds with other patients over their shared life or rehabilitative experiences. This can help improve not only the emotional state of the patient but also those they work with and depend on.

Figure 6. Elements identified by therapists as being crucial to the success of rehabilitation programs

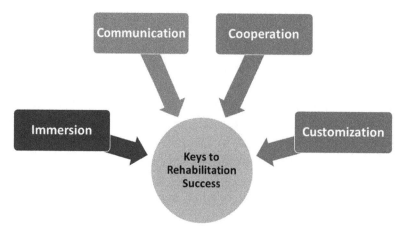

4.2.2. Cooperation

Including elements of cooperation is beneficial for rehabilitation because it provides patients with motivation from others who are in similar situations (i.e., fellow patients). As depression and feelings of helplessness often accompany serious injury, this can help make patients feel as if they are 'not alone' and have a support network. Using cooperation in rehabilitation activities also encourages patients to learn from the people they are interacting with and promotes turn taking, teamwork, and patience.

4.2.3. Customization

Activities should be configurable and have elements of uncertainty. Configurable activities allow therapists to tailor activities to match a patient's motor or cognitive abilities, demographic, background, or specific interests. Activities that contain surprises, uncertainty, and variability can be reused many times throughout a patient's recovery. Even something as simple as allowing a patient to choose the color of their stroke provides the patient with feelings of control over their rehabilitative process.

4.2.4. Immersion

Including positive, salient elements in multi-user activities can help patients to become emotionally immersed. This immersion allows patients to temporarily forget the pain or cognitive deficits they may have and instead focus on the activity at hand, i.e., they can experience and maintain a state of flow (Csikszentmihalyi, 1999). If a patient is working on an activity that has a picture of a loved one, they will likely be more motivated to put in effort and spend more time performing the activity.

Similarly, if patients can become competitively immersed in an activity, they are more likely to try harder and work longer to 'beat their competitor'. Patients can also receive encouragement and motivation from onlookers who are supporting them. Care does however need to be taken to ensure that the patient does not push themselves too far and incur further injury.

4.3. Visualizing Patient Interactions

Across all activities, there are a number of common events that can be recorded and utilized by a therapist to better understand a patient's progress (Table 1). These measures were further refined and four different visualizations were developed to allow for automatic comparisons between current and past performance and enable therapists to store patient-specific activity configurations for later comparison (Figure 7).

The first, a *radial touch map,* displayed the distribution of touch events from the patient's current standing location. This allowed therapists to identify and illustrate issues with flexion and extension. Another visualization, *touch event traces,* provided a 'heat map' style graphic that illustrated the location of each touch event that was generated by the patient along with the touch radius that was recorded, which illustrated the pressure exerted on the screen. This graphic enabled therapists to understand range of motion issues, and also identify areas of neglect that should be targeted in the future. The third visualization provided therapists with an animated rendering of each touch event, enabling therapists to 'scrub' through a session quickly and provide the patient with immediate feedback about their progress. Instead of focusing on the location of each touch event, the last visualization provided therapists with a timeline of the interaction that occurred during the session and allowed them to compare activity and

Table 1. Measures identified across all activities as being important to the monitoring of patient progress

Measure	Associated Rehabilitative Goal
Average touch event radius	Pressure and force exerted, muscle strength
Time of each touch event	Muscle Endurance
Duration of each touch event	Muscle Endurance
Speed of each touch event	Agility, muscle endurance
Time between touch events (i.e., between successive 'touch down' events in a given time period)	Fatigue, cardiovascular endurance, agility, interest, motivation
Number of touch events within a certain spatial location	Range of motion, flexibility, visual-spatial abilities
Time elapsed in activity per day and throughout the week	Interest, motivation, etc.

Figure 7. Examples of the different touch visualizations that were developed. (a) A radial visualization of touch-events, (b) a heat-map-style visualization to understand areas of neglect and range-of-motion issues, c) animated touch event traces, and (d) a touch-event timeline

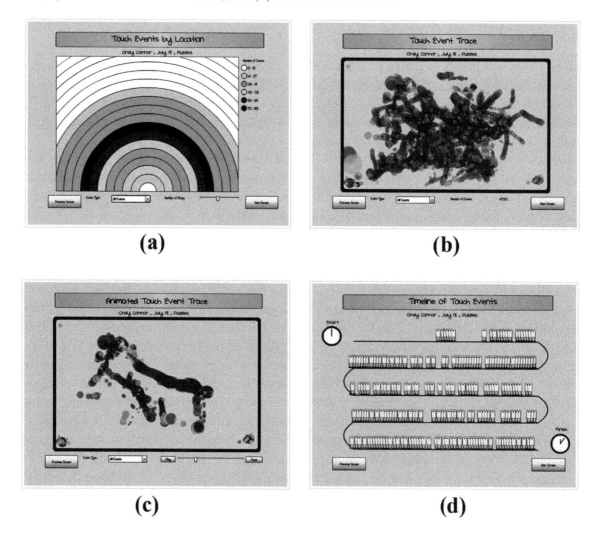

touch durations across multiple sessions. This also allows one to quickly assess each session to understand possible fatigue or motivation factors.

The visualizations allowed therapists to readily evaluate the performance of the patients on the various activities. Additionally, the visualizations supported longitudinal tracking and analysis of patient performance. This feature provided motivation and feedback for the patient as they could see how they were progressing throughout the course of an intervention and receive immediate feedback at the end of their activity or session.

5. KINETICS AND KINEMATICS OF INTERACTIVE SURFACE PHYSICAL THERAPY

It is widely hypothesized that an increase in engagement leads to an increase in activity level and that patients could spend more time performing therapy activities. If this is true, it is of great benefit to therapy programs, as patients often neglect their prescribed activities as they are monotonous and frustrating. As mentioned, therapists have been looking towards virtual reality and tele-rehabilitation (Burdea et al., 2000; Holden et al., 2006, 2007), the Nintendo Wii (Dixon, 2008; Deutsch et al., 2008), and multi-touch tabletops (Mumford et al., 2008, Wall Street Journal, 2015) to increase patient engagement.

While the integration of technology into rehabilitation programs has been widespread, the evidence to support its usefulness has been lacking. Most studies in this area are small case studies, focusing on one or two outcome measures (Deutsch et al., 2008, Burdea et al., 2000, Holden et al., 2006) or a therapist's subjective account of a patient's progress (Halton, 2008). With multi-touch tabletops, there have been no controlled studies comparing patients along multiple quantitative dimensions or directly comparing traditional table-based therapy (i.e., making a puzzle, tracing a picture, touching static targets, etc.) with technology-based approaches. Without such evidence, it is unclear if technology-based rehabilitation is beneficial to patients.

Although technology can make activities more enjoyable, the movements that each activity encourages or requires must be safe and effective. Before widespread adoption of new therapy methods can occur, understanding the changes in movement and force when activities are performed on a different medium (e.g., a multi-touch tabletop instead of a physical table) is an important step.

To understand patient movement while using technology-based rehabilitation, we conducted a lab-based study where we performed a controlled comparison of traditional (table-based) and multi-touch tabletop (technology-based) rehabilitation methods. In this study, we analyzed the hand motion and muscle activation of participants as they completed four activities that were representative of those typically performed in a stroke rehabilitation program. As patient safety is of great concern, we chose healthy individuals as participants. By monitoring the movement patterns and forces exhibited by those who are healthy, we should be better able to understand what impact a change in presentation medium could have on the movement kinetics and kinematics of patients.

5.1. Methods

To analyze the potential benefits of technology-based therapy interventions, a within-subject study design was conducted with able-bodied participants.

5.1.1. Participants

From the general University population, 14 right-handed individuals (7 females and 7 males) participated in our study. Participants had a mean age of 27.9 years ($SD = 12.5$, range 18-77 years) years. Each participant was paid $20 CAD for their time, and did not have prior experience with a multi-touch tabletop, motion capture, or electromyography. The study was approved by the Research Ethics Board at the University of Alberta.

5.1.2. Apparatus

The AirTouch table was used in this study. The upper body movement of each participant was captured using a NaturalPoint 12-camera Optitrack system. Participants wore a motion capture jacket with 19 retro-reflective markers, providing the position of the chest, waist, upper arm, lower arm, and hand at 100 Hz. Surface electromyography (EMG) measured the muscular activity of each participant. Four pairs of electrodes were placed on the skin of the dominant arm (i.e., on the biceps-brachii, on the triceps brachii, on the forearm flexors, and on the forearm extensors). The electrodes were connected to a Bortec AMT-8 amplification system that was then connected to a National Instruments Data Acquisition Card that sampled at 1000 Hz. The EMG signals were filtered using a band-pass filter (20 - 400 Hz), a 60 Hz notch filter, and a Root-Mean-Square filter (with a window size of 300 ms) to remove noise and rectify the signal.

For the traditional, non-interactive activities, a white, corrugated plastic board (91 cm x 61 cm x 0.4 cm) was placed on top of the acrylic surface of the multi-touch tabletop. The repurposing of the multi-touch tabletop in this way allowed participants to remain in the same location and use the same region of interaction across all activities.

5.1.3. Procedure

Participants stood in front of the multi-touch tabletop and performed four activities. Participants performed each activity for 5 minutes, with the order of activities randomized between participants. If participants finished the activity before the allotted time elapsed, the activity was reset and the participant repeated it until 5 minutes elapsed. Resetting the activity was acceptable as we were not concerned with the learnability of the activities or the cognitive strategies employed, and it also reflects a real-world usage scenario. A short 3-minute break was allowed between activities to mitigate possible fatigue effects and allow for the next activity to be set up. Similar to constraint-induced movement therapy (Kunkel et al., 1999; Taub et al., 2004), participants were restricted to use only their dominant (right) arm to complete each activity.

Though some patients may sit at the table in a clinical setting, many stand so that they may work to improve their balance along with upper extremity function. The experiment took approximately 45 minutes to complete.

5.1.4. Activities

Four activities were used in the study (Figure 8). Two of the activities, Touch Tessellation and Match Me, are activities that are currently in use by therapists at the Glenrose Rehabilitation Hospital and re-

Figure 8. Examples of the participant activities. (a) Card Sorting, (b) Grid of Stickers, (c) Touch Tessellation, and (d) Match Me

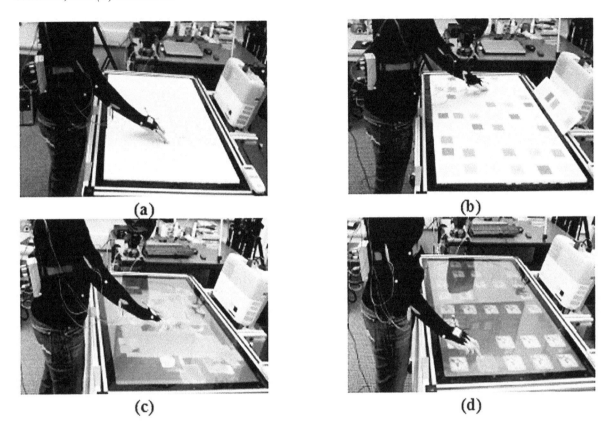

quired participants to interact with the multi-touch tabletop. The other two activities, i.e., Card Sorting and Grid of Stickers, are similar to traditional table-based activities that patients currently perform in therapy sessions and did not make use of the interactive tabletop. While a comparison with 'standardized' activities would seem appealing, the activities and exercises used in therapy programs today vary widely between hospitals and therapists.

- **Card Sorting (Physical):** A deck of miniature playing cards (with face cards removed) was shuffled and placed face up, in a pile, on a white plastic board in a circular area close to participants (Figure 8a). Opposite the cards was a 10 x 4 grid where participants could drag each playing card. Participants sorted the pile (into ascending order, by suit) by sliding each card into the grid.
- **Grid of Stickers (Physical):** This activity used a white plastic board with a 9 x 6 grid containing 45 rectangular stickers (and 9 empty spaces). Five different colors of stickers were used, each numbered sequentially from one to nine (Figure 8b). Participants were required to touch each number in order, cycling through a predefined sequence of colors (i.e., Brown 1, Pink 1, Blue 1, Yellow 1, Green 1, Brown 2, …., Green 9).
- **Touch Tessellation (Digital):** Forty square-shaped puzzle pieces were presented to participants on the multi-touch tabletop. To eliminate the need to rotate tiles, all tiles were presented in the correct orientation (Figure 8c). Participants completed the puzzle by dragging matching pieces

next to each other, causing them to 'snap' together. The finished puzzle was 10 pieces wide x 4 pieces high.

- **Match Me (Digital):** An 8 x 5 grid of tiles was presented on the multi-touch tabletop (Figure 8d). On the underside of each tile was one of 20 images. As participants touched the tiles, they flipped over to reveal an image. Participants touched two images sequentially, trying to find a match. If a match was found, the tiles disappeared from view; if not, the tiles flipped back over and they continued finding matching pairs.

5.1.5. Measures

To assess the potential for technology-assisted rehabilitation, measures of movement (kinematics and kinetics) as well as measures of user-attitude were recorded.

5.1.6. Kinematics and Kinetics

To assess the kinematic components (i.e., those related to spatial movement) of each trajectory (Figure 9), several measures were computed. The quantity of movement was assessed using *total path length,* computed as the sum of the distance between successive points on the trajectory of the hand. Looking at the trajectory distribution and the motion smoothness enabled us to assess the form of participant's movement. The standard deviation of each trajectory was used to compute the *dispersion* of the signal along each axis: left/right (x), up/down (y), and forward/backward (z). The *smoothness* of participant's motion (i.e., the degree to which the trajectory changes direction at each point in time) was computed using the median value of the trajectory's curvature.

To assess the kinetic components (i.e., those related to force production), the *total muscle activity* was computed as the summation of the rectified, filtered signals from the four muscle sites. These measures were chosen based on prior experience analyzing gestures and surgical movement, and represent meaningful simplifications of the complex 3D trajectories. More complex analysis tools (e.g., using HMMs or Dynamic Time Warping) may give more insight, but were beyond the scope of the work.

5.1.7. Motivation and Perceived Usage

The Intrinsic Motivation Inventory (IMI; McAuley et al., 1989) was used to assess participants' subjective opinions towards each of the activities using Likert-type responses to statements such as "I would describe the activities as very interesting". From the responses, scores along four separate dimensions (i.e., interest and enjoyment, effort and importance, mental tension and pressure, and perceived competency) were computed and represent the participants' subjective feelings towards the different activities. Two IMI's were administered, one assessing both of the traditional activities (*Card Sorting* and *Grid of Stickers*) and the other assessing both of the technology-based activities (*Match Me* and *Touch Tessellation*). At the conclusion of the experiment, a semi-structured exit interview was conducted. The following guiding questions were used during the interview and participants were encouraged to engage in open discussion:

- Which activities did you enjoy the most? Which did you enjoy the least?
- If you could change any of activities, what would you change?

Figure 9. Participant P5's trajectories from (a) Card Sorting, (b) Grid of Stickers, (c) Touch Tessellation, and (d) Match Me. The viewpoint is rotated to show movement on and above the tabletop (located at y ≈ 925 mm). Of interest in the graphs is the grid structure visible in the Grid of Stickers and Match Me graphs, the dense region in the Card Sorting corresponding to the initial pile of cards. The density of the trajectory also indicates path length

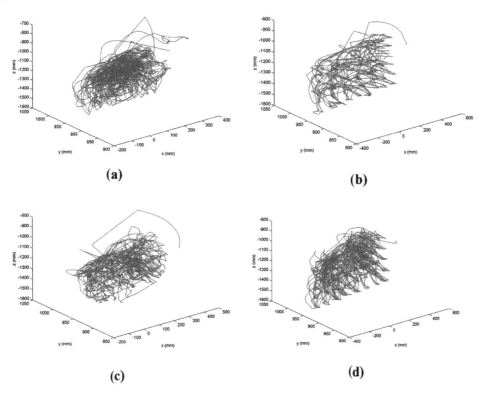

- Which category of activity (traditional or technology) did you prefer?
- Imagine you are in a therapy program. Which of the activities would you prefer to use?

5.2. Results

Herein we detail the quantitative and qualitative results that were attained, first detailing those relating to the Kinematics and Kinetics and then those relating to the preferences of the participants.

5.2.1. Kinematics and Kinetics

The statistical analysis was conducted with Stata on the kinematic and kinetic outcome measures described above. A one-way repeated-measures ANOVA was performed with *Activity* as the main factor (levels: Touch Tessellation, Match Me, Card Sorting, and Grid of Stickers). The ANOVA tests for *total path length*, *x-dispersion*, *z-dispersion*, and *smoothness* were all found to be significant, $p < 0.001$ (Table 2). The y-dispersion was not found to be significantly different between any of the conditions, indicating that the vertical movement of participants' right hand did not vary greatly between activities. The

Table 2. ANOVA Results. The movement data as well as subjective responses were analyzed and are presented separately

	$F_{(3, 39)}$	Significance
Path Length	7.3	$p < 0.001$ ***
EMG Activity	1.99	$p > 0.05$
x-Dispersion	50.32	$p < 0.001$ ***
y-Dispersion	2.66	$p > 0.05$
z-Dispersion	15.63	$p < 0.001$ ***
Smoothness	10.59	$p < 0.001$ ***

total muscle activity was not significantly different between any of the conditions, implying that similar amounts of force were used for all activities.

Post-hoc tests were conducted on the four significant measures using Tukey's HSD (Figure 10). Regarding *total path length*, post-hoc tests revealed the means between the Touch Tessellation and Match Me activities were significantly different ($p < 0.05$) as were the means of the Touch Tessellation and Card Sorting activities ($p < 0.001$). Regarding the *x-dispersion* (left/right), all activities were found to be significantly different from each other ($p < 0.01$ between Match Me and Grid of Stickers, and between Touch Tessellation and Grid of Stickers; and $p < 0.001$ for all other conditions). The post-hoc tests also revealed that the *z-dispersion* (forward/back) of the Touch Tessellation activity was significantly different from all other activities ($p < 0.01$ for Grid of Stickers, $p < 0.001$ for Match Me and Card Sorting). Post-hoc tests also showed that the smoothness of the Card Sorting activity was significantly different from all other activities ($p < 0.01$ for Match Me and Grid of Stickers, $p < 0.001$ for Touch Tessellation).

5.2.2. Motivation and Perceived Usage

The Intrinsic Motivation Inventory responses (Figure 11) were analyzed using Bonferroni-adjusted, Wilcoxon signed-rank comparisons. Participants rated the multi-touch activities (i.e., MatchMe and Touch Tessellation) as significantly more interesting and enjoyable than the traditional activities (i.e., Card Sorting and Grid of Stickers; $Z = 2.79$, $p = .0052$). There were no significant differences along the other dimensions (i.e., effort: $p = .45$, competence: $p = .71$, and tension: $p = .68$). As all four of the activities were quite simple and participants were instructed to perform each activity at their own pace, the lack of statistical differences is unsurprising.

5.3. Discussion

Results from the participant's subjective responses matched well with the presumed benefits of technology-based therapy, however, the motion data presented interesting and surprising results.

5.3.1. Kinematics and Kinetics

The results indicate that technology is not the sole factor determining the quantity of motion. Any differences in *total path length* and *total muscle activity* did not appear to be caused by the use of technology,

Figure 10. The mean kinematic and kinetic results for the four activities (i.e., Card Sorting (CS), Grid of Stickers (GoS), Touch Tessellation (TT), and Match Me (MM)) for the (a) path length, (b) x-Dispersion, (c) z-Dispersion, and (d) smoothness measures

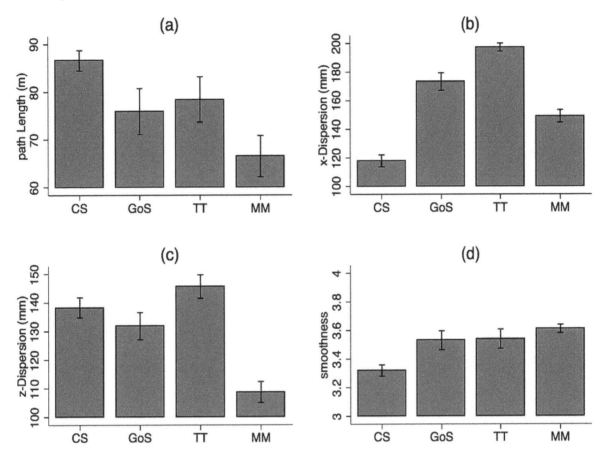

but rather the content of the activity. The *total path length* during the Touch Tessellation activity was significantly lower than the Match Me and Card Sorting activities. We observed that many participants hesitated before reaching for a Touch Tessellation piece. These hesitations led to less frequent movements and thus lower path lengths. Additionally, the Card Sorting activity produced a substantial amount of movement. This is likely because participants did not have to perform a visual search or engage in substantial cognitive processing to find their next target. By designing activities so that targets are easily located and known, thus cutting down on visual search time, we can maximize a patient's movement during therapy sessions.

The analysis of the movement form demonstrates the importance of an activity's spatial layout and a user's strategy. From the dispersion, we see that while most participants kept their hand at approximately the same height above the tabletop, the dispersion of movement along the surface of the table was quite variable. From the *x-dispersion*, we see that all activities produced very different motion, with no clear separation between technology and traditional activities. During Card Sorting, participants often slid cards up the center of the table and then returned their hand to the bottom of the board to get their next card. With Match Me, many participants selected tiles from alternating sides of the table, perhaps think-

Figure 11. The median scores for each of the dimensions of the IMI. The error bars depict the standard error of the mean. The 'Interest' dimension is statistically higher with the technology-based activities (i.e., Match Me and Touch Tessellation) than the traditional activities (i.e., Grid of Stickers and Card Sorting)

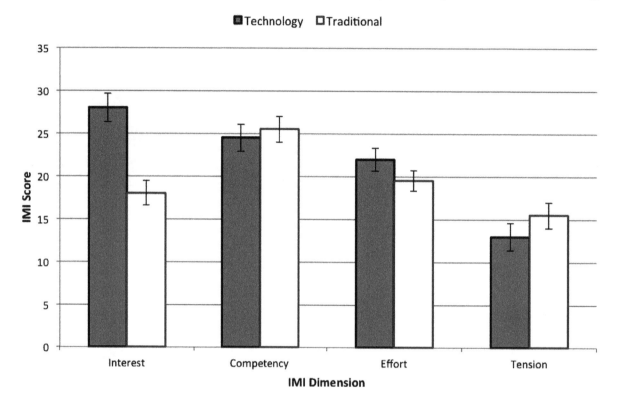

ing that matching pairs would not be placed next to each other (although the tiles were randomized). This led to frequent left-right movements. The small *z-dispersion* for the Touch Tessellation quantifies a strategy that a number of participants used, namely dragging pieces close to themselves so they could more easily see, manipulate, and combine them into smaller groups before they were moved to their final location. This strategy allowed participants to make more efficient movements, leading to small dispersion values. For an activity that emphasizes range of motion, designers should give thought to whether targets are static, dynamic, or user-movable, and what strategies users may employ to complete them.

During Card Sorting, participants made smoother movements, most likely because Card Sorting has a low cognitive load, resulting in continuous, flowing motion. In contrast, the Grid of Stickers required extensive visual search, often leading to 'Aha!' moments. These moments caused participants to touch stickers that were difficult to find quickly, resulting in sharper motion. To minimize intense movements, it may be beneficial to avoid 'surprise' elements that trigger such motion.

5.3.2. Motivation and Perceived Usage

The semi-structured interviews help explain the reasons behind the increased scores of enjoyment and interest. Several participants commented that they enjoyed the technology-based activities more because they contained dynamic elements and feedback about their progress: "hearing the Touch Tessellation tiles click together and having the tiles disappear in front of me was super motivating" (P1). Although the activities were completed individually, many participants mentioned that they took a competitive stance towards completing them, "[the tech] wasn't frustrating at all! For me it was like a competition" (P10). When using the multi-touch tabletop, several participants indicated that they were motivated to accomplish a worthwhile goal: "I like the Touch Tessellation one because you're actually playing a game and trying to finish something instead of just touching stickers" (P3).

These comments suggest that technology-assisted rehabilitation might be more enjoyable because it provides meaningful, achievable challenges and real-time, dynamic feedback to users. The participant's feedback is consistent with beliefs that dynamic gaming elements lead increased enjoyment and adherence to therapy programs. When designing activities for therapy, it is not enough to only rely on the use of technology to increase engagement and adherence. It is important for designers to think carefully about the goals of the activities they are designing and employ feedback at the correct frequency, using the correct medium, and at an appropriate cognitive level. Designers should also work to provide engaging and challenging, yet accomplishable, elements in their activities that are intrinsically motivating to patients.

Other comments alluded to the role that prior exposure with technology had on participants' expectations and experiences with the multi-touch tabletop. Many participants compared the multi-touch tabletop (and its activities) to commercial multi-touch devices: "if you have an iPad you can see that it registers every motion and gesture ... the design of [iPad] games are better" (P13); "I'm just so used to playing those iPhone games" (P12). Many participants expressed that they would definitely prefer to use the multi-touch tabletop in a rehabilitation setting if it was as refined as the commercial products they use every day.

As the quality of commercial technology increases and the budgets for therapy-driven software remain comparatively low, these observations become particularly relevant. The user-facing aspects of therapy software need to be improved to meet the growing expectations and familiarity patients will have with multi-touch technologies. In the near future, many patients will be intimately familiar with software products and video games released by large production studios with equally large budgets. Unfortunately, custom therapy-targeted projects will likely not have these budgets so designers will have to be creative in finding ways to meet such expectations. To create engaging, high-quality games at low costs, designers should leverage existing content and technologies where possible, and use openly available video-game engines to ensure that the rehabilitation games do not feel similar to ad-hoc prototype applications, instead appearing robust, well designed, and thoroughly tested.

Several participants were also quick to cite technology (i.e., the multi-touch tabletop) as the source of any errors that occurred rather than their own actions. As the multi-touch tabletop provides direct-touch interaction, there is a much smaller gulf of execution than with indirect-touch interfaces (Hutchins et al., 1985), causing more ambiguity with regard to the source of errors. During our experiment, the largest sources of frustration were situations in which false touches were being detected and situations where the user received little or no feedback. When this happened, many users were unsure if they were not touching the surface with enough force (even though it was not pressure sensitive) or were not touching in the right location, leading to confusion and annoyance. For example, one participant was "irritated at how the tabletop wasn't too responsive" (P7) and continually exerted more force on the surface. In contrast, none of the participants complained about the mechanics of the traditional activities when they made an error and one participant commented that they "felt [they] could handle the physical materials more easily than the digital ones" (P8). These comments tended to be more frequent amongst the younger users who had existing experience with refined, commercial touch-screens. In contrast, the older users seemed content with the technology, and quickly adapted to any calibration errors.

5.3.3. Guidelines

The study has provided insight into the impact that the design of the activity can have on the movement of the patient. It is not enough to naïvely place targets, as this does not consider all factors of the motion that is used to touch them. While technology-based approaches seem to be more enjoyable for patients, it is essential that the underlying movements actually produce the desired effect and can be performed by users in a reasonable manner. As with most interactive surfaces, it is important that the surface texture of the device does not introduce extra friction that can decrease the fluidity of one's movements (Annett et al., 2014).

To minimize user frustration during input, tabletop activities must have responsive sensing, as users will otherwise become quickly irritated and feel that they are not in control of an activity and potentially their therapy progress. While hardware is a large determinant of the responsiveness and accuracy, some steps can be taken in software to reduce the apparent effects of these parameters. For direct-touch devices with coarse sensing resolution or noisy sensing, on-screen targets can be made larger so that pixel-level accuracy is not required.

Feedforward and feedback is also very important within the design of any technology-based therapy system. Feedback should also be used to indicate the exact location where the user's touch was registered. Providing as much information before and after touch events occur can allow users to adjust their interaction to accommodate for any offsets or input warping and will help reduce the ambiguity caused by positioning errors. The use of the hover-state (Buxton, 1990) may be an important data stream to consider in future rehabilitation-based systems. To mitigate latency issues, developers should ensure that feedback regarding a sensed touch is displayed as soon as possible and not delayed by complex application-specific processing. If complex processing is required, the system should first provide the feedback on where the touch was registered before processing the application-specific response.

6. GENERAL DISCUSSION

The broad scope of the presented work has allowed us to generate insights into the use of technology for rehabilitation and how to best design and implement effective, usable systems. Herein we discuss four of the most prominent factors that need to be considered before one integrates technology-based initiatives or interventions into a rehabilitation program.

6.1. Activity Design

The design of the software activities was found to be very influential in the movements made by participants, as well as for engagement with activities. When designing activities or selecting from pre-made activities, consideration should be given to both of these aspects to ensure maximal benefit for the patient.

A wide range of activities should be available to maximize the chances that patients will be able to select an activity that interests them. Just as people have different preferences for various genres of video games, different patients will prefer different types of activities. Many may not want to play games at all, but might prefer to perform productivity tasks, read books, or communicate with loved ones. While these types of activities were not explored, aside from providing third-party application support, they present interesting and fruitful avenues for future research. Lastly, activities should support end-user customization where possible, allowing the patient to use their own photos and stories and draw upon information from local sources or personal history for content.

Where possible, collaboration or cooperation scenarios should be supported. Some of the activities that were developed (e.g., Touch Tessellation, Pop those Balloons) are inherently multi-player via their support for multi-touch and multiple targets that can be manipulated concurrently. These activities were well received by patients and therapists as the therapist could work with the patient to provide assistance, as well as increasing the social aspect of the activity. For competitive activities more work is needed to ensure skills are balanced and patients with different abilities are able to compete on an even playing field.

6.2. Evaluation Techniques

Robust evaluation techniques are needed in the development of all therapy-focused technology. Currently, clinical trials are out-of-scope and too cumbersome for most developers of therapy-based technology and proxy-evaluations need to be conducted. We presented methodology for one such proxy-evaluation, in which we evaluated both quantitative measures of motion as well as subjective aspects of the experience. It is important for developers to consider both aspects of their proposed intervention, as getting both 'right' is crucial to the success of the therapy sessions.

Future work is needed to reduce the complexity of these evaluations, however. The presented evaluation used optical motion trackers and electromyogram technology, both of which are out-of-reach of many developers. Lower-cost alternatives may be useful in many situations, such as using a Microsoft Kinect to capture and record motion data and using simple force-sensitive-resistors to instrument the user or environment to record kinetic data.

6.3. Necessity for User-Centric, Iterative Prototyping

Integrating the therapists and clients into the development cycle was an important aspect of the success of the technology. The consultations provided opportunities to uncover various usability issues unique to clinical use that would have otherwise gone unnoticed until the time of deployment. These sessions also helped illustrate the importance of simplicity, responsiveness, and ease of use, as therapy sessions are often quite short with little time available to setup, login, and configure systems, tools, or activities that will be used. All of the activity customization that was included in our activities was touch-based and could be modified in-activity in real-time. This allowed for a decreased learning curve on the part of the therapist and increased freedom to change options and parameters on the fly.

Feedback from the therapists drove the design of the data-visualization component of the software. Their input helped understand which useful measures and data were relevant to the successful tracking of patient input. This also helped provide useful and motivating data to the patients to maintain their long-term interest in the activities and ultimately their rehabilitation program.

6.4. Tabletops for Interactive Rehabilitation

Interactive tabletops are a great form-factor for upper-extremity rehabilitation tasks. Their large size supports a wide range of abilities and range of motions from fine motor tasks to large, gross movements that span the width and length of the table. They also provide a familiar form-factor (horizontal surface) which makes affordances such as touching and dragging objects more direct. Lastly, patients are able to use the table for support during standing, if necessary, or can even be seated while using the table. This increases the population that is able to use the table.

The tabletops used in our presented work represented leading-edge technology at the time the work was conducted. Recent advances in commercial displays have provided off-the-shelf solutions which may be better suited for rehabilitation tasks. For instance, SMART Technologies and Microsoft now offer large, high resolution screens (e.g., 55", 65", 84" diagonal size) with touch, stylus, and some tangible input support. These displays can be mounted to actuated stands to allow the angle and height of the screen to be modified, greatly increasing the utility of the hardware. These stands are capable of orienting the screen continuously from horizontal to vertical, providing 90 degrees of rotation. Additionally, the height can be adjusted approximately 75cm, allowing many users to be accommodated. While more expensive, using such commercially available hardware can speed development time and lead to fewer technical issues compared to developing in-house solutions.

The recent developments of touch and stylus-based tablets in the commercial market has opened the possibilities for adapting many of these activities for in-home use. While therapist supervision would be ideal, it is possible that self-guided exercises would be beneficial for patients, especially for developing fine motor control. In addition, there is an existing ecosystem of games and applications that may be usable for patients – perhaps with some adaptations (e.g., larger user interface components) to provide an engaging platform for rehabilitation.

7. CONCLUSION

This work has revealed important insights into multi-touch therapy, activities, equipment, and outcomes. While direct-touch interaction can continue to offer a number of benefits when used in therapy-based activities, there are a number of drawbacks that need to be considered and addressed before rehabilitation facilities should consider developing technology-only interventions and programs. An iterative design process that was undertaken identified many goals, requirements, and guidelines that should be of great benefit to the human-computer interaction and rehabilitation communities.

Given the previous work demonstrating that technology itself is not enough to modify the movement patterns of individuals in therapy programs, it is clear that the benefit of technology lies in its ability to provide responsive, dynamic content. To that end, we have studied user attitudes towards interactive tabletops and found that while users do typically find them more engaging, there are some limitations that must be overcome before they can become truly beneficial for clinical populations. Using our design recommendations, the engagement and enjoyment patients experience during therapy can be improved, and should lead to higher motivation and ultimately compliance and satisfaction with the therapeutic process.

There are several avenues along which this work can be extended. One next step is to refine our activities based on the observations gathered during the current study and perform a long-term study with a patient population. While we expect many of our conclusions and recommendations to generalize to both populations, studying the usage behavior of the target end users (i.e., patients) will likely produce additional insights that will be of great value. Additional future work could also involve studying those aspects of tabletop-based therapy that contribute to success and enjoyment for the end user, for instance, examining the relative importance of customization, dynamic feedback, emotional saliency, and game content.

ACKNOWLEDGMENT

The researchers wish to thank all of their participants as well as their funding agencies: Alberta Innovates: Technology Futures, the Canadian Institutes of Health Research, and the National Science and Engineering Research Council. We additionally wish to thank Gauri Chaggar, Mavis Chan, Phoebe Chen, and Dylan Sheil for their assistance in the creation applications for the rehabilitation suite and with the user studies.

REFERENCES

Accot, J., & Zhai, S. (1999). Performance evaluation of input devices in trajectory-based tasks: an application of the steering law. *Proceedings of the SIGCHI conference on Human Factors in Computing Systems*. doi:10.1145/302979.303133

Al Mahmud, A., Mubin, O., Shahid, S., & Martens, J. (2008). Designing and Evaluating the Tabletop Game Experience for Senior Citizens. *Proceedings of Nordic Conference on Computer-Human Interaction* (pp. 403-406). doi:10.1145/1463160.1463205

Annett, M., Anderson, F., Bischof, W. F., & Gupta, A. (2014). The Pen is Mightier: Understanding Stylus Behavior While Inking on Tablets. *Proceedings of Graphics Interface* (pp. 193-200).

Annett, M., Anderson, F., Goertzen, D., Halton, J., Ranson, Q., Bischof, W. F., & Boulanger, P. (2009). Using a multi-touch tabletop for upper extremity motor rehabilitation. *Proceedings of the 21st Annual Conference of the Australian Computer-Human Interaction Special Interest Group* (pp. 261-264). doi:10.1145/1738826.1738869

Apted, T., Kay, J., & Quigley, A. (2006). Tabletop Sharing of Digital Photographs for the Elderly. *Proceedings of the SIGCHI Conference on Human Factors in Computing Systems* (pp. 781-790). doi:10.1145/1124772.1124887

Augstein, M., Neumayr, T., Ruckser-Scherb, R., Karlhuber, I., & Altmann, J., (2013). The Fun. Tast. Tisch. project: a novel approach to neuro-rehabilitation using an interactive multiuser multitouch tabletop. *Proceedings of Interactive Tabletops and Surfaces* (pp. 81-90).

Augstein, M., Neumayr, T., & Schacherl-Hofer, I. (2014). The Usability of a Tabletop Application for Neuro-Rehabilitation from Therapists' Point of View. *Proceedings of the Interactive Tabletops and Surfaces* (pp. 239-248).

Bauminger-Zviely, N., Eden, S., Zancanaro, M., Weiss, P. L., & Gal, E. (2013). Increasing social engagement in children with high-functioning autism spectrum disorder using collaborative technologies in the school environment. *Autism, 17*(3), 317–339. doi:10.1177/1362361312472989 PMID:23614935

Berger-Vachon, C. (2006). Virtual reality and disability. *Technology and Disability, 18*, 163–165.

Burdea, G., Popescu, V., Hentz, V., & Colbert, K. (2000). Virtual Reality-Based Orthopedic Telerehabilitation. *IEEE Transactions on Rehabilitation Engineering, 8*(3), 430–432. doi:10.1109/86.867886 PMID:11001524

Buxton, W. (1990). A three-state model of graphical input. *Proceedings of the IFIP TC13 Third International Conference on Human-Computer Interaction* (pp. 449-456).

CANSIM – Canadian socioeconomic database from Statistics Canada. Table 105-0203. (2005).

Castle, A. (n. d.). Build your own multitouch surface computer. Retrieved from http://www.maximumpc.com/build-your-own-multitouch-surface-computer/

Chang, Y., Chen, S., & Huang, J. (2011). A Kinect-based system for physical rehabilitation: A pilot study for young adults with motor disabilities. *Research in Developmental Disabilities, 32*(6), 2566–2570. doi:10.1016/j.ridd.2011.07.002 PMID:21784612

Csikszentmihalyi, M., (1997). *Finding Flow*.

Delbressine, F., Timmermans, A., Beursgens, L., de Jong, M., van Dam, A., Verweij, D., & Markopoulos, P. et al. (2012). Motivating arm-hand use for stroke patients by serious games. *Proceedings of the 34th Annual International Conference of the IEEE Engineering in Medicine and Biology Society.*

Deterding, S., Dixon, D., Khaled, R., & Nacke, L. (2011). From game design elements to gamefulness: defining gamification. *Proceedings of the 15th International Academic MindTrek Conference: Envisioning Future Media Environments,* 9-15. doi:10.1145/2181037.2181040

Deutsch, J. E., Borbely, M., Filler, J., Huhn, K., & Guarrera-Bowlby, P. (2008). Use of a Low-Cost, Commercially Available Gaming Console (Wii) for Rehabilitation of an Adolescent with Cerebral Palsy. *Physical Therapy, 88*(10), 1196–1207. doi:10.2522/ptj.20080062 PMID:18689607

Dixon, T., (2008). A Wii Spot of Fun. *Australian Ageing Agenda*, March-April, 28-31.

Domova, V., Vartiainen, E., Azhar, S., & Ralph, M., (2013). An interactive surface solution to support collaborative work onboard ships. In the *Proceedings of Interactive Tabletops and Surfaces,* 265-272.

Dunne, A., Do-Lenh, S., Laighin, G. O., Shen, C., & Bonato, P. (2010). Upper extremity rehabilitation of children with cerebral palsy using accelerometer feedback on a multitouch display. *Proceedings of the Engineering in Medicine and Biology Society* (pp. 1751-1754). doi:10.1109/IEMBS.2010.5626724

Facal, D., Gonzalez, M.F., Martinez, V., Buiza, C., Talantzis, F., Petsatodis, T., Soldatos, J., Urdaneta, E., & Yanguas, J.J., (2009). Cognitive Games for Healthy Elderly People in a Multitouch Screen. *Proceedings of DRT4ALL* (pp. 91-97).

Flynn, S. M., & Lange, B. M. (2010). Games for Rehabilitation, the voice of players. *Proceedings of the 8th International Conference on Disability, Virtual Reality & Associated Technologies* (pp. 185-194).

Gamberini, L., Martino, F., Seraglia, B., Spagnolli, A., Fabregat, M., Ibanez, F.,Alcaniz, M., & Andrés, J. M., (2009). Eldergames project: An innovative mixed reality table-top solution to preserve cognitive functions in elderly people. *Proceedings of Human System Interactions* (pp. 164-169).

Gupta, A., & O'Malley, M. K. (2006). Design of a Haptic Arm ExoSkeleton for Training and Rehabilitation. *IEEE/ASME Transactions on Mechatronics, 11*(3), 280–289. doi:10.1109/TMECH.2006.875558

Halton, J. Virtual rehabilitation with video games: A new frontier for occupational therapy. *Occupational Therapy Now, 9*(6), 12-14.

Han, J.Y., (2005). Low-Cost Multi-Touch Sensing through Frustrated Total Internal Reflection. *Proceedings of User Interfaces and Software Technologies* (pp. 115-118).

Hancock, M., Ten Cate, T., Carpendale, S., & Isenberg, T. (2010). Supporting sandtray therapy on an interactive tabletop. *Proceedings of the SIGCHI Conference on Human Factors in Computing Systems* (pp. 2133-2142). doi:10.1145/1753326.1753651

Holden, M. K., Dyar, T. A., & Dayan-Cimadoro, L. (2007). Telerehabilitation Using a Virtual Environment Improves Upper Extremity Function in Patients With Stroke. *IEEE Transactions on Neural Systems and Rehabilitation Engineering, 15*(1), 36–42. doi:10.1109/TNSRE.2007.891388 PMID:17436874

Holden, M. K., Dyar, T. A., Schwamm, L., & Bizzi, E. (2006). Virtual-environment-based telerehabilitation in patients with stroke. *Presence (Cambridge, Mass.), 14*(2), 214–233. doi:10.1162/1054746053967058

Hutchins, E., Hollan, J., & Norman, D. (1985). Direct manipulation interfaces. *Journal of Human-Computer Interaction, 1*(4), 311–338. doi:10.1207/s15327051hci0104_2

Jacobs, A., Timmermans, A., Michielsen, M., Vander Plaetse, M., & Markopoulos, P., (2013). CONTRAST: gamification of arm-hand training for stroke survivors. In the *Extended Abstracts on Human Factors in Computing System*s (pp. 415-420).

Jorda, S., Geiger, G., Alonso, M., & Kaltenbrunner, M. (2007). The reacTable: exploring the synergy between live music performance and tabletop tangible interfaces. *Proceedings of the Annual Conference on Tangible, Embedded, and Embodied Interaction* (pp. 139-146). doi:10.1145/1226969.1226998

Jung, J., Kim, L., Park, S., & Kwon, G. H., (2013). E-CORE (Embodied COgnitive REhabilitation): A Cognitive Rehabilitation System Using Tangible Tabletop Interface. *Converging Clinical and Engineering Research on Neurorehabilitation* (pp. 893-897).

Khademi, M., Mousavi Hondori, H., McKenzie, A., Dodakian, L., Lopes, C. V., & C Cramer, S., (2014). Comparing direct and indirect interaction in stroke rehabilitation. In the *Extended Abstracts on Human Factors in Computing Systems* (pp. 1639-1644).

Kunkel, A., Kopp, B., Müller, G., Villringer, K., Villringer, A., Taub, E., & Flor, H. (1999). Constraint-induced movement therapy for motor recovery in chronic stroke patients. *Archives of Physical Medicine and Rehabilitation, 80*(6), 624–628. doi:10.1016/S0003-9993(99)90163-6 PMID:10378486

Kwon, G. H., Kim, L., & Park, S., (2013). Development of a cognitive assessment tool and training systems for elderly cognitive impairment. *Proceedings of Pervasive Computing Technologies for Healthcare* (pp. 450-452).

McAuley, E., Duncan, T., & Tammen, V. V. (1989). Psychometric properties of the Intrinsic Motivation Inventory in a competitive sport setting: A confirmatory factor analysis. *Research Quarterly for Exercise and Sport, 60*(1), 48–58. doi:10.1080/02701367.1989.10607413 PMID:2489825

Mumford N., Duckworth, J., Eldridge, R., Guglielmetti, M., Thomas, P., Shum, D., Rudolph, H., Williams, G., & Wilson, P.H., (2008). A virtual tabletop workspace for upper-limb rehabilitation in Traumatic Brain Injury (TBI): A multiple case study evaluation. *Proceedings of Virtual Rehabilitation* (pp. 175-180).

NOR /D. (n. d.). Retrieved from http://labs.nortd.com/

Rand, D., Kizony, R., & Weiss, P. T. L. (2008). The Sony PlayStation II EyeToy: Low-cost virtual reality for use in rehabilitation. *Journal of Neurologic Physical Therapy; JNPT, 32*(4), 155–163. doi:10.1097/NPT.0b013e31818ee779 PMID:19265756

Rizzo, A., & Kim, G. K. (2005). A SWOT analysis of the field of virtual reality rehabilitation and therapy. *Presence (Cambridge, Mass.), 14*, 119–146.

Saposnik, G., Teasell, R., Mamdani, M., Hall, J., McIlroy, W., Cheung, D., & Bayley, M. et al. (2010). Effectiveness of Virtual Reality Using Wii Gaming Technology in Stroke Rehabilitation. *Stroke, 41*(7), 1477–1484. doi:10.1161/STROKEAHA.110.584979 PMID:20508185

Seifried, T., Rendl, C., Perteneder, F., Haller, M., Sakamoto, D., Kato, J., . . . Scott, S. D. (2009). CRISTAL: Control of Remote Interfaced Systems Using Touch-Based Actions in Living Spaces. *Proceedings of SIGGRAPH* (pp. 33-40).

Shaer, O., Kol, G., Strait, M., Fan, C., Grevet, C., & Elfenbein, S. (2010). G-nome surfer: a tabletop interface for collaborative exploration of genomic data. *Proceedings of the SIGCHI Conference on Human Factors in Computing Systems* (pp. 1427-1436).

Taub, E., Uswatte, G., & Pidikiti, R. (1999). Constraint-Induced Movement Therapy: A New Family of Techniques with Broad Application to Physical Rehabilitation--A Clinical Review. *Journal of Rehabilitation Research and Development, 36*(3), 237–251. PMID:10659807

Wall Street Journal. (n. d.). Playing on a tablet as therapy. Retrieved from http://online.wsj.com/article/SB10001424053111903461104576460421541902088.html

Wigdor, D., & Wixon, D. (2011). *Brave NUI world: designing natural user interfaces for touch and gesture*. Elsevier.

ENDNOTES

[1]	There are a number of tutorials available that describe how to construct a multi-touch surface (Castle, 2015; NOR_/D, 2015).

[2]	dynavisioninternational.com

This research was previously published in Virtual Reality Enhanced Robotic Systems for Disability Rehabilitation edited by Fei Hu, Jiang Lu, and Ting Zhang, pages 307-338, copyright year 2016 by Medical Information Science Reference (an imprint of IGI Global).

Chapter 42
Document Management Mechanism for Holistic Emergency Healthcare

M. Poulymenopoulou
University of Piraeus, Greece

F. Malamateniou
University of Piraeus, Greece

G. Vassilacopoulos
University of Piraeus, Greece & New York University, USA

ABSTRACT

A number of recent studies have showed that early and specialized pre-hospital patient management contributes significantly to emergency case survival. Along with the deployment and availability of appropriate emergency care resources, this also requires the availability of timely and relevant patient information to emergency medical service professionals. However, current healthcare information systems are characterized by heterogeneity and fragmentation, hindering emergency care professionals to have access to holistic or integrated patient information from the various organizations that participate in emergency care processes where and when needed. At the same time, many e-health programs have been undertaken worldwide in the area of emergency and unscheduled care with the objective to facilitate sharing of electronic patient information that may be considered important for the delivery of high quality emergency care and, hence, need to be readily available. In this vein, this paper takes a holistic view of the information needed in emergency healthcare and focuses on developing an appropriate tool for providing timely access to holistic care information by authorized users while retaining existing investments. Thus, a special purpose document management mechanism (DMM) is proposed that facilitates creating standardized XML documents from existing healthcare systems and that enables access to such documents at the point of care. For illustrative purposes, the mechanism has been incorporated into a prototype, cloud-based holistic EMS system.

DOI: 10.4018/978-1-5225-3926-1.ch042

INTRODUCTION

The fundamental challenge of a healthcare system is to serve a demand that has unlimited scope for increase with limited resources. Ageing populations, raising expectations and advances in life sciences drive demand for quantity and quality of health services. The difficulties that lie ahead are in reconciling individual needs stemming from those developments with the available financial and non-financial resources (Gooch, Rizk & Vest, 2010). Emergency medical services (EMSs) constitute vital components of healthcare systems as they deal with various kinds of accidents and emergencies, including the most critical acute illness and injury episodes that affect older people, people with chronic diseases and other population groups (Burnside, 2008; Beul & Finell, 2010; Feufell, 2011). Thus, modern health services are expected to provide high quality emergency healthcare in the most cost-effective and appropriate manner.

Conceptually, EMSs are concerned with the provision of both pre-hospital and in-hospital emergency healthcare and their operations typically involve a wide range of interdependent and distributed activities, performed by cooperating individuals (medical, nursing, paramedical and administrative) who differ on levels of background, skill, knowledge and status. As these activities can be interconnected to form emergency healthcare processes within and between the participating organizations (i.e., ambulance services and hospitals), EMSs can be viewed as virtual emergency healthcare enterprises where the cooperative effort of these individuals must be coordinated, aligned, integrated and meshed in order to improve organizational performance (Burnside, 2008; Greenhalgh, 2010). Hence, it is important to define and automate, through suitable information delivery tools, EMS processes, from the time of a call for an ambulance to the time of patient discharge from a hospital, that span organizational boundaries so that to create and empower collaboration and coordination among the participating organizations (Poulymenopoulou, Schooley & Xie, 2011). This paper describes a document management mechanism (DMM) for assembling comprehensive emergency patient information from existing systems and making it readily available to authorized users in the form of standards-based XML documents.

The current state of emergency healthcare delivery is mostly characterized by fragmentation of individual services to patients (e.g. ambulance, health center and hospital services) and by absence of collaboration and coordination among service providers (Poulymenopoulou & Schooley & Remen, 2011). Thus, the various parties involved in emergency healthcare (e.g. ambulance services and hospitals) strive to improve their efficiency, effectiveness and overall performance on their own, based on different perceptions on what the short and long term quality objectives are and on how best to meet them (Xie, 2011). Moreover, while access to integrated medical information is usually supported in all other aspects of healthcare, this is not the case in emergency cases (DePallo, 2011). However, since patients may not be able to recall pertinent medical facts due to new or preexisting conditions, providing emergency professionals with access to important patient medical information is considered important in order to reduce medical errors, such as adverse drug events, as has been demonstrated by several studies (Burnett, Feufell & Remen, 2011; Finnell, 2010). For example, a survey of paramedic self-reported medication errors demonstrated that 9% of respondents admitted to having made errors in the previous 12 months due to a variety of reasons including missing information. As the scope of paramedic practice is continually evolving, and the introduction of new drugs to pre-hospital environment increases, the risk of medication errors may also show a potential to increase (Crossman, 2009). To this end, focusing on the overall EMS performance requires a more holistic view of emergency healthcare delivery by the various parties involved which, in turn, implies that there is a need for integrated patient information in support to EMS processes to reduce errors, limit additional radiation, avoid adverse drug events and eliminate extra costs (Vest & Sicotte, 2010; Feufell, 2011). Indeed, it has been widely recognized that providing timely access to high quality and integrated patient information (e.g. medications, allergies, previous healthcare encounters, hospitalizations) is important in improving medical decision making and in enhancing collaboration and coordination among healthcare providers, both being key determinants for advancing emergency healthcare service performance (Beul & Finell, 2010; Xie & Remen, 2011). Since such information is usually dispersed across heterogeneous information systems of the various healthcare organizations involved, one approach to achieving information integration in support of holistic healthcare is to provide an interoperability platform (Benvoucef, 2011; Lin & Yao, 2012).

A holistic approach to EMS requires coupling among various healthcare organizations (e.g. EMS agencies and hospitals) supported by holistic patient information sharing during EMS process execution in order to enable case transfer to the most appropriate healthcare setting and improved pre- and in-hospital emergency healthcare, resulting in decreased patient morbidity and mortality (Poulymeno-poulou & DePalo, 2011). However, healthcare organizations (including EMSs) typically receive little contextual information about patient health statuses, mainly due to missed holistic care concept and due to heterogeneity and fragmentation of healthcare providers' information systems (Gooch & Rizk, 2010; Feufell & Schooley, 2011).

Although, the need for addressing emergency care holistically has been widely recognized and the advantages of healthcare information integration are clear, divergence still exists about how such integration can be achieved (Greenhalgh, 2010; Poulymenopoulou, 2011). Owing to the different types of services provided by various healthcare organizations and the different nature of healthcare records, full integration may be proved an extremely difficult or infeasible immediate objective and, indeed, an inappropriate long-term objective (Sicotte, 2010; Remen & Rigbya, 2011). Hence, a feasible way forward may be to identify and share the intersection points among the various, interweaved, cross-organizational health processes during EMS delivery.

Recent technological advances have rendered it feasible to share information among disparate and diverse systems through the creation of well-reasoned collaborative architectures (Benvoucef, 2011; Beltran, 2012). The DMM described in this paper supports an extension of the concept proposed by the "Integrating the Healthcare Enterprise (IHE)" technical framework to allow holistic emergency patient information sharing (Aftab, DePalo & IHE, 2011). Hence, it is intended to be used as an integrator among heterogeneous systems to meet the information needs of EMS processes, thus improving emergency healthcare delivery (i.e., resulting in better medical decisions and reducing medical errors) while containing hospitalization (i.e., resulting in fewer hospital admissions) (Finell, 2010; Remen, 2011). The DMM is built on top of an enhanced IHE-based collaborative network among healthcare providers running legacy information systems and uses the IHE profiles to enable sharing of document-based patient information. To illustrate the usefulness of the DMM, an advanced prototype has been incorporated into a cloud-based EMS information system that has been developed in a laboratory environment using the Athens Ambulance Service (AAS) and the "Gennimatas" General Hospital of Athens (GGHA) as the cases in point

HOLISTIC EMERGENCY CARE INFORMATION SHARING

High-quality patient care and optimized healthcare processes require efficient access to all relevant medical data across the continuum of care. Although substantial progress has been made in improving patient information sharing among healthcare providers, whenever and wherever necessary, providing comprehensive patient information still presents a persistent challenge to the emergency healthcare community. In general, the lack of immediate access to comprehensive medical information has been reported to be the source of one-fifth of preventable medical errors while one-seventh of primary care visits is affected by missing medical information (Finel & Greenhalgh, 2010; Feufell & DePalo & IHE, 2011). Emergency care information availability, in particular, may result in confining resource use to serious and life-threatening medical problems, while leaving non-urgent cases to be treated elsewhere, or shortening ambulance response and transfer times (from the time of ambulance request till the time of ambulance arrival at the hospital) in providing most appropriate emergency care to patients on site, en route and at the care facility, and in reducing the number of hospital admissions (Greenhalgh, 2010; Poulymenopoulou & Schooley, 2011). Moreover, in some emergency situations, particularly with un-conscious, incoherent and unaccompanied patients, providing emergency professionals with accurate and comprehensive medical information could make the difference between life and death (Burnside, 2008; Feufell, 2011).

Although the need for addressing emergency care holistically has been widely recognized as a means for advancing effectiveness and efficiency and the advantages of healthcare information integration are clear, there are technical and semantic barriers in achieving information integration since medical information is usually dispersed across heterogeneous information systems of the various healthcare organizations involved (Greenhalgh, 2010; Benvoucef & Bhuvaneswari, 2011; Beltran, 2012). Hence, a feasible way forward is to provide an appropriate interoperability platform that enables the various health information systems to exchange information and use the information that has been exchanged by working together within and across organizational boundaries (Liu, 2009; Googh, 2010; DePalo, 2011). Indeed, systems interoperability is necessary for compiling a rich picture of a patient's care and ensuring it is accessible by EMS professionals as the patient moves through various healthcare settings (e.g., ambulance service and hospital). This enables EMS professionals to have access to longitudinal medical records with full information about each patient, thus supporting them in making fact-based decisions that will reduce medical errors, reduce redundant tests and improve care coordination.

Semantic interoperability takes everything one step further. More than simple message exchange -- or even message exchange with a common field structure definition -- message fields are populated with standard codes enabling interpretation of both the context of messages and the meaning of data content within the message fields (Liu, 2009; Tao, 2011; Yao, 2012). This results in understanding and using information across various healthcare domains, organizations and information systems. One way to achieve semantic interoperability is to introduce a translation layer between disparate systems to map a system's internal codes to standard codes. When information exchange between systems occurs, the standard codes to which the legacy codes have been mapped are used to populate the fields of the messages. Thus, organizations are allowed to continue using their existing codesets, thereby preserving their legacy data. This eliminates the need to update and maintain standard codes in individual systems while each organization has access to all of the codesets contained within the translation layer making the switch from one standard to another relatively uncomplicated.

In the EMS literature, various healthcare organizations have been reported to have documented and mapped their processes in order to evolve existing or legacy information systems into innovative, process-oriented ones despite the significant technical and semantic difficulties (Googh & Rizk, 2010; Poulymenopoulou & Aftab & Benvoucef, 2011). Furthermore, various efforts have been described for creating electronic summary report documents from existing patient information to support information sharing among diverse healthcare organizations. For example, there has been proposed to create electronic summary report documents in general practice record systems in order to make them available to emergency and unscheduled care professionals (Finell & Greenhalgh, 2010; Remen, 2011). Often, such summary reports include demographic data, medicines, allergies and adverse reactions of patients, while missing out additional patient information that may be considered important by emergency healthcare providers (e.g., information created during hospital visits or previous emergency care received) (Burnside, 2008; Beul & Finell, 2010; Feufell, 2011).

In the same vein, a Health Information Exchange (HIE) infrastructure has been proposed as a means for supporting patient information sharing among healthcare organizations with the objective to improve response in individual and public-health emergencies, reduce unnecessary care, decrease the likelihood of adverse events and, in general, improve patient outcomes (Vest & Sicotte, 2010). The HIE infrastructure can be realized through a technical framework, devised by the Integrating the Healthcare Enterprise (IHE) organization, which proposes a set of profiles that can be leveraged for use by healthcare organizations for the purpose of patient information sharing (DePalo & Aftab, 2011). The IHE initiative defines a collaborative framework to seamlessly integrate diverse information systems in the healthcare environment and provides integration profiles, like the IHE cross-enterprise sharing of documents (XDS) profile, for managing the sharing of document-based patient information between healthcare enterprises (IHE, 2011). Specifically, the IHE EMS Transfer of Care (ETC) profile provides a high level model of the EMS workflow specifying the patient information exchange between pre-hospital providers (e.g., EMS agencies and physicians) and emergency care facilities (e.g., hospitals) as well as accessing information available from other sources (e.g., personal health records, hospital and primary care systems) (Feufell & DePalo, 2011).

In the United States, the NEMSIS (National EMS Information System) project proposes the implementation of electronic documentation systems in every EMS system for the creation of a uniform national EMS dataset as well as a national EMS database with aggregated data on a limited number of data elements that describe the entire EMS event from activation of the ambulance service through the release of patient from emergency care. NEMSIS aims at supporting emergency information flow among ambulance services and hospitals. In addition, the integrated data at national EMS database is expected to help evaluating and improving the services provided by EMS collaborative parties (Dawson, 2006).

In essence, the main objective of the above indicative efforts has been to support information sharing among diverse healthcare organizations for the purpose of enhancing collaboration and coordination among EMS process participants by building and making available the richest possible picture of patient condition so that to prescribe the most appropriate medical guidelines, protocols and pathways (Dawson, 2006; Greenhalgh, 2010; Remen & DePalo, 2011). Along this track, the DMM proposed in this paper may be considered as a further attempt to support personalized emergency care delivery by facilitating holistic patient information gathering from existing information systems and making this information available to authorized users in the form of IHE-based XML patient documents anytime, anywhere.

DOCUMENT MANAGEMENT MECHANISM STRUCTURE

As the present paper demonstrates, our main objective has been to develop a DMM in an attempt to close the gaps between disjoined systems and to bridge loosely connected healthcare organizations, thus enabling an unobstructed flow of information that ensures overall data consistency and that eliminates sources of redundant or erroneous emergency care information across organizational boundaries. In fact, the basic motivation for the development of the DMM stems from our involvement in a project concerned with defining, streamlining and automating EMS processes, while providing holistic care information to enhance collaboration and coordination among the various EMS participants. The stringent needs for enabling patient information sharing in real time among disparate healthcare providers, other authorized entities and patients, while ensuring security, privacy and other protections and for preserving investments on existing or legacy systems, motivated this work and provided some of the background supportive information for developing the DMM as an add-on software tool that can be embedded into a holistic EMS system architecture.

As the importance of health information technology continues to be emphasized, organizations will increasingly be faced with the problem of making all of their disparate systems interoperable. Thus, the DMM developed enables semantic interoperability by creating IHE-based XML patient documents from health information stored in existing or legacy systems using unified models such as XML schemas and ontologies. Further, DMM design has taken into account that some healthcare organizations have the in-house expertise to make their systems standards-compliant, but others find the daunting tasks of terminology mapping and maintenance as insurmountable barriers to the adoption and use of standards. By using a translation layer to achieve semantic interoperability between systems, the work of mapping and maintenance can be completed in a more economical and efficient fashion. To this end, the DMM is structured around four modules: the repository module, the ontology module, the service module and the security module. Figure 1 depicts a high level view of the DMM structure.

Figure 1. The document management mechanism

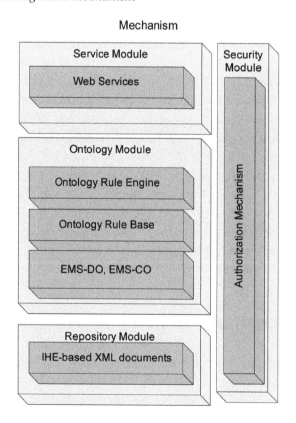

The Repository Module

The repository module stores XML patient documents based on the following XML schemas of the IHE profiles:

- The XML schema of the profile for patient care coordination (PCC) and transport record summary (TRS). This combines data existing in other IHE PCC profiles (e.g. personal health record or HIE system) with the current case data provided by the pre-hospital emergency care provider (i.e. an ambulance service) (DePalo, 2011).

- The XML schema of the IHE specification for emergency department encounter summary (EDES). This is a summary of the current health condition of a patient and a summary of care rendered in the ED of a hospital. This summary is actually an electronic folder that defines a collection of documents from other profiles like ED triage notes, ED nursing notes, ED physician notes and laboratory reports (IHE, 2009).

- The XML schema of the IHE profile for cross-enterprise document sharing (XDS). This is used for creating patient documents to be shared among various healthcare providers, ranging from a private physician office to a clinic to an acute care in-patient facility. It also includes data from existing personal health record systems (IHE, 2011).

Yet another class of documents (XML schema) has been developed as a view of the above, called the holistic emergency care encounter summary (HEC-ES) document class, containing contextually customized data elements, selected from the IHE profiles above, such as: current medications, active problems, allergies, family history, social history, relevant surgical procedures, relevant diagnostic tests and reports and emergency encounter information including emergency contact information, chief complaint, injury incident description, reason for referral, medications given, protocols used, receiving facility, ED diagnoses, assessment and plan and medications administered and at discharge. HEC-ES documents are also stored in the repository module and serve the purpose of enabling EMS profession-als (e.g., medical, nursing and paramedical) get the information they need to make better decisions on a personalized basis with regard to patient care and transfer. Figure 2 shows a class diagram representing a portion of the HEC-ES document XML schema.

The Ontology Module

The ontology module consists of an emergency medicine domain ontology (EMS-DO) and an EMS context ontology (EMS-CO) accompanied by an ontology rule-base and rule-engine.

EMS-DO models emergency medical care domain knowledge and contains: (a) medical concepts such as emergency medical protocols, medical procedures, medical observations, injuries, diseases and drugs which are coded in standard terminology systems such as the Logical Observation Identifiers Names and Codes (LOINC), the International Classification of Diseases (ICD-10) and the Anatomical Therapeutic Chemical Classification System (ATC), (b) data elements such as chief complaints and medications, contained in the IHE-based XML schemas (IHE, 2009; Aftab & IHE, 2011) and (c) relationships be-tween medical concepts and relevant data elements of the IHE-based XML schemas. For example, the

Figure 2. A class diagram representing a part of the HEC-ES document data elements

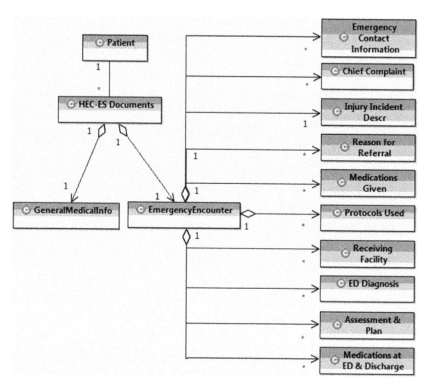

ontology class called "Crushing head injury" represents an injury medical concept which is represented by a code in ICD-10 and associated, through the object property "BelongsToElement", to the ontology class "Injuries" that represents a data element of HEC-ES class.

To facilitate semantic and syntactic integration of medical information contained in existing systems, each participating organization needs to create semantic mappings among the medical concepts used locally and those defined in the EMS-DO ontology. Thus, the patient data retrieved from existing systems is automatically transformed into medical concepts of EMS-DO and, through the EMS-DO relationships, is tag transformed into corresponding XML data elements of the IHE-based documents. Figure 3 presents a portion of the ontology with the data elements used by the HEC-ES document XML schema.

EMS-CO models the operational context with regard to certain parameters such as: patient (e.g., patient identification), EMS professional (e.g., specialty and roles), EMS resource (e.g., ambulance, hospital ED and main medical equipment), location (e.g., incident, ambulance station, hospital ED), time (e.g., time of ambulance arrival/departure at/from place of incident/hospital). In addition, a number of relationships between contextual parameters may be considered such as: the "TransferredBy" relationship between patient and ambulance resource, the "TreatedBy" relationship between patient and EMS professional and the "ManagedBy" relationship between patient and hospital ED resource. For example, through these relationships it can be denoted that a certain patient (patient) has been transferred by a certain ambulance (resource) to a certain hospital ED (resource) which is situated at certain location (location) under the supervision of a certain emergency physician (EMS professional). Figure 4 presents a portion of the ontology that contains certain contextual information.

Figure 3. A part of the EMS-DO with some data elements of the HEC-ES document schema

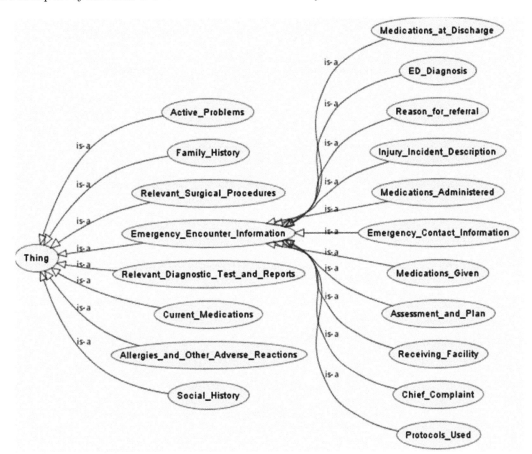

The Service Module

The service module consists of a set of web services. Each event generated by the "ontology rule engine" may result in assigning a role to a user to authorize him/her to invoke one or more web services that are executed through a BPEL-based mechanism. Web services have been developed to perform the following activities:

- **Assign Role:** On the occurrence of certain events designated roles are assigned to users so that to authorize them acquire certain access modes to certain objects (web service invocations or documents).
- **Create IHE Profile Document:** Retrieves emergency case data from existing systems of participating organizations (e.g., ambulance services and hospitals) and consults the EMS-DO to tag the retrieved data into IHE profile documents. Thus, an electronic folder of the above three IHE profile documents is created for each patient where each document corresponds to an emergency encounter of the patient.

Figure 4. A part of the EMS_CO

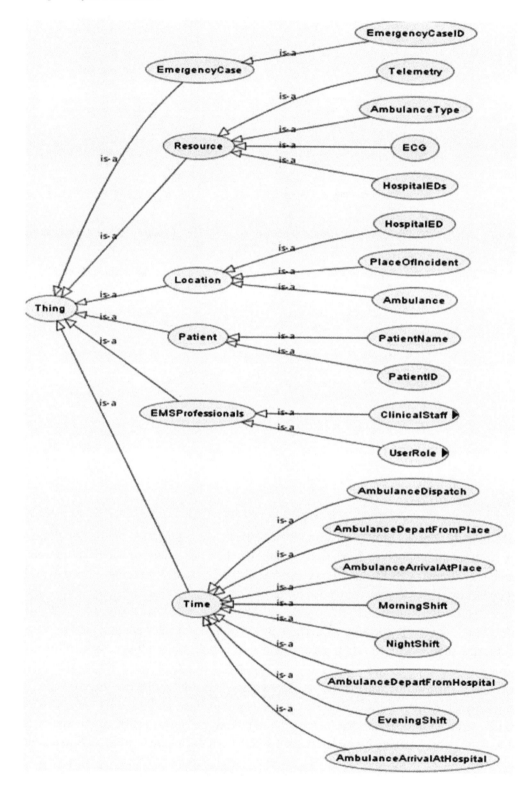

- **Create HEC-ES Document:** Retrieves designated emergency case data elements from IHE profile documents and consults the EMS-DO to tag them into a HEC-ES document for the emergency case under care. This way an electronic folder of HEC-ES documents is created for each patient where each document corresponds to an emergency encounter of the patient.
- **Retrieve HEC-ES Documents:** Retrieves and makes readily available the HEC-ES electronic document folder corresponding to the emergency case at hand.

The Security Module

Health information is highly sensitive and becomes more vulnerable in cases of being transferred through the Internet and stored in central repositories that are accessed by multiple users. Hence, there is a need to implement a holistic information security policy that complies with local needs. DMM contributes to the overall security architecture through an embedded authorization mechanism which implements an attribute-based access control (ABAC) model with regard to web service invocations and associated XML document accesses. An informal review of ABAC concepts is provided in Karp et al (Kuhn, 2010; Jin, 2012).

The ABAC model proposed is based on a recent NIST initiative to integrate roles with attributes, thereby combining the benefits of role-based access control (RBAC) and attribute-based access control (ABAC) to synergize the advantages of each. Thus, motivated by the NIST initiative in extending RBAC through attributes, we integrated attributes into RBAC by allowing dynamic roles (Mohan, 2009; Kuhn, 2010). This approach produces a role-centric, attribute-based access control (RABAC) model which extends the NIST RBAC model with permission filtering policies by using user and context attributes to dynamically assign roles to users in a similar way to attribute-based user-role assignment. Model implementation has been made using the existing standard XACML profile (Bhatti, 2004; Jin, 2012).

Hence, unlike traditional authorization models such as RBAC, the ABAC model incorporated in the DMM is capable of dynamically adjusting user-to-role assignments at run time based on the current context, so that users get appropriate authorizations with regard to web service invocations and associated XML document accesses on the occurrence of certain events. Thus, the model retains the advantages of having broad, attribute-based permissions across web services and XML documents, yet enhanced with the ability to simultaneously support the following features: (a) predicate-based access control, limiting user access to specific XML documents and (b) change of user roles on event occurrences at run time. Figure 5 presents a high level view of a global EMS security architecture emphasizing the DMM component.

Web service invocation and XML document authorization policy is being expressed in terms of authorization rules that define which subject is allowed to invoke which web service, and access which XML documents thereafter, and under what contextual constraints (which are expressed as event occurrences). The authorization mechanism is based on a set of ontology rules that enable inference based on the EMS-CO ontology. Ontology rule reasoning is expressed through the typical logic expression "antecedent ⇨ consequent" indicating that if all atoms in antecedent are true the consequent must also be true (Liu, 2009; Bhuvaneswari, 2011; Yao & Beltran, 2012). The antecedent part receives current contextual information and the consequent part generates contextual events.

Upon performing a certain activity, contextual information is acquired and inserted into the EMS-CO. Then, the rule engine triggers appropriate rules to evaluate conditions and generate event occurrences which, in turn, cause automatic invocations of the "assign role" web service to provide users with the necessary permissions for web service invocations and XML document accesses. For example, an ontol-

Figure 5. A view of the global security architecture

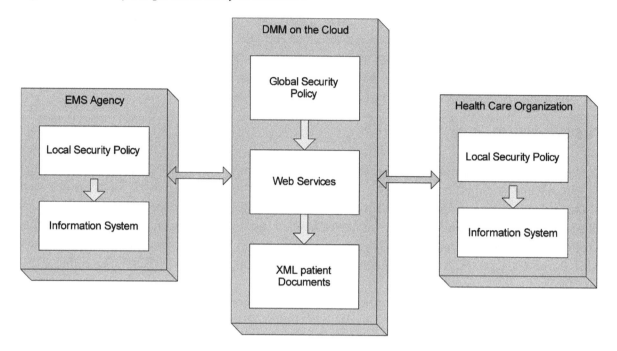

ogy rule may be triggered to result in the occurrence of the event "emergency case assignment to physician" which causes the execution of the "assign role" web service that assigns to a physician the role "therapist physician" for the patient and, hence, authorize him/her to have access to the patient's data. The latter, may be a consequence of an authorization rule dictating that "an ED physician is allowed to invoke the *"Retrieve HEC-ES documents"* web service for one of his/her emergency patients (proximity constraint) while on duty (time constraint) at the hospital ED (location constraint)".

AN ILLUSTRATIVE IMPLEMENTATION

To illustrate the functionality of the DMM, an advanced prototype has been developed and incorporated into an experimental, cloud-based EMS information system which, essentially, supports longitudinal EMS cross-organizational processes enabling authorized EMS personnel (e.g medical, nursing and paramedical) access holistic patient information relevant to emergency care when and where needed.

DMM implementation is based on the assumption that healthcare organizations participating in emergency care processes (e.g., EMS agencies and hospitals) have already in use corresponding information systems to support their emergency activities, such as recording ambulance requests, assigning EMS vehicles to emergency cases, accessing emergency case data by authorized personnel and reporting patient exit from hospital ED. In addition, it is assumed that mobile applications have been developed to enable paramedics exchange emergency case information with EMS agency and hospital information systems. Figure 6 shows an interaction architecture among an EMS information system, a hospital ED information systems, a mobile application and the DMM.

Figure 6. A view of the overall interactions among an EMS information system, a hospital ED informa-tion systems, a mobile application and the cloud-based DMM

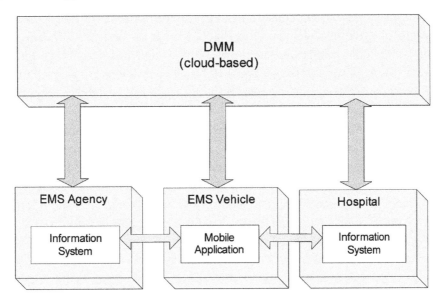

Overall system development was made using the Oracle SOA suite for the web services and BPEL using both static and mobile device clients. The DMM ontologies were encoded in Ontology Web Lan-guage (OWL), that follows an object-oriented approach to describe the structure of a domain in terms of its classes, class properties and class semantic relationships and were created using the Protégé Ontology Editor, Ontology rules and rule reasoning were implemented using the Semantic Web Rule Language (SWRL) and the Jess rule engine, respectively (Yao, 2012).

Regarding emergency healthcare processes, on reception of a request for an ambulance the cor-responding event occurs enabling EMS agency physicians access existing patient information. Then, on ambulance assignment to the emergency case the corresponding event occurs to result in activating DMM and in granting permission to paramedics to access existing patient information. On ambulance arrival at hospital ED the corresponding event occurs to result in creating IHE profile documents related to pre-hospital emergency patient care and in creating an HEC-ES document for the current emergency encounter. Then, authorized ED personnel is enabled to access case information in the form of HEC-ES patient documents. On patient exit from the hospital ED, the corresponding event occurs to result in creating an IHE profile document for in-hospital emergency patient care to the patient and in creating the in-hospital emergency care part of the HEC-ES document for the current emergency encounter.

CONCLUSION

Ultimately, the best emergency care management is propelled by timely access to high quality holistic emergency case information to facilitate delivering personalized and holistic emergency patient care (Burnside, 2008; Rizk & Finell, 2010; Feufell & Schooley & Rigbya, 2011). Hence, holistic information needs be provided in support of emergency healthcare processes using interoperable technology that enables collaboration, coordination and information sharing among the various parties involved. DMM development serves this purpose by enabling the creation and providing readily access to holistic patient information in the form of HEC-ES documents by authorized EMS professionals to enable them make better decisions regarding the management of emergency cases on-site, en-route and at the receiving healthcare facility. The DMM emphasizes interoperability to and standards-based information while preserving investments on existing or legacy systems. Hence, physicians are enabled to have the information they need at the point of care, consumers to have choice and portability, payers to save money and researchers to have better data.

In technical terms, the DMM uses standards-based technologies, presents patient information in standardized form and employs ontologies to enable technical and semantic interoperability of medical information among disparate systems in an enhanced security environment. Furthermore, the DMM has been experimentally implemented and proved to be a stable mechanism with acceptable response times that can be incorporated into EMS information systems to provide holistic information support to authorized EMS professionals where and when needed. Our intention is to provide the DMM as a mobile accessible application on the cloud that can be used in conjunction with real world EMS and hospital information systems. To this end, DMM is undergone a thorough evaluation with regard to system interoperability and performance and, mostly, user acceptance that, among the others might suggest directions for further work on DMM development.

REFERENCES

Aftab, A., & Javed, M. (2011). Implementing integrating the healthcare environment (IHE) using business process execution language (BPEL). *European Journal of Scientific Research, 57*(1), 109–123.

Beltran, V., Arabshian, K., & Schulzrinne, H. (2012). Ontology-based user-defined rules and context-aware service composition system. In *Proceedings of the 8th International Conference on Semantic Web* (pp.139-155). doi:10.1007/978-3-642-25953-1_12

Benyoucef, M., Kuziemsky, C., Rad, A., & Elsabbahi, A. (2011). Modeling healthcare processes as service orchestrations and choreographies. *Business Process Management Journal, 17*(4), 568–597. doi:10.1108/14637151111149438

Beul, S., Mennicken, S., Ziefle, M., & Jakobs, E. (2010). What happens after calling the ambulance: Information, communication, and acceptance issues in a telemedical workflow. In *Proceedings of the International Conference on Information Society* (i-Society) (pp. 111-116).

Bhatti, R., Bertino, E., & Ghafoor, A. (2004). A trust-based context-aware access control model for web-services. In *Proceedings of the IEEE International Conference Web Services (ICWS'04)* (pp. 184-191). doi:10.1109/ICWS.2004.1314738

Bhuvaneswari, A., & Karpagam, G. R. (2011). Ontology-based emergency management system in a social cloud. *International Journal on Cloud Computing: Services and Architecture, 1*(3), 15–29.

Burnett, S., Deelchand, V., Franklin, B., Moorthy, K., & Vincent, C. (2011). Missing clinical information in NHS hospital outpatient clinics: Prevalence, causes,and effects on patient care. *BMC Health Services Research, 11*(114). PubMed

Burnside, J., & Kendall, L. (2008). *Ambulance Service Network. A vision for emergency and urgent care: The role of ambulance services*. Retrieved by July, 2013, from http://www.nhsconfed.org/Publications/Documents/A%20vision%20for%20emergency%20and%20urgent%20care.pdf

Crossman, M. (2009). Technical and environmental impact on medication error in paramedic practice: A review of causes, consequences and strategies for prevention. *Australasian Journal of Paramedicine, 7*(3).

Dawson, D. E. (2006). National emergency medical services information system (NEMSIS). [PubMed]. *Prehospital Emergency Care, 10*(3), 314–316. doi:10.1080/10903120600724200 PMID:16801268

DePalo, P., & Song, Y.-T. (2011). Implementing interoperability using an IHE profile for interfacility patient transport. In *Proceedings of the International Conference on Computers, Networks, Systems and Industrial Engineering, IEEE Internet Computing* (pp. 70-75). doi:10.1109/CNSI.2011.53

Feufell, M., Robinson, F., & Shalin, V. (2011). The impact of medical record technologies on collaboration in emergency medicine. [PubMed]. *International Journal of Medical Informatics, 80*(8), e85–e95. doi:10.1016/j.ijmedinf.2010.09.008 PMID:21036659

Finnell, J., & Overhage, J. (2010). Emergency medical services: The frontier in health information exchange. In *Proceedings of the AMIA 2010 Annual Symposium* (pp. 222-226).

Gooch, P., & Roudsari, A. (2010). Computerization of workflows, guidelines, and care pathways: A review of implementation challenges for process-oriented health information systems. [PubMed]. *Journal of the American Medical Informatics Association, 10*, 2–12. PMID:21724740

Greenhalgh, T., Stramer, K., Bratan, T., Byrne, E., Russell, J., & Potts, H. (2010). Adoption and non-adoption of a shared electronic summary record in England: A mixed-method case study. *British Medical Journal, 340*(jun16 4), c3111. doi: PubMed10.1136/bmj.c3111

IHE - Integrating the Healthcare Enterprise. (2009). *Emergency department encounter summary (EDES)*. Retrieved July, 2013, from http://wiki.ihe.net/index.php?title=PCC_TF-1/EDES

IHE - Integrating the Healthcare Enterprise. (2011). *Cross-enterprise document sharing*. Retrieved July, 2013, from http://wiki.ihe.net/index.php?title=Cross-Enterprise_Document_Sharing

Jin, X., Sandhu, R., & Krishnan, R. (2012). RABAC: Role-centric attribute-based access control. *Lecture Notes in Computer Science, 7531*, 84–96. doi:10.1007/978-3-642-33704-8_8

Kuhn, D., & Richard, D. (2010). Adding attributes to role-based access control. *IEEE Computer Society, 43*(6), 79–81. doi:10.1109/MC.2010.155

Lin, Y.-H., Chen, R.-R., Huey-Ming Guo, S., Chiang, S.-C., & Chang, H.-K. (2012). Sharing personal health information via service-oriented computing: A case of long-term care. [PubMed]. *Journal of Medical Systems, 36*(6), 3563–3571. doi:10.1007/s10916-012-9832-4 PMID:22366977

Liu, S., Ni, Y., Mei, J., Li, H., Xie, G., & Hu, G. et al. (2009). iSmart: Ontology-based semantic query of CDA documents. In *Proceedings of the AMIA Annual Symposium* (pp. 375-379).

Mohan, A., Bauer, D., Blough, D., Ahamad, M., Bamba, B., Krishnan, R., et al. (2009). *A patient-centric, attribute-based, source-verifiable framework for health record sharing.* GIT Center for Experimental Research in Computer Systems, Technical Report No. GIT-CERCS-09-11.

Poulymenopoulou, M., Malamateniou, F., & Vassilacopoulos, G. (2011). Emergency healthcare process automation using mobile computing and cloud services. [PubMed]. *Journal of Medical Systems, 36*(5), 3233–3241. doi:10.1007/s10916-011-9814-y PMID:22205383

Remen, V., & Grimsmo, A. (2011). Closing information gaps with shared electronic patient summaries-How much will it matter? [PubMed]. *International Journal of Medical Informatics, 80*(11), 775–781. doi:10.1016/j.ijmedinf.2011.08.008 PMID:21956001

Rigbya, M., Hill, P., Kochc, S., & Keelingd, D. (2011). Social care informatics as an essential part of holistic health care: A call for action. [PubMed]. *International Journal of Medical Informatics, 80*(8), 544–554. doi:10.1016/j.ijmedinf.2011.06.001 PMID:21724456

Rizk, E. (2010). Holistic care management requires IT integration. [PubMed]. *Managed Care (Langhorne, Pa.), 19*(9), 43–45. PMID:20931892

Schooley, B., Hilton, B., & Abed, Y. (2011). Process improvement and consumer-oriented design of an inter-organizational information system for emergency medical response. In *Proceedings of the 44th International Conference on System Sciences,* (pp. 1-10). doi:10.1109/HICSS.2011.351

Sicotte, C., & Pare, G. (2010). Success in health information exchange projects: Solving the implementation puzzle. [PubMed]. *Social Science & Medicine, 70*(8), 1159–1165. doi:10.1016/j.socscimed.2009.11.041 PMID:20137847

Tao, C., Pathak, J., & Welch, S. (2011). Toward semantic web based knowledge representation and extraction from electronic health records. In *Proceedings of the International Workshop on Managing Interoperability and Complexity in Health Systems* (pp. 75-78). doi:10.1145/2064747.2064765

Vest, J., & Gamm, L. (2010). Health information exchange: Persistence challenges and new strategies. [PubMed]. *Journal of the American Medical Informatics Association, 17,* 288–294. PMID:20442146

Xie, S., & Helfert, M. (2011). *Towards an information architecture oriented framework for emergency response system. International Information Systems for Crisis Response and Management* (pp. 1–5). ISCRAM.

Yao, W., & Kumar, A. (2012). CONFlexFlow: Integrating flexible clinical pathways into clinical decision support systems using context and rules. *Decision Support Systems. Special Issue on Healthcare Modeling, 55*(2), 499–515.

This research was previously published in the International Journal of Healthcare Information Systems and Informatics (IJHISI), 9(2); edited by Joseph Tan, pages 1-15, copyright year 2014 by IGI Publishing (an imprint of IGI Global).

Chapter 43
RFID in Health Care–Building Smart Hospitals for Quality Healthcare

Amir Manzoor
Bahria University, Pakistan

ABSTRACT

RFID is a new technology that is quickly gaining ground in healthcare industry. RFID is being used in many areas of healthcare from asset tracking to patient care to access control. RFID can also be used to provide real-time information for decision support and to create a smart hospital supported by a secure and reliable smart hospital management information system (SHMIS). Such system can enable hospitals dynamically control different objects and transforms operational processes while minimizing any potential risks to patients and staff. The objective of this article is to discuss how RFID can be used to build a smart hospital and how healthcare industry can gain long-term benefits from smart hospitals. Findings indicate that use of RFID to develop smart hospitals require various enablers. There also exist ethical/cultural issues related to smart hospital implementation that require close collaboration among RFID products manufactures and healthcare providers. This article also provides several recommendations for healthcare industry in order gain competitive advantage from the use of smart hospitals.

1. INTRODUCTION

The healthcare industry is one of the largest sectors in many economies (Payton et al., 2011). Healthcare sector in USA created approximately 14.3 million jobs in 2008. This sector was expected to provide an additional 3.2 million jobs by 2018 (United-States-Department-of-Labor, 2010). At present, global healthcare sector is facing many challenges such as increasing operating costs, increasing number of medication errors, and ageing patient population. US healthcare expenses were expected to reach almost 20% of the GNP by 2017. That amounted to an increase of 15% in healthcare expenditure since 1963 (Middleton, 2009; Wurster et al., 2009). In Canada, healthcare expenses were expected to be almost 7.1% of the GNP by 2020, an increase of 1.1% since 2000 (Brimacombe et al., 2001). In Australia, health-

DOI: 10.4018/978-1-5225-3926-1.ch043

care expenses were estimated at 10% of the GNP (GS1-Australia, 2010). Each year, approximately 1.5 million Americans suffered from medication errors and these errors resulted in significant additional healthcare costs (National-Academy-of-Sciences, 2007). A study done in 2002 estimated that the population of people aged 85 and above in western countries would increase by 350% in 2020 (Wiener & Tilly, 2002). Another study estimated that by 2050 the population of older Americans would increase by 135% (Newell, 2011). It is evident that there would be an increased pressure on healthcare expenditure, which will become more complicated given that, due to the economic crisis, several countries are facing critical challenges in providing healthcare services. Healthcare is a very different business due to various reasons. Patients are not typical consumers, they do not always make the decision as to when, and where they will seek which type of care and at what cost. Healthcare providers are not as autonomous as any other typical business could be. Various stakeholders, such as legislators, regulators, and payers often affect both clinical and business decisions of caregivers. For healthcare providers, efficiency is not merely good fiscal practice. It must be a critical component of their mission (Fosso Wamba, Anand, & Carter, 2013; Lefebvre, Castro, & Lefebvre, 2011a).

Healthcare sector today provides strong institutional powers and policies for an effective use of information technology (IT). Healthcare sector considers adoption and effective use of IT a critical goal of modern healthcare system to enable better support service delivery (Menachemi & Brooks, 2006; Payton et al., 2011). IT offer many opportunities for healthcare transformation through business process reengineering. Effective use of IT could provide minimized data-entry errors, real-time access to patient data, improved clinical trials, streamlined processes, increased transparency, reduced administrative overhead, creation of new high-tech healthcare markets and jobs and improved overall healthcare management of individuals (PCAST, 2010; Burkhard et al., 2010). The estimated potential safety savings from adoption and use of interoperable electronic medical records systems in USA was approximately US$142–371 billion (Sherer, 2010). RFID technology is considered the next IT innovation expected to expand healthcare transformation (Fosso Wamba et al., 2008; Ngai et al., 2009a, 2009b; Oztekin et al., 2010a, 2010b; Fosso Wamba & Bgai, 2011). In order maximize efficiency and reduce waste, healthcare providers need to answer some tough questions such as what they have, where they have it, and where it needs to go. In order successfully track equipment and people, healthcare providers need a flexible and scalable system that provides automatic tracking with no dependency on clinical staff. One such system is RFID-bases system. All the capabilities enabled by RFID technology have the potential to facilitate new value creation in healthcare service innovation (Dominguez-Péry et al., 2011). At the moment, many healthcare providers use a manual system for patient care and inventory management. RFID supported by the knowledge reasoning for decision support (KRDS) system can be used to identify, record and ensure an efficient, effective and smooth transition at all stages of patient care (Alharbe, Atkins, & Khalil, 2016).

In short, RFID-enabled healthcare transformation projects, such as smart hospitals, could lead to tremendous benefits. These benefits include improved patient care, improved patient security, and safety, and improved organizational performance (Reyes et al., 2011). Use of RFID in healthcare can enable "new work practices to develop higher order capabilities for improving cost management, enhancing patient safety, and enabling regulatory compliance in hospital settings" (Lewis et al., 2009, p. 8). The high operational and strategic potential of the RFID technology is effective in the healthcare market. The value of the RFID market rose from about $ 5.63 billion in 2010 to almost $ 5.84 billion in 2011(Das & Harrop, 2011). The global market turnover for RFID readers and RFID tags alone was expected to reach $8.9 billion by 2015 (MarketResearch.com, 2011). In 2011, almost 150 million RFID tags were in use in the healthcare supply chain (Pleshek, 2011). The sale of RFID tags and systems was expected to reach almost $ 1.43 billion in 2019, an increase of 51% from 2009. Such an increase is due to the widespread of RFID-enabled healthcare applications, including the item-level tagging of drugs and various medical disposables, real-time locating systems for healthcare staff, patients and assets for improved efficiency and reduced losses, the compliance with safety requirements, and the availability of assets (Harrop et al., 2009). According to a latest study, the global RFID market was valued at US$ 1.9 billion in 2013 and is expected to grow at a CAGR of 13.9% from 2014 to 2040, to reach an estimated value of USD 5.3 billion in 2020. In 2014, North America held largest market share of nearly 51%. The various reasons contributing to this large market share included sophisticated healthcare infrastructure and increasing number of collaborations between medical device industry, regulatory authorities and nonprofit research organizations. It was expected that the increased research spending in the healthcare industry would further drive the RFID market in the years to come. With a CAGR of above 30%, Asia Pacific was one of the most important RFID market. Improved healthcare infrastructure and high economic growth in the countries of Asia Pacific regions were expected to boost the RFID market in the years to come. Furthermore, rising concern for patient safety and tracking of expensive medical devices, were among the key factors attributing to market growth in this region (Grand View Research, 2015).

The objective of this article is to discuss how RFID can be used to build a smart hospital and how healthcare industry can gain long-term benefits from smart hospitals. This article would serve as a good basis for healthcare professionals with limited knowledge of information and communication technologies (ICT) to determine how RFID-integrated smart hospitals can be employed to solve their problems.

2. ROLE OF RFID IN HEALTHCARE

RFID uses radio waves to communicate between an RFID reader (also called RFID interrogator) and an electronic tag affixed to an object. RFID tags (active, passive, or semi-passive) are also called RFID chips or transponders. RFID tags can serve as a digital data store and each tag is encoded with a unique identifier that is tied to a database. Tags can be read using handheld or mobile readers, shelf or tabletop readers, or readers that can be installed at doorways. RFID readers communicate with the tags and retrieve the information to be sent to a host computer. This host computer acts as a RFID middleware and ensures communication between the RFID infrastructure and the different organizational systems (Asif & Mandviwalla, 2005). RFID operates without line-of-sight, provide dynamic item tracking to ensure patient safety, improved supply chain efficiency, improved overall safety, and operational efficiency. RFID systems greatly streamline inventory and asset tracking, virtually eliminating human error. Use of RFID systems provide detailed records of the movement of assets.

3. TOWARDS RFID-INTEGRATED SMART HOSPITAL

A smart, digitized hospital is one wherein data is collated at all important points, stored meticulously, retrieved whenever essential, and analyzed in real-time. This practice shifts the attention for medical equipment and devices management to patient care. This leads to better care services and enhances the brand of the hospital (Dolphinrfid, 2016). RFID-integrated smart hospitals require tagging of many assets and actors of the facilities. For example, the medical equipment must embed RFID tags and the doctors, nurses, caregivers and other staff members wear a smart badge (2) storing their employee ID number.

On arrival, each patient receives a wristband with an embedded RFID tag storing a unique identifier, and some information about him (e.g. a digital picture, a unique patient code, etc.). All the patients' medical histories and other important documents are tagged with self-adhesive RFID labels containing a unique number. All drugs' packages and blood bags contain RFID labels, which should preferably be EPC (Electronic Product Code) compliant. RFID readers are placed at strategic places within the hospital e.g. at entrances and exits of the hospital, operating theaters, and should ideally be placed at every office. The staff members (doctors, nurses etc.) should have a handheld device (e.g. mobile phone) equipped with an RFID reader and possibly with a wireless connection to the web. It is recommended that EPC standards should be used as much as possible.

4. THE SMART HOSPITAL MANAGEMENT INFORMATION SYSTEM (SHMIS)

SHMIS is the backbone of smart hospital. Before developing a SHMIS, the healthcare provider would need its communities of practice (CoPs) and the system developer to identify areas where RFID could be beneficial. Some of these areas may include real-time tracking of both patients and healthcare staff, operation theatre management, bed allocation, monitoring of medical equipment and handling of prescription medications that need authorization before administering to patients.

4.1. Design and Implementation of SHMIS

Many steps are involved in design and implementation of SHMIS. The first step is requirement analysis. Communities of Practice (CoPs) and system developer collaborate to come up with the requirements that SHMIS must fulfill. Some of the important requirements of SHMIS are real-time display of the current location of the object and patient security. The system should have the ability to display, in real time, the location of objects, such as patients, hospital staff, and mobile medical equipment. It is important that SHMIS should have backup functions. Knowledge reasoning for decision support (KRDS) can provide decision-making support to staff. KRDS provides healthcare intelligence by taking into account "what-if" scenarios and real-time decision-making support. Effective knowledge harvesting through interaction with information could provide better decision-making and improve healthcare practice (Ko, 2014).

The SHMIS would be an automatic real-time data collection system that will continuously monitor movements of patients, staff and assets, using RFID technologies to provide optimal real-time information for knowledge management decisions. Some of the important components of this system would include RFID technology, databases, network infrastructure, data visualization, and reasoning technologies. RFID technology includes readers, antennas, and passive tags to collect real-time data from the objects. Databases are used store the data available for KRDS to suggest the best solutions. The database would include object-related information such as where and what the object is, and when it enters and leaves the wards and or departments. The database must be designed to synchronize data from the different tag locations. Reasoning technologies are used to infer and interpret the information in real time, using KRDS (Alharbe, Atkins, & Khalil, 2016).

SHMIS can provide many important functions for hospitals. It can communicate with RFID hardware to receive data from tags in real time. It can also be used to control hardware parameters (e.g. to control which readers should be active). It can record the data received from the RFID and store it in the database. It can also help extract the relevant data from the database. The system would be able to assign a new tag ID to any object. This is important because RFID tags should be removed and disposed once the patient is discharged or the asset is no longer is in use. The system would be able to use sensor data and knowledge harvested from different sources to provide decision support for healthcare professionals. The system would be able to perform real-time analysis of tag data and provide data visualization that would help ensure prompt response for any queries. The system can use algorithms such as Distance Estimators to estimate the distance existing among the different modes (Nebusens, 2010). The interface of the system is very important. The main objective of the interface is to display localization data that include real-time movement records and object's name and type. Depending on the application. the interface would need changes. For example, technical requirements will vary depending on staff numbers, RFID equipment used and the total number of objects that need to be tracked (Alharbe, Atkins, & Khalil, 2016).

Hospital staff often has knowledge of what they do and they can help other staff talk about what they know. Making tacit knowledge explicit can be difficult. Knowledge harvesting is a key part of the KRDS. In a hospital environment, sources of knowledge can be data set and expert knowledge. This knowledge, if properly harvested, can be used to design a rule-based set that will allow quick decisions. Rule-based sets can help store and control knowledge and to interpret information. For example, it could be determined how long a nurse was beside a patient and this time can be compared against certain standards. KRDS can help determine how best to improve and transform expert knowledge for improving future operational and staff performance. It can help reduce the risk of accidental events (Alharbe, Atkins, & Khalil, 2016).

5. BENEFITS OF SHMIS

Following are some of the major benefits healthcare providers can achieve by developing smart hospitals.

5.1. Asset Tracking and Management

Every hospital has high-value assets (such as wheel chairs, IV pumps, instruments, beds, etc.). If these devices move untraceable and we have no clear mechanism to determine their location, hospital staff can be unable to provide timely patient care. The turnover of these assets is essential for efficient operations of healthcare facility. While constant reporting on exact asset location is not required in all cases, but healthcare provider must be able to know the movement and have the ability to track where the asset goes. A wheel chair may cost around $150. However, it could cost $7,000 worth of clinical time per weak and up to 75% of maintenance time to search a wheel chair. To ensure effective performance of medical equipment regular, scheduled maintenance according to manufacturers' specifications is required. A typical hospital bed costs around $1200. Hospitals incur costs when no bed is available and patients spend extra time in an area that required heavy resources (such as ICU) (Motorola, 2013). According to another estimate, there is nearly $4,000 worth of hospital equipment per bed lost or stolen in the average hospital every year (RFID24-7.com, 2015). Most healthcare providers could make their operations better by increasing efficiency, especially in managing vast supplies of medical equipment. It is estimated that on average 15% of a typical hospital's mobile assets are lost or stolen during their useful life. That translates to an average cost of approximately $3,000 per item (Motorola, 2013). RFID is a highly adaptable technology that can be used to track and better manage critical healthcare assets and patients by enabling real-time identification, tracking, and tracing (Symonds et al., 2007; Bendavid et al.,

2010; Fisher & Monahan, 2008). Based on particular needs, RFID-based solutions can include any mix of handheld, mobile, or fixed position readers and RFID tags can be used for virtually any type of item or for people. RFID-based systems can be implemented and be incrementally expanded. RFID tags are widely available, affordable, and inexpensive compared with Real Time Location System (RTLS) tags. RFID technology is a viable mean of checking, tracking, and tracing pharmaceutical products. RFID allows proper management of incident audit trails between the medical equipment and the healthcare staff (Booth et al., 2006). RFID readers doesn't require a line of sight to capture data and their range can be adjusted and modified to meet specific environmental needs and RFID tag types. Since RFID readers are capable of simultaneously capturing the data of multiple assets, the time required to take inventory can be reduced drastically. The RFID readers can be installed at strategic location where there is extensive movement of critical assets to detect and record inventory of such assets. This enables the healthcare provider quickly locate the assets based on their last known location. This quick asset location provides many benefits. These benefits include improved patient care and staff productivity, faster patient and room turnover, improved incremental revenue, tighter asset control, lower replacement costs, reduced patient care delays, reduced capital expenditure, speedy equipment requests, faster equipment delivery, enhanced equipment flow processes, and resource planning. Using data collected using RFID, healthcare providers can easily comply with requirements of the regulatory bodies.

Purdue Pharma L.P., a US-based pharmaceutical company, implemented individual item RFID tagging on its prescription pain relief medicine bottles to follow the products' movements throughout the supply chain (Burt 2005 and Havenstein 2005). Siemens and Isar River University Hospital, Munich, Germany ran a project with RFID tagging of materials to test the use of active and passive RFID tags to track items used during surgery, and to track the surgical process itself to make sure item utilized during surgery are not inadvertently left behind inside a patient's body (Bacheldor, 2007f). The Royal Alexandra Hospital used a hospital-wide RFID asset tracking virtual asset library. The purpose of this library was to improve the use of assets, ensure the medical devices are available when needed, streamline routine scheduled maintenance, and reduce health and safety risks that could result if scheduled inspection plans are not met (Vilamovska et al., 2008; Britton, 2007). Southern Ohio Medical Center deployed a RFID-based asset tracking system to increase its efficiency of asset and equipment tracking. Medline Industries, a US distributor of medical supplies, marketed a RFID-based asset tracking system to detect any surgical asset left behind in patients after an operation. All surgical assets had RFID tags embedded. Hospital personnel passed a handheld wand containing an antenna connected to the RFID interrogator over the patient to pick up the RF signals of any tagged items left in the patient's body. (Sullivan, 2006). US-based Wayne Memorial Hospital deployed RFID technology for real-time asset location tracking and management. Hospital staff was able to keep track of the location and status of tagged assets (such as infusion pumps and wheel chairs) (Bacheldor 2007; RAND Corporation 2009). The UMass Memorial Medical Center (UMMC) in Massachusetts implemented RFID cabinets. These cabinets stored, tracked, and managed the utilization of high cost cardiac rhythm devices and supplies. UMMC was able to achieve approximately 38% reduction in inventory of selected high volume, high cost items (Collette and Johnson 2008). Ter Gooi Hospital employed Wi-Fi-based active RFID tags to track the location of infusion pumps and EKG machines (Wessel, 2007). Benefits from the application included better use of staff time, improved efficiency, and more timely care (Bacheldor, 2007h). Trondheim Hospital deployed an RFID-based uniform-tracking system. The system provided real-time inventory visibility of uniforms. With this system, Trondheim Hospital was able to reduce the space and labor costs with increased inventory accuracy. Texi, a Norway-based solution provider, developed an RFID system for the hospital inventory management where the RFID tags sewn into the garments were read by RFID readers. These RFID readers were installed in inventory closets and bins for soiled garments. The system provided 90% savings in space costs and resulted in an estimated (US$ 6 million) in space saving (O'Connor, 2007). Bon Secours Richmond Health System deployed a RFID enabled mobile asset management system to track and manage critical mobile medical equipment. This system was one of the largest RFID-based asset management system in USA (Vilamovska et al., 2008; Swedberg, 2008b; Harrop et al., 2008).

5.2. Inventory Management

Hospitals have massive inventories of consumables with diverse expiration dates. Because of this, many products are simply thrown away unused. Tagging consumables with RFID allows hospitals to not only eliminate manual inventory processes that waste time, but enjoy greater inventory accuracy and better utilize their consumables. Healthcare providers need to know when various consumables are nearing re-order status, with minimal staff monitoring. Inefficiency also affects inventory management and hospitals often face issues of misplaced, out of stock or expired medical supplies. This happens because no definitive system exists to monitor inventory changes. When there exist high usage levels and access by multiple users, monitoring stock level is often ignored. This absence of monitoring results in inaccurate inventories and unnecessary rush orders to meet patient needs. Many hospitals typically overstock IV because it is a commonly used medical supply often lost or misplaced. This overstocking typically costs hospitals $150,000 per year (Motorola, 2013). Hospitals may overstock other consumables as well such as dressings and instruments. This overstocking could result in tying up an average of 30% of hospital's capital (Motorola, 2013). Multiple RFID tags can be read at once to provide constant monitoring of inventory in a drug or supply cabinet. This way healthcare provider can better manage purchasing, reduce excessive inventories, and reduce delays in patient care. Fixed RFID readers, installed at supply room doors, are able to automatically and continuously record the asset location as it moves from one place to another. Handheld RFID readers provide on-the-spot reading of RFID tags and can be used to count inventory or locate a specific asset that could be misplaced in the supply room. RFID readers are capable of simultaneously capturing data of hundreds of assets. These readers can issue alerts when preset critical levels of inventory are reached. As such, use of RFID tags significantly reduces the time required for taking inventory of all assets in areas such as patient rooms, labs, procedure areas and stockrooms. Another benefit of the real-time, updated, and accurate inventory is to avoid out-of-stock situations for critical supplies needed for patients that would otherwise require rush orders at premium prices. With RFID reader and tagged supplies, items can be automatically dispensed and charged to the patients for proper billing, reduced lost and stolen supplies, reduced replacement costs, and increased revenue by eliminating non-charged consumables. Alerts can be issued to purchasers for expiring products to get timely re-orders. Drugs can be tagged with their national drug codes (NDCs), and LOT numbers. These numbers can be used to specify batch of the drug and drug expiration dates. When RFID is used to track medical inventory, software can issue warning against recalled or expired items. This way healthcare staff can remove compromised items and prioritize use of items that are expiring soon. Use of RFID tags with consumables can allow vendor-managed inventory where vendor would be responsible placing products in the hospital, and retains ownership of the given products until they are used. As such, hospitals can reduce their costs by paying only for this items that were used. In addition, hospitals need to spend less time managing and ordering products (RFID24-7.com, 2015).

DePuy Orthopedics, Inc., is a designer, manufacturer, and distributor of orthopedic devices and supplies. DePuy implemented RFID to track kits of critical operating room products shipped to sales agents and hospitals. Each kit and each part had an RFID tag attached. The system provided improved operational efficiency and labor productivity, time reduction in per-kit processing time and 99.99% read accuracy (ODIN 2008).

5.3. Time Management

Clinical time with patients is a critical resource for hospitals and many a times clinical staff spends too much time on non-patient care activities. Hospital nurses could spend an average of 20% of their time simply searching for portable medical equipment (Motorola, 2013). The ability to locate all hospital equipment in real-time has more benefits than just reducing asset loss. It also allows hospital staff to respond more quickly and accurately to emergencies.

5.4. Patient Tracking

Even with carefully designed plans of patient tracking, mistakes can happen. About 100 babies are switched at birth in U.S. hospitals every year (Motorola, 2013). Many patients need to walk around the facility as part of the recovery process. Many patients are vulnerable (such as people with mental disorders) and such hospitals need to restrict their movement. Practical solutions are required to balance patient freedom with patient safety. Errors in patient identification can lead to medication errors, delay in patient care, and lost valuable clinical time. One solution is RFID tagged wristbands. Patients wear these wristbands to enable positive patient identification (PPID). With positive patient identification, medication and treatment errors are reduced and patient movement can be recorded unobtrusively as they move around the facility. RFID readers are installed at key places to automatically record movement of patients and alerts can be issues to hospital staff in case vulnerable patients leave the designated areas.

Ospedale Treviglio-Caravaggio, an Italy-based hospital, implemented RFID to track admitted patients as they are admitted. Typically, when new patients arrived and admitted, the hospital followed a series of procedures for diagnosis or therapy. The patients were moved from one medical service area to another. This movement was difficult due to the dynamic nature of the system. For example, if x-ray procedure took long time, patients were taken for another procedure. Use of RFID allowed hospital administration to track the location of those patients or the procedures they had undergone (Swedberg, 2008a). Birmingham Heartlands Hospital used RFID-enabled wristbands to track patients and procedures, identify patients, and decrease incidents harmful to patients. (Bacheldor, 2007g). Xtag developed a RFID- based baby tagging system for safety and security. The system could also be used to track wandering patients in elder care facilities. The babies and elder patients wore an RFID bracelet with an embedded battery-powered RFID tag. The Xtag system offered one of the most secure protection system for the prevention of abduction attempts on the market in the world. The RFID tag was tamper proof and generated an alarm if the strap is cut, the tag is slipped of the ankle, the tag is removed underwater while bathing, or if the tag is disguised or damaged. RFID readers were designed to work with existing access control systems and picked up the signal and transmitted location data to the system (Maselli, 2003). ProSolutions, a Canadian firm specializing in RFID systems and integration, developed a RFID-based system (called BlueTag system) that protected newborn babies, Alzheimer's patients, and other individuals staying in hospital. The BlueTag system leveraged active ultrahigh-frequency (UHF) RFID tags embedded in bracelets and is used in 50 maternity wards in 10 countries around the world. (Bacheldor, 2008).

5.5. Smart Operating Theatres

Surgical identification can raise significant problems (Hendrickson, 2004). The most commonly reported surgical errors involved surgery on the wrong body part or site, the wrong patient or the wrong surgical procedure (Fuhrer & Guinard, 2006). In the smart hospital, the hospital staff can use the RFID tag attached with the patient to easily confirm they have the right patient and perform the correct procedure. This could also reduce significantly the risk of litigation resulting from surgery mistakes and the associated costs.

5.6. Healthcare IT Asset Management

Since typical IT equipment in healthcare environments is mobile, the inventory management can be time-consuming and misplaced or stolen equipment can increase costs because hospitals incur costs of hardware and staff costs of searching and re-deploying. There exist very stringent regulatory requirements related to security and control of financial and clinical records. The loss of medical equipment can also result in loss of data and consequently provide severe regulatory implications. Handheld RFID readers can provide a quick and efficient mean for hospital staff to track and manage inventory of equipment. Fixed RFID readers, installed at strategic and high-traffic locations can help keep track of important equipment (such as laptops and workstations on wheels (WOWs)) containing sensitive information.

RFID enable IT asset management provides faster service, improved security, accounting, and helps ensure and demonstrate compliance with HIPAA regulations regarding data security. With an up-to-date and accurate database of assets, hospitals can easily deploy the required upgrades and security updates on the assets. Any interruption in work (due to missing items or data) and time required to take inventory of assets can be effectively optimized.

5.7. File and Data Tracking

Healthcare regulatory requirements to safeguard patient records against loss or unauthorized access (e.g. by visitors, patients and other non-hospital personnel) are stringent and apply to both paper and digital records. There exist a variety of documents and data files that constitute patient records. These documents and data files may include charts, physician and pharmacy orders, and laboratory reports and imaging files. The dilemma here is that these documents must be circulated to be useful. RFID-based security solutions can be deployed to provide limited but secure clinical access on an as-needed basis to patient records while racking access. Handheld RFID readers can be used to locate a misfiled RFID-enabled files and folders minimizing the staff time needed to search for documents. Fixed RFID readers can track the movement of these files and folders around the facility. This feature could also help in forensic investigation. RFID technology is hard to counterfeit and provides greater security for sensitive financial and clinical patient-related information.

Huntsville Hospital used a RFID solution to verify a patient's identity and document the surgical process, from admission to discharge. Passive RFID tags were attached with patients. The objective of the system was to improve efficiency and communication that would directly improve surgical start times (Bacheldor, 2007e). The Emergency Health Centre (EHC) in Houston, Texas deployed a real-time RFID-based location tracking system to improve its patient care. On admission, patients wore RFID-enabled wristbands. These wristbands were tracked by RFID readers to record how much time patients spent to receive the needed medical care. Hospital staff received alerts from the system when beds and rooms were clean and ready for occupation. Emergency medical information service provider MedicAlert Foundation and California State University-Stanislaus (CSU) tested RFID-enabled medical cards to provide a more efficient method of collecting and forwarding patients' health-related data at the point of medical service (Swedberg 2007).

A number of RFID-related software applications were developed in Taiwan. Some of these applications focused on the use of radio frequency identification (RFID) technology to prevent spread of the severe acute respiratory syndrome (SARS) disease. These applications include computerized systems for monitoring the body temperature of healthcare personnel and patients in the hospital, track potential virus carriers and, when necessary, map their movements throughout hospitals and keeping track of people under quarantine in facilities separate from hospitals (Ioan, Turcu, Turcu, & Cerlinc, 2010).

5.8. Anti-Counterfeiting

Drug counterfeiting is an increasing global problem that results in patient's loss of money. Patients not only get inferior, non-economical products but also face significant health threats because these drugs contain dangerous substances. Pharmaceutical companies lose financially due to counterfeit drug trade and governments lose in terms of lost taxes and resources spent to combat counterfeiting. Worldwide counterfeit sales are increasing at about 13 percent annually, which is twice the rate of legitimate pharmaceuticals sales. Counterfeit sales were expected to reach $75 billion mark by 2010 (National Association of Boards of Pharmacy, 2009). RFID technology can help pharmaceutical companies, distributors, and hospitals to combat and deter drug counterfeiting. Counterfeit pharmaceutical products are a major threat to patient safety today. This is because these products may contain hazardous ingredients (Fuhrer &Guinard, 2006) and they may cause important financial losses to pharmaceutical firms (Dahiya, 2008). According to some estimates, almost 10% of pharmaceutical products marketed worldwide in 2010 were counterfeit (Lefebvre et al., 2011b) and resulted in about US$ 75 billion in financial losses by the pharmaceutical industry (Dahiya, 2008). In this context, major US regulatory bodies (e.g., Food and Drug Administration) have issued adoption mandates. These mandates require pharmaceutical firms to adopt a unique identifier (or e-Pedigree) for the tracking and tracing of pharmaceutical products throughout the supply chain. These actions have caused a renewed interest in the adoption and use of RFID technology in healthcare sector. Some studies have even suggested that "RFID is an enabling technology that saves lives, prevents errors, saves costs and increases security. It removes tedious procedures and provides patients with more freedom and dignity" (IDTechEx, 2006, p. 1). Hospital can work with pharmaceutical companies and pharmacies to tag and trace drugs across the supply chain. This way hospitals can assure the authenticity of their drugs. They can also use RFID to gain real-time data on parameters such as temperature and moisture levels, and configure their RFID systems to provide alerts in the case of conditions that could threaten medication quality (RFID24-7.com, 2015).

5.9. Patient Care

RFID technology offers an improved means of reducing errors in patient care, including adverse drug effects, allergies, patient–medication mismatches and medication dosage errors (Thuemmler et al., 2007;

Tu et al., 2009; Aspden, Wolcott, Bootman, & Cronenwett, 2007). RFID technology can enable healthcare stakeholders to monitor all steps related to the patient blood collection and transfusion process, including the identification of blood bags at the collection point, the tracking and tracing of products from the collection point to the healthcare facility, and blood transfusion to a dedicated patient (Najera et al., 2011). Also, this technology makes it easier to manage patients with chronic conditions (Cresswell & Sheikh, 2008; Michael et al., 2008).

In healthcare facility operations, we see growing number of patients who are misidentified before, during or after medical treatment. These patient identification errors can result in improper medication of patients or entirely wrong treatment of patients. There could be inaccurate lab work and results reported for the wrong person, resulting in misdiagnoses related medication errors. Some hospitals are using RFID for correct patient identification and to prevent the above errors. By giving each patient an RFID-enabled bracelet encrypted with confidential medical history and treatment information, medical professionals are able to easily identify patients, access their records, easily see patterns, and update medical information (RFID24-7.com, 2015).

A hospital in Saarbrücken, Germany, used radio frequency technology to track bags of blood to record transfusions and ensure that patients get blood intended specifically for them. This RFID solution added significant security so the hospital can make sure the correct blood product is given to each patient (Wessel, 2006a). Italy's National Cancer Institute in Milan and Ospedale Maggiore hospital in Bologna used RFID technology to increase efficiency and safety in the management of the transfusion process. RFID tags were placed on blood bags and patient wristbands and staffs used handheld computers to register patients upon arrival, verify patient-blood group, and recognize patients and transfusion units at any time (Sini et al, 2008; Wessel, 2006c). Amsterdam Medical Centre used RFID to track and trace medical equipment, monitor the movements of patients and staff, and track and trace blood products. The goal of using RFID was to optimize schedules so more patients could be treated. A RFID-based system was deployed by St Vincent's Hospital, Alabama to provide patient-tracking and real-time clinical information. The system resulted in improved quality of patient care and increased revenues (Bacheldor, 2007b; Gambon, 2006). A concept developed by New Jersey orthopedic surgeon Lee Berger, the noninvasive Ortho-Tag uses radio-frequency identification (RFID) technology designed at University of Pittsburgh to give physicians easy access to information about implants and patients often at the end of a long paper trail (Swedberg, 2008c). Arthur Koblasz developed a body-worn RFID tag. The body-worn RFID tags may include an upper body RFID tag located in a wrist band and a lower body RFID tag located in a sock worn by the monitored person. The RFID instrumentation located in the premises may include one or more antennas located in the floor, door, bed frame, and mattress. The systems may also activate response actions upon detecting specified movements, such as sending an alert message to a patient monitoring system, activating an alarm, activating a camera, and/or playing a recorded message to the person. The purpose was to prevent or detect specific types of movements of the person, such as falls from which the person has not recovered (Koblasz, 2007). The International Medical Centre of Japan implemented a Point of Act System (POAS) to provide real-time input at the point of action. POAS. POAS collected, managed and used consumption data at the point of care (e.g. hospital bed). POAS (Akyama, 2007).

5.10. Medication Error Reduction/ Medication Compliance

According to National Coordinating Council for Medication Error Reporting and Prevention, a medication error is any preventable event that may cause or lead to inappropriate medication use or patient harm while the medication is in the control of the health care professional, patient, or consumer. Such events may be related to professional practice, health care products, procedures, and systems, including prescribing, order communication, product labeling, packaging, and nomenclature, compounding, dispensing, distribution, administration, education, monitoring, and use. Misidentification of drugs can have very serious consequences. One example is accidental administration of a non-prescribed lethal drug dose on a patient that resulted in paralysis. The reason for this incidence was the similar packaging of the drug. RFID can play an important role in reducing these errors. Drugs with RFID tags, can identify drugs so that healthcare staff do not have to rely on packaging to identify drugs. By scanning a drug's tag, all drug-related information can be accessed and verified. The misidentification of blood types is also a danger in health centers because blood transfusions of the incorrect type of blood can result in death. Blood containers with RFID tags can be scanned to verify the type being used is correct. The misidentification of other substances in use in the hospital can be similarly prevented with RFID as well (RFID24-7.com, 2015).

Germany's Jena University Hospital, the largest hospital in the German Federal State of Thuringia, used passive RFID tags to track medication in real-time from the hospital's pharmacy to intensive care and individual patients. Patients wore an RFID bracelet used for digital matching of medication to the individual patient. Handheld scanners read these bracelets and nurses gained instant access to detailed patient information displayed on a screen. The aim of using RFID was to reduce medication errors and improve workflow (Wessel, 2006b, 2007). Jacobi Medical Center in New York used handheld computers match the RFID tags on patients' wrists with bar-coded information on packets of medication to minimize medication errors and provide patients only the medication that has been prescribed to him or her. This system saved nurses time and allowed the nurse more time for direct patient care (Crounse, 2005). Medixine is a Finnish company that specializes in disease management. Medixine developed a system using RFID and mobile phones to make sure Alzheimer's patients take their medication (Collins, 2004a). A European trial, sponsored by Novartis and conducted by ECCT, an Eindhoven-based provider of medical consumer electronic devices, used battery-powered RFID tags embedded within medication blister packs. The trail showed that monitoring patients' compliance with medication prescriptions can help them comply with their medication schedule—thereby improving the benefits of taking the drug (Collins, 2006). A groups of pharmaceutical companies including Merck and Novartis used RFID tags, along with a range of bar code technologies, on individual items to detect dispensing errors and counterfeit drugs before they reached patients (Collins, 2004b). St. Clair Hospital, Pittsburgh, implemented a bar code software system to eliminate medication-dispensing errors (Swedberg, 2005).

5.11. Workflow Improvement

Memorial Medical Center in Long Beach, California implemented a RFID-based people/asset tracking system to improve the operations of its emergency department (Cross, 2006). The new system provided extensive data about emergency department use and patient trends and played key role in the quality improvement initiatives led by the hospital to reduce patients waiting time. This system also provided increased patient safety, better use of staff time, and increased facility capacity (Vilamovska et al., 2008).

US-based Providence Health Center implemented a RFID-based real-time locating system to track patients, staff, and equipment. The objective of the system was to improve its patient and operational processes and tracking of medical devices. RF signals emitted from active RF tags attached with patients/staff/equipment were received by RFID readers. These readers were typically mounted on the walls

(Bacheldor, 2007d). Using a grant from Robert Wood Johnson Foundation, Shelby County Regional Medical Center in Memphis, Tennessee deployed a RFID-based patient tracking system to better manage its overcrowded emergency department. As a result, the typical patient stay time in trauma unit increased from 25% to 80% (Gearon, 2005).

5.12. Improved Staff Utilization

Healthcare staff spend so much of their time searching for equipment and consumables. More than one third of staff spends at least one hour per shift searching for equipment. This is a waste of valuable medical staff. Use of RFID can make hospital operations more efficient and cost-effective. The staff can spend more time with patients to assess their health problems, provide guidance and support, and perform post-operational monitoring. In this way, the staff provides higher quality healthcare for their patients (RFID24-7.com, 2015).

5.13. Improved Access Control

Use of RFID technology in healthcare can restrict access to equipment, medication, or information. This way the security of healthcare facility is improved. This access restriction can be applied to different areas such as pharmaceutical supply rooms and patient records. This can be achieved by using RFID badges programmed with the proper entry codes. With such access control, healthcare facilities can prevent the theft of supplies and drugs. Hospitals can also prevent trespassing into secure, confidential records by unauthorized persons (RFID24-7.com, 2015).

5.14. Temperature Sensing

Storage of various consumables of healthcare facilities (such as pharmaceuticals, tissues, organs, vaccines etc.) requires proper temperatures and humidity levels. This temperature and humidity controls is crucial to healthcare facility operations. Improper storage of a single material can put lives at risk and can result in significant financial and reputation losses. Given the importance of proper storage of consumables, many hospitals continue to rely on time consuming and error-prone manual documentation. RFID-enabled sensors can be placed inside the refrigerators containing consumables. These sensors can transmit radio signals to readers that include environmental data. Using an integrated software, hospital staff can be alerted when the temperature or humidity exceeds the defined threshold levels (RFID24-7.com, 2015).

6. COSTS OF SMART HOSPITAL IMPLEMENTATION

The cost of the RFID technology (tags, readers, middleware, consulting, process design, troubleshooting, training, etc.) will impact return on investment (ROI) and value of RFID implementation. Direct RFID costs include the costs of RFID tags, RFID infrastructure, and RFID middleware. These direct costs are one key barrier to widespread adoption of RFID-integrated smart hospitals. According to Page (2007), the cost of RFID infrastructure can run from $200,000 to $600,000 or more for a facility-wide RFID tracking system in a medium-sized hospital. Davis (2004) reports that the costs for an RFID system can run from $20,000 to over $1 million depending on the size of the area where the technology is deployed and the application. According to Harrop et al., (2008), the prices of RFID tags will fall substantially in the near future. We can also make similar assumptions about prices of RFID infrastructure and middleware. One way to reduced RFID costs is by substituting RFID-designated reader networks with an existing Wi-Fi network (at the cost of worse granularity and network overload), or by using handheld devices at all times (leading to loss of user-friendliness).

7. ISSUES OF SMART HOSPITAL IMPLEMENTATION

There exist many important barriers to wider-scale smart hospital implementation (Ting, Kwok, Tsang, & Lee, 2011; Lefebvre, Castro, & Lefebvre, 2011a; Fosso Wamba, Anand, & Carter, 2013; Middleton, 2009; Buyurgan, Landry, & Philippe, 2013; Garfinkel & Rosenberg, 2006; Wamba, 2012; Ting, Kwok, Tsang, & Lee, 2011; Cheng & Chai, 2012; Yao, Chu, & Li, 2010).

7.1. Privacy, Security, Data Integrity and Legal Issues

RFID-integrated smart hospital implementation raise many issues pertaining to the protection of the privacy, security, integrity, legal issues, and ownership of the data collected through RFID applications. Within and across healthcare sectors, these issues are not addressed either fully or consistently. Benefits of using smart hospitals can be achieved when patients feel confident about security and privacy of the data being transmitted, security of technology, and the related policies (Sotto, 2008). According to Sotto (2008), there can be four categories of privacy concerns with respect to the use of RFID in healthcare. These concerns include the inappropriate collection of health information through RFID technology, the intentional misuse, or unauthorized disclosure of the data by an authorized data holder, the intentional interception of the transmitted/stored in RFID applications information and its subsequent misuse by unauthorized parties, and the unauthorized alteration of the data kept by an RFID application. To resolve the first issue, patients can be allowed to opt out of RFID systems, and by not using RFID chip to store any medical data on the RFID chip. Such data should instead be stored in a secure server in compliance with the Health Insurance Portability and Accountability Act (HIPAA) (Hagland, 2005). Encryption and authentication techniques can be used to address third issue. Halamka et al. (2006) suggests that RFID chips should serve exclusively for identification, and not authentication or access control.

RFID tags are susceptible to many of the same data security concerns associated with any wireless device. Without the manufacturer adding security options, standard RFID technologies are not yet suitable for secure proximity identification in health care applications as they can be subject to skimming, eavesdropping, and relay attacks. An attacker can beat the system by simply relaying the communication between the legitimate reader and token over a greater distance than intended. Passive tags in particular are considered to be promiscuous (automatically yielding their data to any device that queries the tag. This characteristic of tags raise concerns about skimming, interception, interference, hacking, cloning, and fraud, with potentially profound implications for privacy. While a variety of security defenses exist, such as shielding, tag encryption, reader authentication, role-based access control, and the addition of passwords, these solutions can raise complexity and costs. If RFID tags contain personal information, which could include health information, or data linked to personally identifiable individuals, without the proper security or integrity mechanisms in place, privacy interests become engaged. Personal health information is among the most sensitive types of information. As such, it requires stronger justifications for its collection, use and disclosure, rigorous protections against theft, loss and unauthorized use and disclosure, strong security around retention, transfer, and disposal, and stronger, more accountable governance mechanisms (Cavoukian, 2008).

The Unique Device Identifier (UDI) program was created by the U.S. Food & Drug Administration (FDA) to uniquely identify devices in the healthcare supply chain. Medical device manufacturers assign UDI numbers for every version of model of their devices. UDI numbers can be encoded into RFID tags and must also appear in human-readable form. UDI is a standardized numbering system and does not include any RFID specifications. The UDI requirements were developed to improve patient safety. UDI-complied RFID tags can be used to accurately track medical devices, boost the efficiency and effectiveness of device recalls, and simultaneously improve healthcare business processes and supply chain operations. The UDI rollout is in phases with labeling requirements going into effect for some devices in 2014. The program will be expanded to encompass more medical devices each year through 2020.

7.2. Technical Issues

There exist many technical issues related to smart hospital implementation. Some of these issues include the reliability and interoperability of RFID technologies, non-interference of RFID technology with other clinical information systems, and lack of RFID industry standards and best practices. This lack of standardization can also cause interoperability issues for RFID solutions offered by various providers. Practice of non-complying their RFID solutions with current medical regulations (HIPAA) is another barrier to smart hospital implementation (Fisher & Monahan, 2008). Vendors also do not normally tailor systems to specific healthcare provider needs and that could lead to maladaptation of technology. According to Fisher and Monahan (2008), limited standards also limit interoperability between RFID and existing systems in hospital. To solve these issues, European Union (EU) in 2007 adopted formally an ultra-wideband (UWB) frequency range for RFID healthcare application use in EU member countries. A significant implication of this decision was that RFID solution providers using UWB will need to alter their solutions to meet several new frequency limitations.

7.3. Operational/ Managerial Issues

There exist a large number of operational/managerial issues related to RFID-integrated smart hospital implementation. These issues include lack of guaranteed return on investment (ROI), lack of standardization in the risk calculations for identical RFID applications, difficulties in choosing the optimal mix of RFID technologies, lack of RFID best practices, implementation costs, implementation uncertainties, integration of the RFID systems into the existing IT systems, uncertain maintenance costs, and the limited availability of integrated RFID solutions. ROI of RFID implementation may not be guaranteed due to wide variability of RFID technologies and of settings within which they are deployed. Implementation costs and uncertainties are also due to the relatively little experience with RFID-integrated smart hospital implementation (Anand & Wamba, 2013; Buyurgan, Landry, & Philippe, 2013). Lack of RFID best practices is because RFID technology is still relatively a young technology. Some other challenges to RFID implementation include building RFID infrastructure and bundling applications within hospital (Hagland, 2005). According to Dempsey (2005), hospitals also need to understand that there exist different types of RFID and each type has a different place in healthcare. Dempsey (2005) further suggests that RFID implementation can result in various organizational challenges and change in organizational processes.

7.4. Cultural and Ethical Issues

These issues include concerns about the surveillance potential of RFID, lack of understanding of the privacy and security threats associated with RFID-integrated smart hospital, ethical, cultural, and social perceptions about RFID and its functions, and lack of potential patient acceptance due to the factors listed above (Wurster, Lichtenstein, & Hogeboom, 2008). According to Fisher and Monahan (2008), a closer examination is required of the social and organizational factors that contribute to the success or failure of RFID-based systems. The results of this examination should be intertwined in the preparatory work for smart hospital deployment. Expanding capability of interoperable RFID technology is increasing fear of potential privacy threats (Fisher and Monahan 2008). Smart hospital implementation in healthcare has received much attention from those in healthcare community concerned about patient privacy. Boulard (2005) and O'Connor (2005) argues that true threats of RFID-based system implementation related to personal data security and privacy have largely been misunderstood. These misunderstandings have resulted in many anti-RFID movements (Albrecht, 2007) and lobbying initiatives concerned with fear of surveillance threats (Boulard, 2005).

This lack of understanding of the real threats and benefits of RFID-integrated smart hospital implementation can have severe implications for realization of true potential of smart hospitals in improving the safety and quality of healthcare. This issue could become more serious if widespread awareness of RFID-based systems among consumers is not developed in near future. By 2009, only 18% Europeans were aware of RFID (Slettemeås, 2009). This implies that these issues can be harder to overcome among older populations. The acceptance of RFID-based systems by these older populations is key for the success of any RFID-integrated smart hospital implementation. National and global legislation, that addresses the privacy and legal issues, can help achieve this acceptance.

8. PRACTICAL/MANAGERIAL IMPLICATIONS AND RECOMMENDATIONS

Knowing the current state of operation is half the battle in improving it. In a smart hospital, real-time information is collected, stored, and analyzed. The analysis of this information provides the foundation from which healthcare professionals can glean the sort of business intelligence that can optimize workflow, improve utilization of valuable resources, and improve patient care and their outcomes. Smart hospital systems use data from RFID sensors to trigger event notifications, provide situational awareness regarding participant status in a workflow, track and manage assets, and even track and contain disease outbreaks. RFID data from multiple systems can be integrated and streamed in real-time into multiple clinical and administrative databases, and Big Data analysis tools can then be applied to dig deeper meaning from the relationships between seemingly disparate data types.

Healthcare providers can benefit from every extra minute saved by using smart hospital system. RFID tags worn on healthcare professionals ID badges and RFID tags on various assets create a perspective of action and location over time. This gives healthcare providers an objective look at how they're moving their assets/personnel through the hospital and how much time healthcare personals are actually spending with patients versus walking around trying to find needed information and equipment. Adjustments to design or process as a result of this knowledge may help staff feel less pressured as they move through their day, leaving them more capacity to focus on care and minimizing mistakes.

When compared to systems based on similar Automatic Identification and Data Capture (AIDC) technologies (e.g., bar-coding), RFID-based systems present a vast range of advantages including: a unique item/product level identification, no need for line of sight, multiple tags reading, more data storage capability and data read/write capabilities (Asif & Mandviwalla, 2005). However, the high implementation costs of the RFID technology remain a major inhibitor for widespread adoption and use of RFID-based systems (Bensel et al., 2008). Furthermore, the lack of common standard and the low operational performance level of RFID in a harsh environment continue to hamper adoption of RFID-based systems.

RFID-based solutions, such as smart hospitals, provide a justifiable return on investment in many ways including productivity gains from automated workflow, better staffing-to-demand ratio, lower instances of HAIs, reduced staffing turnover and better protection against damages due to improved risk management. One of the most impactful areas may be increasing Medicare reimbursements for care based on patient survey results. This serves as a major incentive for hospitals to do all they can to ensure patients are not only objectively well cared for, but that they are aware of the quality of their care, feel positively about their experience and report as such. The tracking and monitoring in a smart hospital provides an unbiased baseline by which providers can measure their performance and make timely improvements, and serves as evidence of the quality of care provided. It is a transparent model that proves to patients that providers take their perceptions seriously, and aim to excel. It is also a reminder that they must be authentic in their reporting of the care they received. The practical balance of providing quality care efficiently has real impacts on the success of a healthcare organization, but so too does the patient perception of the quality of care.

Legacy information systems may need to be modified to accommodate the smart hospital system, technology, and information. Depending on the operating environment, the intended purposes, the technology contemplated, and the deployment method being considered, RFID-integrated smart hospitals may not deliver sufficient accuracy or performance results to be suitable for mission-critical applications and uses. SHMIS are information systems that automatically capture, transmit, and process identifiable information. Informational privacy involves the right of individuals to exercise control over the collection, use, retention and disclosure of personally identifiable information by others. Such systems inherently pose privacy issues (Garfinkel & Rosenberg, 2006) and warrant a holistic systems approach to privacy. RFID tags contain unique identifiers. RFID tag data can be read at a distance, without line-of-sight even without consent of the individual who may be carrying the tag. This has compelling implications for informed consent. SHMIS can also capture time and location data, upon which item histories and profiles can be constructed, making accountability for data use critical. Healthcare providers need to know what data is collected, how and for what purposes, where it is stored, how it is used, with whom it is shared or potentially disclosed, under what conditions, and so forth. There are inherent tensions between the, at times, competing interests of organizations and individuals over the disposition of the personal health information, especially over the undisclosed or unauthorized revelation of facts about individuals and the negative effects they may experience as a consequence. SHMIS can exacerbate a power imbalance between the individual and the collecting organization (Cavoukian, 2008).

The two major negative implications of SHMIS are the privacy of patient health information (PHI) and system implementation. The SHMIS can be susceptible to privacy and accessibility issues. RFID tags can be secured by using passwords and access codes but it can be costly. The major concern of healthcare industry is how to minimize the cost of ensuring patient privacy at the highest level. In addition, the costs of implementing, operating, and maintaining SHMIS can be significant. SHMIS can be extremely complex to deploy and for a healthcare organization to realize the positive impact of these systems we need investment of significant resources toward the implementation and maintenance of the system (Coustasse, Cunningham, Deslich, Willson, & Meadows, 2015).

Literature identifies many enablers for RFID-integrated smart hospital implementation (Payton, Pare, Le Rouge, & Reddy, 2011; Cao, Baker, Wetherbe, & Gu, 2012; Wamba, 2012; Mehrjerdi, 2010; Wilkerson & McDonald Jr, 2007; Motorola, 2013; Newell, 2011; Ajami & Carter, 2013; Yao, Chu, & Li, 2010). The primary enabler for the use of smart hospital in healthcare delivery is the improvement in the quality of care. This quality of care is associated with implementation and capabilities of RFID. The improvement in the quality of care can be in terms of process control and capacity to support modern medicine practices, reduction of harmful incidents, improved resource use, delivery of safe, fast and unambiguous identification, and the creation of an operationally integrated hospital information system. Some short-term advantages of RFID-integrated smart hospital include distant patient management (at home), biometric data collection, and telemetry and intelligent outpatient care. Given the increasing number of older people in many parts of the world including Europe, these benefits can be promising. RFID is also more efficient as compared to alternative solutions.

Use of smart hospital allows healthcare providers, analysts and researchers to identify a clear business case for specific solutions that meet their needs best. For example, documentary evidence exists that shows good ROI of RFID inventory and asset management applications. Similarly, evidence shows clear benefit of installing real-time location systems for staff, patients and assets within healthcare facilities (Brimacombe, Antunes, & McIntyre, 2001). According to Murphy (2006), real-time RFID systems can provide clinical timesaving of up to two days a week. There are other uses of RFID (such as RFID-supported haemovigilance systems) that help provide positive, correct, patient-procedure and patient medication. All of these lead to improved patient care and bring direct (monetary) and indirect (e.g. reduced liability and additional treatment costs) benefits for healthcare providers. The falling RFID tag prices and vendor initiative for creating interoperable, cost-effective solutions are some other reasons that provide strong case for RFID adoption.

Healthcare is a complex system and, as such, the key to success of smart hospital implementation is the process of implementation itself. One reason for this is that the RFID-integrated smart hospital is a relatively young and still developing technology. In its current state, RFID lacks established best practices and involve multiple technology that differ significantly in their functionality and purpose. Staged implementation is often recommended in case of RFID implementation. A staged implementation involves a well-planned and successful pilot, understanding of various implementation-related issues (such as costs, types of tags, system operation, mix of technologies to be used, understanding of business processes, stakeholder analysis, support from top management, vendor selection, and staff training) (Murphy, 2006).

RFID is technically superior to alternative technologies and provide many significant benefits such as real-time data availability, ability to store more data, security of data using encryption, and user-friendliness. Governments are involved at both national and international level to support RFID-integrated smart hospital implementation. Governments provide various incentives (such as promulgation of explicit patient safety standards for RFID-integrated smart hospital applications, the adoption of quality standards in national healthcare systems, and financial incentives for RFID-integrated smart hospital adoption by healthcare providers (Motorola, 2013).

In the world of healthcare, "the more you know, the better." RFID applications, partnered with data evaluation technology, are a powerful tool in establishing a standard of applied awareness. Hospitals can derive a competitive advantage from this awareness that can dramatically change the way healthcare is deployed and managed to optimize hospital operations and patient outcomes. Smart hospitals can potentially change the delivery of health services in the years to come. One growing concern is the increasing costs of healthcare. Utilization of smart hospital may be a way to control healthcare expenditures.

Group commitment is important for knowledge harvesting but it depends on culture, management style, and communication between staff and management. One such model that can be helpful here is the SECI model of knowledge creation (Andreeva & Ikhilchik, 2011). Currently, majority of the technological components required in building a smart hospital environment are readily available. Many systems are under development both in academia (Fuhrer and Guinard, 2006; Chernbumroong et al., 2010; Ruan et al., 2011; Tsay et al., 2012c; Aminian and Naji, 2013) and industry (Tapia et al., 2012) and commercial systems (Orlov, 2009). Healthcare professionals should understand that building smart hospitals would require knowledge sharing of experience. Without this, it would be very difficult to build a smart and deployable system that provides dynamic control of objects and transform operational processes, while minimizing any potential risks to the objects.

Integration of KRDS module in the SHMIS would help support healthcare tracking and monitoring. KRDS would integrate specific hospital information with functionalities that accept information in formats that are relevant for the hospital (including audio, image, video clips, or text). By providing incentives, users can be encouraged to participate in the process and to increase the usable information for the hospital (Pierson, 2012). The real-time automatic responses or recommendations provided by KRDS can help improve operational and staff performance.

9. FUTURE RESEARCH DIRECTIONS

There is plethora of opportunities for future research in this area. Prior research on IT-enabled firm performance suggests that the role and articulation of 'the underlying mechanisms' through which IT capabilities improve firm performance remain unclear" (Mithas et al., 2011, p. 238). How the management of these new capabilities enabled by smart hospitals should be realized to enhance healthcare performance? This area needs further research.

Fosso Wamba, and Chatfield (2009) found that business value creation and realization from RFID projects was dependent on many contingency factors such as strong leadership, second-order organizational learning, resources commitment, and organizational transformation. Whether these factors are still relevant and the degree to which they still exist in healthcare sector today is a question that needs further research. This question is important given the fact that the context of the healthcare sector today provides high level of complexity (LeRouge et al., 2007). Another area that needs further investigation is technological, organizational and environmental factors that may have an impact on the adoption and use of smart hospital by applying current dominant IS adoption theories (Fichman, 2000).

One of the key challenges of the healthcare sector is the difficulty of measuring the exact healthcare delivery costs to each patient, which allows a comparison of the costs with the outcomes (Kaplan & Porter, 2011). In this context, an area that needs future investigation is the assessment the business value of item level tagging in smart hospitals to evaluate its impact on the healthcare outcome and costs. Furthermore, to understand the influence of different healthcare stakeholders on their peers, it would be interesting to examine the business value from the co-adoption of smart hospitals and other healthcare information systems (e.g., ERP, electronic medical records (EMR) systems etc.). Prior studies on IT adoption (Riggins & Mukhopadhyay, 1994) show a positive correlation between the level of business process reengineering and the use of and value gained from it (Fosso Wamba & Chatfield, 2009). Therefore, additional research is needed to empirically investigate how to reengineer healthcare-related processes (patient, asset and staff) to achieve higher levels of business value from smart hospitals.

Future research should also look at better strategies to incorporate RFID into healthcare processes and operations. Future studies need for example to identify the scope of the smart hospital, then assess the potential impact of the technology in terms of incremental and/or process transformation. This assessment should also include the cascade effect that can be created by applying RFID at certain parts of hospital and/or operations. Developing a holistic performance measurement and management system to assess the value generated by smart hospital should be also included into future research.

It is proven that use of RFID technology can benefit healthcare industry in several areas. However, more research is needed on the governance and standardization of RFID utilization. Another research that could benefit healthcare industry is the research on health information technology and big data management in relation to RFID technology. Future research can also be done on connectivity and interoperability of smart hospitals with other hospitals' and providers' health information systems. Such research will be very important for continued implementation of smart hospitals (Coustasse, Cunningham, Deslich, Willson, & Meadows, 2015).

10. CONCLUSION

This chapter highlights some key requirements, features, and components for the RFID-integrated smart hospitals. Knowledge harvested from healthcare staff, gathered by the KRDS module, combined with the data coming from RFID technologies, can help healthcare organizations make improved decisions. For many healthcare providers, the current challenge is the design of a comprehensive and reliable system. This system would be accessible in real time for various applications and help improve the quality of healthcare services. Such a system would need to take into account multiple environmental factors with emphasis on the human factors.

This article also posits that the realization of the full business benefits from smart hospitals will depend on many enablers namely better healthcare delivery, clear business case for certain RFID applications, smart implementation, technological superiority of RFID applications, and government incentives/support. The article also highlighted several avenues for future research on RFID-integrated smart hospital. It can be said that there is a need for more RFID-integrated smart hospital research. Also, given the sensitive nature of medical information, there is a need for more research on data management, security and privacy issues.

This article contributes to our understanding of smart hospital implementation and its contribution to the efficiency of healthcare. The article also indicates that the policy makers should be aware of the opportunity to use smart hospitals and their policies and strategies should be formulated accordingly. Furthermore, effective use of smart hospitals requires various enablers, most important of which is the government support to use of RFID in healthcare. Furthermore, the ethical/cultural issues related to smart hospital implementation require close collaboration among RFID products manufactures and healthcare providers.

REFERENCES

Ajami, S., & Carter, M. W. (2013). The advantages and disadvantages of Radio Frequency Identification (RFID) in Health-care Centers; approach in Emergency Room (ER). *Pakistan Journal of Medical Sciences*, *29*(1 Suppl.), 443–448.

Alharbe, N., Atkins, A. S., & Khalil, I. (2016). Transforming to a Smart Hospital System: Proposed application in the Medina Maternity and Children's Hospital. *International Journal of Pervasive Computing and Communications*, *12*(4), 503–522. doi:10.1108/IJPCC-07-2016-0037

Aminian, M., & Naji, H. R. (2013). A hospital healthcare monitoring system using wireless sensor networks. *J. Health Med. Inform*, *4*(02), 121. doi:10.4172/2157-7420.1000121

Anand, A., & Wamba, S. F. (2013). Business value of RFID-enabled healthcare transformation projects. *Business Process Management Journal*, *19*(1), 111–145. doi:10.1108/14637151311294895

Andreeva, T., & Ikhilchik, I. (2011). Applicability of the SECI model of knowledge creation in Russian cultural context: Theoretical analysis. *Knowledge and Process Management*, *18*(1), 56–66. doi:10.1002/kpm.351

Asif, Z., & Mandviwalla, M. (2005). Integrating the supply chain with RFID: A technical and business analysis. *Communications of the Association for Information Systems*, *15*, 393–427.

Aspden, P., Wolcott, J., Bootman, J. L., & Cronenwett, L. R. (2007). *Preventing medication errors*. National Academies Press Washington.

Bacheldor, Beth. 2006. Report Sees Sharp Rise in Pharma RFID. *RFID Journal*. (May 8)

Bacheldor, Beth. 2007a. Denver Health Adopting a Hospital-Wide RTLS System. *RFID Journal*. (October 29)

Bacheldor, Beth. 2007b. Health Facility Uses RTLS to Provide 'Concierge' Care. *RFID Journal*. (October 9)

Bacheldor, Beth. 2007c. Pharma RFID Adoption Still Slow. *RFID Journal*. (April 23)

Bacheldor, Beth. 2007f. Siemens Launches RFID Pilot to Track Surgical Sponges, Procedures. *RFID Journal*. (April 24)

Bacheldor, Beth. 2007g. Tags Track Surgical Patients at Birmingham Heartlands Hospital. *RFID Journal*. (April 10)

Bacheldor, Beth. 2007h. Tergooi Hospital Uses RFID to Boost Efficiency. *RFID Journal*. (December 12)

Bacheldor, Beth. 2008. BlueTag Patient-Tracking Comes to North America. *RFID Journal*. (February 13)

Bendavid, Y., Boeck, H., & Philippe, R. (2010). Redesigning the replenishment process of medical supplies in hospitals with RFID. *Business Process Management Journal*, *16*(6), 991–1013. doi:10.1108/14637151011093035

Bensel, P., & Gunther, O. et al.. (2008). Cost–benefit sharing in cross-company RFID applications: A case study approach. *Proceedings of the 29th International Conference on Information Systems (ICIS),* Paris, France (pp. 1–17).

Booth, P., Frisch, P. H., ... (2006). Application of RFID in an integrated healthcare environment. *Proceedings of the Annual international conference of the IEEE Engineering in Medicine and Biology Society. IEEE Engineering in Medicine and Biology Society* (pp. 117–119). doi:10.1109/IEMBS.2006.259389

Boulard, G. (2005). RFID: Promise or Peril? It may be easier than ever to track information, but it is causing concerns over privacy and civil liberties. *State Legislatures Magazine, 31*(10), 22–24. PMID:16397978

Brimacombe, G. G., Antunes, P., & McIntyre, J. (2001). *The future cost of health care in Canada, 2000 to 2020: balancing affordability and sustainability.* Conference Board of Canada.

Britton, J. (2007). An investigation into the feasibility of locating portable medical devices using radio frequency identification devices and technology. *Journal of Medical Engineering & Technology, 31*(6), 450–458. doi:10.1080/03091900701292141 PMID:17994419

Buyurgan, N., Landry, S., & Philippe, R. (2013). RFID Adoption in Healthcare and ROI Analysis. In *The Value of RFID* (pp. 81–96). Springer. doi:10.1007/978-1-4471-4345-1_7

Cao, Q., Baker, J., Wetherbe, J. C., & Gu, V. C. (2012). Organizational Adoption of Innovation: Identifying Factors that Influence RFID Adoption in the Healthcare Industry. Proceedings of ECIS (p. 94).

Cavoukian, A. (2008, January). RFID and Privacy-Guidance for Health-Care Providers. Information and Privacy Commissioner of Ontario. Retrieved from http://www.longwoods.com/articles/images/rfid-healthcare.pdf

Cheng, C.-Y., & Chai, J.-W. (2012). Deployment of RFID in healthcare facilities—experimental design in MRI department. *Journal of Medical Systems, 36*(6), 3423–3433. doi:10.1007/s10916-011-9796-9 PMID:22072278

Chernbumroong, S., Atkins, A. S., & Yu, H. (2010). Document management system using wireless RFID technology for intelligent healthcare operations. *Proceedings of the IADIS International Conference e-Health* (pp. 69–76).

Collins, J. (2004a, November 16). Purdue Pharma Tags OxyContin. *RFID Journal.*

Collins, J. (2004b, November 19). Six U.K. Drug makers Pilot RFID. *RFID Journal.*

Collins, J. (2006, June 20). Novartis Trial Shows RFID Can Boost Patient Compliance. *RFID Journal.*

Coustasse, A., Cunningham, B., Deslich, S., Willson, E., & Meadows, P. (2015, June). Benefits and Barriers of Implementation and Utilization of Radio-Frequency Identification (RFID) Systems in Transfusion Medicine | Perspectives. Retrieved from http://perspectives.ahima.org/benefits-and-barriers-of-implementation-and-utilization-of-radio-frequency-identification-rfid-systems-in-transfusion-medicine/

Cresswell, K. M., & Sheikh, A. (2008). Information technology—Based approaches to reducing repeat drug exposure in patients with known drug allergies. *The Journal of Allergy and Clinical Immunology, 121*(5), 1112–1117.e1117. doi:10.1016/j.jaci.2007.12.1180 PMID:18313132

Cross, M. A. (2006). Keeping the ER on track. *Health Data Management*, *14*(9), 68–69. PMID:17009590

Crounse, B. (2005). RFID: Increasing patient safety, reducing healthcare costs. Retrieved from http://www.microsoft.com/industry/healthcare/providers/businessvalue/housecalls/rfid.mspx

Dahiya, S. (2008). Counterfeit medicines: The global hazard. *Latest Reviews*, *6*(4), 1–4.

Das, R., & Harrop, P. (2011). RFID Forecasts, Players and Opportunities 2011–2021.IDTechEx.

Davis, S. (2004). Tagging along. RFID helps hospitals track assets and people. *Health Facilities Management*, *17*(12), 20–24. PMID:15637841

Dempsey, M. (2005). Weaving through the hopes and hype surrounding RFID. *Biomedical Instrumentation & Technology*, 2005(Supplement), 19–22. PMID:16134535

Dolphinrfid. (2016, September 14). RFID in Healthcare – Creating smarter hospitals. Enhancing quality of healthcare. Saving Lives. Retrieved from https://www.dolphinrfid.com/blog/rfid-in-healthcare-creating-smarter-hospitals-enhancing-quality-of-healthcare-saving-lives/

Dominguez-Péry, C., & Ageron, B., & Neubert, G. (2011). A service science framework to enhance value creation in service innovation projects: An RFID case study. *International Journal of Production Economics*.

Fichman, R. G. (2000). The diffusion and assimilation of information technology innovations. In R. Zmud (Ed.), Framing the domains of IT management: Projecting the future through the past (pp. 105-128). Cincinnati, OH: Pinnaflex Educational Resources, Incorporated.

Fisher, J. A., & Monahan, T. (2008). Tracking the social dimensions of RFID systems in hospitals. *International Journal of Medical Informatics*, *77*(3), 176–183. doi:10.1016/j.ijmedinf.2007.04.010 PMID:17544841

Fosso Wamba, S., Anand, A., & Carter, L. (2013). A literature review of RFID-enabled healthcare applications and issues. *International Journal of Information Management*, *33*(5), 875–891. doi:10.1016/j.ijinfomgt.2013.07.005

Fosso Wamba, S., & Chatfield, A. T. (2009). A contingency model for creating value from RFID supply chain network projects in logistics and manufacturing environments. *European Journal of Information Systems*, *18*(6), 615–636. doi:10.1057/ejis.2009.44

Fosso Wamba, S., Lefebvre, L. A., Bendavid, Y., & Lefebvre, É. (2008). Exploring the impact of RFID technology and the EPC network on mobile B 2B ecommerce: A case study in the retail industry. *International Journal of Production Economics*, *112*(2), 614–629. doi:10.1016/j.ijpe.2007.05.010

Fosso Wamba, S., & Ngai, E. W. T. (2011). Unveiling the potential of RFID-enabled intelligent patient management: Results of a Delphi study. *Proceedings of the 44th Hawaii international conference on systems science*, Koloa, Kauai, Hawaii, USA.

Fuhrer, P., & Guinard, D. (2006). *Building a smart hospital using RFID technologies: use cases and implementation*. Department of Informatics-University of Fribourg.

Fuhrer, P., & Guinard, D. (2006). Building a smart hospital using RFID technologies. *Proceedings of the European conference on eHealth,* Fribourg, Switzerland (pp. 131–142).

GS1-Australia. (2010). Healthcare industry.

Gambon, J. (2006, August 28). RFID Frees Up Patient Beds. *RFID Journal.*

Garfinkel, S., & Rosenberg, B. (2006). *RFID: Applications, security, and privacy.* Pearson Education India.

Gearon, C. (2005) Technology. Behind the hype. *Hospitals & Health Networks, 79*(6), 22, 24.

Grand View Research. (2015, November). RFID in Healthcare Market Size (Industry Report, 2022). Retrieved December 25, 2015, from http://www.grandviewresearch.com/industry-analysis/rfid-in-healthcare-market

Hagland, M. (2005, February). Radianse in the News, Nine Tech Trends: Bar Coding and RFID. Retrieved from http://www.radianse.com/news-hci-feb2005-barcoding.html

Halamka, J., Juels, A., Stubblefield, A., & Westhues, J. (2006). The security implications of VeriChip cloning. *Journal of the American Medical Informatics Association, 13*(6), 601–607. doi:10.1197/jamia. M2143 PMID:16929037

Harrop, P., Das R., & Holland, G. (2009). RFID for Healthcare and Pharmaceuticals 2009–2019. IDTechEx.

Harrop, P. & Crotch-Harvey, T. (2008). RFID for Healthcare and Pharmaceuticals 2008-2018, IDTechEx. Retrieved from http://www.idtechex.com/research/reports/rfid_for_healthcare_and_pharmaceuticals_2008_2018_000146.asp

Hendrickson, D. (2004). Study: RFID in hospitals shows ROI promise. *Mass High Tech: The Journal of New England Technology, 19,* 25–29.

IDTechEx. (2006). Rapid adoption of RFID in healthcare.

Burkhard, R. J., Schooley, B., Dawson, J., & Horan, T. A. (2010). Information systems and healthcare XXXVII: When your employer provides your personal health record—Exploring employee perceptions of an employer-sponsored PHR system. *Communications of the Association for Information Systems, 27,* 323–338.

Ioan, T., Turcu, C., Turcu, C., & Cerlinc, M. (2010). RFID-based Information System for Patients and Medical Staff Identification and Tracking. In C. Turcu (Ed.), *Sustainable Radio Frequency Identification Solutions.* InTech. Retrieved from http://www.intechopen.com/books/sustainable-radio-frequency-identification-solutions/rfid-based-information-system-for-patients-and-medical-staff-identification-and-tracking

Kaplan, R. S., & Porter, M. E. (2011). How to solve the cost crisis in health care. *Harvard Business Review, 89*(9), 46–64. PMID:21939127

Ko, T. (1990). Closing the Knowledge Gap: Internet-based Diabetes Self-Management Support System led by Community Pharmacist.

Lefebvre, É., Castro, L., & Lefebvre, L. A. (2011a). Assessing the prevailing implementation issues of RFID in healthcare: A five-phase implementation model. *Int. J. Electron. Comput. Comm. Tech, 5*(2), 110–117.

Lefebvre, E., & Romero, A., Lefebvre, L. A., & Krissi, C. (2011b). Technological strategies to deal with counterfeit medicines: The European and North-American perspectives. *International Journal of Education and Information Technologies, 5*(3), 275–284.

LeRouge, C., Mantzana, V., & Wilson, E. V. (2007). Healthcare information systems research, revelations and visions. *European Journal of Information Systems, 16*(6), 669–671. doi:10.1057/palgrave.ejis.3000712

Lewis, M. O., Sankaranarayanan, B., & Rai, A. (2009). RFID-enabled process capabilities and its impacts on healthcare process performance: A multi-level analysis. Proceedings of ECIS '09, Verona, Italy.

MarketResearch.com. (2011, January). RFID Readers and Tags – A Global Market Overview. Retrieved from http://industry-experts.com/verticals/other-reports/rfid-readers-and-tags-a-global-market-overview

Maselli, J. (2003, May 27). Xtag Unveils Infant Security System, *RFID Journal.*

Mehrjerdi, Y. Z. (2010). RFID-enabled healthcare systems: Risk-benefit analysis. *International Journal of Pharmaceutical and Healthcare Marketing, 4*(3), 282–300. doi:10.1108/17506121011076192

Menachemi, N., & Brooks, R. G. (2006). EHR and other IT adoption among physicians: Results of a large-scale state wide analysis. *Journal of Healthcare Information Management, 20*(3), 79–87. PMID:16903665

Michael, M. G., Fusco, S. J., & Michael, K. (2008). A research note on ethics in the emerging age of überveillance. *Computer Communications, 31*(6), 1192–1199. doi:10.1016/j.comcom.2008.01.023

Middleton, B. (2009). Re-engineering US health care with healthcare information technology-promises and peril.

Mithas, S., Ramasubbu, N., & Sambamurthy, V. (2011). How information management capability influences firm performance. *Management Information Systems Quarterly, 35*(1), 237–256.

Motorola. (2013). *RFID solutions for healthcare reducing costs and improving operational efficiency.* Retrieved from http://www.motorolasolutions.com/web/Business/Solutions/Industry%20Solutions/RFID%20Solutions/RFID_in_Healthcare/_documents/_staticfiles/Application_Brief_RFID_in_Healthcare.pdf

Murphy, D. (2006). Is RFID right for your organization? Understand your process before implementing a solution. *Materials Management in Health Care, 15*(6), 28–33. PMID:16859241

Najera, P., Lopez, J., & Roman, R. (2011). Real-time location and inpatient care systems based on passive RFID. *Journal of Network and Computer Applications, 34*(3), 980–989. doi:10.1016/j.jnca.2010.04.011

National-Academy-of-Sciences (2007). Preventing medication errors: Quality chasm series.

National Association of Boards of Pharmacy. (2009). National Association of Boards of Pharmacy (NABP), About the issue. Retrieved from http://www.dangerouspill.com/about_the_issue.html

Nebusens. (2010). n-Core platform. Retrieved from www.nebusens.com/index.php/en/

Newell, S. (2011). Special section on healthcare information systems. *The Journal of Strategic Information Systems*, *20*(2), 158–160. doi:10.1016/j.jsis.2011.05.002

Ngai, E. W., Poon, J. K., Suk, F. F. C., & Ng, C. C. (2009a). Design of an RFID-based healthcare management system using an information system design theory. *Information Systems Frontiers*, *11*(4), 405–417. doi:10.1007/s10796-009-9154-3

Ngai, E. W. T., Moon, K. K. L., Riggins, F. J., & Yi, C. Y. (2008). RFID research: An academic literature review(1995–2005) and future research directions. *International Journal of Production Economics*, *112*(2), 510–520. doi:10.1016/j.ijpe.2007.05.004

Ngai, E. W. T., Xiu, L., & Chau, D. C. K. (2009b). Application of data mining techniques in customer relationship management: A literature review and classification. *Expert Systems with Applications*, *36*(2, Part 2), 2592–2602. doi:10.1016/j.eswa.2008.02.021

O'Connor, M.C. (2005, February 17). Surveys Reveal Dubious Consumers. *RFID Journal*.

O'Connor, M.C. (2007, February 6). RFID Tidies Up Distribution of Hospital Scrubs. *RFID Journal*.

Orlov, L. (2009). Living independently group. Retrieved from www.ageinplacetech.com/blog/hohumge-buys-living-independently-group-quietcare

Oztekin, A., Mahdavi, F., Erande, K., Kong, Z. J., Swim, L. K., & Bukkapatnam, S. T. S. (2010a). Criticality index analysis based optimal RFID reader placement models for asset tracking. *International Journal of Production Research*, *48*(9), 2679–2698. doi:10.1080/00207540903565006

Oztekin, A., Pajouh, F. M., Delen, D., & Swim, L. K. (2010b). An RFID network design methodology for asset tracking in healthcare. *Decision Support Systems*, *49*(1), 100–109. doi:10.1016/j.dss.2010.01.007

Page, L. (2007). Testing gives way to implementation. Hospitals tune in to RFID. *Materials Management in Health Care*, *16*(5), 18–20. PMID:17552344

Payton, F. C., Pare, G., Le Rouge, C. M., & Reddy, M. (2011). Health care IT: Process, people, patients and interdisciplinary considerations. *Journal of the Association for Information Systems*, *12*(2), 3.

PCAST. (2010). *Report to the President realizing the full potential of the health information technology to improve healthcare for Americans: The path forward. President's Council of Advisors on Science and Technology (PCAST)*. Executive Office of the President.

Pierson, M. E. (2012). Designing a knowledge harvesting tool: Lessons learned. *Performance Improvement*, *51*(4), 21–27. doi:10.1002/pfi.21258

Pleshek, J. (2011). RFID will see double-digit growth in the healthcare market. *WTNnews.com*. Retrieved from http://wtnnews.com/articles/8824/

Reyes, P. M., Li, S., & Visich, J. K. (2011). Accessing antecedents and outcomes of RFID implementation in health care. *International Journal of Production Economics*.

RFID24-7.com. (2015, September 3). Ten reasons why hospitals deploy RFID. *RFID24-7.com*. Retrieved from http://www.rfid24-7.com/white-paper/ten-reasons-why-hospitals-deploy-rfid/

Riggins, F. J., & Mukhopadhyay, T. (1994). Interdependent benefits from interorganizational systems: Opportunities for business partner reengineering. *Journal of Management Information Systems, 11*(2), 37–57. doi:10.1080/07421222.1994.11518039

Ruan, Q., Xu, W., & Wang, G. (2011). RFID and ZigBee based manufacturing monitoring system. *Proceedings of the 2011 International Conference on Electric Information and Control Engineering (ICEICE)* (pp. 1672–1675). IEEE.

Sherer, S. (2010). Information systems and healthcare: An institutional theory perspective on physician adoption of electronic health records. *Communications of the Association for Information Systems, 27*(7), 127–140.

Sini, E., Locatelli, P., & Restifo, N. (2008). Making the clinical process safe and efficient using RFID in healthcare. *European Journal of ePractice, 2*.

Slettemeås, D. (2009). RFID—the "Next Step" in Consumer–Product Relations or Orwellian Nightmare? *Challenges for Research and Policy, 32*(3), 219–244. doi:10.1007/s10603-009-9103-z

Sullivan, L. (2006). *Medline Markets RFID System for Surgical Sponges*. RFID Journal.

Swedberg, C. (2005, September 12). Pittsburgh Hospital Pilots Hybrid System. *RFID Journal*.

Swedberg, C. (2007, February 16). MedicAlert Aims to RFID-Enable Medical Records. *RFID Journal*.

Swedberg, C. (2008a, January 3). Medical Center Set to Grow With RFID. *RFID Journal*.

Swedberg, C. (2008b, March 18). Surgeon Designs System to Monitor Orthopedic Implants and Promote Healing. *RFID Journal*.

Swedberg, C. (2008c, March 18). Surgeon Designs System to Monitor Orthopedic Implants and Promote Healing. *RFID Journal*.

Symonds, J., & Parry, D. et al.. (2007). An RFID-based system for assisted living: Challenges and solutions. *The Journal on Information Technology in Healthcare, 5*(6), 387–398. PMID:17901606

Tapia, D. I., García, Ó., Alonso, R. S., Guevara, F., Catalina, J., Bravo, R. A., & Corchado, J. M. (2012). Evaluating the n-core polaris real-time locating system in an indoor environment. In *Trends in Practical Applications of Agents and Multiagent Systems* (pp. 29–37). Springer. doi:10.1007/978-3-642-28795-4_4

Thuemmler, C., Buchanan, W., & Kumar, V. (2007). Setting safety standards by designing a low budget and compatible patient identification system based on passive RFID technology. *International Journal of Healthcare Technology and Management, 8*(5), 571–583. doi:10.1504/IJHTM.2007.013524

Ting, S. L., Kwok, S. K., Tsang, A. H., & Lee, W. B. (2011). Critical elements and lessons learnt from the implementation of an RFID-enabled healthcare management system in a medical organization. *Journal of Medical Systems, 35*(4), 657–669. doi:10.1007/s10916-009-9403-5 PMID:20703523

Tsay, L.-S., Williamson, A., & Im, S. (2012). Framework to build an intelligent RFID system for use in the healthcare industry. *Proceedings of the 2012 Conference on Technologies and Applications of Artificial Intelligence (TAAI)* (pp. 109–112). IEEE. doi:10.1109/TAAI.2012.58

Tu, Y.-J., Zhou, W., & Piramuthu, S. (2009). Identifying RFID-embedded objects in pervasive healthcare applications. *Decision Support Systems, 46*(2), 586–593. doi:10.1016/j.dss.2008.10.001

United States Department of Labor. (2010). Healthcare: Career guide to industries U.S.D. o. labor.

Vilamovska, A. M., Hatziandreu, E., Schindler, R., Oranje, C., Vries, H., & Krapels, J. (2008, July). Study on the requirements and options for RFID application in healthcare. Retrieved from http://ec.europa.eu/information_society/activities/health/docs/studies/200807-rfid-ehealth.pdf

Wessel, R. (2006a, February 27). German Clinic Uses RFID to Track Blood. *RFID Journal.*

Wessel, R. (2006b, June 9). German Hospital Expects RFID to Eradicate Drug Errors. *RFID Journal.*

Wessel, R. (2006c, September 26). RFID-enabled Locks Secure Bags of Blood. *RFID Journal.*

Wessel, R. (2007, June 1). Jena University Hospital Prescribes RFID to Reduce Medication Errors. *RFID Journal.*

Wiener, J. M., & Tilly, J. (2002). Population ageing in the United States of America: Implications for public programmes. *International Journal of Epidemiology, 31*(4), 776–781. doi:10.1093/ije/31.4.776 PMID:12177018

Wilkerson, J. L., & McDonald Jr, C. L. (2007). RFID in Healthcare. *The Journal of Organizational Leadership & Business Texas A & M University Tex Ark Ana.*

Wurster, C., & Lichtenstein, B. P., & Hogeboom, T. (2009). Strategic, political, and cultural aspects of IT implementation: Improving the efficacy of an IT system in a large hospital. *Journal of Healthcare Management, 54*(3), 191. PMID:19554799

Wurster, C. J., Lichtenstein, B. B., & Hogeboom, T. (2008). Strategic, political, and cultural aspects of IT implementation: improving the efficacy of an IT system in a large hospital. *Journal of Healthcare management/American College of Healthcare Executives, 54*(3), 191–206.

Yao, W., Chu, C.-H., & Li, Z. (2010). The use of RFID in healthcare: Benefits and barriers. *Proceedings of the 2010 IEEE International Conference on RFID-Technology and Applications (RFID-TA)* (pp. 128–134). IEEE.

ADDITIONAL READING

Means, C. (2008). Mobile technology gets boost with vendor collaboration. Retrieved from http://health-careitnews.eu/content/view/765/45

Southard, P. B., Chandra, C., & Kumar, S. (2012). RFID in healthcare: A Six Sigma DMAIC and simulation case study. *International Journal of Health Care Quality Assurance, 25*(4), 291–321.

Swartz, N. (2005). FDA Okays Implanted Chip for Health Care. *Information Management Journal, 39*(1), 16.

Wamba, S. F. (2012). RFID-enabled healthcare applications, issues and benefits: An archival analysis (1997–2011). *Journal of Medical Systems, 36*(6), 3393–3398.

KEY TERMS AND DEFINITIONS

Active RFID: Active RFID is a method of automatic identification that uses ID tags which are self-powered.

AIDC: Automatic identification and data capture (AIDC) are methods of automatically identifying objects, collecting data about them, and entering that data directly into computer systems. AIDC require no human intervention.

Battery-Assisted Passive RFID: Battery-assisted Passive RFID is a method of automatic identification that uses ID tags that has a small battery on board and is activated when in the presence of an RFID reader.

Counterfeit Medicine: A medicine which is illegal and may be harmful for human health because it may be contaminated, contain the wrong or no active ingredient, or have the right active ingredient but at the wrong dose.

Haemovigilance: Haemovigilance is a system of monitoring, identification, reporting, investigation and analysis of adverse events near-misses and reactions related to transfusion and manufacturing.

Passive RFID: Passive RFID is a method of automatic identification that uses ID tags that uses the radio energy transmitted by the reader.

RFID: RFID (radio frequency identification) is a technology that uses radio frequency signals to uniquely identify an object, animal, or person.

Smart Hospital: A smart hospital is one wherein data is collated at all important points, stored meticulously, retrieved whenever essential, and analyzed in real-time.

This research was previously published in the International Journal of User-Driven Healthcare (IJUDH), 6(2); edited by Ashok Kumar Biswas, pages 21-45, copyright year 2016 by IGI Publishing (an imprint of IGI Global).

Section 4
Utilization and Applications

Chapter 44
Utilisation of Health Information Systems for Service Delivery in the Namibian Environment

Ronald Karon
Namibia University of Science and Technology, Namibia

ABSTRACT

The use of Health Information Systems (HIS) is considered to be a major contributing factor to health-care service delivery. However, the utilisation of HIS which includes use and management is critically challenging in the public health sector in many developing countries. The manifestation of the challenges results in poor service delivery, which includes patient deaths. This is the main motivation for this study, to investigate how HIS can be used to improve service delivering in the hospitals from developing countries perspective. The study was carried out in Namibia, using two hospitals in the public healthcare. The study adopted the qualitative case study. The study revealed that the use of parallel systems, lack of systems integration, lack of portable devices and users' incompetency are some of the factors which impact the use and management of HIS in hospitals.

INTRODUCTION

Maximizing Healthcare delivery through technology integration is such an important topic worldwide as Healthcare is critically important to everyone's life. Healthcare concerns itself with the wellbeing or health of individuals within a community. As such ways in how healthcare service delivery can be improved has been trending globally. Today the incorporation and use of Health Information Systems (HIS) can aid in enhanced healthcare service delivery. Given this importance of healthcare quality, this chapter aimed to investigate the use of HIS in the Namibian public health sector. The objectives of the chapter in attaining the aim was to understand how HIS is utilised by medical practitioner' and administrator', the factors encountered in using the HIS and the impact that the use of HIS has on service delivery within the public health sector.

DOI: 10.4018/978-1-5225-3926-1.ch044

BACKGROUND

The essentiality of maximizing Healthcare quality cannot be over emphasized in our world at present. Kulkarni (2006, p. 8) defined Healthcare as "the prevention, treatment, and management of illness and the preservation of mental and physical well-being through the services offered by the medical and allied health profession". The importance of healthcare continues to receive increasing attention particularly on the aspect of service delivery to the needy. Cline and Luiz (2013) argued that Healthcare service delivery could be improved by incorporating HIS into hospital processes and activities. Dalziel (2008) defines HIS as "a computer program that organizes clinical data through acquisition, storage and distribution of information" (p. 3). HIS functions involves the use of information technology (IT) which basically are the use of computers, telecommunications and other information processing technologies within healthcare organizations to automate the work processes (Kulkarni, 2006).

The need to improve and maintain healthcare service delivery is a global concern. The areas of improvement include hygiene and the production of health environments (Yen-Han, 2013). Healthcare is critical to every nation in that the economic growth and productivity can be negatively hampered should health conditions of communities deteriorate due to poor healthcare services (Vichianin, 2007). According to Xiao (2012), the U.S. government embarked on an effort to increase healthcare quality and minimize healthcare costs by incorporating technology, such as the use of HIS, into the existing healthcare system. Barrette (2011) argued that technology investment in healthcare is escalating, greatly believed to yield enhanced healthcare quality. The Institute of Medicine (IOM) defines healthcare quality as "the degree to which health services for individuals and populations increase the likelihood of desired health outcomes and are consistent with current professional knowledge" (Vichianin, 2007, p. 18).

However in developing countries there are many factors that could have an impact on the utilisation of HIS, more specifically in the public health sector. In Ghana for example there is minimal government contribution and support toward healthcare service delivery efforts (Melesse, 2010). Some other factors include under-resourced facilities or resistance by healthcare professionals to adopt the use of HIS which could be contributed by a lack of understanding about the positive outcomes attributed to the use of HIS within healthcare (Cline & Luiz, 2013). In Namibia, the national health information system (NHIS) was implemented in 1990, soon after the country had its independence. The primary purpose of the NHIS was to provide ample information on a large number of health indicators and to optimize healthcare service delivery (Haoses-Gorases, 2005). The NHIS had since undergone several improvements, in an effort to address the gaps and challenges it is confronted with, such as integration issues.

HIS enables and supports the automation of work processes and activities in hospitals and clinics which adopts practices, such as capturing of patient data electronically instead of the use of a paper-based system. According to Lorenzi and Riley (2004), HIS will allow for easier and faster retrieval and management of patient information when required. The authors further argued that prompt diagnosis will be possible as medical practitioners would have faster access to a patient' medical history which is a support base in determining diagnosis (Lorenzi & Riley, 2004).

The optimisation of functionalities such as the work flow processes using HIS within healthcare would ultimately improve the overall healthcare service delivery (Hersh, 2009). An example is the use of electronic health records (EHRs) in countries, such as the United States of America. Liong (2008) defines an EHR as "...a computerized clinical information system that stores and displays patient information in legible and organized ways, and facilitates the recording and retrieval of clinical information about patients" (p. 1).

It is argued in some quarters that HIS has proven to provide optimal access to healthcare patient records and lowered overall costs within healthcare. An example is the electronic storage of patient data instead of physical files which consume space, facilities and incur administrative costs such as purchasing of files and filing cabinets (Lorenzi & Riley, 2004). However there are certain areas that continue to be challenging the use of HIS in healthcare. This includes privacy and security of patient information on the network. According to Sondheimer et al, (2009) there is a public awareness of the risks or possible loop holes that may lead to the unauthorized access of private information.

Another factor that could influence the use of HIS is nurse's attitude toward the HIS possibly contributed by the generation age gap (Fasolino, 2009). Dalziel (2008) posits that older nurses are prone to have a less positive attitude toward the use of HIS. Furthermore, Jackson (2013) states that there are some challenges attributed to the use of an EHR such as "decreased communication between other disciplines, the quality of care being delivered, and in some cases hindered their work by impairing critical thinking" (p. 4).

The demand for healthcare services will continue to increase as long as there are lives. As such, there is inevitable need for continuous improvement for efficiency and effectiveness of healthcare service to the society at large. The use of HIS is generally accepted as the way through which healthcare operations can be improved (Hersh, 2009). Thus, various stakeholders, namely healthcare experts, policy makers, investors and consumers points to the important role that HIS plays in the healthcare industry (Wu, et al., 2006). Hence the hope that HIS will continue to yield a positive impact if used and managed appropriately (Pisk, 2010).

MAIN FOCUS OF THE CHAPTER

Improper healthcare systems or infrastructures are some possible factors contributing to poor healthcare service delivery, which is especially challenging in the public health sector of developing countries. The manifestation of such challenges results in poor service delivery, which includes patient deaths.

Research Methodology

Based on the aim and objectives of the study the qualitative research method was employed. According to Bricki and Green (2007) a qualitative research focuses on behavioural aspects of specific settings, rather than numeric values. It was thus befitting to adopt the qualitative approach as the research questions sought to understand how and why HIS was used in the delivering of healthcare service. For the study to be specific and in-depth a case study approach was applied. Al-Mutairi and Mohammed (2011) defines a case study as "an empirical inquiry that investigates a contemporary phenomenon within its real-life context, especially when the boundaries between phenomenon and context are not clearly defined" (p. 2). The authors further explained how the case study approach "allows an investigation to retain the holistic and meaningful characteristics of real-life events such as individual life cycles, organization and managerial processes..." (p. 2).

Two public hospitals were selected as cases in the study. Both hospitals are situated in Windhoek, Namibia. The primary rational for had selected the two hospitals include accessibility and functionality. The two hospitals granted access to be used as cases in the study. The core functions of the hospitals are very distinct from each other. Hospital K is a referral, meaning that it is more of a first aid point, where diagnosis is carried out. Thereafter, the patient is referred to another hospital, such as Hospital C. Hospital C is more of a specialist hospital.

The semi-structured interview technique was used for data collection, as interaction was required to obtain individual and group's opinion and perspectives on the use and management of the HIS. The participants were medical practitioners and administrators in the two cases. The interviews were conducted, using the English language and two local Namibian languages, namely Khoekhoe (also known as Nama/Damara) and Afrikaans. This was according to the interviewee's preference. The interviewees from both hospitals were labelled CH001, CH002, etc. and KH001, KH002, etc. respectively. Quotes from the interviewees were referenced in accordance to page and line numbers, E.g. "CH001, 4:88".

As illustrated in Figure 1, at the point of saturation, a total of eleven (11) nurses, four (4) doctors and three (3) administrators (secretaries) were interviewed at the two hospitals. Saturation is at the point where the researcher noticed that there was no new information forth coming from the interviews. Eight (8) nurses were interviewed at Hospital C and three (3) nurses at Hospital K. Doctor's interviewed were two (2) from both hospitals. There were two (2) group interviews conducted with nurses, which ranged from two to three nurses at a time. Both group interviews were conducted at Hospital C. Additionally, two (2) administrative staff members were interviewed at Hospital C and one (1) at Hospital K.

Nurses were interviewed first, followed by the doctors. This order was followed simply to determine or separate the nurses' views and perceptions from that of doctors. This is primarily because nurses are the first contact point for patients. Additionally, the researcher conducted group interviews with nurses mainly because it was impossible to get one-on-one interviews with some of them due to the demanding working environment.

Data Analysis

The data was analysed, using the interpretive technique. Interpretivism relates to understanding and obtaining meaning about objects and subjects of the phenomenon being studied (Noble, 2012). The

Figure 1.

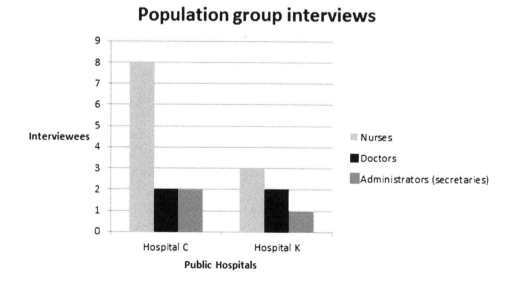

analysis was carried out to examine and understand how HIS was used in the Namibian public health sector. Analysis was performed separately on the two cases using the three research questions below that were designed to attain the objectives and aim of the study.

1. How do the medical practitioners make use of the current HIS for service delivery?

The medical practitioners, which include Nurses and Doctors made use of the HIS in different ways, and for various purposes, more particularly at Hospital C. This was attributed to their different functions and tasks. In order to clearly define how the practitioners used the HIS, the researcher followed and tried to make sense of the process involved in a patient's visit to the hospital.

The nurses are the first contact point with regards to patient care at both hospitals. Patient's first visit to Hospital C begins with registration at reception (CH001, 1:4). Patients are required to provide their demographic details, such as identification number, medical aid number (if available), name, surname, date of birth, residential address and contact number (CH010, 2:64-65). However patients at Hospital C can bypass the registration point and be directly admitted to a ward if it was an emergency. According to one of the nurses, patients can only be referred to Hospital C from two health facilities, "Hospital K and other regions" (CH004-Group, 1:3). A patient is referred from other regions only if the patient cannot be helped at the initial region (CH02, 1:8-9). In cases where a patient is directly taken into a ward the nurses would check for the patient's vital signs, such as blood pressure and thereafter the secretary registers the patient using the HIS. However the HIS neither automatically allocates a doctor nor sends alert messages to specialists on duty. This makes the manual system valid and important. A nurse posited that the "manual file system is used for storing and managing hardcopies of files" (CH001, 2:36). As a result Hospital C operates parallel systems simultaneously, the HIS and the paper based system.

Based patient information obtained, including bio-data, a first time patient is provided with a Medical Registration (MR) number which is automatically generated by the HIS. In addition to the MR number the patient's face is captured using a webcam (CH010, 1:14). The patient's facial image is captured and stored on the system along with the MR number. A card is than produced electronically for the patient, similar to that of a driver's license or identification card. According to a nurse "the MR number also appears on the patient's hospital passport which is in a paper form" (CH010, 2:65-67). Furthermore another nurse stated the importance of a patient's MR number particularly for tracing purposes. The medical staff, more specifically, nurses or secretaries should be able to trace relatives for notification purposes (KH0001, 70:73).

The MR number is a number unique to a patient and when this number is punched into to the electronic system, it displays all medical information of the patient. Medical information such as doctor's appointments or "previous bills and outstanding accounts" can be viewed (CH001, 1:31-32). The MR number is also handwritten on the physical file of a patient by staff on duty at the time. Sometimes, human error occurs as a result, making the process inaccurate. Such human errors can be detrimental as one patient could be mistaken for another.

The MR number does not have authentication, meaning the number can be changed by any individual intentionally or unintentionally (CH003, 1:14). This can have fatal implications as a patient could be mistaken for another. Additionally wrong bills could be sent to patients, as they are generated based on the produced MR number without a validation mechanism. Billing is said to be generated by the accounts office (CH010, 3:79-80).

Doctors at Hospital C can also access patient medical records on the HIS. One of the nurses explained that the doctor uses the MR number to access patients' details (CH010, 2:36-37). For example doctors in the department that deals with HIV make use of the HIS to record patient medical information, for treatment eligibility and their current state of health (CH01, 1:27-30). Every user is assigned login details with little differentiation in accessibility privileges. The doctors attained more access rights and hence could access all patient information, nurses on the other hand could do the same but only to close proximity (CH01, 2:34-36).

When a patient needs to see a doctor, the patient's information is entered by the secretaries and the secretary books the patient for an appointment using the HIS. The doctors can use the HIS system to place medication orders on behalf of patients or instruct a pharmacy at the hospital to prepare medication for a specified patient (CH01, 2:52-54). Laboratory test results could also be retrieved via the HIS but this was not done yet at the time of the study. One doctor explained "It's supposed to be that way but it haven't started working that way, so we are still waiting" (CH01, 2:56-57).

Hospital K on the other hand only utilised a paper-based system. Nurses and doctors including administrators carried out their tasks manually. Upon visiting Hospital K, a patient presents a hospital passport and moves on to pay a service fee at reception. From reception the patient is moved to the casualty area where they wait to be screened by a nurse (KH003, 1:2-3). This is to determine the patients' medical urgency. One of the interviewees explained "the nurse conduct the process of observations, and ask the patient about his or her medical history. Thereafter the nurse recommend whether the patient require the attention of a doctor or not" (KH003, 2:43-45). In case of an emergency, such as vehicle accidents involving several people, the nurse on duty make use of the triage method to determine which of the patients need urgent medical attention. A nurse explained that "the triage method is when you are treating patients according to their situations. For example, a patient with severe bleeding is placed ahead of those without physical injuries" (KH003, 1:15-19).

Patient demographics at Hospital K are recorded in files by nurses or doctors (KH001, 2:46-53). These physical files are stored in a designated storage room at the basement of the hospital (KH0001, 1:23-24). Basically all recording, retrieval, access and storage processes are manual.

2. What are the factors which influence HIS usage for service delivery within the Namibian environment?

There were various factors identified which influenced the use of HIS for service delivery in the two hospitals. The factors ranged from inadequate staff training to not enough computers in the hospital wards.

It was empirically revealed that the use of HIS in Hospital C had some benefits, but at the same time there were concerns on the effective use of the system. According to an interviewed nurse there was a time factor. This includes the time it takes to type patient data on a computer, while dealing with a lot of patients requiring attention in a ward simultaneously (CH008, 2:36-38). It is because the nurses are under staffed and there is a lack of sufficient computers in a ward. Each ward at the Central Hospital only has one computer (CH008, 2:36).

Another factor which influences the use of HIS for healthcare service delivery is the advanced age of some nurses. They are considered to be very slow in typing and affect service when many patients needs to be treated, hence electronic data capturing becomes a hindrance (CH001, 2:73-75). According to one of the nurses HIS training at Central Hospital took only about three to five days, which was considered insufficient by the nurses (CH004-Group, 1:20). Additionally the availability of the HIS was a major concern at the hospital, as a doctors stated that "the system (HIS) is always offline and on (mostly offline) and this type of situation goes for days before it can be fully restored" (CH01, 2:64). The doctor further stated that the template used in the HIS system is inadequate for their department and does not meet the departmental requirements (CH01, 2:65-66).

HIS was not in use at the time of this study at Hospital K but that the medical practitioners were nonetheless being prepared to use HIS to carry out their duties. A secretary that was interviewed at Hospital K stated that "we received two days of training which was very short" (KH0001, 2:46-48).

FINDINGS AND DISCUSSIONS

Based on the analysis of the data presented above, four critical factors were found to influence the use of HIS in the two Namibian public hospitals. The factors are parallel systems, lack of integration, lack of portable devices and human incompetence. The factors are discussed as follows.

Parallel Systems

The HIS and manual system were used in parallel in carrying out the hospital's processes and activities, sometimes, simultaneously at the time of the study. The utilisation of parallel systems at Hospital C was attributed to the fact that the HIS was needed to be fully stable before the manual process could be phased out. As such, the manual system was still considered vital should the use of HIS fail to be efficient in its operation. The plan was to systematically phase out the manual system once the data have been completely captured, processes migrated, and the functions well understood by the users.

Similar to many hospitals, at Hospital C the first point for a patient is at the reception. Patients are required to provide their personal and medical details to the administrator at reception. The patient data is captured on the system and the patient receive a Medical Registration number which is generated by the HIS. The Medical Registration number is a unique medical identifier for the patient which is also recorded on the patient's traditional passport. The Medical Registration number when entered would display all the patient's medical demographics on the HIS. Furthermore, the face of the patient is captured, using a web camera. A hospital card which is similar to a driving license or identification card is issued to the patient to complete the process of registration. This is in an effort to eventually do away with the traditional patient hospital passports that is a shape of a medium sized rectangular booklet, which is prone to wear and tear.

However, patients can bypass the reception point when in critical condition, such as a life threatening situation or unconsciousness. In such cases the patient is sent directly to a ward for first aid attendance by nurses. Depending on the situation and condition of the patient, doctors are assigned. Every ward has one computer and there are administrators assigned to these wards. The administrators are responsible for registering the patient on the HIS, answering telephone calls, filing, etc. this means that a patient can be registered at both the reception point or at the ward.

The nurses are responsible for recording the recovery progress of the patient, using the HIS. The nurses are also responsible for discharging a patient on the system, where in such a case the availability of that particular patient bed will be visible on the system. However, not all the nurses could make use of the system appropriately. Hence majority still relied on the manual process to carry out their tasks. As a result the manual system could be seen as a duplicative effort, causing slower responses to activities.

As empirically revealed, retrieval and access to patients' medical records are faster, when using the HIS. Since patient medical information is contained in the HIS, the billing and payment processes are faster consolidated. Re-registering of patients every time a patient returns to the hospital will not be necessary as patient information that was provided upon first registration is kept on the HIS. Both hospitals have a centralised storage room where all paper files for many years are stored.

Lack of Integration

The HIS was not fully utilised at the time of this research at Hospital C. This was due to integration challenges. The department of HIV for example was one of the affected departments at the Hospital requesting that some of their departmental requirements be met in order to efficiently use the system. This was because of their unique tasks within the health environment, such as counselling of patients before HIV tests. As a result the use of the manual file system continued to be prevalent in the hospital's operations. Some of the doctors indicated that the lack of integration of the systems caused duplication of work load, as the recording of information needed to be done in two different systems. During such a process, accuracy and consistency are not guaranteed because of the double workload.

Lack of Portable Devices

Another challenging factor that the doctors were confronted with is accessibility to the system from anywhere and at any given time. This was primarily to enable the doctors to record patient medical information as they move through the different wards, as well as to access the information outside the hospital for their private scrutiny. This could have been achieved with the use of portable devices. However, the HIS did not accommodate the integration of portable devices such as laptops and smart phones. Additionally the network connection was unstable. The inability to use portable devices once again contributed to a double workload as upon return of the doctors to their offices they had to re-capture the manually recorded patient data on the HIS.

User Incompetency

The competency of the users, which included doctors and nurses, were vital in the effective use and management of the HIS. Nurses at Hospital C were confronted with competency challenges such as lack of familiarity with the computer keyboard causing an inability to type patient medical information accurately and at a faster pace. However this challenge was more prevalent with the older generation of nurses. The implication was that it takes longer to complete registration of patients due to slow typing, thereby causing a delay in responding to urgently needed medical attention by other patients.

The incompetency of users in the use and management of the HIS was also attributed to a lack of proper training. According to some nurses training was offered but for only three to five days. Thus it was considered insufficient to get a grip of the system's functionalities.

With regards to Hospital K, it was established that the patient registration, admission and communication processes were manually done and were not computerized at the time of the study. For example, when a patient gets registered, a file is opened and patient information is recorded therein. The same process applied to patient admissions. Every patient has a hospital passport where medical history is recorded by a nurse or the doctor. Within this operandi, if a nurse intended to communicate a certain diagnose to a doctor, he/she did so by writing on the patient's hospital passport. This system has been there for a very long time and the medical personnel have become very comfortable with it. This has also contributed to the lack of interest in emerging technologies such as the HIS. The four factors are further outlined below with recommendations on how these challenges could be addressed.

Research shows that the above identified factors are commonly faced by most healthcare organisations, especially in developing countries. The use of parallel systems at the one hospital was attributed to the HIS not fully functional and stable at the time of the study and was rather considered to be a pilot run until such a time all major challenges are resolved and full functionality and stability of the system is proven.

The lack of sufficient training contributed to user incompetency which was a major factor that negatively impacted the use of HIS at the Hospital. Nurses and doctors for one had little confidence in using the HIS. It was found that the use of HIS was especially challenging to older Nurses, hence they opted to rather continue using the traditional paper based system. The administrators on the other hand were more optimistic in using the HIS as they claimed would enhance patient information retrieval and billing processes. Training thus was a factor that was necessary in boosting the confidence of the HIS users.

In addition to parallel systems and user incompetency', a lack of portable devices was another factor. Doctors especially indicated that the lack of portable devices caused a double workload since data capturing had to be done manually and needed to be re-captured on the computerised system. Not only was the lack thereof a challenge but that if there were portable devices the integration of these devices to the HIS for remote access would be a challenge.

As such a lack of integration was the final factor. The lack of integration results in ineffective operation of the HIS, causing poor information flow between sectors and units in the healthcare. Unmet user requirements were indicated to be attributing to a lack of integration as different departments have different functions. For example the department of HIV required doctors to take tests and provide counselling and these requirements were different from the doctors doing rounds in the wards.

Based on the outcome of this study, it is evident that to effectively use and manage the HIS for enhanced service delivery the aforementioned challenges need to be addressed. It is recommended that an awareness campaign about the HIS be conducted at the healthcare, as awareness about the system, its functionalities and benefits were lacking. Proper communication about the system functionalities and benefits were necessary. It is suggested that communication about the system be channelled through all levels. More emphasis must be placed on the benefits the use and management of the HIS would bring to healthcare service delivery. In that way all stakeholders, especially the end users of the system would be motivated and buy into the idea of using the system.

Additionally it is suggested that user requirements studies be carried out by the respective IT personnel in the healthcare to ensure that the system meets all departmental user requirements, which would allow for integration of departments and portable devices with the HIS. Training is the underlying success of the effective use of the system. Research showed that older medical practitioners were found to be less enthusiastic about the use of technology in carry out their duties, as such good training would motivate the use of the HIS and dissolve possible barriers in using the system.

CONCLUSION

The wellbeing of a collective of individuals in a nation in terms of health reflects in productivity and economic growth. Therefore healthcare service delivery is vital and can be optimized by introducing HIS in healthcare facilities. HIS allows for manual operational processes in healthcare to be computerised, such as the use of electronic health records (EHR) whereby patient records are electronically produced, stored and retrieved, enabling faster access, bulk storage and accuracy. Readability of electronically recorded patient data as supposed to bad handwriting from some doctors is another advantage.

Many developing countries are challenged with both technical and non-technical challenges as revealed in the analysis of the data for Hospital K and Hospital C in this chapter. The main challenges that were found in the study were the use of parallel systems, lack of integration, lack of portable devices and user incompetency. It was thus recommended that efforts be directed to sufficient training of the HIS users to encourage competency and confidence in using the system. Additionally addressing integration issues was necessary, as the HIS require optimised utilisation to explore its potentials to the fullest in order to improve the service of healthcare to the communities in Namibia. Optimal human interaction with the HIS is vital to avoid redundant Healthcare service delivery. The interaction seemingly had a significant influence on the integration of HIS, which could foster collaboration and consolidation of processes and activities.

It is eminent that research efforts and the practical application thereof be directed toward how Healthcare delivery can be maximised and managed by adopting the use of IT, as sustained community health care development can positively impact the economic growth and productivity of a nation. Thus this chapter aimed to investigate the utilisation of HIS for service delivery in the public health sector from a developing country's perspective.

REFERENCES

Adler-Milstein, J. R. (2011). The use of information technology in US health care delivery. *Proquest Dissertations and Theses*, 1.

Aftahi, S. R. (2013). Spirituality in a heealthcare organization: An exploratory qualitative inquiry. *Proquest Dissertations and Theses*, 52-53.

Akerman, E. A. (2006). Attitudes toward computers and computerization in Canadian critical care nurses. *Proquest Dissertations and Theses*, 1.

Al-Mutairi, M. S., & Mohammed, L. A. (2011). *Cases on ICT Utilization, Practice and Solutions. Tools for managing day-to-day issues.* New York: Information Science Reference. doi:10.4018/978-1-60960-015-0

Al-Mutairi, S. M., & Mohammed, L. A. (2011). *Cases on ICT Utilization, Practice and Solutions. Tools for managing Day-to-Day issues.* New York: Information Science Reference. doi:10.4018/978-1-60960-015-0

Alexander, R. C. (2009). Fostering student engagement in the history through student-created digital media: A qualitative and quantitative study of student engagement and learning outcomes in 6th-grade history instruction. *Proquest Dissertations and Theses*, 62.

Amendola, M. L. (2008). An examination of the leadership competency requirements of nurse leaders in healthcare information technology. *Proquest*, 14.

Amershi, H. (2006). Leading information technology (IT) integration within vancouver coastal health. *Proquest Dissertations and Theses*, 2.

Barrette, E. G. (2011). The impact of health information technology on demand for hospital inpatient services. *ProQuest*, 93-94.

Baumbach, J. (2006). Nurse practitioner utilization of information technology. *Proquest Dissertations and Theses*, 7.

Bogdan, R., Biklen, C., & Knopp, S. (1998). Qualitative research in education. An introduction to theory and methods. Boston: Allyn and Bacon.

Brikci, N., & Green, J. (2007). *A guide to using qualitative research methodology*. Academic Press.

Brown-Davis, C. B. (2009). Managed care and minority healthcare access in Georgia: A qualitative study of the quality and accessibility of care provided to the minority elderly population of Dekalb county. *Proquest Dissertations and Theses*, 12-13.

Chang, J. (2007). Nursing informatics competencies required of nurses in Taiwan: A Delphi method. *Proquest Dissertations and Theses*, 1-2.

Cline, G., & Luiz, J. (2013). Information technology systems in public sector health facilities in developing countries: the case of South Africa. *BMC Medicial informatics and decision making*, 13.

Craig, H. D. (2013). Using Diffusion of Innovation theory to determine Missouri providers' perception of telemedicine. *Proquest Dissertations and Theses*, 10.

Czanderna, K. H. (2013). A qualitative study on the impact of a short term global healthcare immersion experience in bachelor of science nursing students. *Proquest Dissertations and Theses*, 68-69.

Daly, G. (2012). Nursing perceptions of electronic documentation. *Proquest*, 3.

Dalziel, C. A. (2007). Factors that enhance nurses' use of health information systems to support clinical decision-making. *Proquest*, 1.

Dalziel, C. A. (2008). Factors that enhance nurses use of health information systems to support clinical decision making. *Proquest dissertations and theses*.

Dalziel, C. A. (2008). *Factors that enhances nurses use of health information systems to support clinical decision making*. ProQuest Dissertations and Theses.

Dienemann, J., & Castle, B. V. (2003). The impact of healthcare informatics on the organisation. *Jona*, 557-558.

Edwards, D. (2011). Analyzing decision-Making styles and strategic planning techniques for information technology in non-profit organisations. *Proquest Dissertations and Theses*, 24.

Farquharson, P. H. (2009). The perception of information technology investment and its impact on productivity at small private colleges. *Proquest*, 6.

Fasolino, T. (2009). *Nursing related factors influencing medication error incidence on medical surgical units*. Proquest.

Goodwin, C. S. (2013). Healthcare organizational metaphors and implications for leadership. *Proquest Dissertations and Theses*, 1.

Grgurović, M. (2010). Technology-enhanced blended language learning in an ESL class: A description of a model and an application of the diffusion of innovations theory. *Proquest Dissertations and Theses*, 21-25.

Grossman, C. S. (2014). Succession planning and knowledge transfer in higher education. *Proquest Dissertations and Theses*, 70.

Haoses-Gorases, L. (2005). *Utilisation of health information system (HIS) in Namibia: focus on challenges and opportunities faced by health care delivery system*. Academic Press.

Hersh, W. (2009). A stimulus to define informatics and health information technology. *BMC Medical Informatics and Decision Making*, *9*(1), 24. doi:10.1186/1472-6947-9-24 PMID:19445665

Hobbs, S. D. (2007). Clinical nurses' perception of nursing informatics competencies. *Proquest Dissertations and Theses*, 1.

Hofler, L. D. (2007). A case study of the relationship between the North Carolina center for nursing and nursing workforce issues in the state of North Carolina through the lens of planned change. *Proquest Dissertations and Theses*, 33.

Iacono, J., Brown, A., & Holtham, C. (2009). Research methods: A case example of participant observation. *Electronic Journal of Business Research Methods*, 40.

Jackson, A. C. (2014). The effect of suspension as a deterrent to student misconduct. *Proquest Dissertations and Theses*, 110.

Jackson, A. S. (2013). Impact of electronic health records on nurses' information seeking and discriminating skills for critical thinking. *ProQuest*, 4-5.

Jensen, T. A. (2013). Nurses' perceptions of nursing care documentation in the electronic health record. *Proquest Dissertations and Theses*, 1.

Jones, S. M. (2012). The development of trust in the nurse-patient relationship with hospitalized Mexican American patients. *Proquest Dissertations and Theses*, 179.

Jones-Zeigler, C. M. (2011). Computerization in practice: The lived experience of experienced nurses. *Proquest*, 1-2.

Kelley, T. F. (2012). Information use with paper and electronic nursing documentation by nurses caring for pediatric patients. *Proquest Dissertations and Theses*, 15.

Kulkarni, V. A. (2006). *Implementation of electronic health records: Modeling and evaluating healthcare information systems for quality improvements in the U.S. healthcare industry*. Academic Press.

Liong, A. S. (2008, March). *Descriptions of nurses experiences with electronic health records (EHR): A phenomenological study.* Academic Press.

Liong, A. S. (2008). Descriptions of nurses experiences with electronic health records (EHR): A phenomenological study. *Proquest Dissertations and Theses*, 1-2.

Lorenzi, N., & Riley, R. (2004). *Managing technological change: organizational aspects.* New York: Springer. doi:10.1007/978-1-4757-4116-2

Maerten, E. (2009). Study of the first woman president hired by a board of regents in Oklahoma president Emerita of Southwestern Oklahoma state university Dr. Joe Anna Hibler. *ProQuest Dissertations and Theses*, 65-66.

Mallet, R. K. (2014). The influence of organizational subculture on information technology project success in the healthcare sector: A qualitative, multi-case study. *Proquest Dissertations and Theses*, 57.

Mann, C. (2013). Experience of adjunct novice clinical nursing faculty: An interpretive case study. *Proquest Dissertations and Theses*, 88-89.

Melesse, M. (2010). Gender, equity and access to health care: The Case of Ghana's Health Financing Reform. *ProQuest*, 11.

Miller, B. A. (2008). Exploring the use of information technology for enhancing interagency coordination. *Proguest*, 10.

Minor, M. O. (2009). What is the efficacy of using an integrated model in measuring sense of community (SOC) in accelerated degree completion programs? *Proquest Dissertations and Theses*, 8.

Monier, J. P. (2011). Community development in rural America: The power to exchange capital resources in Norton county, Kansas. *Proquest Dissertations and Theses*, 11.

Ngafeeson, M. N. (2013). Understanding user resistance to information technology: Toward a comprehensive model in health information technology. *Proquest Dissertations and Theses*, 113.

Noble, E. (2012). The role mentoring plays in a white female novice teacher's perceptions of her enculturation into a culturally diverse campus. *ProQuest Dissertations and Theses*, 11-12.

Noseworthy, J. (2012). A solitary journey: Interpretive description of women's experiences of perinatal loss in labour. *Proquest Dissertations and Theses*, 40.

Pack, J. (2011). Multiple intelligences and experiential learning styles: A mixed method study of registered nurses' attitudes toward computers and web-based learning. *Proquest*, 1.

Pagano, M. W. (2013). Toward improved security and privacy in modern healthcare. *Proquest Dissertations and Theses*, 10.

Perron, M. D. (2014). Residential substance abuse treatment experiences of baby boomers: A qualitative study. *Proquest Dissertations and Theses*, 6-51.

Perron, M. D. (2014). Residential substance abuse treatment experiences of baby boomers: A qualitative study. *Proquest Dissertations and Theses*, 6-39.

Peterson, L. A. (2006). Information technology use in nursing and nursing education as reported by beginning nurses. *Proquest Dissertations and Theses*, 2.

Peterson, L. A. (2006). Information technology use in nursing and nursing education as reported by beginning nurses. *Proquest*, 2.

Pisk, R. M. (2010). *Physician satisfaction and workflow intergration factors associated with electronic medical record implementation in a pediatric hospital.* Proquest.

Roberts, S. A. (2007). The impact of Information Technology on small, medium, and large hospitals: quality, safety and financial metrics. *Proquest Dissertations and Theses*, 14.

Roberts, S. A. (2007). The impact of Information Technology on small, medium, and large hospitals: quality, safety and financial metrics. *Proquest*, 14.

Rogers, E. M. (1983). *Diffusion of innovations.* New York: Free Press.

Royce, M. (2008). A step beyond inclusion: A case study of what one principle did to improve achievement for students with disabilities. *Proquest Dissertations and Theses*, 63-69.

Sondheimer, N., Katsh, E., Clarke, L., Osterweil, L., & Rainey, D. (2009). *Dispute prevention and dispute resolution in networked.* Academic Press.

Spoelstra, S. (2006). Asking the question: What is organization? *Proquest Dissertations and Theses*, 18.

Thompson, C. D. (2014). Benefits and risks of electronic medical record (EMR): An interpretive analysis of Healthcare consumers' perceptions of an evolving health information systems technology. *Proquest Dissertations and Theses*, 43.

Tian, R. (2013). Effect of work complexity and individual differences on nursing IT utilization. *Proquest Dissertations and Theses*, 19.

Tonge, S. I. (2014). Exploring juvenile delinquency and the justice system: Social workers' perspective. *Proquest Dissertations and Theses*, 55-57.

Tucker, M. T. (2009). Application of the Diffusion of Innovations theory and the health believe model to describe the EMR use among Alabama family medicine physicians: A rural and urban analysis. *Proquest Dissertations and Theses*, 29-34.

Vichianin, Y. (2007). *How to healthcare information and communication technology (HICT) interventions affect access to public sector healthcare delivery in a developing country? A case study of professionals' perception in saraburi province.* Thailand: ProQuest.

Weng, S.-J. (2008). A framework for efficient resource allocation in healthcare. *Proquest Dissertations and Theses*, 1.

Winzenreid, J. E. (2009). Exploring cultural norms and behaviors that define an ethical environment in charitable nonprofit organizations. *Proquest Dissertations and Theses*, 21.

Wu, S., Chaudhry, B., Wang, J., Maglione, M., Mojica, W., Roth, E., et al. (2006). *Systematic review: impact of health information technology on quality, efficiency, and costs of medical care.* Academic Press.

Xiao, N. (2012). Essay on the impact of health information technology on healthcare providers and patients. *ProQuest*, 1-2.

Yen-Han, L. (2013). Healthcare reform in mainland China: The relationship of healthcare reform and economic development in Chinese rural and urban areas. *ProQuest Dissertations and Theses*, 1.

KEY TERMS AND DEFINITIONS

Administrator: A secretary at the reception area of a hospital.

Healthcare: A hospital that provides health related services to a community.

Healthcare Service Delivery: A duty carried out by health professionals at a hospital in meeting medical or health related needs of a patient or community.

Hospital C: A pseudonym for a public hospital in Windhoek, Namibia. It is mainly a specialist hospital.

Hospital K: A pseudonym for a public hospital in Windhoek, Namibia. It is mainly a referral hospital.

Medical Practitioners: Qualified Nurses and Doctors.

MR-Number: Medical Registration number that a patient receives upon first time visit or admission to a hospital.

This research was previously published in Maximizing Healthcare Delivery and Management through Technology Integration edited by Tiko Iyamu and Arthur Tatnall, pages 169-183, copyright year 2016 by Medical Information Science Reference (an imprint of IGI Global).

Chapter 45
Why, What and When in– Home Physiotherapy?

Gabriela Postolache
Universidade de Lisboa, Portugal

Raul Oliveira
Universidade de Lisboa, Portugal

Isabel Moreira
Universidade do Porto, Portugal

Octavian Postolache
Instituto de Telecomunicações, ISCTE-IUL, Portugal

ABSTRACT

In the last decade, rehabilitation process has shifted from medical management to issues that enhance quality of life, community participation, treatment and cost effectiveness. In this context physiotherapists design and implement new and/or tailored interventions that enhance physical and functional abilities, restore, maintain, and promote optimal physical function, wellness, fitness and quality of life. The aim of this review was to assess the extent, content, and outcomes of in-home physiotherapy interventions. A search was conducted in Medline, PEDro, and Cochrane Library and IEEE Xplore. RE-AIM and GRADE guidelines were used to report this review. The findings suggest that in-home physiotherapy tailored specifically to the people needs, functioning and disability has positive results, including patients' engagement in their healthcare. Integration of information and communication technology in-home physiotherapy has great potential to increase accessibility, quality and effectiveness of various interventions provided by physiotherapists.

INTRODUCTION

In-home physiotherapy is rapidly growing, in line with the current shift in emphasis toward: i) patient-centered healthcare, compliant with 4P medicine (personalized, preventive, predictive, participatory medicine) (see Hood & Galas, 2008); ii) self-management for people with long-term and/or chronic conditions, in which greater use of community settings and individual autonomy are being encouraged

DOI: 10.4018/978-1-5225-3926-1.ch045

(see Lommi, Matarese, Alvaro, Piredda, & De Marinis, 2015); iii) healthcare delivery closer to patients' homes - aiming for increasing access to healthcare services, cost-effectiveness, and sustainability of healthcare system (see Coulter, 2005). With advances in information and communication technologies (ICT), dramatic changes are produced in health care provision. There is increasing evidence suggesting great potential of ICT (see list of definitions) to meet healthcare aspirations of patients and citizens (see Coulter, 2005) as: fast access to reliable information about illness and treatment options; attention to physical and environmental needs; participation in health care decision and service developments, etc. ICT through contribution to patient engagement (see Triberti & Riva, 2014a), particularly on patient engagement in physical rehabilitation process (see Triberti et al., 2014) lead to more appropriate health care, tailored treatment, better health outcome and cost effective use of health services (Graffigna & Barello, 2015; Triberti et al., 2014). Home health technologies are now emerging as a distinct segment within the larger ICT market, forecasting the increase of consumers using home health technologies from 14.3 million worldwide in 2014 to 78.5 million by 2020 (Tractica, 2015). This is produced by: rapidly advances in ICT; increased access to Internet - 82,1% of European and 60% American population has now Internet access at home; development of mobile technologies; and increased access to mobile technologies – approximately 80% of Europeans and Americans have active mobile broadband subscriptions (ITU, 2015).

The interest on model, determinants, and technologies for in-home health care has led to a rise in the number of studies addressing the same, or very similar research questions, with a concurrent increase in discordant findings in terms of direction and magnitude of in-home physiotherapy interventions. Differences in scope, methods, and results in studies realized by health care professionals, engineers or information technology specialists cause great confusion, and make it difficult for decision makers to analyze the level of evidence towards finding solutions to improve practice and identify areas where new research is needed.

We investigated the extent (demographic, health, functioning/disability characteristics of patients, level of evidence, amplitude of practice implementation and adoption), content (what type of physiotherapy intervention, in which clinical condition, what technique or technology is used) and outcomes (e.g. balance, posture, coordination) of in-home physiotherapy. The aim of this chapter is characterization of the level of evidence of in-home physiotherapy in various clinical conditions, and on technology use for in-home physiotherapy. We present the framework for the analysis of the level of evidence related with in-home physiotherapy (Study Design and Methodology section) and the results (Main Evidence section) on what and when in-home physiotherapy, emphasizing why in-home physiotherapy may contribute to patient engagement in health care. Ongoing research and trends in technology for in-home physiotherapy are presented in Future Researches section.

BACKGROUND: WHY IN-HOME PHYSIOTHERAPY

In-home health care provided by governmental healthcare services are rapidly growing in industrialized countries, as a result of: i) increase in elderly population, ii) general increase of population with non-communicable, chronic diseases, and iii) epidemiological transition triggered by medical innovation in disease or sickness therapy and treatment (see Omran, 2005). In Europe, all countries are experiencing an ageing of their populations, a trend that is projected to continue until at least the middle of the twenty-first century (Rechel, Doyle, Grundy, & McKee, 2009). Nowadays, in Portugal, elderly population is already around 20%. This adds significant cost to the healthcare system. One study performed in eight countries from Organisation for Economic Co-operation and Development (OECD) found that between one third and one half of total health expenditure was spent on health care for older people (Anderson & Hussey, 2001). In industrialized countries larger proportions of people increased life expectancy, but also larger proportions of patients in these countries live with more than one disease. The monthly costs per patient of co-morbidity increase exponentially, and rise more with mental disorders (Naylor et al., 2012). Most of the subject receiving physiotherapy - elderly population, people with chronic diseases or people with disabilities - often receive a mix of health and social care provided by several formal and informal workers. In this context, to achieve the intent and sustainability of meaningful use of health care services, and to balance rising cost pressure in healthcare system, focus on prevention and prediction became a priority of many health services, particularly in physiotherapy services.

Patient-centered models of health care services were implemented worldwide, in order: to look actively and systematically for conditions in their early stages; to identify factors that are known to be health risk; and to provide tailored, efficient care. Services for continuing care, or long term care are provided in assisted living or nursing home but also at patient home. The Alliance for Home Health Quality & Innovation organization (2014), from U.S.A., that is comprised of home health care providers and organizations committed to advancing research and initiatives on the value of home health care, underlines that *'the value of health care delivery at home will grow because it is a patient-preferred, cost-effective means of delivery high quality care'*.

An important contribution to quality and efficiency of home health care has been the integration of ICT in healthcare services. For instance, various mobile technologies are currently used in-home setting in a broad range of interventions. Most commonly, health professionals use mobile technology for collecting health data; tele-monitoring; management of practice (e.g. schedule of appointments, register of clinical summary of the patient during and after each visit); messaging between health professionals and patients; patient specific health education; better communication with patients (e.g. through interactive communication – video sharing, video games, augmented reality, virtual reality, etc.). Recent studies suggest that mobile technologies present promising opportunities to improve the range, quality and cost-effectiveness of services provided by health professionals (see Nhavoto & Gronlundt, 2014; Berratarrechea et al., 2014). However, demographic, socio-economic and clinical heterogeneity of the patients requiring home health care, in addition to lack of standardization of in-home health services, lack of strong evidence on the optimal model for providing home health care services and optimal model of payment and reimbursement for these services, create a confusing picture regarding in-home healthcare. In-home physiotherapy (also known as domiciliary physiotherapy) as part of home health care services is more challenging, as more uncertainty exists in physiotherapists status and complexity of interventions provided by physiotherapists - some overlapping with other therapies or in-home health services (see Figure 1).

Physiotherapy, also known as physical therapy or kinesitherapy, has different definition worldwide (see Jull, 2013) despite being recognized as the assessment, prevention and treatment of movement disorders as a core of expertise, practice, education and research in physiotherapy. Physiotherapists are often associated with spine and sports injuries treatment although they promote and prescribe physical

Figure 1. Physiotherapy practice and relationships with other health care services

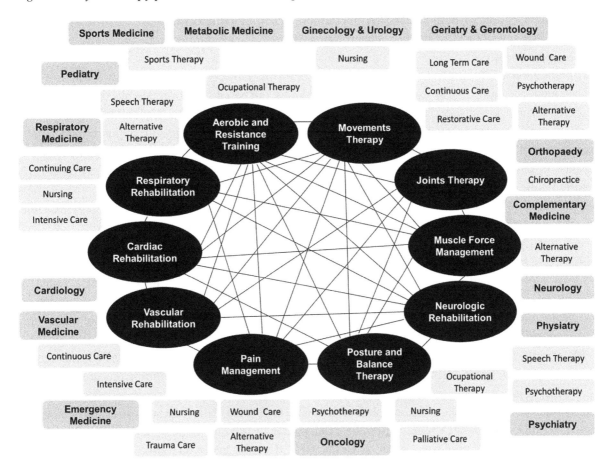

activity programmes in the area of prevention and maintenance, promotion and treatment across lifespan. They are involved in a large variety of healthcare services (e.g. care for the premature babies; care for the children with impaired motor functionalities; rehabilitation of cardiac and respiratory system; therapy for musculo-skeletal disorders; programs for preventions of functional decline in older adults). Physiotherapists can prescribe aerobic and resistance exercise (e.g. for athletes, or people with metabolic diseases like obesity or diabetes), movement therapy (e.g. in upper or lower limbs rehabilitation), joints therapy (e.g. rehabilitation after knee arthroplasty, shoulder dislocation), muscle force management (e.g. strength training, muscle spasticity and rigidity treatment), exercises for neurologic or neuro-motor rehabilitation (e.g. mobility and stability exercises, sensory-motor training, posture and balance training for people with cerebral palsy), therapy for pain reduction (e.g. for rheumatoid arthritis), therapy for vascular rehabilitation (e.g. for therapy for venous or lymphatic edema, physical exercises for people with abdominal aneurism), physical exercises for cardiac rehabilitation (e.g. after cardiac surgery), or respiratory rehabilitation (e.g. after pulmonary surgery), etc. In most countries, patients must have a prescription or referral from a licensed medical doctor before physiotherapy. Some competencies, skills and knowledge of physiotherapists are overlapping with those of others health professionals (e.g. wound care, alternative therapy, occupational therapy) but there are always several differences in the approach and interventions. Physiotherapists can practice either alone or in different teams (see Figure 1) in hospital, primary health centers, private clinics, and community centers. They can be specialized in respiratory physiotherapy, cardiac rehabilitation, woman health, family and community health, in-home physiotherapy, etc.

To our knowledge, adoption of in-home physiotherapy in many countries is currently limited as most physiotherapists and patients are not aware on techniques and benefits of in-home physiotherapy. They perceive various advantages on hospital and clinics setting as: various equipment and multidisciplinary staffing; access to 'expert' support and guideline; facilitation of peer learning and support opportunities; 'economies of scale' when physiotherapy program is delivered in a group setting; safety perception of hospital or clinics environment, and risk of injury in-home setting (although few adverse events were reported until now) (see Gunn, Cattaneo, Finlayson, Freeman, & Sosnoff, 2014).

Various drawbacks of these services, mainly for people that need long term physiotherapy (months, years) were reported: i) programs away from home are unlikely to be frequent enough to provide a sufficient intensity of exercises to improve functionalities or capacities; ii) less accessibility (e.g. when patients live far from the hospital or rehabilitation centers and participation of patients at physiotherapy sessions is constrained by availability of transportation and involved costs); iii) costs of each physiotherapy session; iv) time and energy required for regular attendance, adding an additional burden on people dealing with the challenges of ongoing health conditions. Therefore, in-home physiotherapy may be a solution for the above-mentioned problems.

According to a systematic review based on the analysis of 23 randomized controlled trials and 3 controlled trials (Novak, 2011), strong and moderate evidence supporting in-home physiotherapy was published. Many systematic reviews on various interventions in which physiotherapists may be involved (e.g. stroke rehabilitation, cardiac rehabilitation) have supported that in-home setting physiotherapy have favorable outcomes (Outpatient Service Trialists, 2004; Jolly et al., 2007; Chien, Lee, Wu, Chen, & Wu, 2008; Thomas, Simpson, Riley, & Grant, 2010; Health Quality Ontario, 2013; Crocker et al., 2013; Coulter, Scarvell, Neeman, & Smith, 2013; Siemonsma et al., 2014; Anderson & Taylor, 2014, Chan et al., 2015). However, there are inconclusive data, and some studies showing no positive outcomes for several physiotherapy interventions, mainly when complications or the presence of co-morbidities are also considered in the study (Mehta & Roy, 2011; Al-Jundi, Madback, Beard, Nawaz, & Tew, 2013; Papalia et al., 2013; Valdes, Naughton, & Michlovitzl, 2014). Moreover, it is easy to understand that in-home physiotherapy is not appropriate for every patient. Some patients in need for therapy after hospital discharge may be able to obtain outpatient therapy in-home or clinic environment and adequately meet their needs. Other patients may only need to follow up with their in-home exercises. For some patients, in-home physiotherapy would not offer either quality or effectiveness of traditional physiotherapy. Taking into account the accumulating evidence from the last years, it should be noted that for many patients with multiple chronic conditions or with disabilities, in-home physiotherapy would be cost-effective and adequate care. It is required, therefore, description and comprehensive analysis of evidence related with interventions that are better suited for in-home setting. With rapidly growing of in-home physiotherapy practice as well as changes in health services produced nowadays by ICT integration, the analysis of evidence should be a dynamic process in which various dimensions (e.g. perspectives of patients and physiotherapists on various kind of ICT technologies, usability of new technologies for in-home physiotherapy, effectiveness, wellbeing or quality of life provision) should be integrated.

WHAT AND WHEN IN-HOME PHYSIOTHERAPY: A SYSTEMATIC REVIEW

Study Design and Methodology

Medline via PubMed, PEDro, Cohrane Central Register of Controlled Trials and IEEE/IET Electronic Library were searched from January 2013 up to December 2014 for review of the evidence on technologies and type of physiotherapy that can be applied in-home setting. Search was made by using the following terms: 'in-home physiotherapy', 'in-home rehabilitation', 'balance monitoring' 'Wii,' 'Kinect,' 'exergame,' 'tele-rehabilitation,' 'gait assessment.' To be included, articles had to be available in English; having data and measurements that suggest use or potential use of technique for in-home rehabilitation or physiotherapy. All design studies and all health condition and clinical populations were included. Reference lists from articles meeting the inclusion criteria were checked to ensure all relevant papers were included, and to search for additional studies using 'snowballing' method. Two reviewers used predefined inclusion criteria to select relevant published works and assess their quality using the GRADE - Grading of Recommendations Assessment, Development and Evaluation (www.gradeworkinggroup. org), and RE-AIM - Reach, Effectiveness, Adoption, Implementation and Maintenance (Glasgow, 2013). As the objective of the studies was not measuring the quality of the researches on the new treatment or therapy - for this PEDro scale (www.pedro.org.au) is commonly used - we decided to use a combination of GRADE and RE-AIM guidelines. NVivo10 software was used to manage the data. In our analysis, as trials and works on new technologies for in-home rehabilitation often at *'proof of concept state'* are included, the quality depend on other criteria than PEDro scale, as for example reliability of measurements, feasibility, long-term analysis of functionalities of developed technology, advantages comparing with other technologies, data on safety and adoption of technology. By using RE-AIM analysis of target population, effectiveness of the implemented technique, adoption by target population, staff, setting or institutions, implementation consistency, costs and adaptations made during delivery, maintenance of intervention effects in individuals and settings over time, can be carried out. Figure 2 presents a synthesis of the dimension and definitions of RE-AIM.

Decision on the quality of evidence was based on:

- Effectiveness;
- Potential harm;
- Diagnosis and prognosis potential of the implemented technique for in-home physiotherapy;
- Number of subjects included in the study and description of control condition;
- How clear was the description of the implemented system architecture and experimental protocol, reproducibility of measurements;
- Influence of confounding variables, risk of bias/study limitations;
- Consistency of results, precision of measurements and data reporting.

For decision making on what physiotherapy intervention should be better in-home setting, a Boolean logic (strong evidence or no strong evidence) is more appropriate. Therefore, after multi-dimensional analysis with RE-AIM, the studies were grouped in fewer categories than with RE-AIM, using GRADE guidelines. In this evidence rating scale, the studies should be classified as:

Figure 2. RE-AIM dimension and definitions
(Glasgow, 2013)

REACH

Participation rate among eligible;

Representativeness of settings participating individuals;

Representativeness of participants;

EFFICACY/EFFECTIVENESS

Effects on primary outcome of interest;

Impact on quality of life, negative outcomes;

ADOPTION

Participation rate among possible settings;

IMPLEMENTATION

Extent to which intervention was delivered as intended and adaptation made;

Time and costs of intervention;

than in hospital settings (ref);

MAINTENANCE

(Individual) Longer – term effects of intervention > 6 months;

(Individual) Impact of attrition on outcomes;

(Settings) Sustained delivery and modification of intervention.

- HLE (High Level of Evidence): further research is very unlikely to change the confidence in the estimate of accuracy of measurements;
- MLE (Moderate Level of Evidence): further research is likely to have an important impact on our confidence in the estimate of accuracy of measurement and may change the estimate;
- LLE (Low level of Evidence): further research is very likely to have an important impact on the confidence in the estimate of accuracy of measurement and is likely to change the estimate;
- VLE (Very Low Level of Evidence): any estimate of measurements is very uncertain.

Exclusion criteria for this work were: studies that did not go through a peer-review process for publication; studies published in conference and with a more complete version in a journal - the journal version was included and the conference version was discarded.

Main Evidence

In this chapter we present our results of what and when in-home physiotherapy based on RE-AIM and GRADE classification of 250 studies – pilot study/case report, randomized controlled trials, cohort/ quasi-experimental studies related with in-home physiotherapy. Also, 26 review papers related with in-home rehabilitation or physiotherapy as well as 16 publications on future trials were analyzed for better understanding of the issue, controversies and research trend related with in-home physiotherapy. Systematic reviews and future trials were not included in GRADE and RE-AIM based analysis. In 165 studies, outcomes assessments were based on information and communication technologies – 72 for in-home exercises supervision and assessments, 25 for coordination of movement measurements, 39 for gait assessment and monitoring, 7 for balance assessments and monitoring, 6 for posture and muscle spasticity/rigidity evaluation, 16 for biofeedback (see list of definitions) based therapy.

Table 1 presents the frequency of the studies categorized as having high, moderate or low level of evidence on effectiveness of in-home exercises, where outcomes evaluation was made using scales.

Most studies are related with measurements of in-home exercises effectiveness. Home-based training has shown to increase rehabilitation uptake, and to be safe and effective in improving short-term exercise capacity. Also, the long-term effect of in-home exercises on physical fitness and activity was studied in various clinical frameworks. Most are randomized and controlled studies and with exception of studies included in low level evidence category, they are compliant with RE-AIM criteria. One in 4 of these studies met the criteria for high level evidence and RE-AIM system. There is high level of evidence on effectiveness of tailored exercises for elderly population, for people with multiple sclerosis, Alzheimer disease, cancer, knee rehabilitation after knee arthroplasty (see Table 1).

Positive results were published on a program based on Lifestyle Functional Exercise (LiFE) to engage older people on physical exercising (Burton, Lewin, Clemson, & Boldy, 2013). By using exergame (see Sinclair, Hingston, & Masek, 2007), Nintendo Wii, video training (e.g. DVD video with comprehensive exercise, physiotherapist supervision via videoconferencing or tele-rehabilitation system), or wireless sensors (see Table 2 and Figure 3), the outcomes of in-home exercises were shown to be comparable to the standard in hospital or physiotherapy clinic rehabilitative approach.

This finding suggests that in-home physiotherapy for cardiac rehabilitation or management of functional decline in elderly people can be implemented effectively at home, mainly when co-administered with an integrated tele-rehabilitation service. In a recent study where 307 older adults were recruited from 83 towns, participants in DVD intervention condition demonstrated significant improvements in the Physical Performance Battery, lower extremity flexibility, and upper body strength (McAuley et al., 2013). Range of motion (ROM) for elbow and joint extension significantly increased at 1, 3, and 6 months, while for the wrists joint extension increased significantly at 1 months in comparison to baseline, with detailed one-to one instruction for home based functional training combined with botulin toxin type A injection in upper limb muscles, in a study with 190 post-stroke participants (Takekawa et al., 2013).

For better visualization of data, exergames based on Nintendo Wii, and Kinect technology are separately retrieved in Table 2 and Figure 4. High level of evidence exists on potential of mobile technologies for long term monitoring of Parkinson's disease motor symptom in-home setting (Mhatre et al., 2013; Tzallass et al., 2014). There are high and moderate level of evidence on effectiveness of wearable technologies (e.g. accelerometers, inertial measurement unit – IMU, force sensors) or contactless technologies (e.g. Kinect) for gait assessment and monitoring (see Figure 5). These low cost non-invasive or unobtrusive technologies might be used to deliver tailored in-home physiotherapy.

Small wearable or contactless technologies may greatly contribute for increase effectiveness of in-home physiotherapy both by accurate, real-time assessment and monitoring, as well as a tool for treatment. We include in the category of studies on biofeedback (Lee et al., 2013; Kent, Laird, & Haines, 2015) the development of new technologies for situation dependence cueing (auditory, vibratory or visual cueing) of gait, or freezing episode for Parkinson's disease episode (Zhao, Anhalt, Fietzek, & D'Angelo, 2013; Cinel, Poli, Citi, & Robertson, 2013; Rodger, Young, & Craig, 2014; Imbeault-Nepton & Otis, 2014; Cancela, Morano, Arredondo, & Bonato, 2014; Pepa, Ciabattoni, Verdini, Capecci, & Ceravolo, 2014).

These technologies might be applied in a variety of physiotherapy intervention plan (e.g. prevention of falls in elderly patient, training movements in people with cerebral palsy, Huntington diseases). Moreover, the potential of virtual reality (VR) technologies (see list of definitions) to assist and improve

Table 1. Visual representation of frequency of high, moderate or low level of evidence studies on effectiveness of in-home exercises where outcomes evaluation was made using scales.

	HLE				MLE				LLE		
	RE-AIM		RE-AIM		RE-AIM		RE-AIM				
	2013		2014		2013		2014		2013	2014	
	Number of Studies										Total
	17	17	8	8	23	23	16	16	8	8	80
Condition — Achilles Tendinopathy							1				1
Ageing	3				5		2				11
Alzheimer	1				2						3
Ankylosis Spondylitis	1				1		1				3
Cancer	1		1								2
Cerebral Palsy					1						1
Claudicants							1				1
COPD					1						1
Depression	2										2
Hemofilia							1				1
Hip Rehab			1		1						2
Incontinence	2										2
Ankle Sprain					1						1
Knee Rehab	3		2		2		2				9
Lower Limbs			1		1		1				3
Multiple Sclerosis			2				3				5
Neurogenic Claudication	1										1
Neurological Physiotherapy					1						1
Obesity					1		1				2
Palliative Care			1								1
Parkinson Disease					1						1
Pelvic Girdle Pain	1										1
Respiratory Rehab	1				1		1				2
Stroke					2						2
Temporomandibular Rehab							2				2
Vascular Rehab	1				2						3

rehabilitation techniques and procedures was explored in various studies. VR has been used in several training exercises in-home setting, and has great potential to: incorporate the individual's visual, auditory, touch senses and proprioception for subject engagement; increased adherence to exercise; empowerment; and proactive participation of patients in rehabilitation.

Table 2. Visual representation of frequency of the high, moderate or low level of evidence studies on effectiveness of in-home exercises where outcomes evaluation was made using various portable technologies.

		HLE				MLE				LLE		
		RE-AIM		RE-AIM		RE-AIM		RE-AIM				
		2013		2014		2013		2014		2013	2014	
		Number of Studies										**Total**
		2		6	6	12	12	10	10	1	7	38
Condition	Ageing			1	1			2	2			3
	Ankylosis spondilitis							1	1			1
	Braquial plexus injury							1	1			1
	Cancer					4	4					4
	Cardiac Rehab	2		3	3	1	1					6
	COPD					1	1	1	1			2
	Knee Rehab					1	1	1	1			2
	Metabolic Syndrom			1	1							1
	Parkinson's Disease			1	1	2	2	1	1			4
	Shoulder Rehab					1	1	1	1			2
	Transfemoral Amputation					1	1					1
	Vascular Rehab					1	1	2	2			3

Figure 3. Studies on physical exercises that can be performed in-home by using unobtrusive/contactless technologies

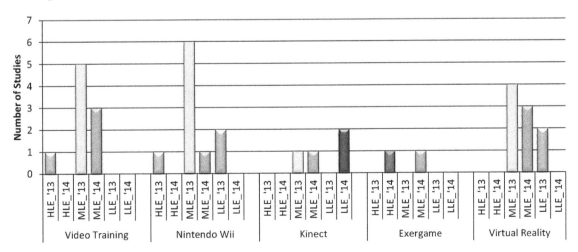

Figure 4. Studies on gait assessment using wearable technologies

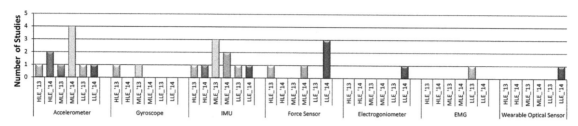
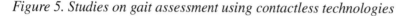

Figure 5. Studies on gait assessment using contactless technologies

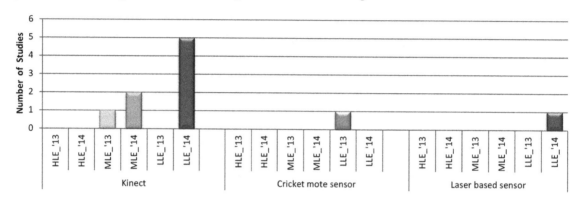

Studies related with tremor evaluation, studies on development of technologies for coordination of movement assessment (e.g. tablet based software for evaluation of Parkinson' disease progression using alternate taping), studies having as main objective evaluation of limbs agility in various clinical context were included in the group of physiotherapy practice related with coordination of movement. New, interesting, techniques, mobile technologies based on accelerometer, inertial measurement unit (IMU), gyroscope, Wii Sports, Kinect are developed and tested for coordination of movement measurements. The majority of these studies are not compliant with RE-AIM (64%), testing being made only for short period of time (e.g. one session, or few days), in a small number of healthy subjects or patients.

By using ICT, physiotherapists can document the effects of interventions with valid outcome tools/ instruments evaluation. However, in the implementation of ICT for tele-rehabilitation, it should be considered that patients with chronic diseases, and/or with disabilities might have greater than expected difficulties in using ICT often due to cognitive impairment or unfamiliarity with technology. Approaches described in the evaluated studies for dealing with such barriers (see Hoerbst & Ammenwerth, 2010; Kaye, Kokia, Shalev, Idar, & Chinitz, 2010; Irizarry, DeVito Dabbs, & Curran, 2015) include: suitable integration of solutions involving patient-caregiver dyads, integration of education to improve health and ICT literacy, better design of technology and careful attention to the safety of technology, adoption and maintenance (see table 3).

The evaluated studies suggest benefits of using ICT for various in-home physiotherapy interventions:

- Tailored program for experiential positions described in Patient Health Engagement Model (Graffigna & Barello, 2015) - blackout, arousal, adhesion and eudaimonic project - can be de-

Table 3. Visual representation of frequency of the high, moderate or low level of evidence studies on in-home physiotherapy interventions

		HL				ML				LL		
		RE-AIM				RE-AIM						
		2013	2014			2013	2014			2013	2014	
		Number of Studies										Total
Muscle		1	1			1	1			2	1	5
Spasticity/Rigidity	Scale	1								2		3
	Sensor					1					1	2
Posture						1		2			1	4
	Accelerometer							1				1
	IMU					1						1
	Kinect							1			1	2
Coordination		1	1	1	1	6	3	9	3	1	7	25
Balance						4	4	3	2	1	1	9
	Scale					1	1	1	1			2
	Nintendo Wii					3	3	1	1			3
	Kinect							1				1
	Virtual Reality									1		1
Biofeedback		1	1			6	4	6	6	1	2	16

signed based on ICT, in order to induce a positive reaction in patients (Triberti & Riva, 2014a) and for cost-effective treatment;

- Context based practice and integration of physiotherapy intervention into real life of subject may be implemented;
- Physiotherapists and subjects can have greater choice over type, planning and progression of exercise activities;
- Shared decision making in care process;
- Subjects can receive personalized advices on home environment modification for safe and better quality of physiotherapy process;
- Family members or other caregivers might be involved directly or through positive technology as source of motivation, support and feedback in rehabilitation process.

FUTURE RESEARCH DIRECTIONS

Main issues that require future research are related with:

- Patient's experience in-home physiotherapy setting (see Triberti et al., 2014);
- Patient health and ICT literacy (see Irizarry et al., 2015);

- ICT literacy of health professionals (see Kaye et al., 2010);
- ICT usability (see Triberti & Riva, 2014b; Irizarry et al., 2015);
- Privacy and security of data (see Coulter & Magee, 2003) in implemented information system for in-home physiotherapy;
- Standards and technologies for integrated, interoperable information systems based on common specifications for technology and end to end services (see Hoerbst & Ammenwerth, 2010);
- Optimal model of physiotherapists endorsement.

Various trials were initiated and will bring within 3-4 years' new evidence for what and when in-home physiotherapy should be to meet personal and provider needs. The analysis of objectives and methodologies of these future trials may foster new research worldwide both for better integration of mobile health and tele-rehabilitation technologies in-home physiotherapy and advancement in physiotherapy practice.

- The potential *identification of functional decline of older adults* registered at the department of emergency for a minor health event, *through a telephone screening process* within four weeks after discharge are investigated (Grimner et al., 2013). This might contribute for early detection of health and medical risk, and identification of subjects for which preventive programs may be more effective.
- Effectiveness of *tailored home based exercise programs for fall prevention* in elderly population (Gschwind et al., 2013), dwelling older with cognitive impairments (Close et al., 2014) or older adults identified as having unsteadiness during turning (Giangregorio et al., 2014) are also ongoing.
- Efficacy and effectiveness of *therapies based on specification of patient participation in everyday activities,* such as therapeutic goal (Barzel et al., 2013), *Tai Chi based exercise program provided via tele-rehabilitation* (Tousignant et al., 2014), *or Nintento Wii Sports* ™ (Adie et al., 2014) are studied in stroke patients.
- The potential of *ICT on behavioural physiotherapy* proposed by Broetz and Birbaumer (2013) for post stroke patients, in which goals, exercises and tasks - based on observation and analysis of daily activities - are setting and anticipated as a "self-control cue"- should be investigated.
- A study on the *engagement on physical exercise* of patients with multiple sclerosis and the feasibility of conducting a full scale clinical and cost-effectiveness trial of a home-based physiotherapist *supported by Wii intervention* ('Mii-vitaliSe') is ongoing (Thomas et al., 2014).
- The effectiveness of *robotic-assisted home therapy* compared with a home exercise program, on upper extremity motor recovery and health-related quality of life for stroke survivors in rural and underserved locations are investigated (Linder et al., 2013). In this trial are also explored whether initial degree of motor function of the upper limb may be a factor in predicting the extent to which patients with stroke may be responsive to home therapy approach.
- A randomized clinical trial evaluating the feasibility of *a home-based exercise program designed to increase physical activity (PA) and reduce the risk of cardiovascular disorders in subjects with human immunodeficiency virus (HIV)* was also initiated (Jaggers et al., 2013).
- *Internet-based multimodal program* - Move it to improve it (Mitii) comprising physical activity *for upper-limb and cognitive training* are evaluated in people with cerebral palsy (Boyd et al., 2013). In addition to better accessibility, the Mitii study aims to test the efficacy and cost-effectiveness of

Mitii program for upper-limb function and motor planning, as well as to investigate neurovascular mechanisms related with upper limb motor function.

- A new program for *cardiac rehabilitation based on tele-guidance for improvement of self-management skills,* like self-efficacy and action planning for independent exercise and, consequently, for long-term engagement on physical fitness and physical activity, was designed and is evaluated (Kraal, Peek, van den Akker-Van Marle, & Kemps, 2013). This is in line with the new proposed model for better management of health care costs in which *quantified self* might be a tool for personalized health care and proactive participation of population in health decisions. In this context, *e-Patients* (see list of definitions) potential for improving quality of care is nowadays analyzed.

- An interesting new technology was described in an article published by Mortazavi et al. (2014) team in which *body-wearable sensors were used for exergame with near-realistic motions.* An enjoyable game is produced by technology that combines acquisition of data related with real world activities, realizes pattern recognition and uses algorithm for serious game. The designed classification algorithm in this work has precision of 77%, compared with 40% precision on current activity monitoring algorithms used for general daily living activities. It is not an optimal precision but it is an important direction of research that should be followed.

- An innovative, *computer-based gaming platform based on instrumentation with a motion-sense mouse which should transform broad range of common objects into therapeutic input devices* was designed and it is being evaluated (Srikesavan, Shay, Robinson, & Szturm, 2013). By using this technology, for control and play of any computer game, algorithm based on acquired movements that replicate common situation in everyday living, can be used. The system was designed for patients with rheumatoid arthritis, or osteoarthritis of the hand, for which training of graded finger mobility, strength, endurance or fine/gross dexterous functions may be realized using personalized objects. *This Internet of Things (IoT) based technology* (see Gubbi, Buyya, Marusic, & Palaniswami, 2013) is in line with trends on smart home technology (see representation from Figure 6, of the emergence, adoption, maturity, and impact on applications of specific technologies which is named *hype cycle,* for 2015). Connecting everyday existing objects and embedding intelligence in-home environment not only harvests information from the inhabitants and home environment, and allows augmented interaction with physical world, but also might provide a context awareness where the context is used to prevent information overload problem and to present *"the 'right' information, at the 'right' time, in the 'right' place, in the 'right' way to the 'right' person"* (Fischer, 2012).

Technology for in-home health care evolve towards continuous monitoring without any manual interventions, thus reducing provider patient interaction and cost while contributing to improvements in the quality of the data. For technology to disappear from the consciousness of the user (Gubbi et al., 2013) is required (1) a shared understanding of the situation of its users and their appliances, (2) software architectures and pervasive communication networks to process and convey the contextual information to where it is relevant, and (3) the analytics tools in the Internet of Things that aim for autonomous and smart behavior.

With move from www (static pages web) to web2 (social networking web) and to web3 (ubiquitous computing web) (Gubbi et al., 2013) health care services will need to adapt in order to create a new model of providing care. Real-time, face-to-face counseling with an expert health provider, and virtual meeting with support group might be provided in-home physiotherapy through ICT. For instance, *Doctor*

Figure 6. Hype cycle for emerging technologies
(Gartner Inc., 2015)

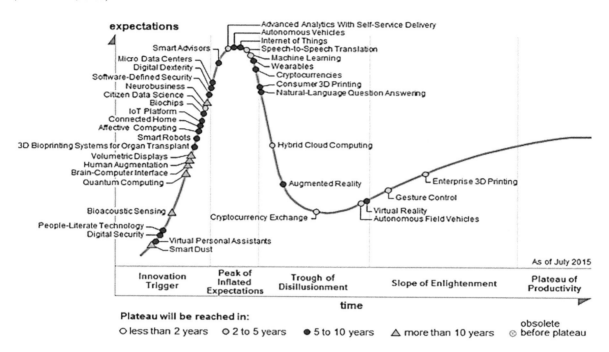

on Demand lets people in U.S.A. to request a rapid video consultation with physician. Prescription can be sent electronically to the patient's nearest pharmacy. The cost for this video consultation can be as little as $40. *MDlive*, a competitor, in U.S.A., also offers quick video consultations, for $49. *Contact a Family* organization (www.cafamily.org.uk) has set up a virtual reality based on their own office where parents of disabled children meet, share information and provide support to each other.

IoT, context awareness, mobile technologies, e-Patients (Ferguson, 2007; Gee, Paterniti, Ward, & Soederberg, 2015; Bujnowska-Fedak & Kurpas, 2015), personal health records (PHRs) (Postolache, Girão, & Postolache, 2013), patient centered medical home (PCMH) (Stange et al., 2010) integrated in electronic health records (EHRs) (Williams & Samarth, 2011) will radically change home health care services, and until an optimal model will be found, cautions and in deep analysis of the advantages and drawbacks of various techniques is need.

It is desirable the development of cost-effective structural *solutions based on hierarchical and adaptive combination of low-cost, non-invasive and unobtrusive technologies capable of performing a wide array of multiple functions for training and care.* The basic idea is to design and develop a sort of 'fractal' and 'hierarchical' elements that can be easily put together to form higher level modules/components (module that build modules) for structural and functional sensing, and tailored rehabilitation. Several ongoing researches might contribute to this trend. The European project EASY-IMP has as main objective development of wearable meta-products for rehabilitation in which the functionalities will be configured by the end-users. This infrastructure will enable creation of new services for smartphone and for EASY users, and 'infinite applications in many target market'. In European research project CareStore an open and flexible infrastructure for facilitating seamless deployment and integration of assisted living devices and applications on heterogeneous platforms without requiring intervention from technical staff is in deployment (Wagner et al., 2013).

Promising, low cost, non-invasive, unobtrusive technologies are continuously presented and comprehensive researches on the effectiveness and large scale implementation of these technologies are required. Each year, many of innovative designs and technologies (e.g. many developed applications based on mobile applications for physiotherapy) with potential gains for health care disappear, as a consequences of low incentive for integration of new technologies, outdate risk-based regulatory framework, inefficient business model, and insufficient training of health professionals and general population for active search and integration of new technologies in daily life. Regulation and standardization of the new technologies for in-home health care is a slow process, and should be adapted to increase velocity of disruptive innovations in-home health care, in order to incorporate elements such as software reliance and cost-benefits analysis.

CONCLUSION

There is no lack of imagination for how to supply in-home physiotherapy and evidence exists on what and when physiotherapy intervention is more suited for better quality of service and cost-effectiveness of intervention. Small-scale efforts, pilot projects, and high level of evidence are increasing. There is a trend toward using feasible and acceptable in-home physiotherapy interventions combined with emerging ICT. Rigorous design of the in-home physiotherapy service incorporating ICT may lead to operational improvement and positive program outcome, augmented physiotherapists-patient relationships, autonomy and engagement of patients in regards to their healthcare. Also, this will provide environment for developing personalized, preventive, predictive and participatory physiotherapy, which will revolutionize healthcare management. ICT for in-home physiotherapy can contribute for integrated care programs (either vertically within healthcare system with continuing care, long-term care and self-management care or horizontal integration self-management care, nursing care, psychotherapy etc.). Training health care teams, informal caregivers and patients, to raise awareness and knowledge on information and communication technologies will greatly contribute for better in-home physiotherapy services and improve quality of life of patients receiving health care in-home setting. Researches should be made: for continuously description of what is known about the safety, feasibility and effectiveness of various in-home physiotherapy interventions; for dynamic adaptation of physiotherapy service in order to integrate multiple types of technologies for person-centered care in-home physiotherapy; and innovative financing mechanisms for in-home physiotherapy tools and services. Collaboration is needed (between public authorities, ICT providers, associations of physiotherapists and other health professionals, patient organizations, reimbursement scheme providers, insurer, medical devices and information technology regulatory organizations) for large-scale deployment of evidenced based in-home physiotherapy, and transferability of the results to other physiotherapy interventions.

REFERENCES

Adie, K., Schofield, C., Berrow, M., Wingham, J., Freeman, J., Humfryes, J., & Pritchard, C. (2014). Does the use of Nintendo Wii Sports improve arm function and is it acceptable to patients after stroke? Publication of the Protocol of the Trial of Wii in Stroke - TWIST. *International Journal of General Medicine*, 7(1), 475–481. doi:10.2147/IJGM.S65379 PMID:25336985

Al-Jundi, W., Madbak, K., Beard, J. D., Nawaz, S., & Tew, G. A. (2013). Systematic review of home-based exercise programmes for individuals with intermittent claudication. *European Journal of Vascular and Endovascular Surgery*, *46*(6), 690–706. doi:10.1016/j.ejvs.2013.09.004 PMID:24076079

Alliance for Home Health Quality & Innovation. (2014). *The Future of Home Health Care Project*. Retrieved August, 2015, from http://www.ahhqi.org/images/pdf/future-whitepaper.pdf

Anderson, G., & Hussey, P. (2001). Comparing health system performance in OECD countries. *Health Affairs*, *20*(3), 219–232. doi:10.1377/hlthaff.20.3.219 PMID:11585171

Anderson, L., & Taylor, R. S. (2014). Cardiac rehabilitation for people with heart disease: An overview of Cohrane systematic reviews. *Cochrane Database of Systematic Reviews*, *12*, CD011273. PMID:25503364

Barello, S., & Graffigna, G. (2015). Patient engagement in healthcare: Pathways for effective medical decision-making. *Neuropsychological Trend*, *17*(17), 53–65. doi:10.7358/neur-2015-017-bare

Barzel, A., Ketels, G., Tetzlaff, B., Krüger, H., Haevernick, K., Daubmann, A., & Scherer, M. et al. (2013). Enhancing activities of daily living of chronic stroke patients in primary health care by modified constraint-induced movement therapy (HOMECIMT): Study protocol for a cluster randomized controlled trial. *Trials*, *14*, 334. PMID:24124993

Beratarrechea, A., Lee, A. G., Willner, J. M., Jahangir, E., Ciapponi, A., & Rubinstein, A. (2014). The impact of mobile health interventions on chronic disease outcomes in developing countries: A systematic review. *Telemedicine Journal and e-Health*, *20*(1), 75–82. doi:10.1089/tmj.2012.0328 PMID:24205809

Boyd, R. N., Mitchell, L. E., James, S. T., Ziviani, J., Sakzewski, L., Smith, A., & Scuffham, P. A. et al. (2013). Move it to improve it (Mitii): Study protocol of a randomised controlled trial of a novel web-based multimodal training program for children and adolescents with cerebral palsy. *BMJ Open*, *3*(4), 4. doi:10.1136/bmjopen-2013-002853 PMID:23578686

Broetz, D., & Birbaumer, N. (2013). Behavioral physiotherapy in post stroke rehabilitation. *NeuroRehabilitation*, *33*, 377–384. PMID:23949069

Bujnowska-Fedak, M. M., & Kurpas, D. (2015). The influence of online health information on the attitude and behavior of people Aged 50. *Advances in Experimental Medicine and Biology*, *861*, 1–17. doi:10.1007/5584_2015_130 PMID:26017724

Burton, E., Lewin, G., Clemson, L., & Boldy, D. (2013). Effectiveness of a lifestyle exercise program for older people receiving a restorative home care service: Pragmatic randomized controlled trial. *Clinical Interventions in Aging*, *8*, 1591–1601. doi:10.2147/CIA.S44614 PMID:24324331

Cancela, J., Moreno, E. M., Arredondo, M. T., & Bonato, P. (2014) Designing auditory cues for Parkinson's disease gait rehabilitation. *Proceedings IEEE Engineering in Medicine and Biology Society* (pp. 5852-5855).

Chan, Y., Wang, T., Chang, C., Chen, L., Chu, H., Lin, S., & Chang, S. (2015). Short-term effects of self-massage combined with home exercise on pain, daily activity, and autonomic function in patients with myofascial pain dysfunction syndrome. *Journal of Physical Therapy Science*, *27*(1), 217–221. doi:10.1589/jpts.27.217 PMID:25642077

Chien, C. L., Lee, C. M., Wu, Y. W., Chen, T. A., & Wu, Y. T. (2008). Home-based exercise increases capacity but not quality of life in people with chronic heart failure: A systematic review. *The Australian Journal of Physiotherapy, 54*(2), 87–93. doi:10.1016/S0004-9514(08)70041-2 PMID:18491999

Cinel, C., Poli, R., Citi, L., & Robertson, D. (2013). An exploration of the effects of audio-visual entrainment on Parkinson's disease tremor. *Proceedings IEEE EMBS Conference on Neural Engineering* (pp. 1562-1565).

Close, J. C., Wesson, J., Sherrington, C., Hill, K. D., Kurrle, S., Lord, S. R., & Clemson, L. et al. (2014). Can a tailored exercise and home hazard reduction program reduce the rate of falls in community dwelling older people with cognitive impairment: Protocol paper for the i-FOCIS randomised controlled trial. *BMC Geriatrics, 14*(89), 1–14. PMID:25128411

Coulter, A. (2005). What do patients and the public want from primary care? *BMJ (Clinical Research Ed.), 331*(7526), 1199–1201. doi:10.1136/bmj.331.7526.1199 PMID:16293845

Coulter, A., & Magee, H. (2003). *The European patient of the future*. McGraw Hill Education.

Coulter, C. L., Scarvell, J. M., Neeman, T. M., & Smith, P. N. (2013). Physiotherapist-directed rehabilitation exercises in the outpatient or home setting improve strength, gait speed and cadence after elective total hip replacement: A systematic review. *Journal of Physiotherapy, 59*(4), 219–226. doi:10.1016/S1836-9553(13)70198-X PMID:24287215

Crocker, T., Young, J., Forster, A., Brown, L., Ozer, S., & Greenwood, D. C. (2013). The effect of physical rehabilitation on activities of daily living in older residents of long-term care facilities: Systematic review with meta-analysis. *Age and Ageing, 42*(6), 682–688. doi:10.1093/ageing/aft133 PMID:24004604

Ferguson, T. (2007). *E-Patients: How they can help us heal healthcare*. Retrieved from http://e-patients.net/e-Patients_White_Paper.pdf

Fischer, G. (2012). Context-Aware Systems -The 'right' information, at the 'right' time, in the 'right' place, in the 'right' way, to the 'right' person. In G. Tortora, S. Levialdi, & M. Tucci (Eds.), *Proceedings of the Conference on Advanced Visual Interfaces (AVI 2012),* Capri, Italy (pp. 287-294). ACM.

Gartner Inc. (2015). *Gartner's 2015 hype cycle for emerging technologies identifies the computing innovations that organizations should monitor*. Retrieved from http://www.gartner.com/newsroom/id/3114217

Gee, P. M., Paterniti, D. A., Ward, D., & Soederberg Miller, L. M. (2015). e-Patients Perceptions of Using Personal Health Records for self-management Support of Chronic Illness. *Computers, Informatics, Nursing, 33*(6), 229–237. doi:10.1097/CIN.0000000000000151 PMID:25899440

Giangregorio, L. M., Thabane, L., Adachi, J. D., Ashe, M. C., Bleakney, R. R., Braun, E. A., & Papaioannou, A. et al. (2014). Build better bones with exercise: Protocol for a feasibility study of a multicenter randomized controlled trial of 12 months of home exercise in women with a vertebral fracture. *Physical Therapy, 94*(9), 1337–1352. doi:10.2522/ptj.20130625 PMID:24786946

Glasgow, R. E. (2013). *Reach, Effectiveness, Adoption, Implementation, and Maintenance (RE-AIM)*. Retrieved from http://www.re-aim.hnfe.vt.edu/presentations/glasgow2013presentation.pdf

Grimmer, K., Luker, J., Beaton, K., Kumar, S., Crockett, A., & Price, K. (2013). Trialing individualized interventions to prevent functional decline in at-risk older adults (TRIIFL): Study protocol for a randomized controlled trial nested in a longitudinal observational study. *Trials, 14*(1), 266. doi:10.1186/1745-6215-14-266 PMID:23962259

Gschwind, Y. J., Kressig, R. W., Lacroix, A., Muehlbauer, T., Pfenninger, B., & Granacher, U. (2013). A best practice fall prevention exercise program to improve balance, strength / power, and psychosocial health in older adults: Study protocol for a randomized controlled trial. *BMC Geriatrics, 13*(1), 105. doi:10.1186/1471-2318-13-105 PMID:24106864

Gubbi, J., Buyya, R., Marusic, S., & Palaniswami, M. (2013). Internet of Things (IoT): A vision, architectural elements, and future directions. *Future Generation Computer Systems, 29*(7), 1645–1660. doi:10.1016/j.future.2013.01.010

Gunn, H., Cattaneo, D., Finlayson, M., Freeman, J., & Sosnoff, J. J. (2014). Home or away? Choosing a setting for a falls-prevention program for people with multiple sclerosis. *International Journal of MS Care, 16*(4), 186–191. doi:10.7224/1537-2073.2014-058 PMID:25694777

Hoerbst, A., & Ammenwerth, E. (2010). Electronic Health Records. A systematic review on quality requirements. *Methods of Information in Medicine, 49*(4), 320–336. doi:10.3414/ME10-01-0038 PMID:20603687

Hood, L. E., & Galas, D. J. (2008). *P4 Medicine: personalized, predictive, preventive, participatory. A change of view that changes everything.* Washington: Computing Community Consortium. Retrieved from http://cra.org/ccc/wp-content/uploads/sites/2/2015/05/P4_Medicine.pdf

Imbeault-Nepton, I., & Otis, M. J. D. (2014). Synchronized walking cadence for TUG in perturbed environments: using Earcon or Tacton cues? *Proceedings of IEEE Internation Symposium on Haptic, Audio and Visual Environments and Games (HAVE)* (pp. 41-46). doi:10.1109/HAVE.2014.6954329

International Telecommunication Union. (2015). *The World Telecommunication/ICT Indicators Database.* Retrieved from http://www.itu.int/en/ITU-D/Statistics/Pages/stat/default.aspx

Irizarry, T., DeVito Dabbs, A., & Curran, C. R. (2015). Patient portals and patient engagement: A state of the science review. *Journal of Medical Internet Research, 17*(6), e148. doi:10.2196/jmir.4255 PMID:26104044

Jaggers, J. R., Dudgeon, W., Blair, S. N., Sui, X., Burgess, S., Wilcox, S., & Hand, G. A. (2013). A home-based exercise intervention to increase physical activity among people living with HIV: Study design of a randomized clinical trial. *BMC Public Health, 13*(1), 502. doi:10.1186/1471-2458-13-502 PMID:23706094

Jolly, K., Taylor, R., Lip, G. Y. H., Greenfield, S., Raftery, J., Mant, J., & Stevens, A. et al. (2007). The Birmingham Rehabilitation Uptake Maximisation Study (BRUM). Homebased compared with hospital-based cardiac rehabilitation in a multi-ethnic population: Cost-effectiveness and patient adherence. *Health Technology Assessment, 11*(35), 1–118. doi:10.3310/hta11350 PMID:17767899

Jull, G., & Moore, A. (2013). Manual Therapy. *Manual Therapy, 18*(6), 447–448. doi:10.1016/j.math.2013.09.006 PMID:24188381

Kaye, R., Kokia, E., Shalev, V., Idar, D., & Chinitz, D. (2010). Barriers and success factors in health information technology: A practitioner's perspective. *Journal of Management & Marketing in Healthcare, 3*(2), 163–175. doi:10.1179/175330310X12736577732764

Kent, P., Laird, R., & Haines, T. (2015). The effect of changing movement and posture using motion-sensor biofeedback, versus guidelines-based care, on the clinical outcomes of people with sub-acute or chronic low back pain-a multicentre, cluster-randomised, placebo-controlled, pilot trial. *BMC Musculoskeletal Disorders, 16*(1), 131. doi:10.1186/s12891-015-0591-5 PMID:26022102

Kraal, J. J., Peek, N., van den Akker-Van Marle, M. E., & Kemps, H. M. (2013). Effects and costs of home-based training with telemonitoring guidance in low to moderate risk patients entering cardiac rehabilitation: The FIT@Home study. *BMC Cardiovascular Disorders, 13*(1), 82. doi:10.1186/1471-2261-13-82 PMID:24103384

Lee, H. N., Lee, S. Y., Lee, Y. S., Han, J. Y., Choo, M. S., & Lee, K. S. (2013). Pelvic floor muscle training using an extracorporeal biofeedback device for female stress urinary incontinence. *International Urogenicology Journal, 24*(5), 831–838. doi:10.1007/s00192-012-1943-4 PMID:23052631

Linder, S. M., Rosenfeldt, A. B., Reiss, A., Buchanan, S., Sahu, K., Bay, C. R., & Alberts, J. L. et al. (2013). The home stroke rehabilitation and monitoring system trial: A randomized controlled trial. *International Journal of Stroke, 8*(1), 46–53. doi:10.1111/j.1747-4949.2012.00971.x PMID:23280269

Lommi, M., Matarese, M., Alvaro, R., Piredda, M., & De Marinis, M. G. (2015). The experiences of self-care in community-dwelling older people: A meta-synthesis. *International Journal of Nursing Studies, 52*(12), 1854–1867. doi:10.1016/j.ijnurstu.2015.06.012 PMID:26296653

McAuley, E., Wójcicki, T. R., Gothe, N. P., Mailey, E. L., Szabo, A. N., Fanning, J., & Mullen, S. P. et al. (2013). Effects of a DVD-delivered exercise intervention on physical function in older adults. *The Journals of Gerontology. Series A, Biological Sciences and Medical Sciences, 68*(9), 1076–1082. doi:10.1093/gerona/glt014 PMID:23401566

Mehta, S. P., & Roy, J. S. (2011). Systematic revie of home physiotherapy after hip fracture surgery. *Journal of Rehabilitation Medicine, 43*(6), 477–480. doi:10.2340/16501977-0808 PMID:21491074

Mhatre, P. V., Vilares, I., Stibb, S. M., Albert, M. V., Pickering, L., Marciniak, C. M., & Toledo, S. et al. (2013). Wii Fit balance board playing improves balance and gait in Parkinson disease. *PM & R, 5*(9), 769–777. doi:10.1016/j.pmrj.2013.05.019 PMID:23770422

Mortazavi, B., Nyamathi, S., Lee, S. I., Wilkerson, T., Ghasemzadeh, H., & Sarrafzadeh, M. (2014). Near-realistic mobile exergames with wireless wearable sensors. *Biomedical and Health Informatics. IEEE Journal of, 18*(2), 449–456.

Naylor, C., Parsonage, M., McDaid, D., Knap, M., Fossey, M., & Galea, A. (2012). *Long-term conditions and mental health. The cost of co-morbidities.* The Kings Fund Report. Retrieved from http://www.kingsfund.org.uk/sites/files/kf/field/field_publication_file/long-term-conditions-mental-health-cost-comorbidities-naylor-feb12.pdf

Nhavoto, J. A., & Gronlund, A. (2014). Mobile technologies and geographic information systems to improve health care systems: A literature review. *JMIR Mhealth and Uhealth, 2*(2), e21. doi:10.2196/mhealth.3216 PMID:25099368

Novak, I. (2011). Effective home programme intervention for adults: A systematic review. *Clinical Rehabilitation, 25*(12), 1066–1085. doi:10.1177/0269215511410727 PMID:21831927

Omran, A. R. (2005). First published 1971). The epidemiological transition: A theory of the epidemiology of population change. *The Milbank Quarterly, 83*(4), 731–757. doi:10.1111/j.1468-0009.2005.00398.x PMID:16279965

Ontario, H. Q. (2013). In-home care for optimizing chronic disease management in the community: An evidence-based analysis. *Ontario Health Technology Assessment Series, 13*(5), 1–65. PMID:24167539

Outpatient Service Trialists. (2004). Rehabilitation therapy services for stroke patients living at home: Systematic review of randomized trials. *Lancet, 363*(9406), 352–356. doi:10.1016/S0140-6736(04)15434-2 PMID:15070563

Papalia, R., Vasta, S., Tecame, A., D'Adamio, S., Maffulli, N., & Denaro, V. (2013). Home-based vs supervised rehabilitation programs following knee surgery: A systematic review. *British Medical Bulletin, 108*(1), 55–72. doi:10.1093/bmb/ldt014 PMID:23690452

Pepa, L., Ciabattoni, L., Verdini, F., Capecci, M., & Ceravolo, M. G. (2014). Smartphone based fuzzy logic freezing of gait detection in Parkinson's disease. *Proceeding IEEE/ASME Conference on Mechatronic and Embedded Systems and Applications (MESA)* (pp. 1-6).

Postolache, G., Girao, P. S., & Postolache, O. (2013). Requirements and barriers to pervasive health adoption. In S. C. Mukhopadhyay & O. A. Postolache (Eds.), *Pervasive and Mobile Sensing and Computing for Health Care. Technological and Social Issues* (pp. 315–352). Springer Verlag. doi:10.1007/978-3-642-32538-0_15

Rechel, B., Doyle, Y., Grundy, E., & McKee, M. (2009). *Policy brief. 10 Health system and policy analysis. How can health system respond to population ageing?* WHO Report. Retrieved from http://www.euro.who.int/__data/assets/pdf_file/0004/64966/E92560.pdf

Rodger, M. W., Young, W. R., & Craig, C. M. (2014). Synthesis of walking sounds for alleviating gait disturbances in Parkinson's. *IEEE Transactions on Neural Systems and Rehabilitation Engineering, 22*(3), 543–548. doi:10.1109/TNSRE.2013.2285410 PMID:24235275

Siemonsma, P., Döpp, C., Alpay, L., Tak, E., van Meeteren, N., & Chorus, A. (2014). Determinants influencing the implementation of home-based stroke rehabilitation: A systematic review. *Disability and Rehabilitation, 36*(24), 2019–2030. doi:10.3109/09638288.2014.885091 PMID:24520957

Sinclair, J., Hingston, P., & Masek, M. (2007). Considerations for the design of exergames. *Proceeding GRAPHITE'07 International Conference on Computer Graphics and Interactive Techniques in Australia and Southeast Asia* (pp. 289-295). doi:10.1145/1321261.1321313

Srikesavan, C. S., Shay, B., Robinson, D. B., & Szturm, T. (2013). Task-oriented training with computer gaming in people with rheumatoid arthritisor osteoarthritis of the hand: Study protocol of a randomized controlled pilot trial. *Trials*, *14*(1), 69. doi:10.1186/1745-6215-14-69 PMID:23497529

Stange, K. C., Nutting, P. A., Miller, W. L., Jaén, C. R., Crabtree, B. F., Flocke, S. A., & Gill, J. M. (2010). Defining and measuring the patient-centered medical home. *Journal of General Internal Medicine*, *25*(6), 601–612. doi:10.1007/s11606-010-1291-3 PMID:20467909

Takekawa, T., Abo, M., Ebihara, K., Taguchi, K., Sase, Y., & Kakuda, W. (2013). Long-term effects of injection of botulinum toxin type A combined with home-based functional training for post-stroke patients with spastic upper limb hemiparesis. *Acta Neurologica Belgica*, *113*(4), 469–475. doi:10.1007/s13760-013-0208-4 PMID:23716062

Thomas, M. J., Simpson, J., Riley, R., & Grant, E. (2010). The impact of home-based physiotherapy interventions on breathlessness during activities of daily living in severe COPD: A systematic review. *Physiotherapy*, *96*(2), 108–119. doi:10.1016/j.physio.2009.09.006 PMID:20420957

Thomas, S., Fazakarley, L., Thomas, P. W., Brenton, S., Collyer, S., Perring, S., & Hillier, C. et al. (2014). Testing the feasibility and acceptability of using the Nintendo Wii in the home to increase activity levels, vitality and well-being in people with multiple sclerosis (Mii-vitaliSe): Protocol for a pilot randomised controlled study. *BMJ Open*, *4*(5), e005172. doi:10.1136/bmjopen-2014-005172 PMID:24812193

Tousignant, M., Corriveau, H., Kairy, D., Berg, K., Dubois, M. F., Gosselin, S., & Danells, C. et al. (2014). Tai Chi-based exercise program provided via telerehabilitation compared to home visits in a post-stroke population who have returned home without intensive rehabilitation: Study protocol for a randomized, non-inferiority clinical trial. *Trials*, *15*(1), 42. doi:10.1186/1745-6215-15-42 PMID:24479760

Tractica. (2015). *Home health technologies, medical monitoring and management, remote consultations, eldercare, and health and wellness applications: Global market analysis and forecast*. Retrieved August, 2015, from https://www.tractica.com/research/home-health-technologies/

Triberti, S., Barello, S., Graffigna, G., Riva, G., Candelieri, A., & Archetti, F. (2014). Evaluating patient engagement and user experience of a positive technology intervention: the H-CIM case. In G. Graffigna, S. Barello, & S. Triberti (Eds.), *Patient Engagement. A consumer Centered Model to Innovate Healthcare* (pp. 66–77). De Gruyter Open.

Triberti, S., & Riva, G. (2014a). Positive technology for enhancing the patient engagement experiences. In G. Graffigna, S. Barello, & S. Triberti (Eds.), *Patient Engagement. A consumer Centered Model to Innovate Healthcare* (pp. 44–55). De Gruyter Open.

Triberti, S., & Riva, G. (2014b). Engaging users to design positive technologies for patient engagement: the perfect interaction model. In G. Graffigna, S. Barello, & S. Triberti (Eds.), *Patient Engagement. A consumer Centered Model to Innovate Healthcare* (pp. 56–65). De Gruyter Open.

Tzallas, A. T., Tsipouras, M. G., Rigas, G., Tsalikakis, D. G., Karvounis, E. C., Chondrogiorgi, M., & Fotiadis, D. I. et al. (2014). PERFORM: A system for monitoring, assessment and management of patients with Parkinson's disease. *Sensors (Basel)*, *14*(11), 21329–21357. doi:10.3390/s141121329 PMID:25393786

Valdes, K., Naughton, N., & Michlovitz, S. (2014). Therapist supervised clinic-based therapy versus instruction in a home program following distal radius fracture: A systematic review. *Journal of Hand Therapy, 27*(3), 165–174. doi:10.1016/j.jht.2013.12.010 PMID:24508093

Wagner, S., Hansen, F. O., Pedersen, C. F., Memon, M., Aysha, F. H., Mathissen, M., & Wesby, O. L. et al. (2013). CareStore Platform for seamless deployment of ambient assited living applications and devices. *Proceedings of International Conference on Pervasive Computing Technologies for Healthcare and Workshops* (pp. 240-243).

Williams, T., & Samarth, A. (2011). *Electronic Health Records for Dummies*. Hobokem, NJ: Wiley Publishing, Inc.

Zhao, Y., Anhalt, F., Fietzek, U. M., & D'Angelo, L. T. (2013). Multi-cue unit: An independent device and actuator of a wearable system for gait-support in Parkinson patients. *Proceedings of IEEE International Conference on Microwaves, Communications, Antennas and Electronics Systems (COMCAS)* (pp. 1-5). doi:10.1109/COMCAS.2013.6685287

KEY TERMS AND DEFINITIONS

Biofeedback: Process that enables an individual to learn how to change body signals for the purposes of improving health and performance. It is necessary a precise measurement of body function and rapidly and accurately "feedback" information to the user. The presentation of this information supports desired function changes. Some recent examples of biofeedback use in physiotherapy are: extracorporeal biofeedback for female stress urinary incontinence, motion-sensor biofeedback in people with low back pain reduced pain and activity limitation.

E-Patients: Also known as Internet patient, is a health consumer who uses the Internet to gather information about a medical condition of particular interest to him, and who uses electronic communication tools (including Web 2.0 tools) in coping with medical conditions. The term encompasses both those who seek online guidance for their own ailments and the friends and family members (e-Caregivers) who go online on their behalf. Tom Ferguson have coined in 2007 E-Patients as individuals who are equipped, enabled, empowered and engaged in their health and health care decisions. E-Patients report two effects of their online health research – 'better health information and services, and different (but not always better) relationship with their doctors". PatientLikeMe, BrainTalk Communities, NeuroTalk are E-Patients social networks. The importance of E-Patients as consumer, curators and creators of information, are recently recognized and investigated. Understanding the frequency and characteristics of pronetariat (term coined by Joel de Rosnay, in 2005) in E-Patient group will be interesting.

Exergame: Term used for video games that are also a form of exercise. In context of health services, the term can be found also as Serious Game or Teragame – software or hardware based on interactive game, designed for the purpose of solving a problem, to train or educate users. Although serious games can be entertaining, their main purpose is more for training or education of the users. Serious game will sometimes deliberately sacrifice fun and entertainment in order to achieve a desired progress by the player. Exergames based on Nintendo Wii ™ technology were among the first games used on rehabilitation.

Various games are now developed for Xbox Kinect technology, for smartphone (e.g. games apps from Google play and ITune store), or commercialized together with software for rehabilitation management (e.g. MIRARehab, BioGaming).

Information and Communication Technologies (ICT): Set of technologies that arise from information and advanced telecommunication and multi-media techniques which allow better communication means, information processing, storing, exchange and dissemination (adapted from OQLF/French wikipedia). ICT stresses the role of unified communications and the integration of telecommunications (telephone lines and wireless communication), Internet, multimedia, computers as well as necessary enterprise software, middleware, storage, and audio-visual systems, which enable users to access, store, transmit, and manipulate information through various means: text, video, audio, human-machine interface, etc.

Internet of Things (IoT): (Sometimes *Internet of Everything*). Was first coined by Kevin Ashton in 1999 in the context of supply chain management. However, in the past decade, the definition has been more inclusive covering wide range of applications like healthcare, utilities, transport, etc. Although the definition of 'Things' has changed as technology evolved, the main goal of making computer sense information without the aid of human intervention remains the same. It means a network of physical objects or "things" embedded with electronics, software, sensors and connectivity that enable it to achieve greater value and service by exchanging data with the manufacturer, operator and/or other connected devices based on the infrastructure of International Telecommunication Union's Global Standards Initiative. Each thing is uniquely identifiable through its embedded computing system, but is able to interoperate within the existing Internet infrastructure. Typically, IoT is expected to offer advanced connectivity of devices, systems, and services that goes beyond machine-to-machine communications (M2M) and covers a variety of protocols, domains, and applications. The interconnection of these embedded devices (including smart objects), is expected to usher in automation in nearly all fields, and expanding to the areas such as smart city.

PHRs: Health data and information related to the care of a patient is maintained by the patient. PHRs can be broadly described as a set of electronic tools that allow consumers to access, coordinate, and control appropriate parts of their health information. PHRs combine not only data, but knowledge and software tools, which motivate patients to become more involved in their healthcare. A PHR should typically present a comprehensive and precise review of the health and medical history of the individual patient through the collection of information from a variety of sources. PHRs, whether through patient portals, electronic downloads onto a personal USB drive, or through a company sponsored Web site (e.g. MyAlert, HealthKit iOS), allow patients timely access to their medical information. According HL7 standard PHRs shall: allow for historical clinical data and current state data management; assist the PHRs account holder to manage his or her compliance with medications and facilitate communication of his or her adherence to designed individuals; manage health education; support wellness, preventive medicine and self-care; support decision making; manage encounters with healthcare providers. Since it is retained, maintained and controlled by the consumer, the PHR positions the consumer at the core of the healthcare process, potentially fostering personal empowerment and facilitating self-management or quantified self, shared decision making and better clinical outcomes.

Virtual Reality (VT): Is computer based interactive, visual, and/or audio, and/or haptic (interaction involving touch), and/or immersive (providing information or stimulation for a number of senses, not only sight and sound, that deeply involve one's senses and may change mental state) simulation of real, imaginary or symbolic environment. The term virtual is used with meaning of digital, immaterial, 'quasi' real. There are many types of VR environments, from simple computer based games played on a computer, tablet, smartphone, TV screen with a mouse or other interface (e.g. MIRARehab, YouRehab, CoRehab, I Am a Dolphin apps developed by John Hopkins Hospital, PocketPhysio, Hand Rehab, Button Board apps for smartphone, Nintendo Wii, Xbox Kinect, PlayStation games, SecondLife) to lifelike scenarios created in a large space in which the user sees the environment all around them (INJOY Quality Cooperation GmbH, Realyz-Mobilyz, CAVE, Icube, SASCube). By contrast, with virtual reality that replaces the real world with a simulated one in augmented reality, real, physical world can be seen directly or indirectly together with augmentation (computer-generation sensory input such as sound, video, graphics, GPS data). For instance, the developed software for Augmedix healthcare service, or Kinesio Capture apps for smartphone use augmented reality. Mixed Reality, a mix of the physical and virtual reality, refers to the merging of real and virtual worlds to produce new environments and visualizations where physical and digital objects co-exist and interact in real time. Windows Holographyc is a mixed reality computing platform developed by Microsoft. Various interfaces were developed for interaction with virtual reality – Leap Motion, Microsoft Kinect, Nimble from Intugine Technologies, Wii Remote, Wii Balance Board, iKids Interactive Zone, Gloveone, Fit Interactive's fitness system 3 Kick, Virtuix Omni, Oculos Rift, Samsung Gear VR, ZSpace, Google Cardboard, Epson Moverio BT-200, Microsoft Hololens).

This research was previously published in Transformative Healthcare Practice through Patient Engagement edited by Guendalina Graffigna, pages 215-246, copyright year 2017 by Medical Information Science Reference (an imprint of IGI Global).

Chapter 46
From Healthcare Services to E-Health Applications:
A Delivery System-Based Taxonomy

Riccardo Spinelli
University of Genoa, Italy

Clara Benevolo
University of Genoa, Italy

ABSTRACT

The increasing adoption of ICT – and especially Internet-based technologies – in healthcare has been very fruitful and has led to the innovative approach to healthcare practice commonly known as e-health. However, the boundaries of this new approach to healthcare are not clear, as it is reflected by the various properties and taxonomies of e-health applications which have been proposed. In this chapter, we first review the definition of e-health and the main taxonomies for its constituents. Then we propose an original taxonomy for e-health applications, based on the structural features of the delivery system of the services which are digitalized: the need for a physical interaction between the subjects involved in the service provisioning and the possibility of delivering the services through Internet-based technology.

INTRODUCTION

The advent of the so-called "ICT revolution" can be undoubtedly considered a turning point in economic history, due to the strong impact it has had on the structure of the economic system and on the way business is done. Many authors – see, among others, Castells (2000), Porter (2001) and Burman (2003) – have theorized the progression from the traditional industrial economic paradigm to the so-called "digital economy", stressing the central role that digital technologies and ICT play in this progression. Underlying this shift in paradigms has been the increasing digitalization of information – that is the process of representing any kind of information as a sequence of *bit*, that is *binary digits* – which has come into conflict with real world processes that remained substantially analog-based (Tocci, 1988) and not always reducible to binary storage. However, modern digital technologies allow for an accurate digitalization of

DOI: 10.4018/978-1-5225-3926-1.ch046

information from many different sources (words, sounds, images, etc.), with minimum loss of the processed information. In other words, more and more typologies of data and information can be properly turned to the digital format or, in short, "digitalized" (Aldrich & Masera, 1999). If digital technologies have enhanced the possibility of processing information more efficiently and effectively, it is thanks to ICT – and especially to Internet-based technologies – that digital information can be transmitted and shared, dramatically increasing its value and its contribution to economic activities.

This process has certainly involved healthcare services too; in fact, the increasing adoption of ICT and Internet-based technologies in that industry has been very fruitful and has led to the innovative approach to healthcare services commonly known as e-health. With respect to this concept, literature is not consistent, as several definitions have been proposed together with just as many taxonomies and classification schemes. Taxonomy studies does not only help to better understand phenomena, but also provide tools to categorize concepts in a field: indeed a taxonomic tool is one of the basic tools in the development of scientific knowledge, as such systems aid in research by helping to identify unexplored phenomena and providing a context for their relationship with other aspects of the environment (Tulu et al., 2007). At present, proposed taxonomies for e-health activities are quite heterogeneous and allow for just a partial view on such a complex phenomenon. As a consequence, to fully appreciate the origins, the structure and the great potential of e-health applications we propose to trace them back to a more general phenomenon, that is the Internet-driven digitalization of services. Healthcare activities, in fact, are part of the wider area of service industries, which have been deeply changed and redesigned by the possibility of performing their delivery through Internet-based technologies.

The main objective of this chapter is therefore to propose an original taxonomy for e-health activities, built around the characteristics of the delivery system of healthcare services; by doing so, it is possible to understand the way in which healthcare activities evolved towards a new digital configuration and to speculate about their potential future development.

To this purpose, we first place the healthcare industry within a wider framework of the digital economy; then we move to a closer analysis of the e-health construct and components. Afterwards we introduce a classification model for services in accordance with their characteristics and their delivery modes. This scheme is then applied to the healthcare industry, to get to a classification scheme which gathers e-health applications into homogeneous groups built around the features of their delivery systems and, consequently, to the way in which they have evolved towards their new digital structure. Finally, we propose some reflections on future technology-driven trends which could affect the healthcare industry.

BACKGROUND

In this section we first present some considerations on the role of healthcare industry within the new economic paradigm of the digital economy, useful to encompass the e-health development within a more comprehensive framework. A definition for e-health is later proposed, which embraces the most relevant elements of this phenomenon; then, the main objectives associated with the development of e-health are illustrated, to show its great potential in terms of efficiency, effectiveness, innovation and relationships. Finally, the issue of e-health taxonomies is introduced.

Healthcare Industry and the Digital Economy

Atkinson and McKay (2007) state that the digital economy "represents the pervasive use of ICT (hardware, software, applications and telecommunications) in all aspects of the economy, including internal operations of organizations (business, government and non-profit); transactions between organizations; and transactions between individuals, acting both as consumers and citizens, and organizations" (p. 7). We certainly recognize the value of this technology-focused definition; nevertheless, the advent of the digital economy has not only a technological origin, but is the result of complex dynamics in the economic system, both on the supply and demand side (Spinelli, 2008), which – together with the innovation in ICT – contribute to shape the new economic paradigm. Consider, in particular, the increasing dematerialization of the economy, namely the complex evolution from material to immaterial, from the preeminence of physical transformation to the prominence of information and knowledge creation; this trend dates back to much earlier than the advent of the ICT revolution: the progressive digitalization of goods and services has historical roots, even if it gained new momentum when ICT made it much easier their transmission and communication. Furthermore, digital technologies – thanks to automation – made information available to manage and govern business processes.

The consequences of the evolution from the traditional to the digital economy are deep and involve almost every aspect of economic activities. In this chapter, the attention is focused on how the development of the digital economy influences one of the most important service sectors that is the healthcare industry.

Over the last decades, the economic scenario and the structural and operative conditions of service firms have deeply changed. First, deregulation, liberalization and globalization processes have had an impact on the general environment; the healthcare industry has been certainly involved in this processes, even if the industry has been "partially protected" by some structural peculiarities (in particular the significant presence of national public operators along with national public policies and regulations) which have kept it somewhat protected from the new and more intense forms of competition. Then, industrialization, digitalization, IT networks, evolution in communication and transport, virtualization and demand-side changes have strongly modified the way of conceiving, producing and delivering services (Javalgi, Martin, & Todd, 2004; Rahman, 2004). In particular, "the industrialization of at least some processes and the digitalization of information [have changed] the options about 'how' to produce and deliver services (e.g. reducing the contact with the consumer) and 'where' (from a distance or across the borders of a country)" (Benevolo & Spinelli, 2011, p. 252).

Given this overall trend of development of the digital economy, its extent is still rather uneven on an industry basis. On industry specificities, Malecki and Moriset (2008, p. 6) use the metaphor of the "pyramid of the digital economy" (see Figure 1) to help identify four distinct groups of industries, that vary in terms of ICT diffusion.

Malecki and Moriset first consider what they call the "spearhead" of the pyramid, that is, the chips and processors industries which produce the basic components of all digital technologies. Below this lies the "core", including the computer and telecommunication industries, which we define as ICT in a narrow sense. The third level, the "main body", includes all fully ICT-enabled industries, that is, those manufacturing and service industries which rely heavily on ICT; we can cite here the great majority of the most relevant industries in the contemporary economy: automotive, high-tech mechanics, media and

Figure 1. The pyramid of the digital economy
Source: Adapted from Malecki and Moriset (2008, p. 6).

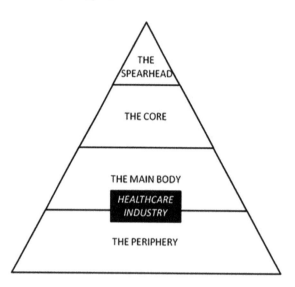

entertainment, business and financial services, and so on. The last group – at the base of the pyramid – is the "periphery", which comprises those sectors not yet or only partially, ICT-enabled or, in other words, where the use of ICT is still limited and not critical. Sectors traditionally included in this group are usually "old economy" ones, such as farming, fishing, mining, forestry or basic consumer and public services. However, examples of intense ICT use are present in these sectors as well, forerunners of a more widespread adoption still in progress. This explains why the boundary between the "main body" and the "periphery" is continuously moving down, as more and more industries reconfigure themselves through greater use of ICT in processes and in organizations.

Those industries belonging to the "spearhead" and the "core" are part of the "engine" of the ICT revolution, as they are the "main actors" of the revolution and drive the process. On the contrary, industries in the "main body" and the "periphery" perceive the ICT revolution as an exogenous factor influencing their general and competitive environment, being, in a way, "victims" of these forces.

In our opinion, the healthcare industry, is progressively entering the "main body" of the pyramid, due to the great changes caused by the pervasive application of ICT: as we are going to analyze in detail in the next sections, the structure of the organizations in this industry is being fundamentally re-shaped; new ways of taking care of the patients are becoming possible; public and private institutions are looking for new and more efficient ways to cooperate; the "consumer" (the patient or a friend or relative) is becoming more and more informed and therefore more active and demanding – in terms of convenience, control and choice (Ball & Lillis, 2001) – in the relationship with the healthcare system. The more innovative components of the industry have already been experiencing such a process, towards the so-called e-health: "ICT has already modified medical practice patterns extensively while facilitating coordination and close cooperation between health care professionals to improve patient management; it is already providing some solutions to the growing need for information and knowledge sharing" (Fieschi, 2002, p. 87). However, the more traditional components too – which are still in the "periphery" of the pyramid – will get soon to a new, more ICT-based, configuration.

Definition, Objectives and Contents of E-Health

Despite the frequency of use of the term, there does not appear to be a general consensus about the meaning of e-health. Many definitions have been proposed, but so far there has not been any universal agreement about what things might be excluded or included within the scope of the term (Showell & Nohr, 2012). Furthermore, terms such as e-health, telemedicine, and telehealth are quite often used interchangeably, although e-health is quickly becoming the most adopted (Fatehi & Wootton, 2012).

In general terms, e-health can be defined as "the use of emerging information and communications technology, especially the Internet, to improve or enable health and healthcare" (Eng, 2001). A more complex and widely accepted definition is provided by Eysenbach (2001), who defines e-health as:

an emerging field in the intersection of medical informatics, public health and business, referring to health services and information delivered or enhanced through the Internet and related technologies. In a broader sense, the term characterizes not only a technical development, but also a state-of-mind, a way of thinking, an attitude, and a commitment for networked, global thinking, to improve health care locally, regionally, and worldwide by using information and communication technology. (p. e20)

The core elements of Eysenbach (2001)'s definition are consistent with the four common perspectives that Sood et al. (2007) find in all 104 definitions of the term "telemedicine" they analyze:

- Medical perspective, which results into mentioning the provision of healthcare services;
- Technological perspective, when the role of ICT is stressed;
- Spatial perspective, which underlines the geographical separation between provider and recipient of medical information;
- Benefits perspective, when the positive repercussions on patients' quality of life are highlighted.

Several more definitions of e-health have been proposed in literature, as Oh et al. (2005) report. Their analysis of 51 definitions confirms that the term e-health encompasses a wide set of concepts, including health, technology, and commerce. A very important conclusion they come to is that "most commonly, the word health [is] used in relation to health services delivery which suggests that eHealth may refer more to services and systems rather than to the health of people"; furthermore, "health, as used in these definitions, usually [refers] explicitly to health care as a process, rather than to health as an outcome".

Moreover, a major importance is given to the communication between the subjects involved in health-care processes: patients and relatives/friends, hospitals, practitioners, local and central public authorities, private corporations, etc. With respect to this topic, we make reference to Pagliari et al. (2005), who – in another review of e-health definitions – find that:

the majority of definitions [...] specify the use of networked information and communications technologies, primarily the Internet, and digital data, thus differentiating eHealth from the broader field of medical informatics, which incorporates 'harder' technologies, such as scanning equipment, and bioinformatics research which tends to take place in isolation and is less directly applicable to health care service delivery. (p. 83)

Our interest in this topic – and the relevance of the study too – is justified by the great potential associated with the adoption of ICT in healthcare services (Commission of the European Communities, 2004; Stroetmann, Jones, Dobrev, & Stroetmann, 2006; WHO, 2006a & 2006b). Healthcare costs are growing at an unsustainable rate throughout much of the world, due to factors such as the aging process of population, the request for better and more effective healthcare services, the introduction of more sophisticated technologies in caretaking processes (Haux et al., 2002). In response, "many governments are taking steps to prod the health care industry to aggressively expand its use of IT" (Kennedy & Berk, 2011, p. 1).

In fact, an increasing number of studies show the potential benefits and limitations of multifunctional clinical ICT systems (Shekelle & Goldzweig, 2009; Buntin et al., 2011); even if data on cost and cost-effectiveness remains limited and a large gap between the postulated and empirically demonstrated benefits of e-health technologies is still present (Black et al., 2011), there is a general consensus that health ICT has the potential to dramatically transform healthcare.

According to the OECD (2010), the use of health information technology can improve the efficiency, cost-effectiveness, quality and safety of medical care delivery. Similarly, Osservatorio ICT in Sanità (2008) proposes another classification of e-health benefits for healthcare organizations, where four main drivers (divided into sub-drivers) of benefit from ICT application to healthcare processes are proposed (p. 19):

- Efficiency, declined into staff productivity, equipment usage, cost control;
- Quality, with respect to diagnosis, cure, clinical risk and processing time;
- Relationship, with both the patient (in terms of service personalization and access) and other organizations;
- Monitoring and control of the healthcare organization, which includes regulations accomplishment and the monitoring of performance and processes.

In our view, five broad inter-related categories of objectives for ICT implementation in healthcare industry arise from the wide literature on e-health (see Figure 2):

1. Reducing operating costs of clinical services;
2. Reducing administrative costs;
3. Increasing efficiency and quality of care;
4. Achieving wider interoperability and integration of health services
5. Enabling entirely new modes of care;

Objective 1 and 2 focus mainly on the efficiency gain obtainable through ICT application to core and ancillary healthcare activities. Nevertheless, this view alone would be quite reductive: "if greater investment in health IT simply automates a broken health care system, vital opportunities for transformation will be missed" (Frisse, 2009, p. w380). Objective 3, on the contrary, is centered on cost-effectiveness, quality and safety and is consequently more demanding than simply cutting expenses. It is worth underlying that this objective jointly focuses on two complementing elements: on the one side, the direct savings and quality improvements obtainable through a new ICT-intensive way of performing health-related activities; on the other side, the equally important indirect savings which derive from the more intensive and effective prevention initiatives which ICT make possible, for example the reduction of the incidence of chronic disease attributable to prevention. Indeed, the payoff of some types of preventive

Figure 2. The main objectives of e-health
Source: Constructed by the authors.

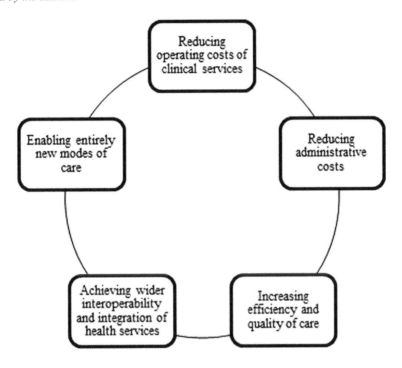

care, such as for diabetes and heart failure, can be very high, as they reduce the need for very expensive and long-term treatments. As regards Objective 4, the coordination and integration of the many subjects involved in the provisioning of healthcare services (patients and relatives, clinicians, hospitals, public administrations, etc.) could guarantee a further increase in both efficiency and effectiveness of the whole process, as "poor care coordination negatively affects patients — particularly those with multiple chronic conditions who account for an overwhelming proportion of [...] health care expenditures (O'Malley, 2011, p. 1090). As Safran (2003) highlights, "the next stage of collaborative business (for healthcare) is where cooperation among customers (individuals, families, and communities), suppliers (pharmaceutical, device manufacturers and medical supply companies), partners (national health systems, insurance companies and payers), and colleagues (physicians, nurses, other care providers, and support personnel) lets companies (health systems) do business in different and better ways" (p. 186). Of particular interest is the possibility of a shift of focus from the hospital to the patient's house as primary place of treatment, through patient empowerment and home monitoring techniques (Alpay et al., 2010). Finally, objective 5 casts light on the most innovative scenario, which is the development of new ways of taking care of people's health – again, with respect to both patient treatment and prevention – thanks to the comprehensive application of ICT to the whole care process, from the administrative side to the clinical one.

The limited consensus on the definition of e-health is reflected in a similarly limited consensus about its constituents: indeed several taxonomies are provided in literature, with the aim of classifying the many applications of ICT to healthcare. Usually the focus is twofold, because – together with actual applications – also potential ones are introduced, which could be consequence of the continuous technology innovation and the gradual overcoming of context-related limitations on the economic, managerial, organizational, legal and social side.

One of the first and more cited taxonomies of e-health applications was created in 2005 by the World Health Organization for the surveys of the *WHO Global Observatory for eHealth*. The list includes the following tools (WHO, 2006a, p. 15):

- Electronic health records, including patient's clinical history, test results, medication, etc.;
- Patient information systems, which contain information about a hospitalized patient and are used to support both the administrative and clinical activities in a hospital;
- Hospital information systems, that support information processing within a hospital in areas such as administration, appointments, billing, planning, budgeting and personnel;
- General practitioner information systems, that support the work of a general practitioner and often link to other health care systems such as billing, GP reimbursement or laboratory results reporting systems;
- National electronic registries, which contain data on specific medical subjects such as births, mortality, cancer, diabetes or other subjects of medical or epidemiological interest;
- National drug registries, containing national pharmaceutical information;
- Directories of healthcare professional and institutions;
- Decision support systems, that is automated or semi-automated systems that support decision-making in a clinical environment;
- Telehealth, which relate with the use of ICT to either support the provision of health care or as an alternative to direct professional care and encompasses telemedicine and the use of remote medical expertise;
- Geographical information systems, which capture, integrate, analyze and display data related to geographic coordinates.

The list does not pretend to be exhaustive but provides a general overview of the various areas in which the application of ICT to healthcare can contribute. Its main limit, in our view, is that tools are listed without a clear classification criterion and the resulting groups are very heterogeneous in width and potentially overlapping.

An alternative proposal is provided by Vincent et al. (2007), who suggest classifying what they call "telehealth technologies" according to the following features:

- The type of telehealth interaction, which indicates whether the patient is with a medical provider and how the communication is structured;
- The location of the controlling medical authority, which distinguishes whether the provider in charge of the patient care is with the patient or away from the patient;
- The urgency of care, which addresses whether the communication is for an emergent or non-emergent health issue;
- The timing of communication, which considers whether the communication is real-time (synchronous) or store-and-forward (asynchronous).

We find the proposed taxonomy quite promising, as it does not simply list applications but provides higher-level classification criteria which make reference to structural features of the adopted technologies and the provided service; by doing this, they introduce a tool that is potentially able to classify new applications which have not been developed yet. However, the chosen criteria seem to suffer from a lack of clarity – especially as regards the differences between the first two of the list – and risk to be only partially effective when trying to classify the wide variety of e-health applications.

Tulu et al. (2005, 2007) adopt a similar methodological approach in their proposed taxonomy for telemedicine activities. Their tool considers three main dimensions, which in turn include several classification criteria:

- Medical dimension, which includes two classification criteria
  - Application purpose (clinical and non-clinical applications)
  - Application area (among the main domains in the medical field such as cardiology, ophthalmology, home care, etc.)
- Delivery dimension, with three criteria
  - Environmental settings (the physical environment that the physician or the patient will be using during the telemedicine event, e.g. hospital, outreach clinic, health center, home, mobile, etc.)
  - Communication infrastructure (wired or wireless, with different technologies and bandwidth)
  - Delivery options (audio, video or data, in a synchronous or asynchronous way)
- Organizational dimension, focused on four areas of interest
  - Human resources
  - IT management
  - Cost, budget and financial issues
  - Legal, procedural and regulations issues

The proposed taxonomy – partially consistent with Vincent et al. (2007)'s one – certainly identifies critical dimensions for classifying e-health applications, but is in our view quite difficult to adopt due to its high level of granularity. Nine criteria are very difficult to jointly manage, so much that the Authors themselves do not consider the organizational dimension in the pilot applications they propose. More generally, the three dimensions are viewed in a hierarchical way, as the classification process should first consider application purpose and area, then move to the delivery dimension and finally focus on the organizational one. From our point of view, such an approach do not provide solution to one of the main aim a taxonomy should have, that is the creation of a finite number of categories into which it should be possible to encompass all the objects we want to classify. Indeed, in the examples the Authors list e-health applications providing a classification on a single criterion at a time, without crossing them.

A different and simpler approach is proposed in the process-centered taxonomy of the Polytechnic of Milan (Osservatorio ICT in Sanità, 2008); according to this classification, three major healthcare macro-processes can be identified, which are increasingly supported by ICT applications:

- Primary processes, directly related to the main steps in the process of caretaking of the patient: admission, diagnosis, treatment and discharge;
- Support processes to caretaking activities, such as quality and risk management, public relations, facility management, programming and controlling, human resource management, etc.;
- Network processes, associated with the whole assistance process in a broad sense; the perspective is the "continuing assistance" view, which goes beyond the moment of hospitalization or of

the treatment for acute disease and includes a continuing relation between the individual and the healthcare system, to exchange information, monitor the patient's health, prevent future disease, support healthier behavior, etc..

Even if conceptually distinct, in practice the three processes are deeply connected and mutually crossing, to such an extent that it would be reductive to identify e-health applications specific for each process, as a great part of the value added by these applications lie exactly in their cross-process nature.

A more recent attempt is made by Bashshur et al. (2011), who talk about "telemedicine" as the wider concept for all ICT application in healthcare. In their taxonomy they distinguish between:

- Telehealth, whose components are health behavior/health education, health & disease epidemiology, environmental/industrial health, health management & policy;
- E-Health, which comprises electronic health record, health information, clinical decision support systems, physician order entry;
- M-Health, which is centered on mobile technologies and encompasses clinical support, health worker support, remote data collection, helpline.

The criterion at the basis of this structure is in our opinion not clearly defined and, furthermore, the classification seems to be by no means exhaustive. On the contrary, the proposed dimensions of the telemedicine concept look quite interesting; the Authors, in fact, find three criteria which can be adopted to distinguish between telemedicine applications:

- **Functionality:** consultation, diagnosis, mentoring, monitoring;
- **Applications:** specialty, disease, site, treatment;
- **Technology:** synchronicity, network, connectivity.

We agree on the value of these criteria which, however, could again result in an excess of granularity when trying to classifying specific applications; furthermore, they could be subject to overlapping, as some complex applications could fall into more categories; finally, they seem to exclude those applications related to support processes in healthcare, which do not correspond to any of the proposed functionalities.

A NEW TAXONOMY FOR E-HEALTH APPLICATIONS

After presenting e-health and the most common categorizations of its activities, we introduce our original taxonomy for e-health applications. Our aim is to overcome the limitations of the proposed classifications, by offering a new one built around the characteristics of the delivery system of the services which are digitalized.

In comparison with its antecedents, our tool shows two strengths. First, it does not simply list and group e-applications but finds classification criteria. Second, while other taxonomies propose a wide set of criteria – very difficult to jointly consider – our choice is to concentrate on just two criteria: they are much simpler to handle and more focused on those aspects we consider critical to achieve the strategic goals of healthcare delivery. Furthermore, these criteria are of "high-level", being related to the characteristics of the provided service and not to very specific technical features of a given application. By doing so, the tool is able to potentially classify not yet developed applications and to trace them back to the more general framework of the digitalization of services; the latter, in particular, is in our view quite relevant, as encompassing e-health development into a more general economic trend – such as service digitalization – can allow for a deeper understanding of its origins, dynamics and potentialities than simply looking at it as the adoption of IT in the health industry.

To this purpose, as aforementioned, we are going to trace e-health back to a more general phenomenon, that is the Internet-driven digitalization of services. To support our taxonomy with a strong knowledge basis, we have consequently performed a deep analysis of the literature on service management and service science (Thomas, 1978; Lovelock, 1983; Lovelock & Wirtz, 2004; Chesbrough H., 2005; Spohrer & Maglio, 2008), which can support us in building a conceptual framework of analysis for the digitalization of services.

First of all, we note that a service is not a physical good, but the output of an economic activity which is characterized by a high degree of intangibility. The distinctive characteristics of services are: intangibility; simultaneous delivery and consumption; contact and interaction between producer and user; perishability; variability; social innovation (Chase, 1978; Normann, 1984; Eiglier & Langeard, 1987; Grönroos, 1990; Lovelock, 1996; Zeithaml & Bitner, 2000). These characteristics are common to all services, but appear with differing intensity according to the kind of service and delivery mode adopted. In the healthcare industry, for instance, public hospitals adopt a different mode of managing and delivering service compared to private hospitals.

Furthermore, every service shows a high degree of complexity, as it is composed by a set of core and additional services: when a customer purchases a service, she actually buys a "package" of core and peripheral attributes (Normann, 1984). The service components may vary in number and be combined in different ways; as a consequence, the service package may be very complex: depending on the pursued strategy and the target customer, every firm offers one or more core services, to which it adds a set of ancillary services which complete the "package". As a consequence service firms, even within the same industry, may differ for several reasons: the service package they offer; the balance between core service and ancillary services; the degree of standardization; the degree of externalization; the delivery mode; the extent of the contact during the delivery, etc. A home-care service, for example, can present various degrees of completeness and personalization, according to the services which are provided, the frequency of the interventions, the kind of staff involved, etc.

Nowadays the role of information and the customer involvement in the delivery system have acquired a crucial role in many services: "today, the more knowledge-intensive and customized the service, the more it depends on client participation and input, whether through clients providing labor, property, or information via organizational or technological value chains" (Maglio & Spohrer, 2008, p. 18). Within this framework, service science aims to respond to the emerging issues related with the intrinsic features of services, to support the search for maximization of service quality and productivity, and to enhance the exploitation of technological and organizational innovation in services (Bitner et al., 2008).

In particular, customer is increasingly considered a resource in action, a co-producer of the service. In healthcare activities this approach is as more relevant as the service delivery system is built around the individual, not only as the receiver of the service but also as co-creator of the value. From this point of view, the customer becomes a part of the service system, defined as "value-co-creation configurations of people, technology, value propositions connecting internal and external service systems, and shared information (e.g., language, laws, measures, and methods)" (Maglio & Spohrer, 2008, p. 18). ICT heavily accelerate this process and sustain such a customer-centered approach.

Posed these premises, we need to focus our attention on those service features which most contribute in identifying different kinds of healthcare services, which have been differently impacted by the advent of the digital economy.

To this purpose, we refer to a model developed by Benevolo and Spinelli (2011). The model was primarily intended to support the analysis of service firms' internationalization according to the characteristics of the services they offer and the supply system they set up, and with a specific focus on the impact on the internationalization processes of the application of internet-based technologies to service delivery systems. Regardless of any reference to those parts of the model more strictly related to the internationalization processes, we consider it useful to adopt the service taxonomy proposed by the Authors when evaluating the impact of ICT on the service delivery; in fact, this part of the model can contribute to casting light on those features of healthcare services which most influenced their evolution towards a new digital configuration in a framework of e-health and which constitute the foundation for our taxonomy.

The aim of Benevolo and Spinelli (2011)'s model is to show the relationship between the characteristics of the service and of its delivery modes, and the way in which the application of Internet-related technologies impacts on the service delivery itself. The Authors focus their attention on a specific group of ICT, which includes those informatics solutions and application platforms based on network technologies: EDI and databases via the Internet, intranet and extranet, website and blogs, marketplaces and e-commerce, live chat, computer reservation systems, etc. Part of the Internet-based technologies (for example, corporate websites or marketplaces) are also Web-based – as they are supported by the system of interlinked hypertext documents which constitutes the World Wide Web – while others (for instance Voice Over IP systems or machine-to-machine communication systems) can do without the Web interface.

Internet-based technologies overcome the limitations, develop the potential and re-define the applicability of the service delivery, reshaping the way in which many services are actually performed and made available to the recepients. Thanks to these technologies it is feasible to create and manage in a more functional way the business processes involving customers, providers, employees, etc.

In the model, services are divided into clusters, designed around two key dimensions. The first dimension is the need of physical co-presence or interaction between producer and user in service delivery. As regards this dimension, the aim is to identify those services in which delivery requires co-presence and interaction (even if from a distance) or a high degree of personalization, which necessarily implies a level of relationship directly related to the need for co-presence (Cho, 2005). Some services require the physical presence of both producer and consumer, such as most personal services. Some others do not: consider, for instance, long-distance services where the contact is not present (such as in telecommunications) or is virtual; or service-embodied goods, where the delivery is mediated by a good (for instance a movie in a DVD) (Bhagwati, 1987). As regards healthcare services, most medical and nurse treatments belong to the first group of services, while other information-intensive services – such as communication, education, and administrative services – belong to the latter group.

The second dimension evaluates the possibility, opportunity and convenience of performing the service delivery through the Internet, that is, replacing the traditional service delivery with Internet-based technologies. The service production and delivery system, as commonly known, consists of two parts: front office and back office, divided by the so-called 'line of visibility' (Eiglier & Langeard, 1987). The front office is the part of the system visible to the customer and where the encounter of customer and personnel/physical support of the service firm takes place, while the back office supports and integrates the front office (Silvestro et al., 1992; Zeithaml & Bitner, 2000). Unlike manufacturing firms – where product and production are conceptually and physically separated – in service firms it is quite difficult to separate the service from its delivery system: the production process of a service partially coincides with its delivery, which in turn becomes a part of the service itself. As a consequence, the transportability of the delivery system is evaluated in terms of replacing the traditional delivery system with an Internet-based one.

When jointly considered, these two dimensions generate four groups of services, as in Table 1, which are now briefly described.

Digital Goods and Services [A]

Digital goods and services are services where the physical co-presence is not required and the service delivery can be performed through the Internet.

They often represent the evolution from service-embodied goods, or services which used to need the support of a physical good to be delivered. Here, technological innovation has acted in two seemingly conflicting ways: firstly, it has supported the "materialization" of services into transferable and tradable goods (for example, recording music on a digital device); later, it has increased the immateriality of services, separating them from physical evidence through digitalization and new Internet-based transferability (Evans & Wurster, 2000; Cho, 2005). In this sense, transferability has been made more pervasive by the possibility of digitalizing and transmitting data, archives, sounds, images, codified knowledge and anything that can be considered "information" (Shapiro & Varian, 1999). Consequently, information-based services are separated from their physical evidence and their delivery can be easily processed through Internet-based technologies. The production of service-embodied goods tends to adopt 'manufacturing' models, exploits new technologies and consequently increases the overall efficiency of sale and delivery. At the same time, consumers are no longer bound to the producer's location and time, as they can buy, receive and consume the service wherever and whenever they like to. Even in these services, however, some sort of interaction with the deliverer or the Internet-based technology may be possible and useful, for ICT allow an unprecedented level of personalization, based on the contact with consumers.

On-Line Delivery [B]

The second group too includes services where the delivery can be performed through the Internet and co-presence is not necessary. In this case, we focus on the evolution of long-distance services, where delivery system is non-transportable but can work from a distance, and the co-presence of both producer and consumer is unnecessary (such as in telecommunications); these services can be delivered via remote communication and strongly benefit from Internet-based technologies.

Table 1. Service delivery and Internet-based technologies

Physical Co-Presence or Interaction/ Personalization	Service Delivery	
	Can be Performed through the Internet	*Cannot be Performed through the Internet*
Necessary	Virtual relationship or reality [C]	Unavoidable "physical-ness" or humanization [D]
Unnecessary	Digital goods and services [A] On-line delivery [B]	

Source: Adapted from Benevolo and Spinelli (2011) © 2011, Inderscience Publishers. Used with permission.

Some of these services originated as digital services to satisfy on-line market needs, which were not, or not fully, satisfied by existing firms (on-line search engines, "wiki" encyclopedias or on-line tourist guides). Others have fundamentally changed their core service and delivery system (on-line insurance companies and banks, live chat services, on-line news and trading). Others have taken advantage of the greater transmission and communication capability and pervasiveness of the new technologies, their lower usage costs, and the opportunity to enrich the service offer with new additional services (digital TV, Web radio, multimedia dictionaries, VOIP) (Benevolo & Spinelli, 2011).

The services presented so far are those where physical presence was unnecessary and delivery was consequently more easily performable through the Internet. Now we are going to introduce the other groups, where co-presence – or at least interaction – is necessary and the need for a greater personalization usually follows.

Virtual Relationship or Reality [C]

In this third group of services, the co-presence and interaction of the producer and the consumer of the service is necessary, but this co-presence can be made virtual by performing the service delivery through Internet-related technologies. The contact degree required for the delivery and how much this can be replaced by a simulation or an Internet-based relationship is crucial. The feasibility of this process is a consequence of the degree of contact required for delivery and of how much this can be replaced by a simulation or an Internet-based relationship. In personal services, a partial replacement for a physical presence and a Web contact is sometimes possible, where a relationship is unnecessary or not critical for service quality.

Unavoidable "Physical-Ness" or Humanization [D]

In this last group, services are included which need co-presence and whose delivery cannot be performed through the Internet. As a consequence, for these services it is not possible to substitute an Internet-based delivery for a traditional one and the direct impact of the digital economy on them is thus indirect. Nevertheless, ICT can play a major role in the delivery of the additional services which precede, follow or accompany the delivery of the core service, thus enriching the traditional service and generating more value for the user (Benevolo & Spinelli, 2011). Consider, for instance, those services assisting the potential consumer in the information-gathering process or in the evaluation of possible options (pre-delivery); those services supporting the sale, the assistance and customer services (post-delivery); those additional services helping the customer during off-line delivery.

Once defined the structure of the matrix, it is possible to place e-health applications on it, in accordance with the features of their delivery system; by doing so, we create various groups of e-health applications which share common structural features and which lead to our proposed taxonomy. The value of this taxonomy is that applications are not grouped on the basis of technological features – which are also exposed to the risk of quick obsolescence – but with respect to the structural characteristics of the services to be digitalized. In other words, we do not gather applications together only because they are delivered through mobile technologies (like the so-called m-health applications); we prefer to put together applications which share a common nature in terms of kind of processes and activities involved. However, as we are going to discuss in the "Future trends" section, it is likely that many services and groups will move on the matrix, because innovation will make available new ways to deliver healthcare services and redefine the borders between necessary and unnecessary co-presence and – even more – between the possibility or not to perform a given service through the Internet.

Moreover, those groups are "open", in the sense that new services could enter them due to important technological innovation which makes it possible their digitalization.

Given the present level of technological development, our classification exercise returns the following four groups of e-health applications:

1. Health information digitalization, transmission and sharing through the Internet;
2. Distance or virtual relationship in the delivery of medical care;
3. Support services to the management of healthcare facilities;
4. Online retrieval of medical data and information for clinicians, patients and the general public.

Figure 3 shows the position on the model matrix of each group, which is later discussed.

Health Information Digitalization, Transmission and Sharing through the Internet [1]

In health care systems, a widely recognized source of inefficiencies is the fragmentation of the care delivery process and the poor transfer of information along the various steps (OECD, 2010, p. 32). The efficient sharing of health information is, however, indispensable for the effective delivery of care (IOM, 2001). "Before the advent of Internet technology, there was no way to escape the inefficiencies of a paper-based system: the piles of prescriptions, forms, and charts, the frustration associated with registering and

Figure 3. Healthcare service delivery and e-health applications
Source: Constructed by the authors.

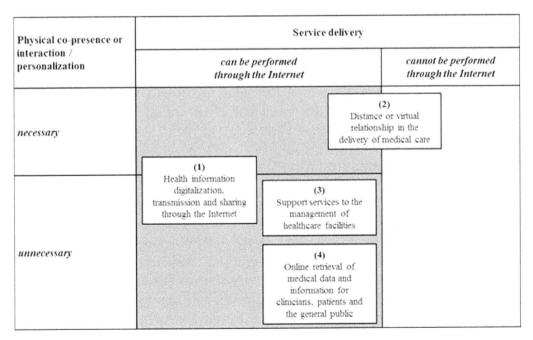

filling in medical histories more than once, the high cost of such inefficiencies" (Ball & Lillis, 2001, p. 5). In group 1 we gather information-centered applications which focus on processes and activities directly related with care provisioning and based on the collection and sharing of information about the patient, her pathologies and therapies. They allow to transfer and share digital data and information via the Internet among doctors and clinicians, within a single healthcare structure or between the several entities involved in the delivery of healthcare services in complex healthcare systems.

In Figure 4 the position of group 1 partially overlaps the border line between necessary and unnecessary physical co-presence of the subjects involved; in our opinion, in fact, the collection of the information to digitalize usually requires a certain physical interaction with the patient, while its transmission and sharing can be generally performed through the Internet without relevant problems.

Among the applications included in this group, the most relevant are patient information systems and electronic health records. These electronic records include patient demographics, progress notes, problems, medications, vital signs, past medical history, immunizations, laboratory data and radiology reports, etc. (HIMSS, 2011) and are used to support both the administrative and clinical activities in a hospital. The electronic health records carry great advantages compared to traditional paper, the main one being that it has evolved from a physical construct into pure information. First, this means that multimedia data can easily be stored in digital archives, something that previously was true only for written data; second, data can be embedded in a portable device the patient can easily carry with her or can be available for access through mobile devices, thanks to cloud storage applications; third, data can be progressively updated, allowing for a complete clinical record of the patient. Furthermore, electronic health records allow for quick and inexpensive communications between doctors or medical centers, especially when a wide set of organizations (hospitals, clinics, long-term care facilities, etc.) are involved in the treatment.

Exploiting the same principle, the results of an exam – for instance an ECG or a radiograph – can be remotely transmitted for analysis by a doctor who is not physically present with the patient. Picture archiving and communication systems (PACS), for example, are computer systems that "replace conventional x-ray film, and greatly improves access to patient information by making it possible for referring clinicians to review their patient's images on PCs from their own offices" (OECD, 2010, p. 36).

Further applications which exploit the digitalization of medical information are the so called e-Prescriptions, that is the computer-based electronic generation, transmission and filling of a medical prescription, and the electronic fit/sick notes, for sick leaves and insurance purposes. In both cases, the information flows becomes quicker, cheaper and more error-free than the traditional paper-equivalent; moreover, these applications allow for a better monitoring of the medical expense by the spender, usually the public entity responsible for the sanitary system.

Distance or Virtual Relationship in the Delivery of Medical Care [2]

In this group, applications are included which focus on the core process of care delivering and consequently require interaction between clinicians and patients. This is the case of those healthcare services, such as diagnostics and treatment, which have traditionally meant local services with high levels of contact and interaction between supplier (the doctor and her team) and consumer (the patient and her family).

Thanks to the advent of the digital economy, the delivery of many of these services can be significantly redesigned and supported by Internet-based technologies. We have especially in mind, for instance, the ubiquitous biometric data measurement and the remote patient monitoring and compliance, that is the mobile real time monitoring of patient vital signs, when patients are continually monitored on health-related parameters with wireless sensors, irrespective of where they happen to be (Van Halteren et al., 2004). Sensors can be embedded on the patient – for instance, in small monitoring devices or in her clothes (Castillejo et al., 2013) – and mobile phones or personal digital assistants (PDAs) with wireless networking capabilities may serve as gateways that process, store, and transfer data to clinicians for further analysis or diagnosis (Bardram et al., 2006). The monitoring device could have multimedia capabilities – allowing for the transmission of audio and video too – or even be coupled with an operating device (for example an insulin pump) which performs a remotely controlled therapy on the patient (Haux et al., 2002, p. 13).

These solutions offer great benefits because they free the patient from the need of being always "within reach" of the doctor, making it possible to remotely monitor a person's health without hospitalization; by doing so they allow for early detection and prevention of diseases by reporting events or changes which could require an intervention by the patient herself, e.g. by taking a medication or ceasing a dangerous behavior, or by a third person, such as a nurse or a doctor. Finally, they represent a tremendous innovation in situations of limited mobility of the patients, such as with remote communities, or in developing countries, since they lack both expert practitioners and health structures on the territory and distances can be significant between patients and hospitals. In this case, patients can be monitored by doctors who are very far away, with a great benefit to the population of disadvantaged countries (Gerber, 2009). Similar considerations could be made as regards specific situations in which continuous monitoring is needed but the presence of a doctor or nurse is unfeasible: we have in mind, for instance, post-partum home recovery, post-discharge home treatments, long-term and chronic home care, etc. In general, these applications could support the development of a more home-based approach to care delivery, with a shift of focus from the hospital to the patient's house as care-delivery place. An example is given by the EU-funded project "GiraffPlus" (www.giraffplus.eu), which has led to the creation of a complex system which can monitor activities in the house using a network of sensors, both in and around the house as well as on the body (Coradeschi et al. 2013). The sensors can measure blood pressure or detect whether somebody falls down. Different services, depending on the individual needs, can be pre-selected and tailored to the requirements of both older adults and health care professionals. At the heart of the system is a unique telepresence robot – Giraff, which lends its name to the project – that uses a Skype-like interface to allow, for instance, relatives or caregivers to virtually visit an elderly person in the home (Frennert & Östlund, 2014).

The last frontier in this virtual relationship regards the treatment step and is represented by tele-surgery via virtual reality 3D systems: in fact, they allow the surgeon to perform the operation from a distance, through an Internet connection by means of a robot-surgeon (Slack, 2007; Zhijiang et al. 2006). As the information flow is bidirectional, the surgeon receives back all the information about the patient (data, images, simulation of the response of the patient's body to the surgeon's actions), without being close to her. This opens the way to a virtual relationship between doctor and patient, with promising consequences for the development of long-distance surgery, which can now be performed regardless of geographical separation; some visionary authors are even imaging space surgery, to support quality of life and medical care in human outposts on the Moon or Mars (Haidegger et al., 2011)!

Nevertheless, the transition to a fully Internet-based delivery is still unfeasible, as some healthcare services require such an intense and personal contact between clinicians and patients which cannot be – and quite often does not even need to be – completely substituted by a virtual surrogate; for this reason, the corresponding box on the matrix overlaps the line between service which can and cannot be delivered through the Internet. In those cases as well when Internet delivery is not possible, Internet technologies can however play a major role in the delivery of the additional services which precede, follow or accompany the delivery of the core service, thus enriching the traditional service and generating more value for the user (Benevolo & Spinelli, 2008). A great part of the medical and nursing activity, in particular, is subject to these limitations: even though part of the traditional set of medical and surgical activities has moved to the Internet in some pioneering experiences, in the vast majority of cases it still has to face the need of a real physical contact with the patient who is going to receive the service. This is certainly relevant for medical activity but may be even more significant for nursing, which in some cases requires a closer contact between the nurse and the patient than the doctor-patient relationship. So long as technological development does not introduce really break-through innovations, it is quite difficult to imagine an Internet-based delivery for nursing services which support the patient in her everyday activities – such as cleaning or feeding – or which relate to applying a medication or dressing a wound. Nevertheless, the development of the digital economy can have a strong indirect impact on this group of healthcare activities as well, if we consider the additional services which always complement the physical performance of the core service. Electronic health records are for instance a powerful tool for constantly accessing and updating the patient's history, so ensuring that the most effective therapy is determined and provided. Similarly, mobile real time monitoring of the patient can limit physical contact to circumstances where it is strictly needed, so allowing the medical staff to concentrate on higher-value creating activities. A doctor who does not have to look for medical examination results but finds them always available on a portable device, can concentrate on diagnosis without losing time; similarly, a nurse who always has access to the prescribed therapies in the patient's file is much less likely to make mistakes or to misinterpret the doctor's instructions (Bates et al, 2001).

Support Services to the Management of Healthcare Facilities [3]

In this third group we gather those applications which aim to support the non-core administrative processes in healthcare facilities. These services do not require a specific interaction of the subjects involved and can consequently be shifted to the Internet to a significant extent. A proper example is given by hospital information systems, enterprise resource planning (ERP) systems that support information processing within a hospital in areas such as administration, appointments, billing, planning, budgeting and personnel; similarly, we can cite LIS (Laboratory Information Systems) and RIS (Radiology Information Systems), which support the management of specific departments. Other areas supported by such applications are, for instance, order management, medication management, disaster recovery, business intelligence, quality management and assessment, etc. Even if not strictly related with the "main" caretaking process, these services are crucial for health organizations, especially in terms of administrative costs and service quality; their impact on the overall efficiency and effectiveness is consequently very strong, as witnessed by the fact that they have long been the main target of investment in IT by healthcare institutions (Osservatorio ICT in Sanità, 2013).

Online Retrieval of Medical Data and Information for Clinicians, Patients and the General Public [4]

In this final group we include those processes and activities which are information-based (as in group 1) but are not directly related with the information generated during the care delivery. In other words, these information-based processes concern ancillary activities such as education, training, knowledge dissemination etc.

A first example is given by online registries, such as national electronic registries (which contain data on specific medical subjects such as births, mortality, cancer, diabetes or other subjects of medical or epidemiological interest), national drug registries (containing national pharmaceutical information) or directories of healthcare professional and institutions (which can support patients and the general public when choosing a clinician or an institution for treatment).

With a closer focus on e-learning and support to clinicians training and education, we can cite Internet-based on-demand clinical case analysis services, such as those developed by MEDgle©. MEDgle is a case analysis engine with a wide range of real-time, predictive health uses. The MEDgle platform is built on top of a large database of relationships between symptoms, diagnoses, drugs, tests, procedures and associated statistical information (MEDgle Inc., 2014). Even if still at the experimental stage, this service could potentially bring valuable support to the medical staff in decision-taking. The user is even excused from the need of acquiring any ICT device or advance infrastructure, as the service is totally web-based and can be accessed from everywhere and by using any kind of Internet-capable device. This last feature is particularly interesting, because it allows for the use of the platform even in extreme situations, such as in a rescue service, when the medical staff is outside the hospital facilities but can access the Internet with portable tools such as an IPad or similar. MEDgle belongs to the family of the Clinical Decision Support Systems (CDSS), a large group of stand-alone or Web-based systems which aim to support the decision-making process of medical staff with inference engines or artificial intelligence software (Garg et al, 2005). The reliability of CDSS is still questioned by the medical community, due to the limit that these technologies face in properly interpreting the whole clinical picture of a patient; nevertheless, the value of the business idea is certainly high and it is probable that, once refined and completely implemented, MEDgle and its competitors will become a useful and reliable support tool for medical staff.

A further research and diagnostic service which is delivered though the Web are bibliographic databases such as MEDLINE© (Medical Literature Analysis and Retrieval System Online), which includes bibliographic information for articles from academic journals covering most of medical science fields. The value added of such a service does not lie only in that the articles are digitalized; more important is the aspect related to the accurate ways in which this knowledge base can be explored, thanks to the connections which are created between the single piece of information and all the rest.

Finally, Internet-based technology can support the development of online professional communities, allowing for virtual consultation and collaboration among doctors, to enhance research and improve healthcare quality through the sharing of best-practices and the opportunities for all the subjects involved to exchange views and disseminate knowledge. This can be particularly useful, for example, in case of public health emergencies, such as epidemics or pandemics like Ebola, that require a strong global sharing of information on how the virus is spreading but also on what cures are being provided and with what results, to improve the treatments and their effectiveness.

FUTURE TRENDS: OPPORTUNITIES AND CRITICAL ISSUES

In this chapter, we have tried to propose a new taxonomy of e-health applications, based on the structural features of the delivery system associated with the services which are digitalized. To this purpose, we have traced back the development of e-health applications to a wider framework of digitalization for services; structural differences among services categories then result into different forms of digitalization and delivery through Internet-based technologies.

As previously stated, our taxonomy presents several advantages over other alternatives, because it is not based on specific technological features but on:

- The structural characteristics of the services to be digitalized;
- The subjects involved and the relationships which are activated in the service delivery;
- The operational potentiality of Internet-based technologies.

However, it is important to speculate on the major trends in the development of e-health, as they could influence the position of the groups on the matrix, moving the borders between necessary and unnecessary co-presence and between possibility or not to perform a given service through the Internet. Hitherto, e-health has not yet revealed all its potential; as reported by Kennedy and Berk (2011), the health care industry "despite being arguably the most information-intensive industry in the world, has been slow to join the digital revolution" and "the transition will be a sea change" (p. 1). Nevertheless the innumerable cases of innovative adoption of ICT – both in the intangible and tangible components of healthcare activities – suggest that the evolution of healthcare activities towards new digital configurations is a structural process already in progress, even if still far from reaching full deployment. On the one side, the adoption, diffusion and pervasiveness of e-health applications could be boosted by technological innovation but also by social and cultural evolution in regards to health services; on the other side, e-health could be restrained by obstacles and limitations of various origins which could even get worse in the future.

In this section, we aim to point out both opportunities and critical issues, trying to highlight the repercussions on our taxonomy.

A significant part of healthcare services are by their nature "high-touch services", due to the need for physical contact and relation, and they are consequently slow in evolving from "low-tech" to "high-tech" configurations, where the use of automatic systems, ICT and other physical supports is more and more significant (Salomann et al., 2006). The progress is therefore not easy, due to cultural, organizational and budget constraints, but the results already achieved suggest that innovation horizons in healthcare are broad and promising. Coming back to the Malecki and Moriset (2008) classification which was presented in the "Background" section, we confirm that the healthcare industry is going to increasingly join the pyramid's "main body", as more and more of its activities will require extensive use of ICT to be performed in innovative and more effective ways, with great benefits for patients, medical staff and national budgets too. More broadly, this trend is stronger when we consider that medical activities in the strict sense of the word are only a part of the complex healthcare industry. Indeed, it includes several service-providing and manufacturing sectors – such as research companies, information providers and diagnostic equipment manufacturers – which are already heavily ICT-enabled and consequently push the "medical core" of the industry towards new digital configurations. While at the beginning of the century the Institute of Medicine (IOM, 2001) could state that the healthcare service delivery remained "relatively untouched by the revolution in information technology that [had] swept nearly every other aspect of society" (p. 15), nowadays the situation has radically evolved and the "revolution" is absolutely in progress.

This is especially true for the "Distance or virtual relationship in the delivery of medical care" group, which will certainly shift leftwards due innovative solutions to substitute a virtual relationship for a physical one in healthcare delivery. The main emerging trend is the shift from a model where the patient "moves towards the cure" (being it at the doctor or at the hospital) to a new one where is the cure to "move towards the patient", thanks to all those technologies which allow to share and transfer health information. As Mukhopadhyay (2015) reports, "the advancement of sensing technologies, embedded systems, wireless communication technologies, nano technologies, and miniaturization makes it possible to develop smart systems to monitor activities of human beings continuously", (p. 1321). In the perspective of the so-called Internet-of-Things, we have especially in mind the further evolution of the aforementioned wearable medical devices, where the interconnection is on a machine-to-machine basis; this means that the first recipient of the transmitted information is not a person but another device, which is programmed to react in a certain way when receiving specific data, such as alarm systems which start other devices up.

These sensors forward their collected data to an M2M device (e.g., a patient's cell phone) that acts as an information aggregator and forwards the data to the M2M application server [...]. The M2M server responds to the collected data by sending alerts and appropriate medical records to medical providers. In emergency situations, an M2M device can directly provide the medical status of a patient en route to the hospital (e.g., in the ambulance), allowing physicians to prepare for treatment in advance of the patient's arrival. (Geng et al., 2011, p. 38)

The device could even be "inside" the patient: this is the case, for instance, of sensors in pills that are swallowed and could automatically send patient information to doctors and nurses; this would allow a sick or elderly person to manage her healthcare from home, rather than in a hospital or nursing home, getting automatic reminders to take medicines or immediate preventive care for changes in health status.

Furthermore, enhanced devices could collect, elaborate and transfer information in real time, enabling faster communications and decision making. and allowing to access information not otherwise available, in terms of width, depth, updating and precision (Safavi, 2014)

This new approach to healthcare delivery would benefit from innovation in georeferencing too: with respect to the objectives of e-health we previously cited, georeference could increase the quality of the assistance and make it feasible to provide healthcare services more integrated and less bounded to physical location.

Big Data is another field of innovation which is certainly going to have a strong impact on healthcare (Srinivasan & Arunasalam, 2013; Liu & Park, 2014; Mancini, 2014; MeriTalk, 2014); as previously mentioned, all the subjects involved in healthcare delivery generate large amount of data, which could be effectively used to reduce the cost of healthcare while improving quality, and supporting prevention and personalization. So far it has been quite difficult to explore them and turn them into valuable information; Big Data solutions now make it possible to exploit the mass of available data in unexperienced manners, offering the potential to improve trial safety, disease surveillance, prescribed treatments, and patient outcomes. Big Data adoption in healthcare is still in its initial stages, but its potential is already beyond doubt.

Nevertheless, the process towards a widespread implementation of e-health practices has to face several obstacles, most of which do not strictly relate to technical matters (Karsh et al. 2010). With respect to technical difficulties, in fact, it is very often just "a matter of time", as continuous innovation is able to progressively overcome them. We are more interested in non-technical questions and – even though a full examination of them is beyond the aim of this chapter – some references cannot be omitted.

A first major barrier concerns the financing of e-health initiatives; purchasing and implementation costs for these projects usually require a significant amount of financing with an uncertain (at least in the short term) assessment of the extent of the achievable benefits and of who is actually benefitting from the gains in efficiency and effectiveness:

one significant barrier to investment in ICTs is the widely recognized fact that any resulting cost savings may not always accrue to the implementer, but may be passed on to a third party. Benefits may appear at one site and in one budget, while a large share of the cost commitments appear at another site and in another budget. (OECD, 2010, p. 46)

Furthermore, there may be lags between ICT investments and benefit realization (Devaraj & Kohli, 2000); quite commonly, the financial benefits are not realized until a level of functionality is reached – a kind of "critical mass" – that allows systems to truly serve the needs of clinicians and system planners. "Until IT investment reaches a threshold, total operating expenses increase in hospitals that have little IT" (PricewaterhouseCoopers, 2007, p. 18). In addition, there are no incentives, and may even be disincentives for care providers to be the first to adopt ICT (Taylor et al., 2005), as commonly happens with radical innovations. At the same, the development of a strong business case is crucial, because – as in Dixon (2007) – it "lowers the risk of adoption, implementation, and use of e-health" (p. 11) and is the first step of an effective roadmap for e-health adoption.

The situation is however extremely varied worldwide. Western countries are certainly dealing with an increase in the elderly share of population and in the diffusion of diseases related to lifestyle and physical inactivity, which result in rapid rises in healthcare costs; furthermore, they have long-established health services and structures, that need deep changes to be converted to ICT adoption; finally, they often face shrinking public budget for healthcare, which make it much more difficult to respond to the challenges that those trends pose. Poorer countries, instead, still have big issues to solve: endemic health problems, undersized structures compared to the needs, chronical lack of resources; as a consequence, they could be excluded from the innovation process for a long time yet. Finally, emerging country are probably those with the greatest potential of adoption: on the one hand, they can count on vast resources, which allow for large budget for healthcare; on the other hand, they are still building their health services and structures: not having to face path dependencies and resistance to change – as we are going to better detail later on – they may be the quickest to efficiently adopt new e-health technologies pervasively.

A second important barrier is associated with organizational factors, both between and within healthcare organizations.

As regards the first aspect, we have to keep in mind that several e-health services involve a plurality of organizations: healthcare systems, indeed, are usually very fragmented, with a multiplicity of public and private providers and payers. This constitutes a significant barrier to the adoption of e-health services, as it implies connecting systems managed by different organizations and with relevant differences as regards the standard and content of the collected data, the transmission protocol, etc. (Kaye et al., 2010). For this reason, a crucial role is played by the organizations for standardization – such as the International Organization for Standardization (ISO) or the Comité Européen de Normalisation (CEN) – which are working, in particular, for the definition of common standards for the Electronic Health Records (Chávez et al., 2009; Moruzzi, 2009). Kennedy and Berk (2011) report about the US experience, where "a host of standards – Including Logical Observation Identifiers Names and Codes (LOINC), Digital Imaging and Communications in Medicine (DICOM), Health Level Seven International (HL7), and Systematized Nomenclature of Medicine Clinical Terms (SNOMED CT) – are allowing for rich information interchange across care settings and are being used by regional health-information organizations [...] to coordinate care across regions, with impressive results" (p.5). The development work on standards is surely critical, but when standards are refined and become more commonplace, the ability to exchange, aggregate, and analyze health care data will increase dramatically. With respect to our taxonomy, this could increase the scope for both the "Support services to the management of healthcare facilities" and the "Health information digitalization, transmission and sharing through the Internet", which strongly rely on shared standards and communication protocols between and within healthcare institutions.

The barrier associated with organizational factors internal to the healthcare organization represents an aspect not yet adequately studied in the literature (Shekelle & Goldzweig, 2009); nevertheless, as previously cited, this topic is crucial and impacts all the categories of e-applications we identified: in particular, the implementation of health information systems (group 3) represents a strong organizational discontinuity and questions consolidated procedures, routines and habits (Gagnon et al., 2005). This opens the door to a vast discussion about leadership and governance for ICT projects (Bernstein, McCreless, & Côté, 2007; Fickenscher & Bakerman, 2011); about technical education and training for doctors and nurses who are asked to use new technologies (Masys, 1998; Ball & Lillis, 2001; Anderson, 2007; Moghaddasi et al., 2012); about how to increase the actual adoption of new systems and overcome the organizational and individual inertia (England, Stewart & Walker, 2000; Gaggioli et al., 2005). Furthermore, we should not forget that high technology cannot do without human skills and capabilities, which must remain absolutely central in the service delivery (Demattè et al., 2007; Freema et al., 2010).

Another big problem is related to privacy, security and legal issues in sharing sensitive patient data in a large and heterogeneous environment through the use of web-based and mobile applications (Berner, 2008; Moruzzi, 2009; Lateef, 2011; Safavi, 2014), as in group 1 ("Health information digitalization, transmission and sharing through the Internet") and in group 4 ("Online retrieval of medical data and information for clinicians, patients and the general public"). Several surveys and studies highlight the concern about the privacy of patients' health information. This concern is well motivated because, "as the contents of electronic health records are shared more widely, the risk increases that stigmatizing disclosures could affect areas such as employment status, access to health insurance and other forms of insurance, and participation in community activities" (OECD, 2010, p. 106). This is certainly a major issue, which is becoming even more important with the advent of Big Data solutions and which needs to be addressed from both the legal and the technical side: from the legal side, to build a regulatory framework (better if on an international scale) for information gathering, storing and sharing; from the technical side, to develop those standards and applications which make possible to match the adoption of e-health practices with the protection of individual rights.

Finally, another issue is also the degree of acceptance of e-health practices by the recipients, that is, the patients and their family. With respect to this topic – crucial in particular for applications in the "Distance or virtual relationship in the delivery of medical care" group – both cultural predisposition and technology acceptance are relevant, especially in older patients (see, among others, Eikelboom & Atlas, 2005; Whitten & Love, 2005); patients have to accept the substitution of a technology-mediated relationship with the medical staff for physical contact and also have to develop such minimum skills which allow them to interact with the devices, such as in the mobile real time monitoring of vital signs. This is a subject that deserves much more attention and could be of major interest not only for medical practitioners but also for engineers and software developers, who have to design those devices. Nevertheless, some studies return quite surprising results, as both patients and their relatives seem to be prepared to take on semi-autonomous telepresence robots but health care providers are not (Frennert & Östlund, 2014). Again, deficiencies in the organization of the introduction of the new approach pose an obstacle and a challenge for the development of modern medical care.

CONCLUSION

Our reflection about e-health applications has tried to trace them back to the more general trend of services digitalization. An original taxonomy has been proposed, which is actually based on the structural characteristics of the delivery systems of the services that are impacted by the Internet technologies. The resulting framework returns an exhaustive picture of e-health applications and allows for some reflections about the evolution of the digital healthcare industry. We believe e-health should not be considered simply a technological innovation, but a paradigm shift which results in a radical redesign of the whole industry. In essence, the adoption of ICT – and especially of Internet-based technologies – triggers a virtuous cycle of innovation: the new opportunities enabled by digital technologies stimulate the creation of original practices and the reconfiguration of the processes; this, in turn, supports the research for latest technologies to apply to healthcare, and so on. Physical limitations – mostly due to the undoubted importance of the physical co-presence of producer (healthcare staff) and user (patient) in many healthcare services – are still present and central. In spite of these obstacles, the future of e-health is nevertheless very promising and will lead to an efficiency gain, together with an increase in the quality of healthcare delivery and practice. As commonly known, health is, in turn, a strong driver of well-being and quality of life (Stiglitz, Sen, & Fitoussi, 2009): as a consequence, the possibility and hope of improving people standards of life strongly rely on e-health applications to turn into reality. This certainly leads to interesting developments in research. New applications are constantly developed and the adoption of ICT in healthcare is increasingly pervasive, rich and deep. It is consequently of undoubted interest to keep on monitoring these innovative activities to track their evolution and to assess the drivers and impediments of e-health development worldwide.

However, a final consideration is worth mentioning: how does the pervasive adoption of ICT in healthcare change the doctor-patient relationship? What remains of non-technological and closely tied to the encounter between people? In our view, empathy remains together with the motivation leading health personnel to take care of patients and, finally, the recognition of the sanctity of the human life. These elements are still, if you will, out of the control and management of technology.

REFERENCES

Aldrich, D., & Masera, P. (1999). *Mastering the Digital Market Place*. New York, NY: John Wiley & Sons.

Alpay, L. L., Henkemans, O. B., Otten, W., Rövekamp, T. A., & Dumay, A. C. (2010). E-health applications and services for patient empowerment: Directions for best practices in The Netherlands. *Telemedicine Journal and e-Health*, *16*(7), 787–791. doi:10.1089/tmj.2009.0156 PMID:20815745

Anderson, J. G. (2007). Social, ethical and legal barriers to e-health. *International Journal of Medical Informatics*, *76*(5), 480–483. doi:10.1016/j.ijmedinf.2006.09.016 PMID:17064955

Atkinson, R. D., & McKay, A. S. (2014). *Digital Prosperity – Understanding the Economic Benefits of the Information Technology Revolution.* Retrieved May 7, 2014 from http://www.itif.org/index.php?id=34

Ball, M. J., & Lillis, J. (2001). E-health: Transforming the physician-patient relationship. *International Journal of Medical Informatics, 61*(1), 1–10. doi:10.1016/S1386-5056(00)00130-1 PMID:11248599

Bardram, J. E., Mihailidis, A., & Wan, D. (Eds.). (2006). *Pervasive Computing in Healthcare.* Boca Raton, FL: CRC.

Bashshur, R., Shannon, G., Krupinski, E., & Grigsby, J. (2011). The taxonomy of telemedicine. *Telemedicine Journal and e-Health, 17*(6), 484–494. doi:10.1089/tmj.2011.0103 PMID:21718114

Bates, D. W., Cohen, M., Leape, L. L., Overhage, J. M., Shabot, M. M., & Sheridan, T. (2001). Reducing the frequency of errors in medicine using information technology. *Journal of the American Medical Informatics, 8*(4), 299–308. doi:10.1136/jamia.2001.0080299 PMID:11418536

Benevolo, C., & Spinelli, R. (2011). International service delivery and Internet-based technologies. *International Journal of Services. Economics and Management, 3*(3), 251–266.

Berner, E. S. (2008). Ethical and legal issues in the use of Health Information Technology to improve patient safety. *HEC Forum, 20*(39), 243–258. doi:10.1007/s10730-008-9074-5 PMID:18803020

Bernstein, M. L., McCreless, T., & Côté, M. J. (2007). Five constants of Information technology Adoption in Healthcare. *Hospital Topics, 85*(1), 17–25. doi:10.3200/HTPS.85.1.17-26 PMID:17405421

Bhagwati, J. (1987). International trade in services and its relevance for economic development. In O. Giarini (Ed.), *The Emerging Service Economy* (pp. 3–57). Oxford, UK: Pergamon Press.

Bitner, M. J., Brown, S. W., Goul, M., & Urban, S. (2008). Services science journey: foundations, progress, and challenges. In B. Hefley & W. Murphy (Eds.), *Service science, management and engineering education for the 21st century* (pp. 227–233). Springer; doi:10.1007/978-0-387-76578-5_35

Black, A. D., Car, J., Pagliari, C., Anandan, C., Cresswell, K., Bokun, T., & Sheikh, A. et al. (2011). The impact of eHealth on the quality and safety of health care: A systematic overview. *PLoS Medicine, 8*(1), e1000387. PMID:21267058

Buntin, M. B., Burke, M. F., Hoaglin, M. C., & Blumenthal, D. (2011). The benefits of health information technology: A review of the recent literature shows predominantly positive results. *Health Affairs, 30*(3), 464–471. doi:10.1377/hlthaff.2011.0178 PMID:21383365

Burman, E. (2003). *Shift!: The Unfolding Internet: Hype, Hope and History.* Chichester, UK: John Wiley & Sons.

Castells, M. (2000). *The Rise of the Network Society.* Oxford, UK: Blackwell Publishers.

Castillejo, P., Martínez, J. F., Rodríguez-Molina, J., & Cuerva, A. (2013). Integration of wearable devices in a wireless sensor network for an E-health application. *IEEE Wireless Communicatons, 20*(4), 38–49. doi:10.1109/MWC.2013.6590049

Chase, R. B. (1978). Where does the customer fit in a service operation? *Harvard Business Review, 56*(5), 137–142. PMID:10239167

Chávez, E., Krishnan, P., & Finnie, G. (2010). A taxonomy of e-health standards to assist system developers. In G. A. Papadopulos et al. (Eds.), *Information Systems Development. Towards a Service Provision Society* (pp. 737–745). New York, NY: Springer US.

Chesbrough, H. (2005). Toward a science of services. *Harvard Business Review, 83*(2), 16–17.

Cho, S.-E. (2005). Developing new frameworks for operations strategy and service system design in electronic commerce. *International Journal of Service Industry Management, 16*(3), 294–314. doi:10.1108/09564230510601413

Commission of the European Communities. (2004). e-Health - making healthcare better for European citizens: An action plan for a European e-Health Area. Luxembourg: Commission of the European Communities.

Coradeschi, S., Cesta, A., Cortellessa, G., Coraci, L., Gonzalez, J., Karlsson, L., . . . Otslund, B. (2013). Giraffplus: Combining social interaction and long term monitoring for promoting independent living. In *Human System Interaction (HSI), 2013 The 6th International Conference on.* IEEE.

Demattè, C., Biffi, A., Mandelli, A., & Parolini, C. (2007). Firms and the Digital Technology in Italy: The Network Moves Forward. In U. Apte & U. Karmarkar (Eds.), *Managing in the Information Economy* (pp. 429–471). New York, NY: Springer. doi:10.1007/978-0-387-36892-4_18

Devaraj, S., & Kohli, R. (2000). Information Technology payoff in the healthcare industry: A longitudinal study. *Journal of Management Information Systems, 16*(4), 41–67. doi:10.1080/07421222.2000.11518265

Dixon, B. E. (2007). A roadmap for the adoption of e-Health. *e-Service Journal, 5*(3), 3–13. doi:10.2979/ESJ.2007.5.3.3

Eiglier, P., & Langeard, E. (1987). *Servuction. Le marketing des services.* Paris, France: McGraw-Hill.

Eikelboom, R. H., & Atlas, M. D. (2005). Attitude to telemedicine, and willingness to use it, in audiology patients. *Journal of Telemedicine and Telecare, 11*(8), S22–S25. doi:10.1258/135763305775124920 PMID:16375788

Eng, T. (2001). *The e-Health Landscape – a terrain map of emerging information and communication technologies in health and health care.* Princeton NJ: The Robert Wood Johnson Foundation. Retrieved May 23, 2014 from http://www.hetinitiative.org/media/pdf/eHealth.pdf

England, I., Steward, D., & Walker, S. (2000). Information technology adoption in health care: When organizations and technology collide. *Australian Health Review, 23*(3), 176–185. doi:10.1071/AH000176 PMID:11186051

Evans, P., & Wurster, T. S. (2000). *Blown to bits. How the new economics of information transforms strategy.* Boston, MA: Harvard Business School Press.

Eysenbach, G. (2001). What is e-health? *Journal of Medical Internet Research, 3*(2), e20. doi:10.2196/jmir.3.2.e20 PMID:11720962

Fatehi, F., & Wootton, R. (2012). Telemedicine, telehealth or e-health? A bibliometric analysis of the trends in the use of these terms. *Journal of Telemedicine and Telecare, 18*(8), 460–464. doi:10.1258/jtt.2012.GTH108 PMID:23209265

Fickenscher, K., & Bakerman, M. (2011). Leadership and governance for IT projects. *Physician Executive, 37*(1), 72–76. PMID:21302752

Fieschi, M. (2002). Information technology is changing the way society sees health care delivery. *International Journal of Medical Informatics, 66*(1-3), 85–93. doi:10.1016/S1386-5056(02)00040-0 PMID:12453562

Freema, W. D., Vatz, K. A., & Demaerschalk, B. M. (2010). Telemedicine in 2010: Robotic caveats. *Lancet Neurology, 9*(11), 1046. doi:10.1016/S1474-4422(10)70261-1 PMID:20965432

Frennert, S., & Östlund, B. (2014). Domestication of a telehealthcare system. *Gerontechnology (Valkenswaard), 13*(2), 197. doi:10.4017/gt.2014.13.02.105.00

Frisse, M. E. (2009). Health Information Technology: One step at a time. *Health Affairs, 28*(2), 379–w384. doi:10.1377/hlthaff.28.2.w379 PMID:19273814

Gaggioli, A., Di Carlo, S., Mantovani, F., Castelnuovo, G., & Riva, G. (2005). A telemedicine survey among Milan doctors. *Journal of Telemedicine and Telecare, 11*(1), 29–34. doi:10.1258/1357633053430476 PMID:15829041

Gagnon, M.-P., Lamothe, L., Fortin, J.-P., Cloutier, A., Godin, G., Gagné, C., & Reinharz, D. (2005). Telehealth adoption in hospitals: An organisational perspective. *Journal of Health Organization and Management, 19*(1), 32–56. doi:10.1108/14777260510592121 PMID:15938601

Gantz, J., & Reinsel, D. (2011). Extracting value from chaos. *IDC iview*, 1-12.

Garg, A. X., Adhikari, N. K. J., McDonald, H., Rosas-Arellano, M. P., Devereaux, P. J., Beyene, J., & Haynes, R. B. et al. (2005). Effects of Computerized Clinical Decision Support Systems on practitioner performance and patient outcomes: A systematic review. *Journal of the American Medical Association, 293*(10), 1223–1238. doi:10.1001/jama.293.10.1223 PMID:15755945

Geng, W., Talwar, S., Johnsson, K., Himayat, N., & Johnson, K. D. (2011). M2M: From mobile to embedded internet. *IEEE Communications Magazine, 49*(4), 36–43. doi:10.1109/MCOM.2011.5741144

Gerber, T. (2009). Health Information Technology: Dispatches from the revolution. *Health Affairs, 28*(2), 390–w391. doi:10.1377/hlthaff.28.2.w390 PMID:19273816

Grönroos, C. (1990). *Service Management and Marketing: Managing the Moments of Truth in Service Competition.* New Britian, CT: Lexington Books.

Gunter, T. D., & Terry, N. P. (2005). The emergence of national electronic health record architectures in the United States and Australia: Models, costs, and questions. *Journal of Medical Internet Research, 7*(1), e3. doi:10.2196/jmir.7.1.e3 PMID:15829475

Haidegger, T., Sándor, J., & Benyo, Z. (2011). Surgery in space: The future of robotic telesurgery. *Surgical Endoscopy, 25*(3), 681–690. doi:10.1007/s00464-010-1243-3 PMID:20652320

Haux, R., Ammenwerth, E., Herzog, W., & Knaup, P. (2002). Health care in the information society. A prognosis for the year 2013. *International Journal of Medical Informatics, 66*(1-3), 3–21. doi:10.1016/S1386-5056(02)00030-8 PMID:12453552

HIMSS – Healthcare Information and Management Systems Society. (2014). *Electronic health record (HER)*. Retrieved on May 16, 2014 from http://www.himss.org/ASP/topics_ehr.asp

Holler, J., Tsiatsis, V., Mulligan, C., Avesand, S., Karnouskos, S., & Boyle, D. (2014). *From Machine-to-machine to the Internet of Things: Introduction to a New Age of Intelligence*. Oxford, UK: Academic Press.

IOM – Institute of Medicine. (2001). *Crossing the Quality Chasm: A New Health System for the 21st Century*. Washington, DC: National Academy Press.

Javalgi, R. G., Martin, C. L., & Todd, P. R. (2004). The export of e-services in the age of technology transformation: Challenges and implications for international service providers. *Journal of Services Marketing, 18*(7), 560–573. doi:10.1108/08876040410561884

Karsh, B. T., Weinger, M. B., Abbott, P. A., & Wears, R. L. (2010). Health information technology: Fallacies and sober realities. *Journal of the American Medical Informatics Association, 17*(6), 617–623. doi:10.1136/jamia.2010.005637 PMID:20962121

Kaye, R., Kokia, E., Shalev, V., Idar, D., & Chinitz, D. (2010). Barriers and success factors in health information technology: A practitioner's perspective. *Journal of Management & Marketing in Healthcare., 3*(2), 163–175. doi:10.1179/175330310X12736577732764

Kennedy, S., & Berk, B. (2011), Enabling E-Health: A revolution for informatics in health care. *BCG Perspectives*. Retrieved on June 17, 2011 from www.bcgperspectives.com

Lateef, F. (2011). The practice of telemedicine: Medicolegal and ethical issues. *Ethics & Medicine, 27*(1), 17–25.

Liu, W., & Park, E. K. (2014). Big Data as an e-Health Service. In *Computing, Networking and Communications (ICNC), 2014 International Conference on*. IEEE. doi:10.1109/ICCNC.2014.6785471

Lovelock, C. H. (1983). Classifying services to gain strategic marketing insights. *Journal of Marketing, 3*(47), 9–20. doi:10.2307/1251193

Lovelock, C. H. (1996). *Service Marketing* (3rd ed.). London: Prentice Hall International.

Lovelock, C. H., & Wirtz, J. (2004). *Services Marketing: People, Technology, Strategy* (5th ed.). Upper Saddle River, NJ: Prentice Hall.

Maglio, P. P., & Spohrer, J. (2008). Fundamentals of service science. *Journal of the Academy of Marketing Science, 36*(1), 18–20. doi:10.1007/s11747-007-0058-9

Malecki, E. J., & Moriset, B. (2008). *The Digital Economy: Business Organization, Production Processes, and Regional Developments*. Oxon, UK: Routledge.

Mancini, M. (2014). Exploiting big data for improving healthcare services. *Journal of e-Learning and Knowledge Society, 10*(2), 23-33.

Masys, D. (1998). Advances in Information Technology. Implications for medical education. *The Western Journal of Medicine*, *168*(5), 341–347. PMID:9614791

MEDgle Inc. (2014). *The details*. Retrieved on May 15, 2014 from http://www.medgle.com/front.jsp?t ask=technology&section=details

MeriTalk. (2014). *The Big Data Cure*. Retrieved on January 25, 2015 from http://www.meritalk.com/ bigdatacure

Moghaddasi, H., Asadi, F., Hosseini, A., & Ebnehoseini, Z. (2012). E-health: A global approach with extensive semantic variation. *Journal of Medical Systems*, *36*(5), 3173–3176. doi:10.1007/s10916-011-9805-z PMID:22113437

Moruzzi, M. (2009). *E-health e fascicolo sanitario elettronico*. Milano, Italy: Il Sole 24 Ore.

Mukhopadhyay, S. (2015). Wearable sensors for human activity monitoring: A review. *IEEE Sensors Journal*, *15*(3), 1321–1330. doi:10.1109/JSEN.2014.2370945

Normann, R. (1984). *Service Management Strategy and Leadership in Service Business*. Chichester, UK: John Wiley & Sons.

O'Malley, A. S. (2011). Tapping the unmet potential of health information technology. *The New England Journal of Medicine*, *364*(12), 1090–1091. doi:10.1056/NEJMp1011227 PMID:21428764

OECD – Organisation for Economic Co-operation and Development. (2010). *Improving Health Sector Efficiency. The Role of Information and Communication Technologies*. Paris, France: OECD.

Oh, H., Rizo, C., Enkin, M., Jadad, A., Powell, J., & Pagliari, C. (2005). What is eHealth (3): A systematic review of published definitions. *Journal of Medical Internet Research*, *7*(1), e1. doi:10.2196/jmir.7.1.e1 PMID:15829471

Osservatorio ICT in Sanità – School of Management of the Politecnico di Milano. (2008). *ICT e innovazione in sanità: nuove sfide e opportunità per i CIO*. Milano: Politecnico di Milano, Dipartimento di Ingegneria gestionale.

Osservatorio ICT in Sanità – School of Management of the Politecnico di Milano. (2013). *ICT in sanità: perché il digitale non rimanga solo in agenda*. Milano: Politecnico di Milano, Dipartimento di Ingegneria gestionale.

Pagliari, C., Sloan, D., Gregor, P., Sullivan, F., Detmer, D., Kahan, J. P., & Mac Gillivray, S. et al. (2005). What is eHealth (4): A scoping exercise to map the field. *Journal of Medical Internet Research*, *7*(1), e9. doi:10.2196/jmir.7.1.e9 PMID:15829481

Porter, M. (2001). Strategy and the Internet. *Harvard Business Review*, *79*(2), 63–78. PMID:11246925

PricewaterhouseCoopers. (2007). *The Economics of IT and Hospital Performance*. Retrieved July 14, 2011 from http://www.pwc.com/us/en/healthcare/publications/the-economics-of-it-and-hospital-performance.jhtml

Rahman, Z. (2004). E-commerce solution for services. *European Business Review*, *16*(6), 564–576. doi:10.1108/09555340410565396

Safavi, S., & Shukur, Z. (2014). Conceptual privacy framework for health information on wearable device. *PLoS ONE*, *9*(12), e114306. doi:10.1371/journal.pone.0114306 PMID:25478915

Safran, C. (2003). The collaborative edge: Patient empowerment for vulnerable populations. *International Journal of Medical Informatics*, *69*(2), 185–190. doi:10.1016/S1386-5056(02)00130-2 PMID:12810122

Salomann, H., Kolbe, L., & Brenner, W. (2006). Self-services in customer relationships: Balancing high-tech and high-touch today and tomorrow. *E-Service Journal*, *4*(2), 65–84. doi:10.2979/ESJ.2006.4.2.65

Shapiro, C., & Varian, H. R. (1999). *Information Rules: A Strategic Guide to the Network Economy*. Boston, MA: Harvard Business School Press.

Shekelle, P., & Goldzweig, C. L. (2009). *Costs and Benefits of Health Information Technology: An Updated Systematic Review*. London, UK: The Health Foundation.

Showell, C., & Nohr, C. (2012). How should we define eHealth, and does the definition matter?. *Quality of Life through Quality of Information, 180*, 881-884.

Silvestro, R., Fitzgerald, L., Johnston, R., & Voss, C. (1992). Towards a classification of service processes. *International Journal of Service Industry Management*, *3*(3), 62–75. doi:10.1108/09564239210015175

Slack, C. (2007). The robot surgeon. *Proto Magazine*. Retrieved May 17, 2014 from: http://www.protomag.com/assets/the-robot-surgeon?page=1

Sood, S., Mbarika, V., Jugoo, S., Dookhy, R., Doarn, C. R., Prakash, N., & Merrell, R. C. (2007). What is telemedicine? A collection of 104 peer-reviewed perspectives and theoretical underpinnings. *Telemedicine Journal and e-Health*, *13*(5), 573–590. doi:10.1089/tmj.2006.0073 PMID:17999619

Spinelli, R. (2008). The digital economy: A conceptual framework for a new economic paradigm. *The Journal of Business*, *8*(1/2), 53–59.

Spohrer, J., & Maglio, P. P. (2008). The emergence of service science: Toward systematic service innovations to accelerate co-creation of value. *Production and Operations Management*, *17*(3), 238–246. doi:10.3401/poms.1080.0027

Srinivasan, U., & Arunasalam, B. (2013). Leveraging big data analytics to reduce healthcare costs. *IT Professional*, *15*(6), 21–28. doi:10.1109/MITP.2013.55

Stiglitz, J. E., Sen, A., & Fitoussi, J.-P. (2009). *Report by the Commission on the Measurement of Economic Performance and Social Progress*. Retrieved on January 25, 2015 from http://www.stiglitz-sen-fitoussi.fr/en/index.htm

Stroetmann, K. A., Jones, T., Dobrev, A., & Stroetmann, V. N. (2006). eHealth is Worth it. The Economic Benefits of Implemented eHealth Solutions at Ten European Sites. Luxembourg: Commission of the European Communities.

Taylor, R., Bower, A., Girosi, F., Bigelow, J., Fonkych, K., & Hillestad, R. (2005). Promoting Health Information Technology: Is there a case for more-aggressive government action? *Health Affairs*, *24*(5), 1234–1345. doi:10.1377/hlthaff.24.5.1234 PMID:16162568

Thomas, D. R. E. (1978). Strategy is different in service businesses. *Harvard Business Review*, *56*(4), 158–165.

Tocci, R. (1988). *Digital System- Principles and Applications* (4th ed.). Englewood Cliffs, NJ: Prentice-Hall International.

Tulu, B., Chatterjee, S., & Laxminarayan, S. (2005). A taxonomy of telemedicine efforts with respect to applications, infrastructure, delivery tools, type of setting and purpose. In *Proceedings of the 38th Hawaii International Conference on System Sciences*. IEEE. doi:10.1109/HICSS.2005.56

Tulu, B., Chatterjee, S., & Maheshwari, M. (2007). Telemedicine taxonomy: A classification tool. *Telemedicine Journal and e-Health*, *13*(3), 349–358. doi:10.1089/tmj.2006.0055 PMID:17603838

Van Halteren, A., Bults, R., Wac, K., Konstantas, D., Widya, I., Dokovsky, N., & Herzog, R. et al. (2004). Mobile patient monitoring: The MobiHealth system. *The Journal on Information Technology in Healthcare*, *2*(5), 365–373.

Vincent, A., Cusack, C. M., Pan, E., Hook, J. M., Kaelber, D. C., & Middleton, B. (2007). A new taxonomy for telehealth technologies. In *AMIA Annual Symposium Proceedings*.

Whitmore, A., Agarwal, A., & Da Xu, L. (2014). The Internet of Things—A survey of topics and trends. *Information Systems Frontiers*, 1–14.

Whitten, P., & Love, B. (2005). Patient and provider satisfaction with the use of telemedicine: Overview and rationale for cautious enthusiasm. *Journal of Postgraduate Medicine*, *51*(4), 294–299. PMID:16388172

WHO – World Health Organisation. (2006a). eHealth Tools and Services. Needs of the Member States. Geneva, Switzerland: WHO.

WHO – World Health Organisation. (2006b). *Building Foundations for eHealth. Progress of Member States*. Geneva, Switzerland: WHO.

Zeithaml, V. A., & Bitner, M. J. (2000). *Service Marketing: Integrating Customer Focus across the Firm*. New York, NY: McGraw Hill.

Zhijiang, D., Zhiheng, J., & Minxiu, K. (2006). Virtual reality-based telesurgery via teleprogramming scheme combined with semi-autonomous control. *Proceedings of the 27th Annual International Conference*. Engineering in Medicine and Biology Society.

KEY TERMS AND DEFINITIONS

Big Data: A new generation of technologies and architectures, designed to economically extract value from very large volumes of a wide variety of data, by enabling the high velocity capture, discovery, and/or analysis (Ganz & Reinsel, 2011).

Digital Economy: The pervasive use of ICT in all aspects of the economy, including internal operations of organizations; transactions between organizations; and transactions between individuals and organizations (Atkinson & McKay, 2007).

E-Health: The use of emerging information and communications technology, especially the Internet, to improve or enable health and healthcare (Eng, 2001).

Electronic Health Records: A systematic collection in digital format of health information about an individual patient (Gunter & Terry, 2005).

E-Prescriptions: Computer-based electronic generation, transmission and filling of a medical prescription, and the electronic fit/sick notes, for sick leaves and insurance purposes.

Georeferencing: The act of assigning locations to pieces of information, objects or individuals.

Internet of Things: A paradigm where everyday objects can be equipped with identifying, sensing, networking and processing capabilities that allow them to communicate with one another and with other devices and services over the Internet to accomplish some objective (Whitmore et al. 2014).

M2M: Solutions that allow communication between devices of the same type and specific application, all via wired or wireless communication networks (Holler et al., 2014)

RFID (Radio Frequency Identification): A technology that uses electronic tags placed on objects, people, or animals to relay identifying information to an electronic reader by means of radio wave.

Wearable Technology: A category of technology devices that can be worn by a consumer and that incorporates computer and advanced electronic technologies.

This research was previously published in Reshaping Medical Practice and Care with Health Information Systems edited by Ashish Dwivedi, pages 205-245, copyright year 2016 by Medical Information Science Reference (an imprint of IGI Global).

Chapter 47
Healthcare Services Delivery in India:
Special Reference to Mother and Child Health

Ajith Paninchukunnath
KIIT School of Rural Management, India

ABSTRACT

This chapter deals with innovation in healthcare services. Addressing the healthcare needs of consumers in the lower middle and lower class of Indian society demands innovative approaches. Child and maternal health demands special focus as the infant mortality rate of India is higher than the world average as well as the Asia-Pacific average. After giving a brief description about the need for innovation, healthcare innovation, and secondary care hospitals, the chapter introduces the reader to an innovative secondary healthcare service provider in India. The innovative approach adopted by this organization is making maternal and child care more affordable while maintaining good quality. Service innovations can provide value for money as well as value for many.

INTRODUCTION

This chapter has multiple objectives. In the initial part, it will deal with the healthcare service scenario in India and the role of service innovation in addressing healthcare challenges in emerging economies. The next part deals with definition of innovation, frugal innovation and healthcare innovation. The chapter will move on with four types of innovation, hierarchy of service innovation and basic elements of service design. In the remaining part, the author discusses the healthcare needs of mother and child especially with a focus on infant mortality. The entry of a new service provider which addresses the needs of mother and child using a frugal innovation model is highlighted. Merrygold Health Network which is an innovative Social Franchising Program in India providing essential health care services to the poorer sections in the society is briefly described. The chapter concludes by highlighting how the learning from this chapter, in devising new solutions to address healthcare service challenges, can be adopted in other emerging economies.

DOI: 10.4018/978-1-5225-3926-1.ch047

BACKGROUND

Healthcare Services in India

India has the second largest population in the world. In terms of revenue and employment, healthcare is one of India's largest service-sector industries. Indian healthcare industry is poised to double from $60 billion to $120 billion by 2015, growing at a 15 per cent CAGR (Rao, 2012). According to rating agency Fitch, the Indian healthcare sector is expected to reach US$ 100 billion by 2015 from the current US$ 65 billion, growing at around 20 per cent a year (Dutt, 2012). Though the forecasts may vary, the factors driving the growth in the sector are very clear. They include increasing population, growing lifestyle related health issues, cheaper costs for treatment (especially for foreign patients), improving health insurance penetration, increasing disposable income, thrust in medical tourism, government initiatives, focus on Public Private Partnership (PPP) models and the Government of India's decision to increase health expenditure to 2.5 per cent of GDP by the end of the 12th Five Year Plan (2012-17), from the existing 1.4 per cent. According to a report by McKinsey Global Institute (2007), health care spending in India is expected to touch 13% of average household income by 2025 from 7% in 2005.

Three broad components of healthcare sector are; healthcare delivery, pharma products, and medical equipment. Healthcare delivery, comprising primary, secondary and tertiary care facilities, constitutes 77% of the total market. Pharma and medical equipment segments constitute 14% and 5% respectively. India has an additional requirement of 0.8 million doctors and 1.7 million nurses, apart from facing a significant shortage of paramedics. Forty five per cent of the population travels more than 100 km to access tertiary level of medical care. Poor accessibility, accountability and affordability of healthcare services are key constraints that make the idea of 'health for all' just a dream (Rao, 2012). Seventy five per cent of Indian allopathic doctors are practicing in urban areas where as nearly 70% of Indians live in rural areas. The Central Government had introduced Rashtriya Bal Swasthya Karyakram (RBSK, meaning National Child Health Programme), under the National Rural Health Mission (NRHM), which is an initiative for Child Health Screening and early intervention. A total of 270 million children, between birth and 18 years, would be checked for birth defects, diseases, deficiencies, and developmental delays. Children who are diagnosed with any of the specified illness would be treated free of cost, including surgery, under the NRHM. Despite significant efforts to improve child healthcare, the infant mortality rate in the country is still an area of grave concern (Banerjee, 2013). Another area of equal concern is the maternal health. Maternal and child health are the most sensitive markers of the robustness of health delivery as a whole in any given country. Any well-functioning health system should not allow deaths of mothers and children from causes which are easily preventable.

Levels of Healthcare in India

Health service delivery in India is characterized by a three-tier system (see Figure 1). At the lowest level are the sub centers (each covering a population of about 5,000). Only paramedical staff is available in these sub centers. The first points of contact with a doctor are the primary health centers (each covering about 30,000 people). Community health centers provide secondary care and are organized at the block levels. The sub divisional hospitals and district level hospitals constitute the higher tiers. In principle, the sub centers, primary health centers (PHCs), and community health centers (CHCs) are required to handle the preventative aspects of health care, institutionalize deliveries, treat minor diseases, and act as

Figure 1. Three tier system of healthcare in India
Source: Developed by Author

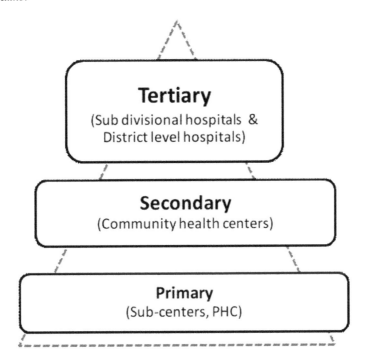

referral centers. The subdivision and district level hospitals would then treat major ailments as referral hospitals (Rao & Choudhury, 2012). According to Ministry of Health and Family Welfare-Government of India, there are 1,48,124 Sub Centres, 23,887 PHCs and 4,809 CHCs functioning in the country as on March 2011.

A study by Muralidharan, Chaudhury, Hammer, Kremer, and Rogers (2011) shows that the national average absence rate for PHC and CHC medical providers is over 39 percent. The absence rate for doctors exceeded 43 percent. In 7 states, more than 40 percent of facilities surveyed had no doctor in attendance at the time of the visit as reported by the study. Such high absence rate is a clear indicator of low quality health care available at many of the PHCs and CHCs in India, making consumers seek alternate service providers mostly in the private sector.

Secondary Care Hospitals in India

According to Rao (2012) secondary care hospitals are mid-sized (100-150 bedded) hospitals offering secondary care and basic diagnostic and pharmacy facilities. Such hospitals can be upgraded to incorporate some elements of tertiary care. They generally focus on specialities like general medicine, general surgery, obstetrics & gynecology, pediatrics, orthopedics and trauma, ophthalmology, ENT, dental surgery, endocrinology, and critical care. Such hospitals are easily replicable, scalable, flexible, and more affordable. Capital and overhead costs are lower than typical multi-speciality hospitals, workflows are standardized, operational management is easier, and outreach, penetration and patient loyalty higher. The total market for secondary care services in India currently stands at Rs 42,000 crore, and is expected to reach Rs 261,000 crore by 2020. One of the main driving forces for this market is the fact that 80 per cent of ailments can be catered by secondary care. India is likely to see aggressive activity and investment in this market by corporate groups, especially in tier II and tier III cities. To serve consumer segments such as lower-middle income, urban poor and rural population, secondary care hospitals with one speciality focus is more suitable.

Innovation and Healthcare

Innovation is not creativity. Creativity is about the big idea. Innovation is about executing it, and making money out of that idea. It's about making the right resource allocations, building the right team, and getting the product to the market (Govindarajan, 2011). Innovation can be anything as long as it is about new ways of creating value; value for your customers, vendors, employees, shareholders, or even the society (see Figure 2). According to Jane Stevenson, Vice Chairman, Board & CEO Services at Korn/Ferry International, innovation is creating unique value that generates growth or commercial success. Innovation is powered by a thorough understanding, through direct observation, of what people want and need in their lives and what they like or dislike about the way particular products are made, packaged, marketed, sold, and supported (Brown, 2008).

Leaders who look at innovation as a principal source of differentiation and competitive advantage would do well to incorporate design thinking into all phases of the innovation process (Brown, 2008). Strategic innovation, which is a must for all marketing firms in today's market place, in developing markets is fundamentally different from what occurs in developed economies. It is not about locating new consumers (assuming the products and services are affordable), there are plenty of under and non-consuming customers to tap. More often, it involves adapting existing products to customers with fewer resources or different cultural backgrounds and creating basic market ingredients such as distribution channels and customer demand from the ground up (Anderson & Markides, 2007; Paninchukunnath, 2010).

Frugal Innovation and Healthcare

The meaning of word 'frugal' is - practicing or marked by economy, as in the expenditure of money or the use of material resources, living without waste, not costly, meager etc. The root of the word is from Latin "frglis" which means virtuous or thrifty. Frugal innovation results in great value- no-frills, good quality, functional products that are also affordable to the customer with modest means (majority of the rural consumers). Frugal innovation is also called "constraint-based" innovation.

Figure 2. Defining innovation (Source: Developed by Author)

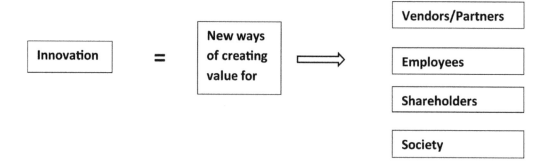

The term 'Frugal Engineering' was coined by Carlos Ghosn the chief executive of Renault and Nissan, to describe the automotive engineering that went into Tata Motors' Nano. Others have described similar ideas under terms such as reverse innovation, "Gandhian innovation" or even "Indo-vation" (Kumar & Puranam, 2012)

Tata itself sometimes refers to its low-cost innovations as Gandhian engineering in honor of India's independence leader Mahatma Gandhi, a renowned proponent of self-sufficiency. Thus "frugal engineering" is achieving more with fewer resources. Innovation goes beyond invention and engineering to aspects like benefit, utility, value and customer acceptance. Frugal innovation is innovation designed to be inexpensive, robust and easy to use. It also means being sparse in the use of raw materials and their impact on the environment (see Figure 3). Howard (2011) described frugal innovation as offerings which are; low-cost, ingenious, rapidly produced and with a low carbon footprint.

Thus frugal innovation can be defined as – A zero-based approach to solving customer's problem by arriving at homegrown solutions/offerings which are simple, sustainable and extremely affordable leading to fast adoption by target customers.

Simplicity requires a deep understanding of consumers, their needs and their habits. Simplicity and "good enough" products deliver higher value because they are designed to do one thing exceptionally well (functional specialization), rather than doing multiple things in a mediocre fashion.

The last century has produced a proliferation of innovations in the health care industry aimed at enhancing life expectancy, quality of life, diagnostic and treatment options, as well as the efficiency and cost effectiveness of the healthcare system (Varkey, Horne, & Bennet, 2006). According to Omachonu and Einspruch (2010) healthcare innovation can be defined as;

The introduction of a new concept, idea, service, process, or product aimed at improving treatment, diagnosis, education, outreach, prevention and research, and with the long term goals of improving quality, safety, outcomes, efficiency and costs.

As per Omachonu and Einspruch (2010), healthcare organizations serve six distinct purposes – treatment, diagnosis, prevention, education, research and outreach (see Figure 4). In serving these purposes, healthcare organizations must effectively manage quality, costs, safety, efficiency and outcomes. At the very core of healthcare innovation are the needs of patients and the healthcare practitioners and providers who deliver care. Quite often, healthcare organizations arrive at innovation by relying on new or existing technology. When successful, healthcare innovation focuses on three areas the most – (a) how

Figure 3. Frugal innovation (Source: Developed by Author)

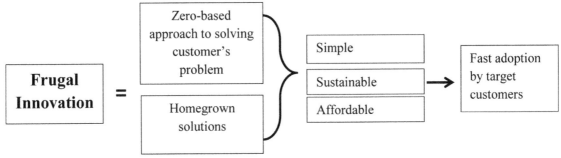

Figure 4. A conceptual framework for innovation in healthcare - Adapted from Omachonu and Einspruch (2010)

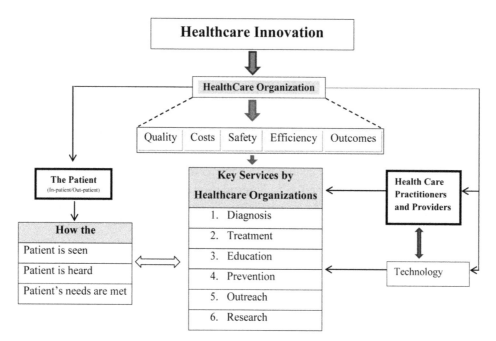

the patient is seen, (b) how the patient is heard, and (c) how the patient's needs are met. The adoption of innovation by the healthcare practitioners and providers of the healthcare organization is the first step to deliver innovative healthcare solutions. According to Berwick (2003) health care innovation is hard, but dissemination is even harder.

Four Types of Innovations

Stevenson and Kaafarani (2011) identified four core types of innovations. They are as follows (Refer Figure 5);

1. **Transformational:** These innovations are disruptive and change society. This kind of innovation brings the highest risk and reward. Very often, the people who drive this kind of innovation don't even realize the core benefits as the time-to-marketplace is long. Internet took forty years to become commercially viable in the marketplace.

2. **Category:** Customers' needs or insights drive these innovations. Often, category innovations come out of transformational innovation. eBay created a new online auction category that leveraged a transformational innovation – the Internet. Category innovation involves either a breakthrough in applications, or in markets served. This type of innovation is strongly guided by a valid business model. While still risky, category innovation has significantly lower risk than transformational innovation, and is generally sustainable over time. Internet banking, debit card are other examples of category innovation.

Figure 5. Four types of innovations (adapted from Stevenson and Kaafarani, 2011)

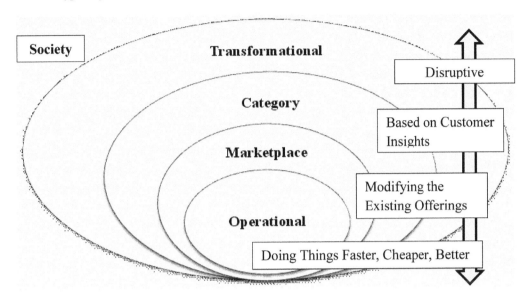

3. **Marketplace:** This could include new packaging or ingredients that give an existing product a fresh appeal. Examples include Proctor & Gamble's single-use sachets for shampoo and detergent, or Coca-Cola's hot canned drinks in vending machines in Japan. Marketplace innovation is great for building increased market share or for keeping a more mature product ahead of the competition.

4. **Operational:** This type of innovation is about doing things faster, cheaper, better. It is focused on new ways to build or deliver products and achieve strong bottom line results. This type of innovation demands a lot of internal focus. Operational excellence and flexibility is a must to deliver operational innovation.

Hierarchy of Service Innovation

Service design encompasses a number of elements: customers, service concept, service encounters, and service delivery system. Service design acts as an integrator of these components. The purpose of service design is to have processes that consistently deliver high quality services to drive customer satisfaction and retention, whilst maintaining process efficiency (Johnston & Clark, 2005). Designing a service product is a complex task. It requires good understanding of how the core and supplementary services should be combined, sequenced, branded and delivered to create a value proposition that meets the needs, wants and preferences of target market segments. New service development demands that marketers adopt innovative approaches.

Service innovation can occur at many different levels. It's important to recognize that not every type of innovation has an impact on the characteristics of the core product or results in a significant change in the customer's experience. The word "new" is popular in marketing because it's a good way to attract people's attention. However, there are different degrees of "newness" in new service development. In fact, we can identify seven categories of new services, ranging from major innovations to simple style changes (Lovelock, Wirtz, & Chatterjee, 2011).

1. **Major Service Innovations:** Are new core products for markets that have not been previously defined. They usually include both new service characteristics and radical new processes. Examples include FedEx's introduction of overnight, nationwide, express package delivery in 1971, the advent of global news service from CNN, and eBay's launch of online auction services.

2. **Major Process Innovations:** Consist of using new processes to deliver existing core products in new ways with additional benefits. For example, the University of Phoenix competes with other universities by delivering undergraduate and graduate degree programs in a nontraditional way. It has no permanent campus; instead its courses are offered online or at night in rented facilities. Its students get most of the core benefits of a college degree in half the time and at a much lower price than other universities. The existence of the Internet has led to the creation of many start-up businesses employing new retailing models that exclude the use of traditional stores, saving customer's time and travel costs. Often, these models add new, information-based benefits such as greater customization, the opportunity to visit chat rooms with fellow customers, and suggestions for additional products that complement what has already been purchased.

3. **Product Line Extensions:** Are additions to current product lines by existing firms. The first company in a market to offer such a product may be seen as an innovator, but the others are merely followers who are often acting defensively. These new services may be targeted at existing customers to serve a broader array of needs, designed to attract new customers with different needs, or both. Starbucks, known for its coffee shops, has extended its offerings to include light lunches. Major computer manufacturers like Compaq, Hewlett-Packard, and IBM are going beyond their traditional business definitions to offer integrated "e-solutions" based on consulting and customized service. Telephone companies have introduced numerous value-added services such as caller ID, call waiting, and call forwarding. Cable television providers are starting to offer broadband Internet access. Many banks sell insurance products in the hope of increasing the number of profitable relationships with existing customers. American Express, too, offers a full range of insurance products, including auto, home, and umbrella policies. And at least one insurance company State Farm Insurance as gone into the banking business, relying on its well-established brand name to help draw customers.

4. **Process Line Extensions:** Are less innovative than process innovations. But they do often represent distinctive new ways of delivering existing products, either with the intent of offering more convenience and a different experience for existing customers or of attracting new customers who find the traditional approach unappealing. Most commonly, they involve adding a lower-contact distribution channel to an existing high-contact channel, as when a financial service firm develops telephone-based or internet-based services or a bricks -and -mortar retailer adds catalog sales or a Web site. For example, Barnes and Noble, the leading bookstore chain in the United States, added a new Internet subsidiary, BarnesandNoble.com, to help it compete against Amazon.com. Such dual-track approaches are sometimes referred to as click and mortar. Creating self-service options for customers to complement delivery by service employees is another form of process line extension.

5. **Supplementary Service Innovations:** Involve adding new facilitating or enhancing service elements to an existing core service, or significantly improving an existing supplementary service. Low-tech innovations for an existing service can be as simple as adding parking at a retail site or agreeing to accept credit cards for payment. Multiple improvements may have the effect of creating what customers perceive as an altogether new experience, even though it is built around the same

core. Theme restaurants like the Rainforest Cafe are examples of enhancing the core with new experiences. The cafes are designed to keep customers entertained with aquariums, live parrots, waterfalls, fiberglass monkeys, talking trees that spout environmentally related information, and regularly timed thunderstorms, complete with lightning.

6. **Service Improvements:** Are the most common type of innovation. They involve modest changes in the performance of current products, including improvements to either the core product or to existing supplementary services. For instance, a movie theater might renovate its interior, adding ergonomically designed seats with built-in cup holders to increase both comfort and convenience for customers during the show or an airline might add power sockets for laptops in its business-class cabins.

7. **Style Changes:** Represent the simplest type of innovation, typically involving no changes in either processes or performance. However they are often highly visible, create excitement, and may serve to motivate employees. Examples include repainting retail branches and vehicles in new color schemes, outfitting service employees in new uniforms, introducing a new bank check design, or making minor changes in service scripts for employees.

Service Design

Service innovations will be successful with effective designing of services so that service delivery can happen as required by consumers. As per Frei (2008), a service design has four core elements namely; (1) the offering, (2) the funding mechanism, (3) the employee management system and (4) the customer management system. Getting all of them right and aligning them well is crucial for the success of any business. The design is good when the managers are clear about the preferences of target customers and have decided the attributes which the service organization will excel at and the ones in which they will remain weak. Frei (2008) argues that service excellence can be achieved by clearly deciding the attributes on which company will not do well.

Here, the offering refers to the company being able to not only understand the need of the customers, as is often sufficient in regard to physical products, but more importantly the experiences customers wish to gain from the service. By funding mechanism, the author refers to not only setting the price at a sustainable level, but also forming the payment in such a way that it creates minimal negative connotations to the customer. In addition, operators within rather saturated markets such as the insurance business should have a clear understanding of the key points for incurring costs and in the optimal case invest in a new service aspect which, in fact will lower the overall costs of delivering the service as a whole. An employee management system is particularly relevant in the service context, as services are characteristically very labor intensive. Finally, customer management translates into transferring some of the key, or bottleneck, elements of the service delivery process to be handled by the customers.

Healthcare Needs of Mother and Child

Healthcare, one of the basic needs of human beings is not delivered cost effectively for majority of Indians. The cost of healthcare at private hospitals is not affordable to lower middle class and lower class consumers. In the government hospitals, there is under investment and under management. The district hospitals, primary health centers (PHCs) and community health centers (CHCs) are understaffed and overworked. The KPMG study (2011) highlighted the lack of health care infrastructure in the country and noted that maternity was the second most common reason for hospitalization in India, next only to acute infection. The quality of ante-natal care and the number of institutional deliveries in the country were also found to be quite low. Importantly, the utilization of services from non-governmental medical care institutions was found to be expanding at the rate of 30% annually.

India's health achievements are low in comparison to the country's income level. According to UNDP's Human Development Report 2010, in a set of 193 countries, while India ranked 119th on the human development index, it ranked 143rd in infant mortality rate, and 124th in maternal mortality rate (Rao & Choudhury, 2012).

The latest bulletin of the Sample Registration System (SRS) released by the Registrar General of India (RGI) shows that India's infant mortality rate (IMR) has come down by three points from 47 to 44 deaths per 1,000 live births during 2011. IMR for rural areas has dropped by three points from 51 to 48 deaths per 1,000 live births while the urban rate now stands at 29 from the previous 31. Among the states, Goa and Manipur have the lowest IMR of 11, followed by Kerala with 12 deaths per 1,000 live births. Madhya Pradesh has the highest IMR of 59 per 1,000 live births followed by Uttar Pradesh and Odisha with 57 each. Assam, Chhattisgarh, Rajasthan and Meghalaya have IMRs higher than the national average of 44. The SRS is a large-scale demographic survey for providing reliable annual estimates of birth rate, death rate and other fertility and mortality indicators at the national and sub-national levels. The field investigation consists of continuous enumeration of births and deaths in selected sample units by anganwadi workers and teachers (Joshi, 2012).

The under-five mortality rate (U5MR) in Asia and the Pacific was reduced from 86 per 1,000 live births in 1990 to 49 per 1,000 in 2009 (see Figure 6). While this is an impressive improvement, many countries are unlikely to achieve Millennium Development Goal 4 (MDG-4), which targets a two-thirds reduction in U5MR between 1990 and 2015. India's U5MR is higher than Asia-Pacific and World averages. This is an area which requires immediate attention by government and private healthcare institutions.

CASE 1: LIFESPRING HOSPITALS FROM INDIA (AFFORDABLE AND ACCESSIBLE MATERNAL CARE MODEL)

Introduction about LifeSpring

LifeSpring was formed as a Private Limited Company in 2008. It is a 50/50 joint venture between HLL Lifecare and the Acumen Fund. HLL Lifecare is a government of India enterprise (Mini Ratna Company under the Ministry of Health & Family Welfare) providing contraceptives and other health care products and services and the Acumen Fund is a U.S.-based social venture capital firm. The two partners jointly invested about US$4 million in the venture. LifeSpring is formally registered in Kerala, India. The company's corporate headquarters is located in Hyderabad, India (Pingali, 2010).

The Board consists of six directors (including the Chairman), with two Directors each from HLL Lifecare and Acumen Fund, and two Independent Directors with extensive industry experience. LifeSpring's management team consists of professionals with a blend of different backgrounds and expertise, recruited from India and the US. Mr. Anant Kumar, who is the CEO, has worked extensively in areas of social & rural marketing. Mr. M. Ayyappan is the Founder Chairman of LifeSpring Hospitals Pvt. Ltd.

LifeSpring offers pre-natal, delivery and post-natal services both for outpatients and inpatients. It also offers laboratory, pharmacy and family planning services. In addition, it has a community outreach

Figure 6. Infant mortality rate, Asia and the Pacific, 1990 and 2009
Source -The United Nations Economic and Social Commission for Asia and the Pacific (ESCAP) – [http://www.unescap.org/ stat/data/syb2011/I-People/Child-health.asp]

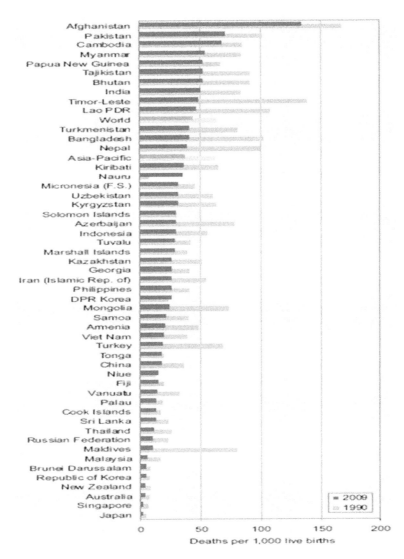

program to educate the surrounding communities on maternity and related health issues. Each hospital is typically a 20-bed facility and has one general ward and two to three deluxe rooms.

Goal of the Company - Serving the Unserved Market

The mission of LifeSpring is to be the leading health care provider delivering high-quality, affordable core maternal health care to low-income mothers across India. LifeSpring offers an alternative to resource constrained government hospitals and higher priced private hospitals. With 80 percent of all health care expenditures in India being out-of-pocket, the goal is;

1. To operate small sized maternity hospitals in the proximity of urban slums, catering to pregnant women whose husbands work in the informal sector and who have no health coverage.
2. To provide core maternal healthcare (antenatal and postnatal, normal and caesarian deliveries, and family planning services) at an affordable price. LifeSpring's prices are 30 to 50 percent lower than market rates). A normal delivery at LifeSpring costs Rs. 4,000. LifeSpring also provides pediatric care (including immunizations), diagnostic and pharmacy services, and health care education to the communities in which its hospitals are located.
3. To maintain a very high level of quality control (clinical and operations), continuously benchmarked with the best health systems in the world.
4. To serve its "patients" as customers, and treat them with respect and dignity.

Services by LifeSpring Hospitals

LifeSpring Hospitals provide outreach, outpatient and inpatient care (see Figure 7) as explained below:

Community Outreach

LifeSpring focuses on community outreach programs to educate the surrounding communities about women's health. Outreach workers and nurses based in each hospital go door-to-door within LifeSpring's communities to educate women and key decision-makers about women's health and maternity issues. LifeSpring's outreach workers and nurses follow-up with each new mother and baby, at the customer's house. The outreach workers and nurses ensure that mother and child are doing well and encourage them to come for follow-up visits with LifeSpring's doctors. Outreach workers and nurses are also available to answer any questions the customer may have.

Prenatal Care

LifeSpring provides prenatal care throughout the length of a woman's pregnancy, from the time she seeks pregnancy confirmation through delivery. LifeSpring's doctors and outreach workers promote prenatal care, as women who see a health care provider regularly during pregnancy have healthier babies, are less likely to deliver prematurely, and are less likely to have other serious problems related to delivery. LifeSpring's suggested schedule for prenatal care visits for a low-risk woman with a normally progressing pregnancy is:

*   **Weeks 4 to 28:** 1 visit per month (every 4 weeks.)
*   **Weeks 28 to 36:** 2 visits per month (every 2-3 weeks.)
*   **Weeks 36 to birth:** 1 visit per week.

LifeSpring Hospital offers high quality prenatal care and consultations with gynecologists. Diagnostic services and a pharmacy are also available to outpatients.

Deliveries

LifeSpring's core inpatient service is normal and caesarean deliveries in general ward. Delivery package includes hospital stay, medicines, doctor's charges and any government supplied free vaccination.

Postnatal Care

After the birth of the baby, LifeSpring Hospitals offer postnatal care services to mother and child. LifeSpring has a team of gynecologists and pediatricians to care for mothers and their babies post-delivery. They provide mothers and their families with medical advice on caring for their newborn, including the baby's vaccination schedule. Additionally, the outreach workers visit each and every woman post-delivery to enquire about the health of mother and baby. LifeSpring's flagship hospital, Moula Ali, provides free vaccinations to babies, through its partnership with the government of Andhra Pradesh.

Innovative Business Model (By a Secondary Care Hospital)

LifeSpring's twin focus on reducing costs and improving volumes help its hospitals become profitable in two years. Mr. Kumar, who is the driving force behind the organization, opened the first 20-bed low-cost LifeSpring hospital in 2005. This was the pilot phase at Moula Ali, a low-income suburb of Hyderabad. The hospital broke even in just 18 months. This was achieved with the support of the management at HLL Lifecare (Kumar, 2011).

LifeSpring developed a low-cost, no-frills maternal care model focusing on service specialization, high asset utilization and para-skilling (the breaking down of a complex process into multiple simple tasks that can be performed by less skilled professionals). The model was designed keeping in mind the core customer base: the bottom 60% of the Indian population with a monthly household income of US$60 to US$140. Most of LifeSpring's customers at present are employed in the informal sector. Each consultation with a LifeSpring doctor is priced at Rs. 80 (~$1.45 USD) and pediatricians cost Rs.100 (~$1.82 USD). A normal delivery costs Rs. 4000 (~ $ 73 USD) and a caesarean delivery costs Rs. 9000 (~ $ 164 USD) in the general ward.

A tiered pricing model helps its commercial viability. Women, for instance, can choose to give birth in a general ward, semi-private room or private room. Rates will rise accordingly. LifeSpring's general

Figure 7. Services by lifespring hospitals (source: developed by author)

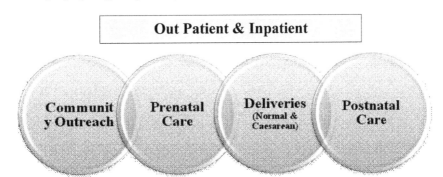

ward, which makes up 70 per cent of each hospital, is 30-50 per cent cheaper than comparable market rates; its private room is at par with the rest of the market. Normal deliveries, that costs Rs. 4000 (~ $ 73 USD), includes the cost of a two-day stay in the hospital and medicines. The cost of caesarean operation, that costs Rs. 9000 (~ $ 164 USD) at LifeSpring, is just a fifth of what is charged by private hospitals. While that is more than the official rate at public hospitals, which are supposed to be free though they often require undisclosed payments, these are still only about a sixth of the price at a private clinic (Joshi, 2012).

LifeSpring is a major nonmedical service innovation. The innovation is mainly at the business model and management level than at the medical level. The key innovative aspects (see Figure 8) are given below:

1. **High Throughput:** LifeSpring operates at a much higher volume (outpatient and deliveries) than traditional players, which spreads its fixed costs over a larger number of customers. LifeSpring hospitals complete 100-120 deliveries per month compared to 30-40 in similarly sized hospitals.

2. **No Frills Model:** LifeSpring provides services that are required by most of its customers while refraining from making investments in additional infrastructure required by very few of its customers.

3. **Service Specialization:** LifeSpring's specialization in core maternal healthcare allows its processes to become standardized and repeatedly performed by its clinical staff. These processes are replicated across all hospitals, facilitating LifeSpring's expansion.

4. **Maximising Asset Utilisation:** LifeSpring hospitals operate in clusters. By setting multiple hospitals in a city, some of the expensive resources (ambulances, back-end operations) are shared across hospitals.

5. **Collaboration:** Collaboration with pediatric hospitals to provide intensive care for the 2%-3% of the new born babies has helped not only in keeping the initial capital costs low, but also in reducing operating expenses related with hiring full-time pediatricians and pediatric nurses.

Key Stakeholders of the Healthcare Innovation Process

Balancing the demands of different stakeholders while introducing an innovative solution is not easy. Some of the needs, wants and expectations of the key stakeholders are given below (see Table 1).

Figure 8. The lifespring hospitals model (source: developed by author)

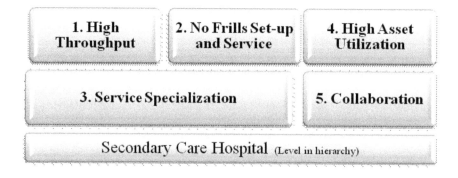

Table 1. Expectations of stakeholders (source: developed by author)

Stakeholders	Needs, Wants & Expectations
Spouse, Parents	Safety of mother and child, Safe delivery, Good care, Affordable, Awareness
Mother	Safe delivery, Good care and attention, Awareness, Accessibility
Child	Good care, Registration of birth, Birth certificate, Immunization
Management of LifeSpring	Profitability, Improved outcomes, Customer satisfaction, Achieving the mission, Growth of firm, Positive word of mouth
Regulatory Agencies/Govt.	Reduced risks and improved patient safety, Reduction in IMR and maternal deaths
Employees	Regular payment of salary, Training, Safe and clean working environment
Society/Nation	Achieve MDG 4&5 (Child Health and Maternal Health)

Strategy for Low Cost but High Quality

Twin focus on reducing costs and improving volumes helps the individual hospitals to become profitable in less than two years.

Managing Costs

LifeSpring hospitals operate in leased premises to keep project costs lower than traditional hospital models. Operating out of leased premises, flexi-staffing (an optimum patients-to-staff ratio is maintained on the basis of the number of deliveries done) and short-term transfers to sister facilities have also helped to keep the costs down. Following the success of its pilot hospital, LifeSpring's business model is designed such that each hospital could become operationally profitable within 18 months.

Higher Volume

LifeSpring operates at a much higher volume for outpatient care and deliveries than traditional players. A LifeSpring hospital typically completes 100 to 120 deliveries per month compared with 30 to 40 in similarly sized hospitals. The scale helps spread the company's fixed costs over a larger number of customers.

Quality

LifeSpring's hospitals are ISO-certified with strict clinical guidelines. More than 150 processes related to clinical and operational protocol are followed at LifeSpring. A partnership with the Cambridge-based Institute for Healthcare Improvement (IHI) is also in place. IHI's expertise in clinical quality improvement has helped LifeSpring decrease rates of maternal and neonatal morbidity, improve clinical protocol adherence and strengthen a culture of safety in all hospitals. In addition to clinical outcomes, quality improvement initiatives have simultaneously increased operational efficiency, leading to a reduction in operating costs.

LifeSpring established a protocol for employee-customer relations: The CARES (courteous, attentive, respectful, enthusiastic and safe) staff protocol played an important role in overcoming local families' distrust of institutional health providers and in building trust. LifeSpring employed a five-pillar metric to gauge its performance and sustainability in terms of growth, finance, customer satisfaction, clinical quality and talent (Joshi, 2012).

Promotion

LifeSpring has also adopted an innovative approach to reach out to its target audience. Its marketing team utilizes the clinical health information management system to track pregnant women in the communities it serves. Realizing that the real decision makers are usually the pregnant woman's mother, mother-in-law or husband, the hospital's campaigns address these decision-makers through orientation programs, health camps and other initiatives. Community outreach workers are employed at each LifeSpring hospital for executing these marketing initiatives. The outreach workers mostly come from the very communities that they serve.

Network and Long Term Plans

LifeSpring currently operates 12 hospitals in the city of Hyderabad. LifeSpring plans to set up 100 hospitals across India in the next 5 years. Currently LifeSpring is a private, for-profit company. It is looking to go public in five years.

Impact on Market

Among the customers of LifeSpring, 52% had previously delivered at home or in a public hospital, and 48% have husbands who work in the informal sector. LifeSpring is bringing down the cost of healthcare in the market by forcing other private players to remain competitive. It works as a catalyst to improve the quality of healthcare being delivered by other providers in the market. LifeSpring also brings out substantial saving to its customers, as they pay a much lower price for their healthcare than they would otherwise have been forced to pay. Its chain of hospitals is reducing the burden on resource-constrained government hospitals. LifeSpring will significantly lessen the burden of rising health costs on the nation's low-income communities, increasing their disposable income. When the out of pocket money spent on healthcare is less, low-income households can use the saved money to meet some of their other unmet needs. As of June 2012, more than 16,000 healthy babies have been delivered across all LifeSpring Hospitals.

LifeSpring was honoured with World and Business Development Awards. These awards are organized by the UN Development Program, the International Business Leaders Forum and the International Chamber of Commerce. The purpose of these awards is to raise awareness among governments, donors and other stakeholders, of the positive impact that inclusive business models can have on the progress towards the Millennium Development Goals (MDGs). The awards ceremony was part of the special focus on the MDGs during the opening week of the United Nations' General Assembly in New York. LifeSpring has also received an award from Frost & Sullivan, a business research and consulting firm, for the "Mother and Child Healthcare Provider of the Year" and from ET Now "leap of faith award" under the healthcare category.

CASE 2: BIRTH OF A NEW ENTITY UNDER PPP MODEL FOR MOTHER AND CHILD HEALTH

State Innovations in Family Planning Project Services Agency (SIFPSA), Government of Uttar Pradesh (UP), India and United States Agency for International Development (USAID) in collaboration with Hindustan Latex Family Planning Promotion Trust (HLFPPT), a not for profit trust promoted by Hindustan Latex Limited, India, launched Merrygold Health Network (MGHN) on 23rd August 2007. UP with 16% of the Indian population (Census, 2011) is the most populous state of India. The MMR in UP is 359, second highest rate after the state of Assam with 390 (SRS, 2007-09).

Merrygold Health Network is an innovative Social Franchising Program in India providing essential health care services to the poorer sections in the society. The program is being implemented through a Public Private Partnership (PPP) in an endeavor to make health care services accessible for the underprivileged. MGHN aims at creating access to low cost good quality Maternal and Child Health (MCH) services by networking with private health service providers as franchisees.

The project has a hub and spoke design with Level 1 franchisees (Merrygold) established at district levels as the hub connected to level 2 and level 3. Level 2 comprises of fractional franchisees (Merrysilver) established at subdivision and block level. Level 3 (merryAYUSH) comprises of providers like auxiliary nurse midwives (ANMs), and ASHA (Accredited Social Health Activist) workers. It acts as the first point of contact with the community. Level 3 also provides referral support to Merrysilver and MerryGold hospitals. Emphasis is on affordable pricing, quality assurance, customer servicing and efficient service delivery through standardized operating protocols.

With 70 Merrygold hospitals, 371 Merrysilver clinics and 10,814 Merrytarang members functioning currently in 36 districts of UP, it is the single largest health network in the state. It has provided safe delivery service to 1,37,830 women till August 2012. Since its inception in 2007, Merrygold have been continuously endeavoring to scale new heights in provision of quality maternal & child care health services. Over the years, MGHN aims at covering the entire state of UP in India.

Creating a Culture of Innovation

According to the Korn Ferry Institute, there is a need to create a culture of innovation that makes a difference in the workplace and ultimately, the whole business. Given below are the various activities service managers have to implement in their organization for creating a culture of innovation. The nine recommendations are from the paper titled - Asia's innovation imperative (Stevenson, n.d.).

1. **Foster a Customer-Focused Culture:** Create an environment that makes it obvious that everyone ultimately reports not to the internal hierarchy, but to your company's customers. Empower employees at all levels, even the CEO, to think about how they can fill customer's as yet unmet needs.
2. **Celebrate Creativity and Learning:** Most commercial successes come after learning from approaches that didn't initially work. Make sure you celebrate these true progress points on the path to success.
3. **Take a Portfolio Approach to Managing Innovation:** Make sure you have the right mix of each type of innovation from both an opportunity and a risk perspective.

4. **Link your Business Strategy to the Types of Innovation that Best Exploit your Capabilities:** Then ensure you have connected the right type of leadership and culture to the opportunities you have identified.

5. **Know what Type of Innovation Leaders you Have:** Put them in situations that maximize their odds for success. For example, if you put an operational innovation leader into a role that requires category innovation, the odds for success are very low.

6. **Incubate Innovation:** Protect it—especially the transformational variety—from mainstream corporate culture or the traditional success metrics will kill it before it takes off.

7. **Use Marketplace Innovation as a Training Ground:** It is lower risk, and it allows leaders to build confidence before taking on category innovation challenges.

8. **Use Compensation and Other Reward Systems to Encourage Creativity:** Rewarding any talent that finds new ways to help the company to reach a common goal is a sure way to enhance innovation success. On the other hand, a fear-based culture will kill innovation every time.

9. **Reward Teamwork:** Innovation is a team sport, and nothing spurs it on more than when new ideas are shared and utilized broadly.

LEARNINGS AND MANAGERIAL IMPLICATIONS

Lessons for Healthcare Managers in India

The components of service design namely the offering, the funding mechanism, the employee management system and the customer management system of LifeSpring Hospitals are well aligned. Within the Indian context, secondary care institutions are the most suited to address the challenge of inclusive healthcare delivery. Tertiary care institutions are very capital intensive. Primary care organizations cannot address a large number of medical needs. Secondary care institutions, especially the ones which have specialized in one, two or a maximum of three medical specialties are the most suited to penetrate the bottom of the pyramid. They are less capital intensive and can address a large number of medical needs apart from effectively doing the work of primary care institutions.

Managers of the existing tertiary and primary care institutions need to understand and appreciate the unique strengths of secondary care institutions. Introduction of many secondary care hospitals with specialization in various domains of medical specialty can effectively address the challenge of affordable and accessible health care especially at the BOP and rural areas of India. Government can also promote secondary care institutions by giving fast track clearances for new projects, tax incentives during the initial years of a new project establishment or by partnering with private players through PPP models.

Lessons for Other Emerging Markets

LifeSpring hospitals are a major service innovation as a new offering to the market place. It is for the first time in India that a dedicated low cost model of secondary care hospital chain is introduced to address the healthcare needs of mother and child. Through its process-driven model, each LifeSpring Hospital is easily replicable in other locations, ensuring scalability and supporting rapid expansion. With a dual goal of fulfilling its social mission while achieving financial sustainability, LifeSpring hospitals is a good model for providing high quality health services to the poor in emerging markets. Making healthcare inclusive is a major hurdle for many emerging economies.

LifeSpring's focus on a particular niche - maternal and child care - cuts down on the need for many specialist doctors and also on the range of equipment needed (Joshi, 2011a). Specialising in in-patient gynecology and obstetrics leads to easy standardisation. It has over 90 standard procedures, including standardised surgery kits and clinical protocols. LifeSpring uses a narrow range of drugs and equipment for large numbers of repeat procedures and thus purchases standard equipment and generic medicines in bulk. LifeSpring's highly standardised processes allow for quality control and easy routines and replication by lesser-skilled hospital employees.

LifeSpring doctors earn fixed salaries rather than the variable consulting fees of their private clinic peers. Doctors nevertheless have strong non-monetary incentives to stay, like less administrative duties and more clinical practice. LifeSpring hires less qualified auxiliary nurse midwives (ANMs) rather than graduate nurse midwives (GNMs). The former are trained as birth attendants. But because the ANMs are less qualified, they are less costly to employ than GNMs, whose degrees are more advanced and expensive to attain. Moreover, the attrition rate of ANMs is low as well (Joshi, 2011b).

LifeSpring's innovation lay in figuring out how to deliver world-class care at a price that many of the poor could afford and that also made economic sense. Maintaining hygiene, privacy, transparent and economic pricing, and retaining skilled medical personnel allowed LifeSpring to position themselves as a trusted provider of consistently high-quality package of maternity services to low-end markets. LifeSpring's high throughput/high asset use model is vastly more productive than that of its counterparts, allowing it to become profitable quickly and sustain itself. LifeSpring presents a scaleable model for healthcare because it services densely-populated peri-urban areas, filling gaps left by the alternately dismal and highly exclusive maternity care services preceding it and awakening latent demand for trustworthy, credible healthcare services. Its no-frills approach allows for minimum costs and optimum asset utilisation, as well as highly standardised and replicable processes. Its strongly customer-centric positioning and strategic retention of skilled staff is also the key to the sustainability of this model.

Lessons for Developed Markets

The cost of healthcare is very high in many developed countries. Clear focus on few specialties and understanding the target market well can contribute to reducing the cost of healthcare service delivery. Over focus on tertiary care and super-speciality hospitals to address even small, minor or routine healthcare needs can be very costly approach. A large number of medical interventions can be effectively handled by small secondary care hospitals which are much easier to set up and manage. The focus on one, two or three specialities can further make the processes simple and faster contributing to better customer outcomes, customer satisfaction and bottom line of the organization.

CONCLUSION

India faces several challenges in healthcare industry such as improving access, affordability and quality. The health care system is seriously broken despite the existence over many decades of primary, secondary and tertiary health centres and public hospitals open to all. India has one of the most fragmented and commercialized healthcare systems in the world.

Private expenditure on health is among the highest in the world. About 60% of all the hospitals in India are private. With the high economic growth and emergence of the famed Indian middle class, 20th century models of health care will not deliver the care India need in the 21st century. Health care, far from helping people rise out of poverty, has become an important cause of household impoverishment and debt. India has among the highest rates of infant mortality and maternal deaths in childbirth.

Innovation is about looking ahead, and helping people believe that they can make a difference. Innovation is a team activity, it has to be integrated into the fabric of the company. Innovative solutions have to be identified to address the healthcare challenges especially of lower middle class and lower class consumers of society. Secondary care hospitals are the most suited to make modern healthcare more accessible and affordable to Indian consumers, especially for those at BOP. India needs strategies that are customized to address its needs and in alignment with the financial resource available. This calls for rigorous participation from both the public and the private sectors. We need to improve our management capacity and the health system should not be doctor dependent. We should focus on task-shifting, where nurses and paramedics are trained to handle work efficiently. Innovation in management of healthcare is the way forward rather than depending only on medical technology to make healthcare more accessible and affordable. LifeSpring, a secondary care hospital based at Hyderabad, India has developed an innovative and sustainable model to address some of the current challenges in healthcare inclusion.

By building an affordable hospital system with uncompromising quality and a focus on new mothers as consumers, LifeSpring has changed the way we think about what low-income women should expect when it comes to reproductive health care. LifeSpring's business model on the operations and marketing side make it an excellent double bottom line business (people and profit). A healthy India is crucial for the country to make the most of its demographic advantage and to sustain economic prosperity. Innovative approaches by organizations like LifeSpring should be encouraged by government for making healthcare more accessible and affordable to the BOP. LifeSpring's focus on providing benefits to a neglected but important target segment has made healthcare more inclusive in India. Sustainable innovations in health care delivery models, as introduced by LifeSpring, can make 'health for all' in emerging markets like India a reality.

REFERENCES

Anderson, J., & Markides, C. (2007). Strategic innovation at the base of the pyramid. *MIT Sloan Management Review*, *49*(1), 83.

Banerjee, S. (2013). *Infant mortality an area of concern*. Retrieved February 9, 2013, from http://www. thehindu.com/news/national/sonia-launches-national-child-health-screening-programme/article4386001. ece

Berwick, D. M. (2003). Disseminating innovations in health care. *Journal of the American Medical Association*, *289*(15), 1969–1975. doi:10.1001/jama.289.15.1969 PMID:12697800

Brown, T. (2008). Design thinking. *Harvard Business Review*, *86*(6), 84–92. PMID:18605031

Census. (2011). Retrieved November 13, 2012, from http://censusindia.gov.in/2011-prov-results/prov_results_paper1_india.html

Dutt, S. (2012). *Making India an evolved healthcare market.* Retrieved November 3, 2012, from http://www.financialexpress.com/news/making-india-an-evolved-healthcare-market/976447

Frei, F. X. (2008). The four things a service business must get right. *Harvard Business Review*, *86*(4), 70–80. PMID:18435008

Govindarajan, V. (2011). *Jugaad: A model for innovation.* Retrieved November 30, 2012, from http://forbesindia.com/article/defining-debates-of-2011/vijay-govindarajan-jugaad-a-model-for-innovation/25512/1?id=25512&pg=1#ixzz1k6iaUBif

Howard, M. (2011). Will frugal innovation challenge the west? *Market Leader*, *3*, 53.

Johnston, R., & Clark, G. (2005). *Service operations management: Improving service delivery* (2nd ed.). Harlow, UK: FT Prentice Hall.

Joshi, M. (2012). *India's infant mortality rate drops.* Retrieved November 30, 2012, from http://www.topnews.in/health/indias-infant-mortality-rate-drops-217258

Joshi, S. (2011a). *A sixfold path to sustainable and inclusive innovations.* Retrieved February 25, 2013, from http://www.causebecause.com/news-detail.php?NewsID=285

Joshi, S. (2011b). *A spring of hope.* Retrieved January 5, 2012, from http://www.business-standard.com/article/management/a-spring-of-hope-111110700084_1.html, 12

KPMG. (2011). *Emerging trends in healthcare.* Retrieved December 2, 2012, from http://www.kpmg.com/IN/en/IssuesAndInsights/ThoughtLeadership/Emrging_trends_in_healthcare.pdf-

Kumar, A. (2011). *A better way to do healthcare.* Retrieved February 25, 2012, from http://www.hosmacfoundation.org/Pulse/Hosmac_Pulse_September_2011.pdf

Kumar, N., & Puranam, P. (2012). Frugal engineering: An emerging innovation paradigm. *Ivey Business Journal, 76*(2).

Lovelock, C., Wirtz, J., & Chatterjee, J. (2011). *Services marketing: People, technology, strategy* (7th ed.). Delhi: Pearson.

McKinsey Global Institute. (2007). *The 'bird of gold': The rise of India's consumer market.* Retrieved November 5, 2012, from http://www.mckinsey.com/locations/india/mckinseyonindia/pdf/India_Consumer_Market.pdf

Ministry of Health and Family Welfare. (n.d). Retrieved November 5, 2012, from http://mohfw.nic.in/

Muralidharan, K., Chaudhury, N., Hammer, J., Kremer, M., & Rogers, F. H. (2011). *Is there a doctor in the house? Medical worker absence in India.* Retrieved December 24, 2012, from http://www.economics.harvard.edu/faculty/kremer/files/Is%20There%20a%20Doctor%20in%20the%20House%20-%2012%20April%202011.pdf

Omachonu, V. K., & Einspruch, N. G. (2010). Innovation in healthcare delivery systems: A conceptual framework. *The Innovation Journal: The Public Sector Innovation Journal, 15*(1).

Paninchukunnath, A. (2010). Rural marketing in India and the 3P framework. *SCMS Journal of Indian Management, 7*(1), 54–67.

Pingali, P. (2010). *Affordable, high quality core maternal healthcare for low-income women in India.* Retrieved January 20, 2013, from http://www.cha ngemakers.com/browse/human-rights-peace/gender-equity?page=8

Rao, M. (2012). *Forecasts for Indian healthcare.* Retrieved December 3, 2012, from http://www.expresshealthcare.in/201201/market24.shtml-

Rao, M. G., & Choudhury, M. (2012). *Health care financing reforms in India* (Working Paper No: 2012-100). Retrieved December 13, 2012, from http://www.nipfp.org.in/newweb/sites/default/files/wp_2012_100.pdf-

SRS. (n.d.). Retrieved February 13, 2013, from http://planningcommission.nic.in/data/datatable/0904/tab_145.pdf

Stevenson, J. (n.d.). *Asia's innovation imperative.* Retrieved July 26, 2013, from http://www.kornferryasia.com/leadership/Asia's%20innovation%20imperative.pdf

Stevenson, J., & Kaafarani, B. (2011). *Breaking away: How great leaders create innovation that drives sustainable growth and why others fail.* New York: McGraw Hill.

Varkey, P., Horne, A., & Bennet, K. E. (2008). Innovation in health care: A primer. *American Journal of Medical Quality, 23*, 382–388. doi:10.1177/1062860608317695 PMID:18820143

KEY TERMS AND DEFINITION

Acceptability: The extent to which the firm's total product offering meets and exceeds customer expectations.

Accessibility: The extent to which customers are able to readily acquire and use the product.

Affordability: The extent to which customers in the target market are able and willing to pay the product's price.

Asset Light: Managing the service business by leasing or renting the various fixed and capital assets rather than owning them by the service organization.

Frugal Innovation: A zero-based approach to solving customer's problem by arriving at homegrown solutions/offerings which are simple, sustainable and extremely affordable leading to fast adoption by target customers.

Healthcare Innovation: The introduction of a new concept, idea, service, process, or product aimed at improving treatment, diagnosis, education, outreach, prevention and research, and with the long term goals of improving quality, safety, outcomes, efficiency and costs.

No-Frills Model: Services are designed and delivered with more focus on features which are basic and essential for service delivery for target customers. Value added services and augmented services are either not provided or are provided on payment of additional price.

Public Private Partnership (PPP): An emerging model of providing services under which the government organizations partner with private organizations in developing or delivering services to target customers.

This research was previously published in Innovations in Services Marketing and Management edited by Anita Goyal, pages 170-189, copyright year 2014 by Business Science Reference (an imprint of IGI Global).

Chapter 48
A Demand–Driven Cloud–Based Business Intelligence for Healthcare Decision Making

Shah Jahan Miah
Victoria University, Australia

ABSTRACT

Technology development for process enhancement has been a topic to many health organizations and researchers over the past decades. In particular, on decision support aids of healthcare professional, studies suggest paramount interests for developing technological intervention to provide better decision-support options. This chapter introduces a combined requirement of developing intelligent decision-support approach through the application of business intelligence and cloud-based functionalities. Both technological approaches demonstrate their usage to meet growing end users' demands through their innovative features in healthcare. As such, the main emphasis in the chapter goes after outlining a conceptual approach of demand-driven cloud-based business intelligence for meeting the decision-support needs in a hypothetical problem domain in the healthcare industry, focusing on the decision-support system development within a non-clinical context for individual end-users or patients who need decision support for their well-being and independent everyday living.

INTRODUCTION

Health organizations have randomly been made substantial investments in improving their processes through assistance of new technology over the past decades. As their technological intervention, most of the cases they aim at developing ways to delivering timely and accurate health or medical information to the right people, at a right time, to enable and enhance various operational and strategic decision-making (Carte et al. 2005). In particular on decision support aids previous studies suggest two main emphasizes on developing technological intervention to provide better decision support mechanisms. First emphasis goes on such decision support system that helps various practitioners in a clinical environment in relation to information management perspective. On the other hand, second emphasis goes on decision support

DOI: 10.4018/978-1-5225-3926-1.ch048

system development within a non-clinical context for individual end-users or patients who need decision support for their well-being and independent every-day living.

Developing intelligent decision support systems within the medical domain for improving clinical activities is not a novel research area. Over the past decades many studies have identified different problems of intelligent solution developments for different purposes. Examples includes Zhuang, Wilkin & Ceglowski (2013) for pathology test ordering; Corchado, Bajo, Paz & Tapia (2008) for monitoring Alzheimer patients; Lin, Hu & Sheng (2006) for lower back pain diagnosis and Haghighi et al. (2013) for the improvement of emergency management systems. These studies employ various intelligent techniques to improve clinical practices for medical professionals. However, the intelligent systems design should not only focus on the problem analysis and relevant technology design for process improvement, but also focus to meet the client's domain-specific on-site information demands within the new technological provisioning platform that would provide better user-access and flexibility (Miah, 2012a). Other line of relevant studies highlight their interventions on non-clinical care domain, for example the study on home based care delivery (Barjis, Kolfschoten & Maritz, 2013), web-based patients intervention (Liang et al. 2006) and wireless patient monitoring (Varshney, 2008). These studies compliment the research done in the direction of telemedicine or telehealthcare domain for decision support (Karim & Bajwa, 2011). Drawing from this the key focus of this chapter goes on how an approach of demand-driven cloud-based Business Intelligence (BI) can be conceptualized to benefit of end users for their well-being and independent every-day living through the application of new technological provisioning platform such as cloud computing.

The importance of decision support systems (DSS) have increasingly identified as an enabler to the achievement of medical industry's strategic and operational objectives over the many decades. DSS promises to provide timely and relevant information in addition to analytical capabilities to assist effective decision-making (Turban & Aronson, 2001). Keen & Scott Morton (1978, p 1-2) identified four major characteristics of DSS:

- Impact on decision in which there is sufficient structure for computer and analytic aids to be of interest,
- Payoff is in extending the range and capability of decision process to help improve effectiveness,
- The relevance for users is in the creation of a supportive tool, under their own control, and
- Applications are no routine as needed.

As the demand of DSS to support effective decision making have increased, so have the terms used to describe them: data warehousing, knowledge management, data mining, collaborative systems, online analytical processing, with Business Intelligence tending to encompass all (Gibson et al, 2004). Business Intelligence (BI) can be considered as the combination of processes and technologies to assist in decision making for managers and end users. The BI systems have been well-recognized for enhancing the effectiveness of information management and decision making. It is suggested that BI provides comprehensive decision support mechanism to meet all levels of demands for decision makers through applications such as decision support systems, query and reporting, online analytical processing (OLAP), statistical analysis, forecasting, and data mining (Stasieńko, 2010).

The advantage of cloud computing is that it is capable to offer a cloud-based (e.g. Internet or web-based provisioning) decision support service to meet the health professionals and end users decision needs. Other known benefit is that it can bring access and service flexibility both for service users and service providers (Miah, 2012b). With the benefit, it is important to understand and develop conceptual approach for designing the service delivery technology. In this chapter, our study is relevant to such a service design, namely an intelligent DSS application for the provision of cloud computing. As such, this book chapter will analyze current decision support issues of health organizations and professionals in order to develop a demand-driven cloud-based BI solution approach. The chapter will also identify fundamental issues in developing such a combined decision support mechanism by employing ontology and rules-based techniques. The mechanism could ensure decision support processes for management of information from three particular views such as professionals-oriented, patient-care oriented and organization and government settings oriented to their decision making aid.

BACKGROUND

Healthcare data provides wide variety of purposeful meanings to influence on decisions making. In health informatics, the need of decision making has generally been addressed for various practitioners as professional users (such as patients, hospital carers and healthcare professionals) as well as end users (such as patients and private and government health organizations). Health organizations and professionals nowadays are suffering from difficulties to effectively manage, process, and use the bombarded health information which has influence on their decisions making. They use various piecemeal e-health approaches for retrieving, displaying, analyzing, transferring and sharing such a huge amount of information offline and online to meet their regular demands of decision support.

Jackson (2009) mentioned that the current economic crisis is having a severe impact on many healthcare providers as "the financial market's decline has reduced available investment income funds that offset declining reimbursements and falling philanthropic donations" and "the rising unemployment associated with the downturn has lowered admissions and elective procedures and increased uncompensated care" (pp.3). Jackson (2009) also described that continuing rising costs for qualified personnel in almost every roles within a healthcare provider's organization and the cost of supplies essential to the delivery of care have been of significant strategic issue in terms of implementing and monitoring continuous improvements in patient safety and quality of care delivery. This problem became a common headache all over the world. Patient groups also deliberately suffer from the dilemma as it is more than a simple matter of having more information systems available to resolve the delivery issue of appropriate care and decision support process to targeted stakeholders.

Web services are Internet-based application components provide universally available standard interface for various users. With enormous development of the Internet and the web service technologies over the past decade, web services have been very successful in e-commerce, e-business, artificial intelligence (AI), and service computing. They have also offered a number of strategic advantages such as mobility, flexibility, interactivity and interchangeability in comparison with traditional services (Hoffman, 2003). Web services are Internet-based application components that have been offered provisions to deliver healthcare information in a better accessible way and much more affordable way. The newly rising Cloud computing have also been used as a modern architecture of shared computing service in many areas for minimizing labor and implementation expenses (Santos, Gummadi & Rodrigues, 2009). However, the use of cloud based services for the effective decision making of multiple parties is still largely overlooked given its potential benefits. The service is mainly supported through computing utility rental by service providers. After the introduction of web-based utility services by Amazon.com, many web service providers became increasingly interested in the cloud-computing platform for launching new services to meet clients' demands as the cloud-based provision involves minimal labor and implementation expense (Santos et al. 2009). Nurmi, Wolski, & Grzegorczyk (2010) described an open-source software framework for cloud computing in which computing resources are considered as an Infrastructure as a Service. Santos et al. (2009) addressed requirements of confidentiality and integrity in data access and process in order to deliberately propose a trusted cloud computing platform for facilitating a closed box execution and storage in a virtual environment (p.2). This implies that the cloud-based provision must provide secure functionalities with a concurrent trusted storage facility. However, it is important to bring new insights that could improve the decision-making process within the provider communities as well as end users. As mentioned earlier BI techniques help create timely, accurate, and integrated knowledge that transforms healthcare with important outcomes including higher quality services, patient satisfaction, operational efficiency and financial and operational performance (Jackson, 2009; Stasieńko, 2010). In the same way, it is important to formalize the growing requirements of new problem-specific intelligent application design with better service benefits in terms of providing domain-specific decision support to the decision makers through cloud-based functionalities. This is the central motivation of the chapter.

MAIN FOCUS OF THE CHAPTER

The section introduces cloud computing as a central topic and how it can be used in healthcare decision making. This section also describes the targeted decision support in the three particular perspectives such as professionals-oriented, patient-care oriented and organization and government settings oriented to their decision making aid. The main aim is to identify relevant need of decision support technologies in order to reinforce cloud computing-based decision support mechanisms to professionals and end users in delivering the health or medical decision services.

As outlined in many latest journal articles cloud computing is still a developing paradigm. The definition attributes, and characteristics of the cloud computing provisions will be evolving over time. In a literature review, Vaquero, Rodero-Merino, Caceres & Lindner (2008) found more than 20 definitions of cloud computing as of significance definitions containing the essential characteristics. Based on the study Vaquero et al. (2008, p. 51) provided a definition as follows:

Clouds are a large pool of easily usable and accessible virtualized resources (such as hardware, development platforms and/or services). These resources can be dynamically re-configured to adjust to a variable load (scale), allowing also for an optimum resource utilization. This pool of resources is typically exploited by a pay-per-use model in which guarantees are offered by the Infrastructure Provider by means of customized Service-Level Agreements.

This implies that clouding computing is about the way of use to meet demands of users and organizations. The basis of the demand is service oriented rather than process or product oriented requirements. Kuo (2011) suggested three typical models of cloud computing from a service point of view such as: software, platform, and infrastructure. They are namely: Software as a service (SaaS), Platform as a service (PaaS) and Infrastructure as a service (IaaS). In SaaS, software applications are accommodated by a cloud service provider and made available to users and organizations over the Internet. Platform as a service refers to operation platforms or system environments that are hosted on cloud and accessed through users' browser. With PaaS, organizations can employ and develop various web based applications without installing any tools on their local computer, and then deploy those software applications without any specialized maintenance and administrative requirements. Finally, with IaaS, the computing equipment such as hardware, servers, and networking components are hosted for cloud users to use for business support operations, such as for storage, manipulation and processing. The provider of cloud service owns the equipment and is responsible for accommodating, operating, and maintaining the technology. Cloud user typically pays on a per-use basis such as per transactions (Kuo, 2011).

According to IBM & Juniper Networks Solutions (2009) and Kuo (2011) there are models of cloud computing from a deployment point of views (Kuo, 2011). These are as follows:

- **Public Cloud:** A cloud service provider makes resources such as applications and storage environment available over the Internet on a per-use basis. For instance, the Amazon Elastic Compute Cloud (EC2) (as cloud service) allows users to rent virtual computing resources on which to operate their own applications. The cloud service runs within Amazon's network infrastructure and data centers and allows users and public organizations to pay only for what they use.
- **Private Cloud:** A cloud infrastructure is operated solely for sole organization. In this case the proprietary networks such as data center provide hosted services to a certain group of users. For instance, Microsoft Azure enables customers to develop the foundation for a private cloud using windows server with the dynamic data center toolkit (Kuo, 2011).
- **Community Cloud:** A cloud infrastructure is shared by several organizations with common concerns such as security requirements, policy and compliance considerations. For instance, the Google GovCloud provides the Los Angeles City Council with a segregated data environment to store applications and data that are deliberately accessible only to the city's agencies (Kuo, 2011).
- **Hybrid Cloud:** This type of cloud infrastructures contains more than one cloud (e.g. private, public, community). In this cloud service, an organization provides and manages some resources within its own data center and has others provided externally. For example, IBM collaborates with Juniper Networks to deliver a hybrid cloud infrastructure to users and their organizations to extend their private clouds to remote servers (IBM & Juniper Networks Solutions, 2009).

Cloud Computing in Healthcare Decision Support

Many health professionals and experts believe that the cloud computing technologies can improve healthcare services by changing the face of current static health information technology, although it is still emergent to its widespread adoption in many aspects. The potential benefits of cloud computing have been reported in many studies to improve healthcare services. Studies proposed different frameworks to improve health care service (for example the study by Wang & Tan, 2010). Rolim et al. (2010) described a cloud computing solution to automate the process of collecting patients' vital data via a network of sensors connected to legacy medical devices. This system is used to deliver the data to a medical center's cloud for storage, processing, and distribution. Rolim et al. (2010) suggested that the system provides users at anytime from anywhere, real-time data collecting, eliminates manual collection work and the possibility of typing errors, and eases the deployment process. This system mainly makes healthcare data available for the medical professionals. Rao et al. (2010) reported a pervasive cloud initiative called "Dhatri", which integrates the cloud computing functionalities with wireless technologies to enable physicians to access patient health record at anytime from anywhere. Koufi et al. (2010)

proposed a cloud-based solution for emergency medical system for the Greek National Health Service that integrates the emergency system with personal health record systems to provide physicians with easy access to patient records. It implies that cloud computing has been considered as effective solution platform to create automated information support in healthcare sector.

The key functionalities of cloud computing is that it is demand-oriented, self-managed and based on self-service Internet infrastructure that enables the user organizations to access computing resources. It can be seen as an out-sourced infrastructure for computing services as a new model of employing information technologies resources. As mentioned earlier, it is yet to have useful functionalities in this service so relevant decision makers in this sector can have better option to use this as decision support technology. For example, functionalities of DSS can be on cloud for the decision support aid of government and healthcare professionals in healthcare organisations. In designing DSS Haghighi et al. (2013) proposed ontology based knowledge repository for putting appropriate knowledge reasoning with better interpretations for individual's decision support in medical emergency management. For well-defined domains, it is claimed that ontology, as a conceptual modeling technique, has the potential to improve the structuring of knowledge in decision making aid. Apart from this, healthcare sector requires continuous and systematic innovation in order to remain cost effective, efficient, and timely, and to provide high-quality services (Kuo, 2011; Koufi et al., 2010). As indicated in many studies promising innovations through the use of cloud computing have been demonstrated to improve the decision support provisions to targeted user groups. In the scope of this chapter, three particular perspectives are only focused such as professionals-oriented, patient-care oriented and organization and government settings oriented that could help create a platform to support automated data gathering in decision making aid.

Professionals Oriented Decision Support

Clinical decision support systems (CDSS) are one of the appropriate examples of professionals oriented decision support. CDSS analyses medical data to help professionals make clinical decisions. The system commonly used for the support of medical business management. Rouse (2010) suggested that CDSS provide supports for physicians, nurses and other health care professionals to prepare a diagnosis and to review the diagnosis as a means of improving the final medical result and its interpretations. Within the approach most of the cases data mining techniques are used to examine the patient's medical history in conjunction with relevant clinical research, in order to predict potential events, which can range from drug interactions to disease symptoms. Under this specific class of DSS, many example studies exist that are used to provide help decision support to medical professionals. Zhuang, Wilkin & Ceglowski (2013) for pathology test ordering; Corchado, Bajo, Paz and Tapia (2008) for monitoring Alzheimer patients; Lin, Hu & Sheng (2006) for lower back pain diagnosis; and Haghighi et al. (2013) for emergency management.

Zhuang, Wilkin & Ceglowski (2013) described a decision support framework that assists general practitioners (GPs) in ordering pathology tests effectively. The study developed a concept of an integrated intelligent approach that combines knowledge discovery and case-based reasoning technique to capture the contextual requirements for an evidence-based and situation-relevant solution. The key innovation of Zhuang's et al. (2013) approach is that the approach helps GPs to have new understanding about the use of pathology tests by discovering and extracting practical and relevant knowledge from past pathology request data, from both patient-centric and clinical situation-centric perspectives. The approach provides guidance for practitioners through fulfilling ordering needs as it is situation oriented. As diagnostic support tool, Lin, Hu & Sheng (2006) described an intelligent DSS approach to support clinicians' diagnosis of lower back pain (LBP), a usual medical problem that requires appropriate responses to several challenging characteristics. It is because the diagnosis process of LBP required highly specialized knowledge that involves a complex anatomical and physiological structure (Lin et al. 2006). Lin's et al. diagnosis support approach is used multiple complementary methods to acquire the targeted knowledge from two highly experienced domain experts who practice in different clinics and used verbal probability estimation to capture uncertainty. Based on that, they developed a voting scheme for knowledge inference on the basis of consensus. However, Lin's et al. (2006) web-based approach is designed for the clinicians only that consist of a knowledge base, an inference engine, a case repository, and two interfaces for convenient system access and update.

Patient Care Oriented Decision Support

Liang, Xue & Berger (2006) suggested that web-based decision support mechanism has received considerable attention in the healthcare arena for patients specially for transforming healthcare, since Web technologies have been introduced. This decision support approach shares knowledge about providing tailored interventions to individual patients. As part of providing healthcare support the approach helps patients with chronic diseases make decisions about their medication persistency through motivating patients to continue taking their medications. The approach is developed as an initiative in fulfilling consumers' increasing requests of health-related information specific diseases and treatments, especially to support delivery of health services such as behavioral interventions (Liang et al. 2006). Corchado, Bajo, Paz &Tapia (2008) introduced intelligent decision support for monitoring Alzheimer patients' health care in execution time in elderly residences. The AGALZ (Autonomous aGent for monitoring ALZheimer patients) is an autonomous deliberative case-based planner tool designed to plan the nurses' working time dynamically, to maintain the standard working reports about the nurses' activities, and to guarantee that the patients assigned to the nurses are given the right care.

Barjis, Kolfschoten & Maritz (2013) introduced a healthcare decision support recently for providing home-based healthcare services to patients. The approach can be seen as a patient monitoring systems for fulfilling the requirements of medical staff (nurses, doctors) to decide on the course of intervention or further treatment based on the vital signs of the rural patients on a regular basis. The decision support approach provides patient information flow from home-based care workers to a local clinic or hospital, where the information is presented on a desktop computer used by clinic nurses and doctors for monitoring the patients' health and speeding up decision making (Barjis et al. 2013). The proposed system by Barjis et al. has been tested through a proof of concept prototype, which is applied in practice and generating data for evaluation.

Organization and Government Settings Oriented Decision Support

Organizations and governments also seek for decision support aids in improving healthcare service delivery. E-health systems can be seen as appropriate examples of organization and government oriented decision support approach. For example, Shavit (2009) identified the need of government decision making in the allocation of public resources for improving health focusing on needs of the population. The study identifies the importance of analyzing range of technological interventions available for characterizing the need in order to meet the demand of national health goals. Similarly, Moisil & Jitaru (2006) reported on government initiatives of e-health situation in Romania. Barjis, Kolfschoten & Maritz (2013) introduced a healthcare decision support recently for administering home-based healthcare services. From an organizational point of view the approach can be viewed as a patient monitoring systems for fulfilling the requirements of medical staff (nurses, doctors) to decide on the course of intervention in service delivery to mass people. The intervention can be described as further treatment of the rural patients that are tele-monitored by the healthcare organization. Eichler et al. (2004) identified issues of healthcare resource allocation decision making. The study provides an overview of the development of debate on thresholds, reviews threshold figures in relation to cost per unit of health gain, currently proposed for resource-allocation decisions in addition to explore how thresholds may emerge. Eichler's research contributes to the need of transparent and consistent decision-making for government organizations. De Meo et al. (2008) described a decision support approach aiming to support government agency decision makers to design new services tailored to citizen profiles in a complex and distributed e-government scenario. The approach is used to meet design need of citizen's expected access highly personalized services which has been at the basis of many public services such as health education and public housing.

PROPOSED CONCEPTUAL APPROACH

To meet the demand from the perspectives of patient-care, practitioners and organization or government oriented decision support, our study outlines a combined intelligent system approach. Our approach is influenced by a "one-size-fits-all" approach of De Meo et al. (2008), which has been of interest at the basis of many public healthcare services. The proposed conceptual approach of intelligent system focuses on extending a DSS approach introduced by Miah, Kerr & von-Hellens (2013) for the decision support aid of government professionals, domain experts and end users in the rural business context. An Ontology based knowledge repository has been employed for putting appropriate knowledge reasoning with better interpretations for individual's decision support. For well-defined domains, it is claimed that ontology, as a conceptual modeling technique, has the potential to improve the structuring of knowledge. Ontology refers to a particular view of the properties that comprise the problem domain, and how those properties relate to each other (Gennari et al. 2003). The use of ontology to model knowledge can lead towards the development of a solid, contextually relevant cognitive base that enables effective knowledge representation for a specific problem domain (Evermann, 2005). This can result in a useful knowledge-based platform for the development of a contextually relevant knowledge-base. The ontology has been extensively used for DSS developments, such as in the domain of medical emergency management for mass gatherings (Haghighi et al. 2013). The study by Haghighi et al. (2013) used ontology to resolve inconsistencies of terminology to enhance communication support among medical emergency personnel. Our study uses such domain ontology for better knowledge management in decision support across users and organisations, in terms of providing common vocabulary for effective knowledge sharing to different group of users.

The approach works in three layers of functional processes in that it allows three groups of users' decision support as it is important to recognize different classes of user as defined by specific industry requirements and the relevant managerial responsibility. Whilst scientifically informed domain models will be built by healthcare professionals, the choice and focus of these is a policy matter, and their use and customization is an end-user or patients matter. The first (layer at left-hand side in Figure 1) is an authorization layer for organizational users such as healthcare/government managers who allocate resources to assign one or more healthcare professionals to specific domain (e.g. diseases knowledge and relevant expertise). The second layer (middle) allows access to the knowledge acquisition component of the system where the healthcare professionals/experts on particular diseases (targeted domain) will develop decision-making rules and identify cases through the inference engine calibrations using real data on specific diseases. Findings suggested that most intelligent systems simply use rules-based methodology although they may employ various AI techniques varying from agent-based to case-based decision support approaches (Miah, Kerr & Gammack, 2009). However, a set of expert rules for decision making can be determined from domain experts, which are then used to generate the target-relevant rules (such as business logics) of decision support to the end users decision making requirements. This layer employs rules and case based reasoning for providing advisory and monitoring services. The final layer (right-hand side) allows patients access to the system, thus enabling them to achieve their advisory support specific to their own disease management through the support of healthcare information that will be delivered. The authorization layer is required to control resources allocations and to provide accountability in healthcare. The last two layers, namely knowledge acquisition from the specific health service domain (e.g. diseases domain) and specific options to diseases management for targeted patient groups are essential to identify decision support functionality. Figure 1 shows the overall conceptual model in which the three functional processes are given for the three user layers.

For the patient's layer of advisory functionalities, we employ the MYCIN (an earlier expert systems (1970) developed at Stanford for medical professionals to diagnose and recommend treatment for certain blood infections) concept to functionalize the patient's need. The four metaphorical stage tasks are: 1)

Figure 1. The overall architecture of the combined decision support approach

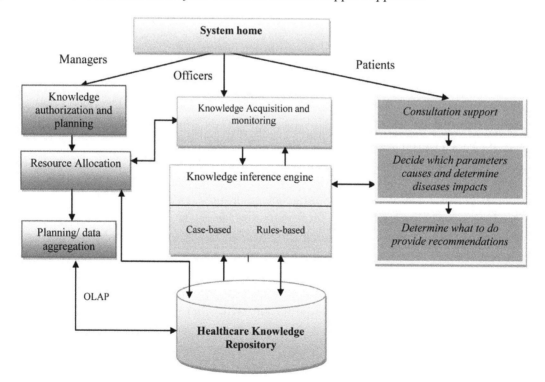

decide which organisms, if any, cause significant disease; 2) determine the likely identify of the significant organisms; 3) decide which drugs can be potentially used and finally; 4) select the best drug or set of plan for drugs. We utilized this metaphor in providing advisory support to specific patients groups. Figure 2 illustrates the possible architectural consideration of the proposed DSS on cloud.

In the cloud based architectural design, the proposed DSS on cloud is based on private and public cloud using hybrid cloud deployment in that the strategy is to share technologies for application servers, however the storage server can still seat at their own premises. Hybrid cloud deployment can offer an unprecedented opportunity to reduce the cost of IT, while improving functionalities of cloud services by employing DSS provisions to meet decision support requirements. In the aspect of the proposed DSS on hybrid cloud, ontology based knowledge will be hosted on public cloud to provide voculabury consistency specially to enhance communication support among medical emergency personnel and meeting their domain need. Database will be still located at private cloud, considering its sensitivity of privacy and security concerns. The ontology layer will integrate the business logics and inference rules of the targeted specific domain in order to display data according to user requests. Our study uses the ontology for better knowledge management in decision support across users and organisations, in terms of providing common vocabulary for effective knowledge sharing to different group of patients/users. However, health organization should outline their strategic planning to examine user and service delivery factors such as information demands, targeted users, information service delivery procedure, technologies, standard rules and policy in healthcare information delivery, and relevant government regulations that may have impact to achieve the goal of implementing such cloud based services. It is important to consider these factors prior to moving the service into the cloud within a non-clinical context for individual end-users or patients who need decision support for their well-being and independent every-day living. In the proposed model it is explained how the government managers and healthcare professional can coordinate and help provide decision support information to patient groups. The proposed conceptual approach attempts to provide an initial decision support solution basis for cloud based platform for potential users.

Figure 2. Proposed DSS design clusters on cloud computing

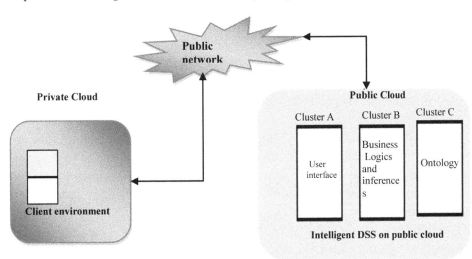

FUTURE RESEARCH DIRECTIONS

The chapter introduced an emergent approach of cloud based intelligent application design. The solution concept is provided within the context of a combined problem space for healthcare service delivery. Based on a literature analysis while the finding presented in this chapter was to create an initial basis of a concept on a review of relevant research, it only represents an early stage research of innovative systematic solution development in the targeted application area. Further research will be required for designing specific knowledge repository through appropriate domain ontology development methodology that will be capable of working with contemporary technological provision. The interactive user's provision in cloud based application design can also be a challenge relevant to healthcare industries in terms of security, ethics and privacy issues. In this purpose, user specific provision considering appropriate ethical and privacy legislations are required to define and implement further for each user groups within their community settings for enabling better decision making or action taking through effective collaboration. An in-depth evaluation study will also be required for system integration and acceptability considering a wide range of healthcare or medical support situations and to ensure compatibility of different technological components within an operating environment.

Further to evaluate the conceptual approach of the solution framework, a test environment for such solution design will be required for ensuring appropriate information generation according to the stakeholder's requirements. This test will also help identify technical difficulties of the intelligent technique and various process-oriented challenges associated with practice and protocol standard in healthcare industries.

CONCLUSION

The chapter discussed a theoretical foundation of creating a new combined intelligent system to meet the demand of industry and new technological interventions of outlining a cloud-based solution for healthcare management. We reinforced the requirement from a management of information from three particular views such as professionals-oriented, patient-care oriented and organization and government settings oriented to their decision making aid. We have demonstrated the requirements of a comprehensive approach design in a targeted problem area in which decision making needs of coordination and cooperation among different groups are identified. A combined solution model was introduced as an example, was previously demonstrated its usability in rural industry for the need of decision making coordination. However, healthcare professionals at any problem domain may have different requirements of decision making that may be used different management concerns, however the main concerns of resource allocation and organization of knowledge domain can be ultimately similar and it is not covered in this chapter. Many organizations may not have appropriate resources and infrastructure associated with healthcare management. Although the cloud-based solution can support flexibility and easier access to real-time data, it involves security and privacy of information and data resources including access control policy concerns.

The collaboration of cloud computing in healthcare industry can be seen as a big step for the healthcare delivery since computing era began. The cloud computing can be a potential answer to enable many services in healthcare organizations that may improve clinical and non-clinical services, especially through the use of intelligent applications. Although intelligent techniques have grown to a sophisticated level, the combination of these services with cloud-based computing is still in an emergent stage. Many relevant tools and technologies are still being developed. The topic area introduced in the chapter for the aid of decision support of targeted professionals' decision making is still just a concept. There is a need for considerable research on initial design and testing prior to implementation of the relevant technology in practice and need to suit the standard protocol of industry. The author attempts to bring a multidisciplinary application area of intelligent cloud techniques to enhance readers' knowledge and understanding in the field.

REFERENCES

Barjis, J., Kolfschoten, G., & Maritz, J. (2013). A sustainable and affordable support system for rural healthcare delivery. *Decision Support Systems*. doi:10.1016/j.dss.2013.06.005 PMID:23729945

Carte, T. A., Schwarzkopf, A. B., Shaft, T. M., & Zmud, R. W. (2005). Advanced business intelligence at cardinal health. *MIS Quarterly Executive*, *4*(4), 413–424.

Corchado, J. M., Bajo, J., de Paz, Y., & Tapia, D. I. (2008). Intelligent environment for monitoring Alzheimer patients, agent technology for health care. *Decision Support Systems*, *44*, 382–396. doi:10.1016/j.dss.2007.04.008

De Meo, P., Quattrone, G., & Ursino, D. (2008). A decision support system for designing new services tailored to citizen profiles in a complex and distributed e-government scenario. *Data & Knowledge Engineering*, *67*, 161–184. doi:10.1016/j.datak.2008.06.005

Eichler, H. G., Kong, S. X., Gerth, W. C., Mavros, P., & Jönsson, B. (2010). Determinants of continuous usage intention in web analytics services. *Electronic Commerce Research and Applications*, *9*, 61–72. doi:10.1016/j.elerap.2009.08.007

Evermann, J. (2005). Towards a cognitive foundation for knowledge representation. *Information Systems Journal*, *15*, 147–178. doi:10.1111/j.1365-2575.2005.00193.x

Gennari, J. H., Musen, M. M., Fergerson, R. W., Grosso, W. E., Crubezy, M., & Eriksson, H. et al. (2003). The evaluation of Protégé: An environment for knowledge based systems development. *International Journal of Human-Computer Studies*, *58*, 89–123. doi:10.1016/S1071-5819(02)00127-1

Gibson, M., Arnott, D., & Carlsson, S. (2004). Evaluating the intangible benefits of business intelligence: Review & research agenda. In *Proceeding of the Decision Support in an Uncertain and Complex World: The IFIP TC8/WG8.3 International Conference*, (pp. 295-305). Preto, Italy: IFIP.

Haghighi, P. D., Burstein, F., Zaslavsky, A., & Arbon, P. (2013). Development and evaluation of ontology for intelligent decision support in medical emergency management for mass gatherings. *Decision Support Systems*, *54*, 1192–1204. doi:10.1016/j.dss.2012.11.013

Hoffman, K. D. (2003). Marketing + MIS = e-service, e-services: A cornucopia of digital offerings ushers in the next net-based evolution. *Communications of the ACM*, *46*(6), 53–55. doi:10.1145/777313.777340

IBM and Juniper Networks Solutions. (2009). *Website IBM and Juniper networks: Delivering solutions that transform your networking infrastructure.* Retrieved from ftp://public.dhe.ibm.com/common/ssi/ecm/en/jns03002usen/JNS03002USEN.PDF

Jackson, L. (2009). *Leveraging business intelligence for healthcare providers* (Oracle White Paper). Redwood Shores, CA: Oracle Corporation.

Jiang, S., Fang, L., & Huang, X. (2009). An idea of special cloud computing in forest pests control. *Lecture Notes in Computer Science, 5931,* 615–620. doi:10.1007/978-3-642-10665-1_61

Karim, S., & Bajwa, I. S. (2001). Clinical decision support system based virtual telemedicine. In *Proceedings of 2011 Third International Conference on Intelligent Human-Machine Systems and Cybernetics.* Academic Press.

Keen, P. G. W., & Morton, M. S. (1978). *Decision support system.* Reading, MA: Addison Wesley.

Koufi, V., Malamateniou, F., & Vassilacopoulos, G. (2010). Ubiquitous access to cloud emergency medical services. In *Proceedings of the 2010 10th IEEE International Conference on Information Technology and Applications in Biomedicine (ITAB).* Corfu, Greece: IEEE.

Kuo, A. M. H. (2011). Opportunities and challenges of cloud computing to improve health care services. *Journal of Medical Internet Research, 13*(3), e67. doi:10.2196/jmir.1867 PMID:21937354

Liang, H., Xue, T. Y., & Berger, B. A. (2006). Web-based intervention support system for health promotion. *Decision Support Systems, 42,* 435–449. doi:10.1016/j.dss.2005.02.001

Lin, L., Hu, P. J. H., & Sheng, O. R. L. (2006). A decision support system for lower back pain diagnosis: Uncertainty management and clinical evaluations. *Decision Support Systems, 42,* 1152–1169. doi:10.1016/j.dss.2005.10.007

Miah, S. J. (2012a). The role of end user in e-government application development: A conceptual model in the agricultural context. *Journal of Organizational and End User Computing, 24*(3), 69–85. doi:10.4018/joeuc.2012070104

Miah, S. J. (2012b). Cloud based DSS development for emergency medical professionals. In *Multidisciplinary computational intelligence techniques: Applications in business, engineering and medicine* (pp. 47–60). Hershey, PA: IGI Global. doi:10.4018/978-1-4666-1830-5.ch004

Miah, S. J., Kerr, D., & Gammack, J. (2009). A methodology to allow rural extension professionals to build target-specific expert systems for Australian rural business operators. *Journal of Expert Systems with Applications, 36,* 735–744. doi:10.1016/j.eswa.2007.10.022

Miah, S. J., Kerr, D., & von-Hellens, L. (2013). A collective artefact design of decision support systems: Design science research perspective. *Information Technology & People, 27*(3).

Moisil, I., & Jitaru, E. (2006). E-health progresses in Romania. *International Journal of Medical Informatics, 75,* 315–321. doi:10.1016/j.ijmedinf.2005.08.013 PMID:16275159

Nurmi, D., Wolski, R., Grzegorczyk, C., Obertelli, G., Soman, S., Youseff, L., & Zagorodnow, D. (2010). The eucalyptus open-source cloud-computing system. In *Proceedings of 9th IEEE/ACM International Symposium on Cluster Computing and the Grid*. IEEE. Retrieved on 22 April, 2011, from http://www.cca08.org/papers/Paper32-Daniel-Nurmi.pdf

Park, J., Kim, J., & Koh, J. (2010). An e-health platform for the elderly population: The butler system. *Electronic Commerce Research and Applications*, 9, 61–72. doi:10.1016/j.elerap.2009.08.007

Rao, G. S. V. R. K., Sundararaman, K., & Parthasarathi, J. (2010). Dhatri: A pervasive cloud initiative for primary healthcare services. In *Proceedings of the 2010 14th International Conference on Intelligence in Next Generation Networks (ICIN)*. Berlin, Germany: IEEE.

Rolim, C. O., Koch, F. L., Westphall, C. B., Werner, J., Fracalossi, A., & Salvador, G. S. (2010). A cloud computing solution for patient's data collection in health care institutions. In *Proceedings of the 2nd International Conference on eHealth, Telemedicine, and Social Medicine*. New York, NY: IEEE.

Rouse, M. (2010). *Definition of clinical decision support system (CDSS)*. Retrieved from http://search-healthit.techtarget.com/definition/clinical-decision-support-system-CDSS

Santos, N., Gummadi, K. P., & Rodrigues, R. (2009). *Towards trusted cloud computing*. Retrieved on 22 April, 2011, from http://www.mpi-sws.org/~gummadi/papers/trusted_cloud.pdf

Stasieńko, J. (2010). Business intelligence as a decision support system. In G. Setlak & K. Markov (Eds.), *Methods and instruments of artificial intelligence* (pp. 141–148). Rzeszow, Poland: Academic Press.

Turban, E., & Aronson. (2001). *Decision support systems and intelligent systems* (6th Ed.). Hoboken, NJ: Prentice Hall, Inc.

Vaquero, L. M., Rodero-Merino, L., Caceres, J., & Lindner, M. (2008). A break in the clouds: towards a cloud definition. *ACM SIGCOMM Computer Communication Review*, 39(1), 50–55. doi:10.1145/1496091.1496100

Varshney, U. (2008). A framework for supporting emergency messages in wireless patient monitoring. *Decision Support Systems*, 45, 981–996. doi:10.1016/j.dss.2008.03.006

Wang, X., & Tan, Y. (2010). Application of cloud computing in the health information system. In *Proceedings of the 2010 International Conference on Computer Application and System Modeling (IC-CASM)*. New York, NY: IEEE.

Zhuang, Z. Y., Wilkin, C. L., & Ceglowski, A. (2013). A framework for an intelligent decision support system: A case in pathology test ordering. *Decision Support Systems*, 55, 476–487. doi:10.1016/j.dss.2012.10.006

ADDITIONAL READING

Buzolic, J., Mladineo, N., & Knezic, S. (2009). Decision support system for disaster communications in Dalmatia. *International Journal of Emergency Management*, 1(2), 191–201. doi:10.1504/IJEM.2002.000520

Cox, P. G. (1996). Some Issues in the Design of an Agricultural Decision Support Systems. *Agricultural Systems*, *52*, 355–381. doi:10.1016/0308-521X(96)00063-7

Evermann, J. (2005). Towards a cognitive foundation for knowledge representation. *Information Systems Journal*, *15*, 147–178. doi:10.1111/j.1365-2575.2005.00193.x

Fischer, G. (1999). Domain-Oriented Design Environments: Supporting Individual and Social Creativity. In J. Gero & M. L. Maher (Eds.), *Computational Models of Creative Design IV* (pp. 83–111). Sydney, Australia: Key Centre of Design Computing and Cognition.

Haghighi, P. D., Burstein, F., Zaslavsky, A., & Arbon, P. (2013). Development and evaluation of ontology for intelligent decision support in medical emergency management for mass gatherings. *Decision Support Systems*, *54*, 1192–1204. doi:10.1016/j.dss.2012.11.013

Hayman, P. T., & Easdown, W. J. (2002). An ecology of a DSS: reflections on managing wheat crops in the North-eastern Australian grains region with WHEATMAN. *Agricultural Systems*, *74*, 57–77. doi:10.1016/S0308-521X(02)00018-5

Mackrell, D., Kerr, D. V., & von Hellens, L. (2009). A qualitative case study of the adoption and use of an agricultural decision support system in the Australian cotton industry: the socio-technical view. *Decision Support Systems*, *47*, 143–153. doi:10.1016/j.dss.2009.02.004

Maio, C. D., Fenza, G., Gaeta, M., Loia, V., & Orciuoli, F. (2011). (in press). A knowledge-based framework for emergency DSS. *Knowledge-Based Systems*.

Marston, S., Li, Z., Bandyopadhyay, S., Zhang, J., & Ghalsasi, A. (2011). Cloud computing — The business perspective. *Decision Support Systems*, *51*, 176–189. doi:10.1016/j.dss.2010.12.006

McCown, R. L. (2002). Changing systems for supporting farmer's decisions: problems, paradigms, and prospects. *Agricultural Systems*, *74*, 179–220. doi:10.1016/S0308-521X(02)00026-4

Miah, S. J. (2008), An ontology based design environment for rural decision support, Unpublished PhD Thesis, Griffith University, Brisbane, Australia.

Miah, S. J. (2009). A new semantic knowledge sharing approach for e-government systems, 4th IEEE International Conference on Digital Ecosystems, Dubai, UAE, pp. 457-462, 2010.

Miah, S. J. (2012). An Emerging Decision Support Systems Technology for Disastrous Actions Management. In S. J. Miah (Ed.), *Emerging Informatics - Innovative Concepts and Applications* (pp. 101–110). Rijeka, Croatia: InTech Open Access. doi:10.5772/2393

Miah, S.J., Kerr, D., & Gammack, J. (2009). A methodology to allow rural extension professionals to build target-specific expert systems for Australian rural business operators, Journal of Expert Systems with Applications, (36), pp. 735-744.

Michalowski, W., Rubin, S., Slowinski, R., & Wilk, S. (2003). Mobile clinical support system for pediatric emergencies, Decision Support Systems, 36 (2), 161-176 Microsoft Azure Services, Retrieved on 12, January, 2012 from URL: http://www.microsoft.com/azure/default.mspx

Mirfenderesk, H. (2009). Flood emergency management decision support system on the Gold Coast, Australia. *Australian Journal of Emergency Management*, *24*, 2.

Mirfenderesk, H. (2009). Flood emergency management decision support system on the Gold Coast, Australia, The Australian Journal of Emergency Management, Vol. 24 No. 2, May 2009

Muntermann, J. (2009). Towards ubiquitous information supply for individual investors: a decision support system design. *Decision Support Systems*, *47*, 82–92. doi:10.1016/j.dss.2009.01.003

Nurmi, D., Wolski, R., Grzegorczyk, C., Obertelli, G., Soman, S., Youseff, L., & Zagorodnow, D. (2010). The Eucalyptus Open-source Cloud-computing System, the 9th IEEE/ACM International Symposium on Cluster Computing and the Grid, retrieved on 22 April, 2011, from http://www.cca08.org/papers/Paper32-Daniel-Nurmi.pdf

Otten, J., Heijningen, B., & Lafortune, J. F. (2004) The virtual crisis management centre. An ICT implementation to canalise information, International Community on Information Systems for Crisis Response (ISCRAM2004) Conference, 3–4 May 2004, Brussels, Belgium.

Qin, J., & Paling, S. (2001). Converting a controlled vocabulary into an ontology: the case of GEM. *Information Research*, *6*(2), 1–11.

Vouk, M.A. (2008). Cloud Computing – Issues, Research and Implementations, Journal of Computing and Information Technology – CIT, 16 (4), 235–246

KEY TERMS AND DEFINITIONS

Case-Based Method: Case-based method uses case based reasoning (CBR) that is the process of solving new problems based on the solutions of similar past problems.

Clinical DSS: CDSS provide supports for physicians, nurses and other health care professionals to prepare diagnosis and to review the diagnosis as a means of improving the final medical result and its interpretations.

Cloud Computing: Cloud computing can be seen as a large pool of easily usable and accessible virtualized resources. The key functionalities of cloud computing are demand-oriented, self-managed and based on self-service Internet infrastructure that enables users to access computing resources.

Business Intelligence: Business Intelligence (BI) can be considered as a combination of processes and technologies to assist in decision making for managers and end users.

Decision Support Systems: Decision Support Systems (DSS) is a computer-based application that provides information support to various organizational decision-making activities. This application enables the management, operations, and planning levels of an organization and help to make decisions for effective businesses.

Rules-Based Method: Rule-based methods use rule discovery or rule extraction from data. This method is one of the data mining techniques aimed at understanding data structures to provide comprehensible description.

This research was previously published in the Handbook of Research on Demand-Driven Web Services edited by Zhaohao Sun and John Yearwood, pages 324-339, copyright year 2014 by Information Science Reference (an imprint of IGI Global).

Chapter 49
Effect of Mobile Phone SMS on M-Health:
An Analysis of Consumer Perceptions

Mahmud Akhter Shareef
North South University, Bangladesh

Jashim Uddin Ahmed
North South University, Bangladesh

Vinod Kumar
Carleton University, Canada

Uma Kumar
Carleton University, Canada

ABSTRACT

This chapter is engaged in identifying consumer perceptions regarding short message service (SMS) of the mobile phone as an alternative service delivery channel for Mobile-health (M-health) and study-ing the cultural impact of this change. In this connection, the Unified Theory of Acceptance and Use of Technology (UTAUT) model was used as the theoretical base to perceive consumer perceptions about M-health. The authors have performed an empirical study of diabetic patients in Bangladesh and Canada. Path analysis was conducted on the results of both samples. Analysis results confirmed that the UTAUT model fits quite nicely in predicting consumer perceptions of M-health-driven mobile technology. It also acknowledged that differences in cultural traits have an impact on consumer behavior.

INTRODUCTION

Globalization, economic development, regular monitoring of the human development index, health consciousness, and soaring life expectancy are factors that voluntarily and forcibly push and diffuse the healthcare service system worldwide. Many consumers are now extremely concerned about better service quality of the healthcare system as they are not satisfied with the present health service delivery

DOI: 10.4018/978-1-5225-3926-1.ch049

system. In this context, health service providers, including physicians, are very interested in exploring the integration and application of different technological interfaces of information and communication technology in the service delivery system of modern healthcare. One of many possible opportunities to be applied in the service delivery of healthcare, which many practitioners are recently exploring, is the application of a mobile phone-based message system, such as short message service (SMS), as the newest addition to the service delivery system of better quality healthcare. In this present effort to reveal the effectiveness of modern technology on the healthcare system, the current study is engaged in identifying customer perceptions of SMS as a service delivery channel for modern healthcare, which we termed here as Mobile-health or M-health.

Mobile-health or M-health can be defined as providing right healthcare service at right time continuously to any remote patients without hampering their regular lifestyle. In this service system patients' physical presence in hospitals, clinics, and/or doctors chambers is not required. They will be communicated through ICT-driven wireless systems, software, and health monitoring devices. Several wireless communication systems can be used for medical professionals' interaction with patients like, any kind of smartphones, body sensors containing accelerometers, pedometers, electrocardiograms, pulse oximeters, blood-glucose meters, weight scales, etc. Other required technologies may include SMS, multimedia messaging service (MMS); remote communicators and location tracking technology like radio frequency identification (RFID); GPS etc.; data processing tools like personal data assistant (PDA), pocket PC, palm and laptop as well as wireless network like the WiFi Internet network. Through sensor, the patient's health conditions will be monitored, recorded, and analyzed. And then through connected smartphone, essential information will be continuously transferred to medical professionals from a remote place. Medical professionals will receive any data, related to patients' health condition, through their laptop, tablet PC, PDA, or other wireless-based Internet communication. This communication will be a continuous regular pattern; however, if urgent advice is required due to any deteriorating health conditions of the patients, two-way communication will be established through SMS from physicians.

M-health researcher Kahn et al. (2010) illustrated: "Innovative applications of mobile technology to existing healthcare delivery and monitoring systems offer great promise for improving the quality of life." Since the beginning of modern information and communications technology (ICT), wireless communication, electronic health recording, and monitoring devices predominate in a major driving role of the technological and social beliefs of consumer decision-making processes and their complex buying behavior. This is composed of the cognitive, affective, and conative, or behavioral, components of attitude, which play a significantly comprehensive role in accepting an ICT-driven healthcare system. Theorizing this integrated health and technological adoption behavior for consumer complex buying behavior has the potential to help us discover better future designs of a culture and market economy governed by ICT for an innovative and revolutionary M-health system.

Consumers generally are not engaged in buying or pursuing M-health as a regular product. Its purchase frequency, oriented with only a small number of patients, is insignificant to general consumers. In the M-health service system, self-service technology is predominant and this needs extensive self-explanatory skills. From the perspective of a health-concerned matter, M-health-related issues potentially deserve a higher consideration from consumers in the light of usage (Yu et al., 2006). Therefore, the systematic adoption of M-health necessitates a complex buying behavior, and consumers must integrate several different ideas to justify their decision to receive M-health services.

The worldwide proliferation of mobile phone SMS as the service delivery channel contains several issues, challenges, barriers, and limitations. Many researchers (He et al., 2007; Moynihan et al., 2010; Muk, 2007; Srisawatsakul & Papasratorn, 2013; Zhang & Mao, 2008; Zhang & Li, 2012) have asserted from extensive empirical studies that service delivery to the intended segments of customers through messaging on a mobile phone SMS will be successful if it can capture the ubiquitous opportunities of wireless devices such as providing time, location, and customer-context-based messages of service. The findings of the studies suggested that service delivery through mobile phone SMS could be accepted among consumers if it can maintain continuous connectivity with reliability. The authors also affirmed that for the most effective SMS interactivity, authenticity of information and delivery of the correct content to the right customer is important. It is especially important in M-health, as the content of healthcare is extremely important and privacy is a prevalent factor in this context. As a result, consumers will perceive service delivery through SMS of their mobile phone as an effective service delivery channel if it can deliver trustworthy, personalized information, at any time and in any location. To reveal the effectiveness of M-health service delivery through mobile phone SMS, understanding customer perceptions about adopting this new trend of service delivery channel is potentially important; however, researchers have not comprehensively examined the possibility of adding this service delivery channel in M-health.

Consumer behavior about any ICT-related adoption cannot be generalized, as cultural traits have a significant impact on consumer attitudes toward ICT. This argument is justified by many researchers who conducted research on the impact of the cultural differences in consumer attitudes (Jamieson, 2012; McDonald & Dahlberg, 2010). Irani et al. (2007) claimed that ICT adoption behavior is highly controlled by socio-psychological traits which signify the impact of culture. With reference to the study of Goodman and Green (1992), where ICT adoption behavior for Middle Eastern countries was explored, Ein-Dor et al. (1993) acknowledged that any attempt to theorize consumer behaviors cannot be generalized without comparing the cultural differences among consumers of different nations. Other researchers, like Kettinger et al. (1995) and Winsted (1997), investigated consumer behavior for ICT in the USA and some Asian countries and finally concluded that a trend could be generalized considering the effect of impulsive cultural differences. Tajfel's social identity theory (1972) identified that behavioral and social differences among cultures have potential implications for modeling consumer behaviors. The theory of planned behavior (Ajzen, 1991) suggested that there were different beliefs concerning an attitudinal, subjective norm and behavioral control in predicting behavioral intention and actual behavior. Several researchers, such as Straub et al. (1994), while verifying the technology adoption model (TAM) (Davis, 1989) among consumers of three different countries (Japan, Switzerland, and the United States), postulated that those beliefs predicting actual behavior might not be similar among consumers of different countries having observable dissimilarities in cultural traits. Donthu and Yoo (1998) analyzed the cultural influences on service perception among the consumers of four countries – Canada, India, UK, and USA – and noted significant differences in perceiving service quality among consumers who had different cultural traits.

This current study is engaged in identifying consumer perceptions regarding the SMS of mobile phones as an alternative service delivery channel for M-health and studying the cultural impact of this type of service delivery.

Theoretical Model

Before reacting to any system, consumers first expose themselves to the new system and attempt to decide if it is acceptable or not. If they find the new system to be favorable in terms of their intention, they try to create their motive for the system as acceptable, i.e., to perceive it positively. Perception can be defined as the process by which individuals receive information, organize it, and then interpret their sensory impressions in order to impart significant meaning to the system. This project has two significant issues: one is M-health and the other one is the SMS of mobile phones as the service delivery channel.

About SMS-based connectivity, many researchers have identified that SMS provides additional values, such as perceived usefulness to recipients, which is deemed as a significant driving factor for positive perception about the system (Carroll et al., 2007; Cheng et al., 2009). They revealed that consumer perceptions of usefulness, enjoyment, and cost effectiveness are important factors for them to create a positive perception about any system if it is delivered through mobile phone-based SMS as an alternative service delivery system. Researchers (Turel et al., 2007; Zhang & Mao, 2008) also identified that users have a positive attitude toward wireless information like SMS (Trappey & Woodside, 2005) and thus willingness to be exposed (Zhang & Mao, 2008; Zhang & Li, 2012), because it can provide process, socialization, and content motivations. The findings of several studies (Qureshi et al., 2012; Srisawatsakul & Papasratorn, 2013) of the effect of SMS on consumer perceptions indicated that since SMS-based service delivery has many interactive; personalized; and time, place, and context-based benefits, customers have appreciated SMS.

To examine and conceptualize consumer perceptions about M-health where service is being delivered through mobile phone-based SMS, the authors used the Unified Theory of Acceptance and Use of Technology (UTAUT) (Venkatesh et al., 2003) model. According to the UTAUT model, performance expectancy, effort expectancy, social influence, and facilitating conditions are the four potential constructs to explain user perception and acceptance behavior.

Performance expectancy (PE): Venkatesh et al. (2003) developed this construct from the integrated paradigms of different behavioral theories based on system usefulness, and defined it as "the degree to which an individual believes that using the system will help him or her to attain gains in job performance" (Venkatesh et al., 2003). We propose based on UTAUT, that,

H_1: Performance expectancy (PE) has a positive influence on customer perceptions of SMS (PER) as a service delivery channel for M-health.

Effort expectancy (EE): This formative construct of the UTAUT model captures integrated notions of ease of use and is defined as "the degree of ease associated with the use of the system." The effect of this construct has been proposed as,

H_2: Effort expectancy (EE) has a positive influence on customer perceptions of SMS (**PER**) as a service delivery channel for M-health.

Social influence (SI): SI has captured the overall influence of society on creating consumer perceptions; it is defined as "the degree to which an individual perceives that important others believe he or she should use the new system." We have proposed this construct in this theoretical development process as,

H_3: Social influence (SI) has a positive influence on customer perceptions of SMS (**PER**) as a service delivery channel for M-health.

Facilitating conditions (FC): For M-health, SMS-based service delivery can facilitate the system as an alternative service delivery channel. It is defined as "the degree to which an individual believes that an organizational and technical infrastructure exists to support use of the system."

H_4: Facilitating conditions (FC) has a positive influence on customer perceptions of SMS (PER) as a service delivery channel for M-health.

Research Methodology

For M-health, we designed a hybrid model of an ICT-driven health service delivery system for diabetic patients. The system is illustrated as follows:

Diabetic patients would wear a hospital-provided sensor system as a wristband and this sensor system would be connected to the patients' smartphone. Through analytical software added to the smartphone, the patient would be directly connected with and continuously monitored by health professionals of any hospital. Health professionals would periodically monitor patient health-related data, which is transmitted directly and continuously to their personal laptop or any hand-held computing system. Whenever the medical professionals find that any diabetic-related parameters have dropped to the danger limit they alert the patient by sending SMS to the patients' smartphone for regular instructions and tips. This remote health service delivery system through SMS is considered here as M-health.

To capture consumer perceptions and explore the effect of culture on the perception process of SMS as a service delivery channel for M-health, the study was conducted in Bangladesh and Canada among diabetic patients. All other measuring items were extracted directly from the UTAUT model and then revised to align the measuring items with the notion of M-health and SMS as the service delivery channel. The scale items of the four constructs were measured by a five-point Likert scale ranging from 1 (strongly disagree) to 5 (strongly agree). Diabetic patients of these two countries who are now taking diabetic monitoring services almost every week from direct presence in any healthcare service provider facility were presented with the proposed hybrid model of M-health. They were asked to respond to the questionnaire based on their perceptions of seeking that alternative healthcare service through SMS operated by mobile phone from any remote locations.

The same procedure was used to collect data from patients in Canada and Bangladesh. For Bangladesh, the survey was conducted in Dhaka City among registered diabetic patients in the Bangladesh Institute of Research and Rehabilitation in Diabetes, Endocrine and Metabolic Disorders (BIRDEM). The total number of respondents was 127. The same questionnaire was distributed in Ottawa, Canada, at two different centers in the diabetes management community program. 115 responses were collected from Ottawa.

Results and Discussions

Since the measuring items are extracted directly from the UTAUT model, we did not conduct any factor analysis; rather we directly conducted path analysis following structural equation modeling (SEM). However, before that we verified the reliability of the constructs through Cronbach's alpha for the two samples. Since the coefficient alpha for all the constructs varied from 0.801 to 0.923, the constructs' reliability (Nunnally & Bernstein, 1994) was approved.

The path diagram displays factor loadings for the independent variables. After several iterations with inclusion of several error covariants among the determinants of perception, the authors accepted the final model for the Bangladeshi and Canadian sample as shown in Figures 1 (Consumers' Perception of M-health through SMS, Path coefficients, Bangladesh) and 2 (Consumers' Perception of M-health through SMS, Path coefficients, Canada) respectively.

The standardized path coefficients, Chi-Square statistic, degree of freedom (df), p-value, and RMSEA are also shown in Figures 1 and 2, which are the final cause and effect relationship between the independent constructs and perception of M-health conducted through SMS for Bangladesh and Canada.

Figure 1. Consumers' Perception of M-health through SMS (Path coefficients) (Bangladesh)

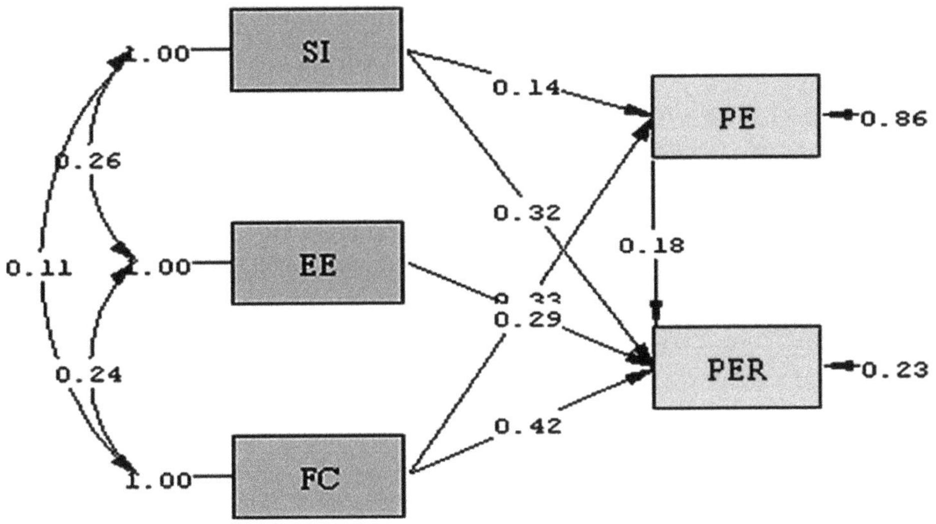

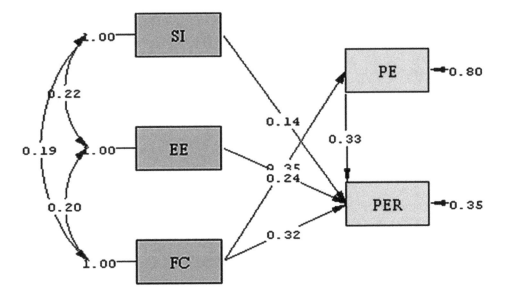

Figure 2. Consumers' Perception of M-health through SMS (Path coefficients) (Canada)

The $\chi2$ statistic of 6.85 and 5.36 for Bangladesh ((df = 4, p-value 0.224976) and Canada respectively (df = 4, p-value 0.111239) indicates that the null hypothesis of the model is a good fit for the data, or at least cannot be rejected. The root mean square error of approximation (RMSEA) (0.045 and 0.061 for Bangladesh and Canada respectively) is quite reasonable as goodness of fitness (Kline, 2005, pp.133-144). Other fit measures such as CFI, IFI, RFI, GFI, AGFI, NFI, and NNFI are verified (all range from 0.97 to 0.99), which indicate that the model fit compares reasonably with the literature (Segars et al., 1993; Chau, 1997).

The results show that the UTAUT model could perfectly predict consumer perceptions for M-health, which is primarily operated through mobile phone-based SMS. All the independent variables are found significant at 0.05 level. For Bangladeshi consumers, FC is the most important attribute (path coefficient 0.42) to impart a positive perception about M-health service operated through SMS. SI is the second most (path coefficient 0.32) important construct to create a positive impression for M-health. Load coefficients for EE and PE are 0.29 and 0.18 respectively. Other than these regular relations captured by the UTAUT model, two new relations emerged from the LISREL analysis for the proper fit of the model as per sample. Other than the predicted relations of FC and SI to perception, these two constructs also influence PE. It indicates that if the supporting environment and condition is well organized and consumers feel the normative effect of using M-health through the SMS of a mobile phone, they find a higher performance of this new technology-driven health service system. Overall, ancillary systems of M-health in particular have immense support from consumers in perceiving the M-health system conducted by mobile phone SMS to be reliable, trustworthy, and effective and thus they find that the system has a high performance.

In contrast, for Canada the magnitude of the effects of different constructs on developing a positive perception about M-health conducted by mobile phone SMS has some differences from that of Bangladeshi consumers. For Canadian diabetic patients who seek or maintain connectivity with M-health service through the SMS of mobile phones, the expected performance (PE) of this particular remote control service is the most important reason (path coefficient 0.33) to create a positive perception about this service. Overall, ancillary support (FC) is the second most vulnerable issue (path coefficient 0.32) for them to develop positive perception. Two other constructs, ease of system use (EE) and the normative influence of society (SI), are also important predictors for pursuing a positive perception about the system. The load coefficients for EE and SI are 0.24 and 0.14 respectively. Again, for Canadians the integrative effect of the ancillary system (FC) of M-health service has a positive impact on PE, which leads to creating a positive perception about this service where SMS plays the key connectivity between the service provider and service recipient.

The results indicate significant differences of consumer perceptions of M-health operated through mobile phone-based SMS between Canada and Bangladesh. It reflects and provides exploratory justification for the claim that culture has a significant impact on forming perceptions about the M-health service system where connectivity is controlled through the remote SMS of mobile phones. As a developing country where the medical service system is not well organized and reliable, when the physical presence of medical professionals is absent, consumers might not expect this system to be reliable. So they might not expect this system to perform well. So, for them, the ancillary system which ultimately supports the total design and implementation of M-health through SMS of a mobile phone is the most vulnerable issue of concern. If they are confident of the FC of this system, they develop a positive perception of the system. For Bangladeshi users the normative influence of the society has an impact on the perception of the M-health system as a high performance system. In a developing country, this finding can be justified for a new technology-driven system as an alternative to traditional brick and mortar healthcare services. When diabetic patients use a wrist band directly connected with doctors through a smartphone and receive continuous feedback through SMS from doctors, so that they do not need to go to a medical center and can continue their daily life without hampering their regular jobs, they find this revolutionary remote control medical service system to be a matter of social prestige. So for both Canada and Bangladesh, this SI construct is an important factor for a positive perception of the system.

SI also has an impact on the construct PE for Bangladeshi consumers. This concept is well supported by the construct subject norm of the theory of planned behavior (TPB) (Ajzen, 1991) and the construct of the image of diffusion of innovation theory (DOI) (Moore & Benbasat, 1991).

Theoretical and Managerial Implications

This exploratory study has potential contribution in the advancement of revolutionary health service delivery system through modern ICT. Both the academics and practitioners can be benefited from the findings of this study. UTAUT model is suggested to assume consumers behavior for ICT. Although, M-health is a very new and exploratory research issue, this study revealed that this model can also be used to conceptualize consumers behavioral intention for seeking M-health through mobile phone SMS. This theoretical identification can provide deep insight for the researchers, practitioners, and policy makers to advance this new kind of health service delivery system for all patients living in remote areas. Practitioners and policy makers can be assured that creating reference group and pushing this new trend of service through them can be an effective idea to positively motivate general consumers. Like all ICT related consumers behavior, M-health adoption is also highly dependent on how easy it is to use. For reliability, this apparently virtual service system must be authentically supported by required policies and arrangements.

It is identified that patients' perception about M-health delivered through mobile phone SMS is notably different for Canadian and Bangladeshi consumers. From cultural perspective, social influence (SI) is an important issue to pursue behavioral intention (Ajzen, 1991). For Bangladeshi patients, in seeking M-health through mobile phone SMS, they are highly motivated by reference group and social norms, where as for Canadian patients, although significant, surrounding social influence has the least impact on consumers perception about M-health delivered through mobile phone SMS. It reflects the impact of culture on consumers' behavior. Several researchers (Ein-Dor et al., 1993; Espinoza, 1999; Pavlou & Chai, 2002; Shareef et al., 2011) who conducted research on consumers' behavior for ICT adoption acknowledged that culture has significant impact on consumers' behavior.

CONCLUSION AND FUTURE RESEARCH DIRECTION

Beginning in the last century, the substantial advancement and revolutionary accomplishments of the healthcare service system helped consumers to create enormous expectations in identifying and accepting new healthcare services (Kahn et al. 2010). As an essential, precious, and emergency product, consumers demand healthcare services to be flexible, accessible, available, and compatible with a maximum price-value trade-off. They also prefer to streamline their high expectations for cost-effectiveness, quality, efficiency, life-pattern-congruency from health professionals (Wu et al. 2007). However, and not specifically for ICT, consumers desire a competent service compatible to a modern-day life pattern. It needs to be dynamic, flexible, and an easy-going medical service which would at the same time pressure all the stakeholders in a healthcare service system to incorporate and integrate the core characteristics of a wireless communication system in the selection of delivery of healthcare services to the patients.

The research had two objectives. As the first goal, the authors attempted to identify the causes which can induce consumers to have positive perceptions about M-health driven by the SMS of mobile phone.

In this connection, the UTAUT model was used as the theoretical base to perceive consumer perceptions about M-health. The authors have conducted an empirical study among diabetic patients in Bangladesh and Canada. Path analysis has been conducted for both samples. The results confirmed that PE, FC, SI, and EE are the significant constructs for capturing consumer perceptions about M-health conducted by the SMS of mobile phones. Therefore, the UTAUT model fits quite nicely in predicting consumer perceptions for M-health-driven mobile technology. Nevertheless, the degree of convergence and magnitude of effect of different constructs in learning consumer perceptions for M-health are potentially different for Bangladeshi and Canadian consumers. This identification reflects the cultural effects on the consumer perception process for an ICT-driven, M-health system that is predominantly controlled from remote places.

Several researchers (Espinoza, 1999; Irani et al., 2007; Posey et al., 2010; Shareef et al, 2014), in exploring the impact of culture on consumer behavior for ICT-driven service, acknowledged this finding. Pavlou and Chai (2002) addressed consumer adoption behavior for Chinese and USA consumers, and, in the light of Hofstede's (2001) cultural dimensions, revealed that any attempt to formulate a standardized ICT-related consumer behavior model is impractical. The authors asserted that culture, indeed, has potential implications for consumer attitudes and behavioral norms. Tajfel (1972), in a social identity theory, strongly asserted that social identity, which is potentially governed by cultural traits, has a substantial impact on paradigms of consumer behavior. Technological, behavioral, and social beliefs of the system's functional, organizational, and professional benefits will render it congruent with a life pattern comprising an attitude toward using it. However, this research has been conducted in only two countries. To justify the cultural impact on perception process of consumers, future researchers can conduct similar research in several countries having significant differences in cultural traits.

REFERENCES

Ajzen, I. (1991). The Theory of Planned Behavior. *Organizational Behavior and Human Decision Processes, 50*(2), 179–211. doi:10.1016/0749-5978(91)90020-T

Carroll, A., Barnes, S. J., Scornavacca, E., & Fletcher, K. (2007). Consumer perceptions and attitudes towards SMS advertising: Recent evidence from New Zealand. *International Journal of Advertising, 26*(1), 79–98.

Chau, P. Y. K. (1997). Reexamining a Model for Evaluating Information Center Success: Using a Structural Equation Modeling Approach. *Decision Sciences, 28*(2), 309–334. doi:10.1111/j.1540-5915.1997.tb01313.x

Cheng, J. M. S., Blankson, C., Wang, E. S. T., & Chen, L. S. L. (2009). Consumer attitudes and interactive digital advertising. *International Journal of Advertising, 28*(3), 501–525. doi:10.2501/S0265048709200710

Davis, F. D. (1989). Perceived Usefulness, Perceived Ease of Use and User Acceptance of Information Technology. *Management Information Systems Quarterly, 13*(3), 319–340. doi:10.2307/249008

Donthu, N., & Yoo, B. (1998). Cultural Influences on Service Quality Expectations. *Journal of Service Research, 1*(2), 178–186. doi:10.1177/109467059800100207

Ein-Dor, P., Segev, E., & Orgad, M. (1993). The Effect of National Culture on IS: Implications for International Information Systems. *Journal of Global Information Management, 1*(1), 33–44. doi:10.4018/jgim.1993010103

Espinoza, M. M. (1999). Assessing the cross-cultural applicability of a service quality measure A comparative study between Quebec and Peru. *International Journal of Service Industry Management, 10*(5), 449–468. doi:10.1108/09564239910288987

Goodman, S. E., & Green, J. D. (1992). Computing in the middle east. *Communications of the ACM, 35*(8), 21–25. doi:10.1145/135226.135236

He, D. H., & Lu, Y. B., (2007). *Consumers Perceptions and Acceptances towards Mobile Advertising: An Empirical Study in China.* IEEE.

Hofstede, G. (2001). *Culture's Consequences* (2nd ed.). Thousand Oaks: Sage.

Irani, Z., Love, P. E. D., & Montazemi, A. (2007). e-Government: Past, present and future. *European Journal of Information Systems, 16*(2), 103–105. doi:10.1057/palgrave.ejis.3000678

Jamieson, K. (2012, October 15-17). *SMS Advertising: A Cross-national Study on Acceptance and Response.* Proceeding of the 13th West Lake International Conference on Small and Medium Business, (WLICSMB 2011). Hangzhou, China.

Kahn, J. G., Yang, J. S., & Kahn, J. S. (2010). 'Mobile' Health Needs and Opportunities in Developing Countries. *Health Affairs, 29*(2), 252–258. doi:10.1377/hlthaff.2009.0965 PMID:20348069

Kettinger, W. J., Lee, C. C., & Lee, S. (1995). Global measures of information service quality: A cross-national study. *Decision Sciences, 26*(5), 569–588. doi:10.1111/j.1540-5915.1995.tb01441.x

Kline, R. B. (2005). *Principles and Practice of Structural Equation Modeling.* NY: The Guilford Press.

McDonald, J., & Dahlberg, J. (2010, March 8-10). US Consumer Attitudes Toward And Acceptance Of SMS Mobile Text Advertising, *Proceeding of the 4th International Technology, Education and Development Conference (INTED).* Valencia, Spain.

Moore, G., & Benbasat, I. (1991). Development of an Instrument to Measure the Perceptions of Adopting an Information Technology Innovation. *Information Systems Research, 2*(3), 173–191. doi:10.1287/isre.2.3.192

Moynihan, B., Kabadayi, S., & Kaiser, M. (2010). Consumer acceptance of SMS advertising: A study of American and Turkish consumers. *International Journal of Mobile Communications, 8*(4), 392–410. doi:10.1504/IJMC.2010.033833

Muk, A. (2007). Consumers' intentions to opt in to SMS advertising - A cross-national study of young Americans and Koreans. *International Journal of Advertising, 26*(2), 177–198.

Nunnally, J. C., & Bernstein, I. H. (1994). Psychometric Theory. New York: McGraw-Hill.

Pavlou, P. A., & Chai, L. (2002). What Drives Electronic Commerce across Cultures? A Cross-Cultural Empirical Investigation of the Theory of Planned Behavior. *Journal of Electronic Commerce Research, 3*(4), 240–253.

Posey, C., Lowry, P. B., Roberts, T. L., & Ellis, T. S. (2010). Proposing the online community self-disclosure model: The case of working professionals in France and the U.K. who use online communities. *European Journal of Information Systems*, *19*(2), 181–195. doi:10.1057/ejis.2010.15

Qureshi, I. M., Batool, I., & Shamim, A. (2012). Consumer Perception In Response To E-Marketing Stimuli: The Impact of Brand Salience, *Actual. Problems of Economics*, *2*(4), 137–143.

Segars, A., & Grover, V. (1993). Re-examining Perceived Ease of Use and Usefulness: A Confirmatory Factor Analysis. *Management Information Systems Quarterly*, *17*(4), 517–527. doi:10.2307/249590

Shareef, M. A., Kumar, U., Kumar, V., & Dwivedi, Y. K. (2011). E-government Adoption Model (GAM): Differing Service Maturity Levels. *Government Information Quarterly*, *28*(1), 17–35. doi:10.1016/j.giq.2010.05.006

Shareef, M. A., Kumar, V., Dwivedi, Y. K., & Kumar, U. (2014). Global Service Quality of Electronic-Commerce. [IJICBM]. *International Journal of Indian Culture and Business Management*, *8*(1), 1–34. doi:10.1504/IJICBM.2014.057947

Srisawatsakul, C., & Papasratorn, B. (2013). Factors Affecting Consumer Acceptance Mobile Broadband Services with Add-on Advertising: Thailand Case Study. *Wireless Personal Communications*, *69*(3), 1055–1065. doi:10.1007/s11277-013-1065-4

Straub, D. W. (1994). The Effect of Culture on IT Diffusion: E-Mail and FAX in Japan and the U.S. *Information Systems Research*, *5*(I), 23–47. doi:10.1287/isre.5.1.23

Tajfel, H. (1972). La Categorisation Sociale (Social categorization). In S. Moscovici (Ed.), *Introduction a La Psychologie Sociale, 1* (pp. 272–302). Paris: Larousse.

Trappey, R. J., & Woodside, A. G. (2005). Consumer responses to interactive advertising campaigns coupling short-message-service direct marketing and TV commercials. *Journal of Advertising Research*, *45*(4), 382–401.

Turel, O., Serenko, A., & Bontis, N. (2007). User acceptance of wireless short messaging

Turel, O., Serenko, A., & Bontis, N.services. (2007, January). Deconstructing perceived value. *Information & Management*, *44*(1), 63–73. doi:10.1016/j.im.2006.10.005

Venkatesh, V., Morris, M. G., Davis, G. B., & Davis, F. D. (2003). User Acceptance of Information Technology: Toward a Unified View. *Management Information Systems Quarterly*, *27*(3), 425–578.

Winsted, K. F. (1997). The service experience in two cultures: A behavioral perspective. *Journal of Retailing*, *73*(3), 337–360. doi:10.1016/S0022-4359(97)90022-1

Wu, J.-H., Wanga, S.-C., & Lin, L.-M. (2007). Mobile computing acceptance factors in the healthcare industry: A structural equation model. *International Journal of Medical Informatics*, *76*(1), 66–77. doi:10.1016/j.ijmedinf.2006.06.006 PMID:16901749

Yu, P., Wu, M. X., Yu, H., & Xiao, G. C. (2006, June 21-23). The Challenges for the Adoption of M-Health. *IEEE International Conference on Service Operations and Logistics and Informatics (SOLI 2006)* (pp. 181-186). Shanghai, China. doi:10.1109/SOLI.2006.329059

Zhang, J., & Mao, E. (2008). Understanding the acceptance of mobile SMS advertising among young Chinese consumers. *Psychology and Marketing*, 25(8), 787–805. doi:10.1002/mar.20239

Zhang, R. J., & Li, X. Y. (2012). Research on Consumers' Attitudes and Acceptance Intentions toward Mobile Marketing. In L. Hua (Ed.), *2012 International Conference on Management Science & Engineering* (pp. 727-732). doi:10.1109/ICMSE.2012.6414259

ADDITIONAL READING

Archer, N. (2007). Mobile eHealth: Making the Case. In I. Kushchu (Ed.), Mobile Government: AN Emerging Direction in E-government (pp. 155-170). Hershey, PA: IGI Publishing.

Assael, H. (1995). *Consumer Behavior and Marketing Action* (5th ed.). Cincinnati, Ohio: ITP, South-Western College Publishing.

Bloch, P. H., & Marsha, L. R. (1983). A Theoretical Model for the Study of Product Importance Perceptions. *Journal of Marketing*, 47(3), 69–81. doi:10.2307/1251198

Cadogan, J. (2010). Comparative, cross-cultural, and cross-national research: A comment on good and bad practice. *International Marketing Review*, 27(6), 601–605. doi:10.1108/02651331011088245

Kotz, D., Avancha, S., & Baxi, A. (2009). A Privacy Framework for Mobile Health and Home-Care Systems. SPIMACS'09. Chicago, Illinois, USA.

Kumar, V., Kumar, U., Shareef, M. A., Chowdhury, A. H., & Sharan, V. (2013). Developing Citizen-centric Service: Adoption Behavior for Mobile Health. *Proceedings of the Administrative Sciences Association of Canada Conference*. Calgary, Alberta, Canada.

Mallat, N. (2007). Exploring consumer adoption of mobile payments – A qualitative study. *The Journal of Strategic Information Systems*, 16(4), 413–432. doi:10.1016/j.jsis.2007.08.001

Mattila, A. S. (1999). The role of culture in the service evaluation process. *Journal of Service Research*, 1(3), 250–261. doi:10.1177/109467059913006

McSweeney, B. (2013). Fashion Founded on Flaw - The Ecological Mono-Deterministic Fallacy of Hofstede, GLOBE, and Followers. *International Marketing Review*, 30(5), 483–504. doi:10.1108/IMR-04-2013-0082

Meingast, M., Roosta, T., & Sastry, S. (2006). Security and privacy issues with health care information technology, *Proceedings of the 28th IEEE EMBS Annual International Conference*, August, DOI doi:10.1109/IEMBS.2006.260060

Michael, R. T., & Becker, G. S. (1973). On the New Theory of Consumer Behavior. *The Swedish Journal of Economics*, 75(4), 378–396. doi:10.2307/3439147

Miyazaki, A. D., & Fernandez, A. (2001). Consumer Perceptions of Privacy and Security Risks for Online Shopping. *The Journal of Consumer Affairs*, 35(1), 27–44. doi:10.1111/j.1745-6606.2001.tb00101.x

Nelson, K. G., & Clark, T. D. Jr. (1994). Cross-Cultural Issues in Information Systems Research: A Research Program. *Journal of Global Information Management, 2*(4), 19–29. doi:10.4018/jgim.1994100102

Neslin, S., & Shankar, V. (2009). Key Issues in Multichannel Customer Management: Current Knowledge and Future Directions. *Journal of Interactive Marketing, 23*(1), 70–81. doi:10.1016/j.intmar.2008.10.005

Payan, J., Svensson, G., & Hair, J. (2010). A "cross-cultural RELQUAL-scale" in supplier distributor relationships of Sweden and the USA. *International Marketing Review, 27*(5), 541–561. doi:10.1108/02651331011076581

Robertson, T. S. (1974). A Critical Examination of Adoption Process Models of Consumer Behavior. In J. N. Sheth (Ed.), *Models of Buyer Behavior.*

Shareef, M. A., Archer, N., & Dwivedi, Y. K. (To be published in 2015). An Empirical Investigation of Electronic Government Service Quality: From the Demand Side Stakeholder Perspective. Total Quality Management & Business Excellence.

Shareef, M. A. & Dwivedi, Y. K. (To be published in 2015). A Bird Eye View of Existing Research on Consumer Behavior in the Context of SMS Based Marketing, The Marketing Review, 15(1),

Shareef, M. A., Kumar, V., Dwivedi, Y. K., & Kumar, U. (2014). *Citizen Attitudes toward Service Delivery through Mobile-Government (mGov): Driving Factors and Cultural Impacts, Information Systems Frontiers.*

Shareef, M. A., Kumar, V., & Kumar, U. (Forthcoming). Predicting Mobile Health Adoption Behavior: A Demand Side perspective. *Journal of Customer Behavior.*

Shareef, M. A., Kumar, V., Kumar, U., & Dwivedi, Y. K. (2014). Factors affecting citizen adoption of transactional electronic government. *Journal of Enterprise Information Management, 27*(4), 385–401. doi:10.1108/JEIM-12-2012-0084

Shareef, M. A., Kumar, V., Kumar, U., & Dwivedi, Y. K. (To be published in 2015). Consumer online purchase behaviour: perception versus expectation. International Journal Indian Culture and Business Management.

Sun, G., D'Alessandro, S., Johnson, L. W., & Winzar, H. (2014). Do we measure what we expect to measure? Some issues in the measurement of culture in consumer research. *International Marketing Review, 31*(4), 1–38. doi:10.1108/IMR-03-2012-0055

Swoboda, B., Pennemann, K., & Taube, M. (2012). The Effects of Perceived Brand Globalness and Perceived Brand Localness in China: Empirical Evidence on Western, Asian, and Domestic Retailers. *Journal of International Marketing, 20*(4), 25–77. doi:10.1509/jim.12.0105

Taylor, S., & Todd, P. (1995). Decomposition and crossover effects in the theory of planned behavior: A study of consumer adoption intentions. *International Journal of Research in Marketing, 12*(2), 137–155. doi:10.1016/0167-8116(94)00019-K

Vallerand, R. J. (1997). In M. Zanna (Ed.), *Toward a Hierarchical Model of Intrinsic and Extrinsic Motivation* (Vol. 29, pp. 271–360). Advances in Experimental Social Psychology New York: Academic Press. doi:10.1016/S0065-2601(08)60019-2

Venkatesh, V., Davis, F. D., & Morris, M. G. (2007). Dead or Alive? The Development, Trajectory and Future of Technology Adoption Research. *Journal of the AIS*, *8*(4), 268–286.

Venkatesh, V., Thong, J. Y. L., & Xu, X. (2012). Consumer Acceptance and Use of Information Technology: Extending the Unified Theory of Acceptance and Use of Technology. *Management Information Systems Quarterly*, *36*(1), 157–178.

Wu, I.-L., Li, J.-Y., & Fu, C.-Y. (2011). The adoption of mobile healthcare by hospital's professionals: An integrative perspective. *Decision Support Systems*, *51*(3), 587–596. doi:10.1016/j.dss.2011.03.003

KEY TERMS AND DEFINITIONS

Consumer: In this article, actually, patients are terms as consumers. Generally consumers can be defined as anyone who use any products or services.

Culture: Culture, in this article, is defined as overall traits of any society or nations which can distinctly identify their characteristics to develop a unique identity.

Mobile-Health or M-Health: Can be defined as providing right healthcare service at right time continuously to any remote patients without hampering their regular lifestyle. In this service system patients' physical presence in hospitals, clinics, and/or doctors chambers is not required. They will be communicated through ICT-driven wireless systems, software, and health monitoring devices.

Perception: It is a process by which individuals organize and interpret their sensory impressions in order to give meaning to their environment or any objects.

Short Message Service: Any message delivered through mobile phone is termed as "short message service" (SMS).

UTAUT Model: The full name of UTAUT Model is Unified Theory of Acceptance and Use of Technology (UTAUT) (Venkatesh et al., 2003) model. According to the UTAUT model, performance expectancy, effort expectancy, social influence, and facilitating conditions are the four potential constructs to explain user perception and acceptance behavior.

This research was previously published in the Handbook of Research on Cultural and Economic Impacts of the Information Society edited by P.E. Thomas, M. Srihari, and Sandeep Kaur, pages 284-296, copyright year 2015 by Information Science Reference (an imprint of IGI Global).

Chapter 50
Telemedicine in Low Resource Settings:
A Case for Botswana

Kagiso Ndlovu
University of Botswana, Botswana

Kabelo Leonard Mauco
Boitekanelo College, Botswana

Ryan Littman-Quinn
Botswana- UPenn Partnership, Botswana

ABSTRACT

Telemedicine is a means to support health-care provision utilizing information and communication technology (ICT) tools and telecommunication services. This chapter focuses on telemedicine practices in low resource settings, referencing key telemedicine initiatives in Botswana. Telemedicine is highly practiced in the developed world, and recently there is an increasing interest in the developing world. Current literature suggests telemedicine as an important tool for improving healthcare delivery for low resource settings. Hence the authors' interest in exploring the current status of telemedicine practices with reference to telemedicine projects from low resource settings such as Botswana. The chapter reveals that telemedicine in such settings is mainly implemented through mobile phones, also known as mobile health (mHealth). In this chapter, the authors discuss factors influencing successful implementation of telemedicine solutions in Botswana. Furthermore, the chapter discusses telemedicine implementation challenges in each of the projects and presents possible mitigation strategies. The chapter concludes by affirming the feasibility of successfully practicing telemedicine in low resource settings; notwithstanding challenges such as lack of legal and eHealth frameworks in most developing countries.

DOI: 10.4018/978-1-5225-3926-1.ch050

INTRODUCTION

One of the global health challenges in the 21st century is the ability to reach and maintain the highest available level of health for all humankind throughout their lifespan. Such a vision has been expressed by the World Health Organization (WHO) in its health-for-all strategy in the 21st century (WHO, 1997). According to the World Health Organization (WHO) report on the second global survey on electronic health (eHealth), telemedicine as a term is traced as far back as the 1970s, and it literally means "healing at a distance" (WHO, 2009). The report further mentions telemedicine as a solution utilizing information and communication technologies (ICT) to improve patient outcomes by increasing access to care and medical information. The WHO acknowledges that there is no one definition of telemedicine and indicates existence of one hundred and four (104) peer-reviewed definitions of the word. WHO adopted the following broad descriptions of telemedicine (WHO, 2009, p. 9):

The delivery of health care services, where distance is a critical factor, by all healthcare professionals using information and communication technologies for the exchange of valid information for diagnosis, treatment and prevention of disease and injuries, research and evaluation, and for the continuing education of health care providers, all in the interests of advancing the health of individuals and their communities.

According to WHO, the terms telemedicine and telehealth are in most cases used interchangeably in various texts and the following four key elements are essential for telemedicine to occur (WHO) 1998):

1. Provision of clinical support.
2. Overcoming geographical barriers and connecting users not in the same physical location.
3. Utilization of various types of ICT tools.
4. A focus on the improvement of health outcomes.

Realizing the WHO vision of making high-quality healthcare available to all is incredibly difficult if not impossible. This is a result of the fast-growing burden of new disease patterns, and socioeconomic issues that have widened the gap in health status among countries. Traditionally, the main challenge to achieving equitable access to health care has been that the clinician and the patient must be present in the same place and at the same time. Advances in ICT for both developed and developing worlds, however, have created unprecedented opportunities for overcoming this by increasing the number of ways in which healthcare services can be delivered.

Telemedicine has also been defined as *the delivery of health care and the exchange of health-care information across distances* (Craig & Patterson, 2005, p. 4). Craig and Patterson (2005) further indicate that the prefix 'tele' derives from the Greek for 'at a distance'; hence, more simply, telemedicine can also mean medicine at a distance. Telemedicine encompasses the whole range of medical activities including diagnosis, treatment and prevention of disease, continuing education of health-care providers and consumers, research and evaluation (Craig & Patterson, 2005).

According to a study by Craig and Patterson (2005), the first public health surveillance networks were in the middle ages, when information about bubonic plague was transmitted across Europe by such means as bonfires. The study further indicates that during the mid-19th century, developments in national postal services provided the means by which more personal health-care delivery at a distance could be performed. Furthermore, the practice of physicians providing diagnosis, and directions for a cure, was established at that time.

In its modern form, telemedicine is said to have started in the 1960s, and it was mostly driven by the military and space technology sectors (Craig & Patterson, 2005). Examples of early technological milestones in telemedicine include the *use of television to facilitate consultations between specialists at a psychiatric institute and general practitioners at a state mental hospital, and the provision of expert medical advice from a major teaching hospital to an airport medical centre* (Craig & Patterson, 2005, p. 5).

The common factor for all telemedicine applications is that a client of some kind (e.g. patient or healthcare worker) obtains an opinion from someone with more expertise in the relevant field, when the parties are separated in space, in time or both. Telemedicine episodes therefore may be classified on the basis of: the interaction between the client and the expert and the type of information being transmitted. The type of interaction is usually classified as either store-and-forward (also called asynchronous) or real time (also called synchronous) (Allely, 1995). Store-and-forward, or asynchronous, telemedicine involves the exchange of pre-recorded data between two or more individuals at different times. For example, the patient or referring health professional sends an e-mail description of a medical case to an expert who later sends back an opinion regarding diagnosis and optimal management (Allely, 1995). In contrast, real time, or synchronous, telemedicine requires the involved individuals to be simultaneously present for immediate exchange of information, as in the case of videoconferencing (Allely, 1995). In both synchronous and asynchronous telemedicine, relevant information may be transmitted in a variety of media, such as text, audio, video, or still images. These two basic approaches to telemedicine are applied to a wide array of services in diverse settings, including teledermatology, telepathology, and teleradiology.

Most developing countries also known as low resource settings, are faced with a severe shortage of specialized medical personnel coupled with upcoming ICT infrastructures (Littman-Quinn, Mibenge, Antwi, Chandra, & Kovarik, 2013). In the recent past, most governments in the developing world have come to recognize the value of investing in ICT tools to boost various sectors one of which entails provision of healthcare (Microsoft Whitepaper, 2004). Low resource settings are countries typically characterized by lack of funds to cover healthcare costs, on individual or societal basis, which leads to limited access to medication, equipment, supplies, devices and less developed infrastructure such as electrical power, transportation, controlled environment/buildings.

The situation in low resource settings has resulted in prolonged waiting times, congestion at healthcare facilities and high mortality rates due to disease complications while travelling long distances to receive healthcare or standing in long queues waiting for specialized medical attention (Littman-Quinn et al., 2013). The practice of telemedicine therefore presents a potential solution towards improving healthcare service delivery in these settings by eliminating distance barriers and improving access to medical services that would often not be consistently available in distant rural communities.

In the interest of advancing telemedicine access in low resource settings, a number of pilot telemedicine projects as well as research on telemedicine have been conducted. Challenges encountered as well as possible mitigation strategies employed to overcome the challenges have also been documented (Wootton & Bonnardot, 2015). The documented research is critical for improving telemedicine awareness amongst various stakeholders, and contributing to better ways of telemedicine implementation in low resource settings.

The main goal of this chapter is therefore to showcase what is obtained in the practice of telemedicine solutions in the context of Botswana's mobile telemedicine projects. By so doing, the chapter brings out the key opportunities and challenges and articulates best practices in overcoming or mitigating challenges in implementing telemedicine for low resource settings. The chapter also showcases the current status of knowledge development in the implementation of telemedicine solutions given that this field is in its nascent stage. The findings provide insight into the issues pertinent to successful implementation and scale-up of telemedicine solutions in a low resource setting.

BACKGROUND

Access to specialized healthcare continues to be a major challenge across the developing world, also known as low resource settings (Naicker, Plange-Rhule, Tutt, & Eastwood, 2009). The term "low-resource settings" covers mostly low-income countries, and also includes regions in middle-or high-income countries where under-served populations have difficulties in accessing medical specialists (Wootton & Bonnardot, 2015). Healthcare challenges faced in low resource settings are mostly brought about by the limited number of specialized medical doctors when compared to those in the developed world. A 2009 study reveals that there are 57 developing countries with a critical shortage of healthcare workers, a deficit of 2.4 million doctors and nurses (Naicker et al., 2009). The study further indicates that Africa has 2.3 healthcare workers per 1000 population, compared with America, where there are 24.8 healthcare workers per 1000 population (Naicker et al., 2009). The 2006 WHO report reveals an estimated shortage of almost 4.3 million doctors, midwives, nurses and support workers worldwide (WHO, 2006). According to the report, shortage of healthcare personnel is most severe in the poorest countries, especially in sub-Saharan Africa, where health workers are most needed (WHO, 2006). Table 1 shows a summary of global estimated averages for regional healthcare workforce distribution.

In the context of Botswana, healthcare human resource development has been a priority in national development plans with the aim of increasing both the numbers and the skill mix. By 2013, the health workforce had therefore steadily increased with doctor to patient ratio at 1:924 and nurse to patient ratio at 1:203. The hospital bed density stood at 1.81 bed/1000 population (CSO, 2010). Despite Botswana's sparse population distribution, health facilities are accessible to over 90% of the population. About 84% of the population lives within a 5km radius and about 95% live within a 8 km radius from a health facility. For rural areas, the corresponding figures are 72% and 89% for the 5 km and 8 km standards respectively (CSO, 2010).

Table 1. Global health workforce by world health organization region

Region	Total Number (Millions)	Density Per 1000 Population
Africa	1.64	2.3
Eastern Mediterranean	2.10	4.0
Southeast Asia	7.04	4.3
Western Pacific	10.07	5.8
Europe	16.63	18.9
America	21.74	24.8
Rest of the World	59.22	9.3

Source: World Health Organization Report 2006. Available at www.who.init/whr/2006/en/. Last accessed 29 September 2016

The World Health Organization (WHO) in its second global survey on eHealth, mentions Information and Communication Technologies (ICTs) tools as having great potential to address some of the challenges faced by both developed and developing countries in providing accessible, cost effective, high quality health care services. WHO emphasizes the practice of telemedicine and its reliance on ICTs to overcome geographical barriers and increase access to health care services benefiting rural and underserved communities in developing countries ((WHO), 2010).

Previous studies conducted also demonstrated that if implemented appropriately and successfully, the benefits to patients who engage in telemedicine encounters could include reduced disease morbidity, decreased spending and time away from work, and improved treatment outcomes due to more rapid diagnosis and therapy (Castro, Miller, & Nager, 2014). Similarly, the benefits to clinicians who engage in telemedicine practices could include development of skills and knowledge as a result of interactions with the medical specialist, hence acquiring knowledge for future disease management. Telemedicine therefore has the potential to increase efficiency and reduce unnecessary or inappropriate referrals, hence an entire healthcare system can benefit from the reduction in costs that would have been spent on automobiles and petrol, wasted resources, clinic congestion, and poor health outcomes that negatively influence economic progress (Castro et al., 2014).

Despite the above benefits, telemedicine implementation challenges for many developing countries are still high (Sood et al., 2008). In many of these countries, implementers of healthcare information technology based solutions are faced with complex challenges such as inadequate funding, lack of resources and weak healthcare infrastructure. In addition, some of these economies may have just a rudimentary application level of healthcare technology. In a study by Sood et. al. (2008) which examined challenges faced by the healthcare workforce toward the implementation of the electronic medical record (EMR), many of the clinical workforce in developing countries were considered computer illiterate (Sood et al., 2008). Some telemedicine programmes in low resource settings, such as the telemedicine project at the Aravind Eye Hospital in Tamil Nadu, India, reported some challenges including equipment failure, power problems, remote management and training difficulties, theft of equipment, and transportation problems (Brewer et al., 2006).

Hence for the developing world, many initiatives usually die out, or fade away after pilot project runs and in many cases very few initiatives are locally sustained. Therefore, proper planning prior to implementation of telemedicine innovations is required in low resource settings much as it is in the developed world. Developing countries need to learn from the mistakes of the developed world, potential barriers also need to be considered in order to ensure successful implementation of future telemedicine projects in low resource settings.

A 2013 study conducted in the United States (US) presented the following telemedicine adoption challenges in the developed world (Dantu & Mahapatra, 2013), which developing countries could learn from:

Individual Factors

Dantu and Mahapatra (2013), indicate that for successful adoption of technology in any organization, it is important for end users to accept it. They further highlight that lack of acceptance by key stakeholders, particularly physicians could be a major obstacle to telemedicine adoption. They conclude by mentioning that "individual concerns about loss of face-to-face interaction in a healthcare setting, skepticism about potential usefulness, and perceived incompatibility between telemedicine technology and organizational routines also affect telemedicine adoption" (Dantu & Mahapatra, 2013).

Institutional Factors

Another factor affecting telemedicine adoption according to Dantu & Mahapatra (2013, p. 5), is *making sure multiple organizations that are formally or informally affiliated with one another come together to provide necessary care to remote patients.* They allude to the fact that, *in the healthcare ecosystem, payment or reimbursement to the care providers for their services is made by private insurance companies or through government programs, such as, Medicare and Medicaid in America and that currently, reimbursements by Medicare are not consistent across various types of telemedicine services.* They state that reimbursement policies have not been standardized among various private payers and though Medicare currently reimburses some of the telemedicine services, not all types of services are reimbursed (Dantu & Mahapatra, 2013). Several other studies are said to have also found out that a key reason for the slow adoption of telemedicine is inconsistent standards in the reimbursement mechanism for care provided using telemedicine technologies (Baker & Bufka, 2011; Ghosh & Ahadome, 2012; Grigsby, Brega, Bennet, & Devore, 2007; Najjar & Bourquard, 2012; Silva, Farrell, Shandra, Viswanathan, & Schwamm, 2012; Whitten, Buis, & Love, 2007). Hence, providers and administrators are reluctant to adopt telemedicine due to a lack of clear guidelines on reimbursement.

Regulatory Factors

Dantu & Mahapatra (2013) allude to the fact that the healthcare sector is heavily regulated. Hence, care providers need to be licensed to provide care meaning health care institutions must comply with numerous regulations to operate. In contrast, policies and guidelines for licensing physicians to use telemedicine technologies for care delivery are still under development (Dantu & Mahapatra, 2013). The reality on the ground is that physicians providing care using telemedicine are subject to same licensing regulations as physicians providing care in-person. Licensing and credentialing process is very complicated and expensive. Dantu & Mahapatra (2013) indicate that there are restrictions for providing service across state lines. For example, physicians providing care through telemedicine from out of state have to obtain full licensure from the state where the service is being provided. In addition, apart from provider licensure, the equipment used in telemedicine also has to be approved by the appropriate regulatory agency. The process involved in getting licensure and the penalties associated with malpractice or violation of any regulation is said to scare providers away from adopting telemedicine (Dantu & Mahapatra, 2013).

Technological Factors

According to Dantu & Mahapatra (2013), another barrier to telemedicine adoption is the issue of interoperability of the numerous healthcare systems. They emphasise the importance for various IT systems to communicate with each other seamlessly (Dantu & Mahapatra, 2013). In the health care system, multiple organizations – physicians, hospitals, insurance companies, etc. get involved in the care delivery process. Each of these organizations has their own information systems that store patient health information. When multiple organizations come together to provide patient care, perfect communication among various systems is crucial for the provision of patient care. Interoperability is *the ability of health information systems to work together within and across organizational boundaries in order to advance the effective delivery of healthcare for individuals and communities* (HIMSS, 2005, p. 1). In order for health care organizations to adopt telemedicine technology, it is imperative for different systems used by these organizations to interact with each other smoothly. Adoption of telemedicine is also hindered because of lack of interoperability standards.

Another challenge has to do with proper exchange of data between various IT systems within and across organizations. In the case of telemedicine, ways to store and transmit data need to be considered depending on the type of service provided, that is, if providers require to store large image files and video files of patients. Hence, robust telecommunication lines, high speed Internet connections, power backups, and IT systems that are properly tested in the rural community settings would be required for transmitting information back and forth between the patients and the provider. Lack of proper communication infrastructure and performance issues with technology can affect adoption of telemedicine (Kang et al., 2010).

Standardized, secure, timely, and accurate data is also paramount to the success of care delivery. When dealing with patient health information, security of data is imperative. Data security refers to *the technical and procedural methods by which access to confidential information is controlled and managed* (Abdelhak, Grostick, & Hanken, 2014, p. 209). Standardization of data would be required for interoperability of various IT systems used in a healthcare setting. Privacy is concerned with an individual's right to share their personal information selectively (Abdelhak et al., 2014). Laws protect patients by providing guidelines for privacy and confidentiality of medical data. Lack of data standards and security measures to protect patient privacy impede the adoption of telemedicine technologies (Ackerman, Filart, Burgess, Lee, & Poropatich, 2010). In order to provide useful results, new IT systems must be compatible with the existing technology and processes of an organization. In a complex healthcare ecosystem where multiple professionals and specialists come together to provide patient care, compatibility of telemedicine technologies with existing systems becomes even more significant. Adoption of telemedicine depends on its fit with existing organizational routines and practices (King, Richards, & Godden, 2007), and its compatibility at the individual, process, and organizational levels (Al-Qirim, 2007; Vuononvirta et al., 2009). Usability of the technology and glitches in the IT systems also influence the adoption of telemedicine technologies.

According to a study conducted by the U.S. Military, usability, technical problems, and limitations are cited as factors that impede the use of teledermatology systems (Stronge, Nichols, Rogers, & Fisk, 2008).

Despite the aforementioned human and technical challenges surrounding telemedicine implementation in developed countries as well as in low resource settings, this has not deterred implementers from continuing to explore telemedicine pilot projects.

TELEMEDICINE PRACTICES IN LOW RESOURCE SETTINGS

As new technologies evolve, new ways of implementing telemedicine in low resource settings are being considered (Graschew & Roelofs, 2011). Modern telemedicine practices in the developing world have come to entail application of telemedicine techniques in medical fields such as dermatology, radiology and dentistry, referred to as teledermatology, teleradiology and teledentistry respectively. All of these medical specialties involve visual inspection, hence their relevance for telemedicine uptake.

As opposed to the traditional telemedicine practices, current telemedicine trends in low resource settings involve the use of electronic medical health records (EMHR) (HealthIT.gov, 2015). The EMHR creation, storage and dissemination over an IT infrastructure is facilitated by software platforms known as electronic medical health record systems (EMHRS). An EMR is simply a replica of the paper based patient health record. An example of an EMR system commonly adopted in Botswana is the Integrated Patient Management System (IPMS) by Meditech (Botswana Ministry of Health, 2015). The IPMS is an information system that enhances information sharing between healthcare providers across multiple sites. At the centre of the IPMS system is a life-long electronic health record for every patient that can be accessed from any facility using the system throughout the country, irrespective of where the patient was treated. Patients therefore can move from one hospital to another and their medical records will always be available to authorized providers, for example, the Medical Practice Management (MPM) module for HIV management (Botswana Ministry of Health, 2015). Most EMRs in low resource settings are constrained by the weak ICT infrastructure, hence their full potential is hardly experienced.

Despite the limitations incurred while implementing EMR solutions in low resource settings, recent telecommunication developments have presented an avenue to leverage on for healthcare service delivery. Mobile telecommunication technologies such as short message service (SMS), unstructured supplementary service data (USSD), mobile data, and the development of intuitive smartphone mobile applications are now on the rise and easily accessible by most people in low resource settings (Hampton, 2012). The practice of medicine and public health supported by mobile telecommunication services is also known as mobile health (mHealth). mHealth solutions are supported by mobile devices such as mobile smartphones, handheld tablets and laptops. Several studies conducted in low resource settings suggest mHealth solutions as effective as other forms of telemedicine interventions (WHO, 1998; Littman-Quinn et al., 2013; Wootton & Bonnardot, 2015).

TELEMEDICINE PRACTICES IN BOTSWANA

This section presents the state of telemedicine in a low resource setting such as Botswana, highlighting some important mHealth pilot projects which led to the roll-out of the first mobile telemedicine project in Botswana, also known as Kgonafalo.

Botswana exists as a landlocked country sharing boundaries with the Republic of South Africa, Namibia, Zambia and Zimbabwe. It covers a total land area of 582,000 square meters. Botswana has a population of about 2 038 228 with an annual growth rate of 1.9% according to 2011 Population and Housing Census. Health care in Botswana is delivered through a decentralized mode with primary health care being the pillar of the delivery system. Botswana has an extensive network of health facilities (hospitals, clinics, health posts, mobile stops), which are clustered in 27 health districts. There are 3 national referral hospitals, 15 district hospitals, 17 primary hospitals, 290 clinics, 349 health posts and 900 mobile stops. A complex network of largely public and autonomous private care providers working across the country provides healthcare services. The Government of Botswana fully understands and appreciates the developmental importance of ICTs to increase access to, and availability of life-enriching information and services. In addition, Botswana's telecommunication industry has grown over time. In 2010, there were 137,400 land-line phones and 2.4 million mobile phones in Botswana, making mobile phones over 95% of the telephones in use (Central Intelligence Agency, 2016; International Telecommunication Union, 2016). Over the past few years, the Botswana Telecommunications Corporation Limited and private telecommunications providers have expanded mobile telecommunications services to rural underserved communities and 95% of Botswana's population has access to Global System for Mobile communication (GSM) mobile phone networks. GSM refers to the digital mobile telephony system widely used in Europe and the other parts of the world (International Telecommunication Union, 2007). In Botswana, 36% of rural households use mobile phones, whilst in urban villages, towns, and cities, usage is at 89%, 93% and 94% respectively (Central Statistics Office, 2011; Orange Foundation, 2016).

Prior to 2009, the Botswana Ministry of Health (MoH) as the main policy setting and healthcare implementation organization, maintained 37 health information systems. However, in 2009, a systems rationalization exercise was undertaken to reduce the number of isolated health information systems from their initial 37 to the current 12 systems. The 12 systems include one Public Health system, two HIV clinical support systems, two systems for Monitoring and Evaluation under the Department of Health Policy Development, Monitoring and Evaluation (DHPDME), two systems under Clinical Services, three systems under the Drug and Regulatory Unit, one central system at the MoH, that is, IPMS and one HIV and Aids system supported by the National Aids Coordinating Agency (NACA).

Botswana's health ICT solutions include mHealth solutions piloted over time by various stakeholders. These mHealth pilot projects have reached different levels of success and challenges, most of which were lessons learnt leading to the scale-up of Botswana's first mobile telemedicine project. The following section summarises some of Botswana's mHealth pilot projects motivated by health challenges and also served as proof of concepts.

Tuberculosis (TB) Contact Tracing

Tuberculosis (TB) contact tracing is typically conducted in resource-limited settings with paper forms, but the approach is limited by inefficiencies in data collection, storage, and retrieval and poor data quality (Ha et al,2016). In Botswana, the TB Contact Tracing (TBCT) project has been supported by the Botswana-UPenn Partnership in collaboration with the Ministry of Health. The project evaluated a mobile health (mHealth) approach to TB contact tracing that replaced the paper form–based approach for a period of 6 months. For both approaches, a comparison of the time required to complete TB contact tracing and the quality of data collected was made. For the mHealth approach, the Computer System Usability Questionnaire was also administered to 2 health care workers who used the new approach, and operational considerations for implementation were identified and addressed. Compared to the paper form–based approach, the mHealth approach reduced the median time required to complete TB contact tracing and improved data quality.(Ha et al.,2016) The mHealth approach also had favorable overall rating, system usefulness, information quality, and interface quality scores on the Computer System Usability Questionnaire. Overall, the mHealth approach to TB contact tracing improved on the paper form–based approach used in Botswana. The average time to complete Contact Tracing (per contact) was 5 minutes when using the paper-based approach and 3.2 minutes when conducted using the mHealth solution.

With the paper form–based approach, 12/113 (10.6%) contacts of adult TB cases and 45/57 (78.9%) contacts of pediatric TB cases had ≥ 1 missing or illogical values for start and stop dates. In contrast, no contacts of adult or pediatric TB cases had missing or illogical values with the mHealth approach. Furthermore, the mHealth approach had favorable overall rating (2.1/7.0), system usefulness (1.6/7.0), information quality (2.6/7.0), and interface quality (2.3/7.0) scores (Ha et al.,2016 p. 4).

Based on the study findings, the new TBCT mHealth approach may be suggested as a potential solution for TB contact tracing efforts in other resource-limited settings.

MDR-TB mHealth Clinical Support

The multidrug resistant (MDR) TB mHealth pilot project came as a variation of the TBCT project also supported by the Botswana-UPenn Partnership in collaboration with the Ministry of Health. The main goal addressed by the MDR-TB pilot project is to close the communication gap between TB clinicians and medical officers (MOs). In this study MOs are equipped with mobile tablets loaded with medical application resources, MDR-TB resources, case sharing applications and a closed-user group (CUG) calling package all targeted to improving communications among TB clinicians. Treatment of MDR-TB is said to be complex and expensive compared to other forms of TB (Marks, Flood & Seaworth et al, 2014).The foreseen benefits from the study were that clinicians would have easy access to MDR-TB guidelines for prevention, monitoring and treatment of the disease.

According to the head of the TB Programme at BUP, the MDR-TB pilot study was conducted partially and was never concluded and evaluated. This was mainly due to budget constraints and some technical delays.

Tuberculosis (TB) mHealth for Training, Monitoring, and Evaluation

An ongoing project supported by the Botswana-UPenn Partnership and funded by the President's Emergency Plan for AIDS Relief (PEPFAR) is the TB PEPFAR mHealth for Training, Monitoring and Evaluation. This project is aimed at training TB/HIV clinicians in Botswana at 62 sites, monitor improvements on training, and collect public health data at all of the 62 sites. SMS technology has been used to send short weekly quizzes to the trainees requesting them to dial a USSD short code to answer the short quiz. As the clinicians answer the questions, the next menu screen will explain whether they provided a correct or incorrect answer, as well as giving them any relevant educational information. The questions will emphasize important learning points and also assess knowledge retention. The answers are fed into a database and providers are targeted for more training or a site visit depending on the false answer rates. The system will be rolled out in parallel with TB training across all participating sites, and users register for the service during their first training.

According to the head of the TB Programme at BUP, major milestones of the TB PEPFAR project so far is the conversion of paper based evaluation forms to digital forms. The USSD evaluations are currently being tested with end-users for their feedback. The mHealth solution encountered some challenges mainly to do with technical errors on the USSD quizzes leading to frequent time-outs. Suggestions have been made to expand the use of the mHealth solution in other trainings with the Ministry of Health once the TB project has been successful.

Television White-Space (TVWS) Pilot Project

TVWS is an ongoing pilot project undertaken by the Botswana Innovation Hub, Microsoft, University of Pennsylvania, and Global Broadband Solution to deliver telemedicine services through broadband internet connection to health posts and clinics outside the capital city Gaborone at far off towns and villages such as Lobatse, Francistown and Maun where there are few or no medical specialists. The Ministry of Health and Botswana Communications Regulatory Authority (BOCRA) both have separately considered that there is need within the health sector to improve broadband connectivity especially for outreach health centres and facilities so as to improve health care service delivery and monitoring. The TVWS project was launched in March 2015, following several months of discussions and planning involving all key partners. While the project funding officially started in January 2015, Phase 1 started in March 2015 with the ceremonial launch of the project in Lobatse. The project was initially funded to be implemented in two phases, with the thought that if the first two phases were successful, a new contract would be negotiated for a third phase. The project partners agreed to conduct a pilot project to deliver eHealth services to regions in Botswana with limited access to broadband and adequate specialized health care services using a new cutting edge technology for the delivery of broadband. The technology is utilizing dynamic spectrum access over unused spectrum across television spectrum band, what is commonly referred to as TV White Space.

Project Kgolagano has been successful in delivering broadband internet over the TVWS and in the process, helping deliver healthcare needs in the town of Lobatse and its catchment area. The telemedicine program is expected to reap economic and social benefits, and the project includes a monitoring and evaluation function to document the socio-economic impact on the communities involved. A total of 50 visits were registered using the TVWS connectivity at one of the Lobatse clinics. From the 50 cases at Lobatse, 10 were consulted by the Botswana-UPenn Partnership (BUP) specialist based at Princess Marina Hospital (PMH) at the time utilizing the TVWS connectivity. These consultations were supported using normal Skype application since the Skype for Business platform was not ready for use at the time. In order to enforce confidentiality, there were no patients identifiers on the pictures discussed during the normal Skype sessions.

A total of 106 cases were registered from the Cervical Cancer clinics at the city of Francistown using the TVWS connectivity during phase 2 of the project. Francistown clinic statistics at Nyangabwe Referral Hospital (WHC) were 51 records and Donga Clinic (WHC) having 55 patient records. These are patients registered and administered using platforms utilizing the TVWS connectivity.

As stated earlier it was envisaged that a third phase might be considered. However, the inherent complexity of coordinating activities of multi-stakeholders in different time zones, within a dynamic health care system not only impacted implementation speed, but also necessitated the need to streamline some of the clinical consultations.

Peek Botswana Project

Another ongoing mHealth pilot project is Portable Eye Examination Kit (Peek) Botswana. According to the Director of the Health Informatics Program at BUP, the Peek Vision technology provides people in remote parts of the world with access to clinically approved eye tests to help combat blindness in developing countries. It provides a low cost device for managing and monitoring the treatment of patients, even in the remotest of settings. Seeing is Believing (Standard Chartered Bank Botswana), Peek Vision, Botswana Ministry of Health (MoH), Botswana Ministry of Education (MoE), Botswana Optometrists Association (BOA), and Botswana-UPenn Partnership (BUP) have partnered to implement Peek Vision School Screening in the Goodhope subdistrict (a village in the southern district of Botswana) as Phase 1 of the national implementation of Peek Botswana.

Since the commencement of the phase 1 in July 2016, 12,800 school children have been screened at 49 schools, of which 848 required refractive services which were provided by MoH and the Botswana Optometrists Association (BOA). An additional 93 children required medication and 63 required ophthalmic services which are being provided at Good Hope Hospital and Scottish Livingstone Hospital in Molepolole.

Some of the challenges encountered during implementation of the PEEK Vision project included participants' incompetency in using smartphones since most were using smartphones for the first time. Another challenge was to do with mobile data bundles getting exhausted quickly. The PEEK platform also experienced a few bugs which presented minor hiccups in the program, and lastly the logistics of getting participants to the training site on schedule was another issue.

Kgonafalo Mobile Telemedicine Scale-Up Project

Since 2009 until 2012, the Botswana government through the Ministry of Health (MoH) in collaboration with the Botswana-UPenn Partnership, conducted pilot studies on an mHealth solution in four medical specialties: Oral Medicine, Dermatology, Radiology and Women's Health (Cervical Cancer Screening) Ndlovu, K., Littman-Quinn, Q., & Kovarik, C. (2014). The main purpose of the mobile telemedicine pilot project was to develop a 'store and forward' telemedicine solution that will be used to facilitate referral/consultancy communication between healthcare workers at district hospitals and clinics for the specialties of oral medicine, dermatology, women's health (cervical cancer screening) and radiology.

All the above mentioned clinical specialties involve visual inspection. Hence, during the project pilot phase, clinicians were equipped with smart phones with a built-in camera and data enabled subscriber identity module (SIM) cards provided by the Orange Foundation of Botswana. The organizational structure of each mobile telemedicine project includes an in-country specialist, an international specialist, a national specialty manager, a referral site coordinator and the referring health care workers. The processes are as follows:

- Healthcare worker collects pertinent clinical history and associated images pertaining to a complex patient case.
- Collected history and images are sent via mobile phones directly by a healthcare worker to an in-country remote specialist for consultation.
- In-country specialist uses the information to diagnose the illness and recommend an appropriate course of treatment.
- In-country specialist could forward the case to an international specialist for further input and collaboration.

A total of 696 cases were successfully managed through the use of mobile telemedicine in the pilot studies. 27 health care providers were trained on how to use mobile telemedicine and they benefited through their day-to-day interaction with the system. The Ministry of Health saved some costs which could have been incurred through referral processes. Table 2 below summarises benefits and findings from pilot studies (Ndlovu et al., 2014).

Some implementation challenges encountered during Kgonafalo pilot project were both technical and social, both internal and external to the projects' environments. Internal technical challenges include application software bugs, SIM card and mobile device malfunctions, smartphone battery power problems, lack of local hardware and software maintenance support, and lastly hackers attacking telemedicine servers (Ndlovu, Littman-Quinn, & Kovarik, 2014).

Following successful pilot study results in 2012, the MoH embarked on a nation-wide scale-up of the mobile telemedicine solution also known as "Kgonafalo". The Botswana MoH further adopted mobile telemedicine into its long term eHealth strategy. Kgonafalo's sustainability milestones included the de-

Table 2. Benefits and findings from the pilot study

Benefits	Pilot Study Findings
Reduction in waiting times for hospital Treatment	All patients were attended remotely by a specialist
Cost saving during referrals	Projected ~P3 750,000 saved per year in the first year of implementation (According to UB and Wharton Business research)
Patient's long distance travel reduction	~P187.50 saved per patient per visit
Health care workers involved in the project gain more knowledge as they interact with the telemedicine solution	27 health care workers trained and gained more clinical knowledge through interaction with the telemedicine system

velopment and signing of a Memorandum of Understanding (MOU) between the Botswana government and private telecommunications partner, the publication and awarding of the government tender to a local IT company, and the development and signing of a Memorandum of Agreement between the Ministry of Health Clinical Services department and the tender winner. The initial system scale-up occurred in 2014 and to ensure project's sustainability, the system was aligned with the national ehealth strategy as well as being locally owned. The initial scaleup phase included Gaborone and nearby villages. That was to be followed by sites in the central district such as Mahalapye, Serowe then going north east to Selibe Phikwe and Francistown facilities and lastly Maun and the surrounding areas. The Kgonafalo system was envisaged to store patient data and generate relevant reports for various management needs. The system is to interface with the current MOH Integrated Patient Management System (IPMS).

CONSIDERATIONS FOR TELEMEDICINE PILOT PROJECTS

Prior to piloting each of the mentioned telemedicine projects in Botswana, some considerations were made. The Ministry of Health (MoH) has a draft eHealth Strategy document developed in 2014 in consultation with the WHO eHeatlh Strategy Toolkit. Prior to 2014, the MoH made reference to the national ICT policy known as Maitlamo to advise its eHealth systems implementations. The Maitlamo policy had its own limitations in that it was entirely a technical document which did not say much about handling of an electronic health record, standards or legal issues around eHealth records. This negatively affected the success of most pilot telemedicine projects as most users and stakeholders were reluctant to adopt such initiatives without proper guiding policies on the ground.

Another important consideration made during Botswana's telemedicine pilot projects was to have clearly stated end-user requirements from the start of each project. This facilitated telemedicine solutions which were acceptable to users. However, even with stated end user requirements, there were requests to make changes, resulting in delayed implementation and project completion time. End-users were sensitized on the costs attached to frequently changing requirements. The following requirements solicitation methods were used during telemedicine pilot projects in Botswana: one-on one interviews, group interviews, questionnaires, prototyping, and use cases.

Another important consideration had to do with engaging all potential partners. Public Private Partnerships were key in influencing the success of most telemedicine pilot projects in Botswana where multiple stakeholders were engaged. Where applicable, Memorandum of Agreements (MOAs) provided a legal ground.

In all the pilot projects highlighted above, an experienced project manager was engaged. This was key to the establishment of a committed and well-coordinated team. Although not all pilot projects were a success in the end, the presence of a project manager assisted in getting work done as intended.

Due to lack of a comprehensive eHealth strategy in Botswana, the legal and ethical aspects of telemedicine were not fully considered at the time of piloting most of the telemedicine projects. The legal and ethical considerations include the responsibilities and potential liabilities of the health professional, the duty to maintain the confidentiality and privacy of patient records, and the jurisdictional problems associated with cross-border consultations. These are key issues to consider as they could negatively affect the success of any telemedicine project.

RECOMMENDATIONS FOR SUCCESSFUL TELEMEDICINE IMPLEMENTATION

Some of the challenges experienced during implementation of the mHealth pilot projects in Botswana are similar to those experienced in the developed world as previously highlighted by Dantu & Mahapatra (2013). Although telemedicine is a relatively new field especially for low resource settings, it is important for any telemedicine solution to be adequately provided for in terms of human resources and the requisite technology. Research has also shown that senior management buy-in and end-user acceptance of any telemedicine intervention is key for successful implementation (Littman-Quinn et al., 2013; Ndlovu et al., 2014; Wootton & Bonnardot, 2015).

There is an urgent need for training and education of both care providers and patients. Many patients and providers' concerns, skepticism about usefulness of telemedicine, diminishing quality of communication in clinical settings, lack of compatibility between telemedicine technologies and organizational routines, can be overcome with proper training and education. Health care administrators need to design appropriate training mechanisms to promote telemedicine awareness among providers and patients. It is not easy to change routines overnight. However, with proper education and training, it is possible to influence changes in routines for better care delivery. Many nurses, physicians, and even patients believe that providing patient care requires physical presence rather than high-technology devises. Therefore it should be understood that telemedicine is one of the many mechanisms to provide care, and it may not be an appropriate medium in situations where physical presence is required.

Interoperability among various IT systems is another important factor for low resource settings. Due to the funding situation in low resource settings, a lot of eHealth solutions are imposed and accepted leading to future incompatibility challenges. The effective exchange of confidential patient information securely among various entities in the health system is imperative. This improves care quality and reduces cost by controlling redundancies. Electronic health record systems in hospitals, clinics, and physician offices must interoperate with existing telemedicine systems in order to have more impact of telemedicine solutions. Consistent standards for both data and software applications are required for seamless exchange of data among various systems (Ackerman et al., 2010; Ghosh & Ahadome, 2012).

The privacy and protection concerns towards patients' information, and providers' fear of malpractice liability could be overcome by developing sophisticated IT systems to protect confidential patient data (Ackerman et al., 2010). Government and regulatory agencies must develop necessary legal framework to encourage providers to open up to telemedicine interventions.

Successful development of any technology solution is also dependent on clearly stated user requirements. If user requirement are not clearly outlined, even though there is adequate budget to support the project or management is in support of the project, the solution developed will not be accepted hence the telemedicine solution will not be a success.

Telemedicine solutions require the support of multiple stakeholders and therefore the engagement of all relevant stakeholders is critical. There should be skilled software developers who design and implement the solution on stable technology platforms. The engagement of an experienced project manager could also contribute to the success of a telemedicine solution. Project managers are the drivers of any project and they should be engaged on the basis of previous track records in project management. An experienced, committed and well-coordinated team is vital for the development success of any telemedicine solution

According to Stanberry (2006), another important consideration is the legal and ethical aspects of telemedicine. *These include the responsibilities and potential liabilities of the health professional, the duty to maintain the confidentiality and privacy of patient records, and the jurisdictional problems associated with cross-border consultations. There is also the issue of reimbursement for care provided using a telemedicine service. Telemedicine allows the transmission of health information across the borders of nation states. Cross-border telemedicine services have begun, particularly in specialties such as teleradiology, but questions of jurisdiction and registration have yet to be answered definitively. While this may be true of many of the legal and ethical aspects of telemedicine generally, it is also the case that health-care professionals who undertake telemedicine in a prudent manner will minimize the possibility of medicolegal complications* (Stanberry, 2006 p. 166).

The mHealth pilot projects conducted in Botswana provides an insight into the country's degree of readiness to successfully adopt telemedicine solutions. The challenges encountered by the project implementers suggests that a lot of work needs to be done before Botswana can be considered to be e-health ready. A number of challenges were encountered in implementing the mHealth solutions, most of which centered on the unavailability of a definitive national eHealth strategy. At the forefront of any telemedicine solution development, should be effective policies for clinical data collections, storage and dissemination utilizing telecommunication networks. A country's eHealth strategy is one key document as it outlines a clear roadmap to which all telemedicine solution developments should be in alignment with. Without clear guidance, projects are likely to fail or be unsustainable in the long term.

FUTURE OF TELEMEDICINE

The field of telemedicine in low resource settings presents significant research and application opportunities. Future opportunities include efficient telemedicine use for educational purposes as well as using telemedicine data for decision support systems. Research is currently focused on making traditional medical instruments such as the stethoscope, microscope, ultrasound scanner, etc., compatible with mobile operation systems such as android or iOS (Prieto-Egido, Simó-Reigadas, Liñán-Benítez, García-Giganto, & Martínez-Fernández, 2014). In this way, developing countries could take advantage of the products developed in the industrialized countries. The success and future of telemedicine is dependant on using as much in-country expertise as possible as well as integration of telemedicine solutions into core EMR systems available.

CONCLUSION

Telemedicine has proven to be effective and achievable in low resource settings as in the developed world. However, the success of telemedicine implementation and adoption is dependent upon a number of factors. First, key stakeholders' buy-in from at all levels is of utmost importance. Without adequate support and engagement of all key stakeholders throughout the telemedicine solution design, development and implementation, there is a high risk of failure. Telemedicine adoption continues to face numerous challenges. Based on a review of literature, the authors have identified several factors that impede the adoption of telemedicine technologies beyond the pilot phase and recommended possible ways for resolving them. Telemedicine, as part of a public health program, has the potential to save lives of millions of people living in low resource settings by bringing them closer to the much needed healthcare services. Pilot studies conducted already demonstrated with evidence the greater potential of telemedicine towards improvement of patients' outcomes.

REFERENCES

Abdelhak, M., Grostick, S., & Hanken, M. A. (2014). *Health information: management of a strategic resource*. St. Louis, MO: Elsevier Health Sciences.

Ackerman, M. J., Filart, R., Burgess, L. P., Lee, I., & Poropatich, R. K. (2010). Developing next-generation telehealth tools and technologies: Patients, systems, and data perspectives. *Telemedicine Journal and e-Health*, *16*(1), 93–95. doi:10.1089/tmj.2009.0153 PMID:20043711

Al-Qirim, N. (2007). Championing telemedicine adoption and utilization in healthcare organizations in New Zealand. *International Journal of Medical Informatics*, *76*(1), 42–54. doi:10.1016/j.ijmedinf.2006.02.001 PMID:16621682

Allely, E. B. (1995). Synchronous and asynchronous telemedicine. *Journal of Medical Systems*, *19*(3), 207–212. doi:10.1007/BF02257174 PMID:7643019

Baker, D. C., & Bufka, L. F. (2011). Preparing for the telehealth world: Navigating legal, regulatory, reimbursement, and ethical issues in an electronic age. *Professional Psychology, Research and Practice*, *42*(6), 405–411. doi:10.1037/a0025037

Brewer, E., Demmer, M., Ho, M., Honicky, R., Pal, J., Plauche, M., & Surana, S. (2006). The challenges of technology research for developing regions. *IEEE Pervasive Computing / IEEE Computer Society [and] IEEE Communications Society*, *5*(2), 15–23. doi:10.1109/MPRV.2006.40

Castro, D., Miller, B., & Nager, A. (2014). Unlocking the potential of physician-to-patient telehealth services. *The Information Technology & Innovation Foundation*. Retrieved from http://www2.itif.org/2014-unlocking-potential-physician-patient-telehealth.pdf

Central Intelligence Agency. (2016). *World Factbook*. Retrieved from https://www.cia.gov/library/publications/the-world-factbook/geos/bc.html

Central Statistics Office. (2010). *Health Statistics Report*. Gaborone: Government Printers.

Central Statistics Office. (2011). *Botswana Transport and Communications Statistics*. Retrieved from http://www.cso.gov.bw/templates/cso/file/File/Botswana%20Transport%20and%20Communications%20 Stats%20Brief%202011%20April%2026%202012.pdf

Craig, J., & Patterson, V. (2005). Introduction to the practice of telemedicine. *Journal of Telemedicine and Telecare, 11*(1), 3–9. doi:10.1177/1357633X0501100102 PMID:15829036

Dantu, R., & Mahapatra, R. K. (2013). Adoption of Telemedicine-Challenges and Opportunities. *Proceedings of the Nineteenth Americas Conference on Information Systems.*

Ghosh, R., & Ahadome, T. (2012). *Telehealth's promising global future*. Retrieved from www.analytics-magazine.org/januaryfebruary-2012/508-telehealths-promising-global-future

Graschew, G., & Roelofs, T. A. (Eds.). (2011). *Advances in telemedicine: Applications in various medical disciplines and geographical regions*. Rijeka: Intech. doi:10.5772/1863

Grigsby, B., Brega, A. G., Bennet, R. E., & Devore, P. (2007). The slow pace of interactive video telemedicine adoption: The perspective of telemedicine program administrators on physician participation. *Telemed e-Health, 13*(6), 645-656.

Ha, Y. P., Tesfalul, M. A., Littman-Quinn, R., Antwi, C., Green, R. S., Mapila, T. O., & Kovarik, C. L. et al. (2016). Evaluation of a Mobile Health Approach to Tuberculosis Contact Tracing in Botswana. *Journal of Health Communication, 21*(10), 1115–1121. doi:10.1080/10810730.2016.1222035 PMID:27668973

Hampton, T. (2012). Recent advances in mobile technology benefit global health, research, and care. *Journal of the American Medical Association, 307*(19), 2013–2014. doi:10.1001/jama.2012.4465 PMID:22665083

HealthIT.gov. (2015). *Benefits of EHRs*. Retrieved from www.healthit.gov/providers-professionals/electronic-medical-records-emr

HIMSS. (2005). *Interoperability Definition and Background*. Retrieved from www.himss.org/content/files/AUXILIOHIMSSInteroperabilityDefined.pdf

International Telecommunication Union. (2007). *WSIS Stocktaking and Partnerships: Activity Details*. Retrieved from http://www.itu.int/wsis/stocktaking/plugin/documents.asp?project=1327569411&lang=en

International Telecommunication Union. (2016*). ICT Data and Statistics: Free Statistics on mobile cellular Subscriptions*. Retrieved from http://www.itu.int/ITU-D/ict/statistics

Kang, H. G., Mahoney, D. F., Hoenig, H., Hirth, V. A., Bonato, P., Hajjar, I., & Lipsitz, L. A. (2010). In situ monitoring of health in older adults: Technologies and issues. *Journal of the American Geriatrics Society, 58*(8), 1579–1586. doi:10.1111/j.1532-5415.2010.02959.x PMID:20646105

King, G., Richards, H., & Godden, D. (2007). Adoption of telemedicine in Scottish remote and rural general practices: A qualitative study. *Journal of Telemedicine and Telecare, 13*(8), 382–386. doi:10.1258/135763307783064430 PMID:18078547

Littman-Quinn, R., Mibenge, C., Antwi, C., Chandra, A., & Kovarik, C. L. (2013). Implementation of m-health applications in Botswana: Telemedicine and education on mobile devices in a low resource setting. *Journal of Telemedicine and Telecare*, *19*(2), 120–125. doi:10.1177/1357633X12474746 PMID:23454821

Marks, S. M., Flood, J., Seaworth, B., Hirsch-Moverman, Y., Armstrong, L., Mase, S., & Sheeran, K. et al. (2014). Treatment Practices, Outcomes, and Costs of Multidrug-Resistant and Extensively Drug-Resistant Tuberculosis, United States, 20052007. *Emerging Infectious Diseases*, *20*(5), 812–821. doi:10.3201/eid2005.131037 PMID:24751166

Microsoft. (2004). *ICT as enablers of development: A Microsoft white paper*. Retrieved from http://www.academia.edu/5272661/icts_as_enablers_of_development_a_microsoft_white_paper

Ministry of Health. (2015). *eHealth stratergy of Botswana 2016-2020*. Final draft. Author.

Naicker, S., Plange-Rhule, J., Tutt, R. C., & Eastwood, J. B. (2009). Shortage of healthcare workers in developing countries-Africa. *Ethnicity & Disease*, *19*(1), 60.

Najjar, J., & Bourquard, J. (2012). High-tech health care: Lawmakers are building up telehealth by breaking down barriers. *State Legislatures*, *38*(10), 26. PMID:23547325

Ndlovu, K., Littman-Quinn, Q., & Kovarik, C. (2014). Scaling up a mobile telemedicine solution in Botswana: Keys to sustainability. *Front Public Health*, *2*, 275. doi:10.3389/fpubh.2014.00275 PMID:25566520

Orange Foundation. (2016). *Coverage*. Retrieved from http://www.orange.co.bw/mobile/coverage.php

Prieto-Egido, I., Simó-Reigadas, J., Liñán-Benítez, L., García-Giganto, V., & Martínez-Fernández, A. (2014). Telemedicine networks of EHAS foundation in Latin America. *Frontiers of Public Health*, *2*(188). doi:10.3389/fpubh.2014.00188 PMID:25360436

Silva, G. S., Farrell, S., Shandra, E., Viswanathan, A., & Schwamm, L. H. (2012). The status of telestroke in the United States a survey of currently active stroke telemedicine programs. *Stroke*, *43*(8), 2078–2085. doi:10.1161/STROKEAHA.111.645861 PMID:22700532

Sood, S. P., Nwabueze, S. N., Mbarika, V. W., Prakash, N., Chatterjee, S., Ray, P., & Mishra, S. (2008). *Electronic medical records: a review comparing the challenges in developed and developing countries*. Paper presented at the Hawaii International Conference on System Sciences. doi:10.1109/HICSS.2008.141

Stanberry, B. (2006). Legal and ethical aspects of telemedicine. *Journal of Telemedicine and Telecare*, *12*(4), 166–175. doi:10.1258/135763306777488825 PMID:16774696

Stronge, A. J., Nichols, T., Rogers, W. A., & Fisk, A. D. (2008). Systematic human factors evaluation of a teledermatology system within the US military. *Telemedicine Journal and e-Health*, *14*(1), 25–34. doi:10.1089/tmj.2007.0016 PMID:18328022

W. H. O. (1997). *Health for all policy for the 21st century*. Geneva: World Health Organization.

W. H. O. (1998). *A health telematics policy in support of WHO's health for all strategy for global health development*. Geneva: World Health Organization.

W. H. O. (2006). *The World Health Report 2006-working together for health*. Retrieved from www.who.int/whr/2006/en/

W. H. O. (2009). *WHO Library cataloguing in Publication Data, Telemedicine: opportunities and developments in member states*. Geneva: World Health Organization.

Whitten, P., Buis, L., & Love, B. (2007). Physician-Patient e-Visit Programs. *Disease Management & Health Outcomes*, *15*(4), 207–214. doi:10.2165/00115677-200715040-00002

W.H.O. (2010). *Telemedicine: opportunities and developments in member states: Report on the second global survey on eHealth*. Geneva: World Health Organization.

Wootton, R., & Bonnardot, L. (2015). Telemedicine in low-resource settings. *Frontiers in Public Health*, *3*(3). doi:10.3389/fpubh.2015.00003 PMID:25654074

ADDITIONAL READING

Adambounou, K., Adjenou, V., Salam, A. P., Farin, F., N'Dakena, K. G., Gbeassor, M., & Arbeille, P. (2015). A low-cost tele-imaging platform for developing countries. *Telemedicine in Low-Resource Settings*, 57.

Alajlani, M., & Clarke, M. (2013). Effect of culture on acceptance of telemedicine in Middle Eastern countries: Case study of Jordan and Syria. *Telemedicine Journal and e-Health*, *19*(4), 305–311. doi:10.1089/tmj.2012.0106 PMID:23540280

Andronikou, S. (2015). Pediatric teleradiology in low-income settings and the areas for future research in teleradiology. *Telemedicine in Low-Resource Settings*, 68.

Delaigue, S., Morand, J.-J., Olson, D., Wootton, R., & Bonnardot, L. (2015). Teledermatology in low-resource settings: the MSF experience with a multilingual tele-expertise platform. *Telemedicine in Low-Resource Settings*, 88.

Jefee-Bahloul, H. (2014). Use of telepsychiatry in areas of conflict: The Syrian refugee crisis as an example. *Journal of Telemedicine and Telecare*, *20*(3), 167–168. doi:10.1177/1357633X14527709 PMID:24814471

Jefee-Bahloul, H. (2015). Telemental health in the middle East: overcoming the barriers. *Telemedicine in Low-Resource Settings*, 53.

Jennett, P., Jackson, A., Healy, T., Ho, K., Kazanjian, A., Woollard, R., & Bates, J. et al. (2003). A study of a rural communitys readiness for telehealth. *Journal of Telemedicine and Telecare*, *9*(5), 259–263. doi:10.1258/135763303769211265 PMID:14599328

Joseph, V., West, R. M., Shickle, D., Keen, J., & Clamp, S. (2011). Key challenges in the development and implementation of telehealth projects. *Journal of Telemedicine and Telecare*, *17*(2), 71–77. doi:10.1258/jtt.2010.100315 PMID:21097563

Patterson, V. (2015). Telemedicine for epilepsy support in resource-poor settings. *Telemedicine in Low-Resource Settings*, 8.

Wootton, R., Liu, J., & Bonnardot, L. (2015). Assessing the quality of teleconsultations in a store-and-forward telemedicine network. *Telemedicine in Low-Resource Settings*, 104.

Xue, Y., Liang, H., Mbarika, V., Hauser, R., & Schwager, P. (2014). *Understanding Healthcare Professionals' Resistance of Telemedicine: an Empirical Study in Ethiopia.* Paper presented at the PACIS.

Zolfo, M., Arnould, L., Huyst, V., & Lynen, L. (2005). Telemedicine for HIV/AIDS care in low resource settings. *Studies in Health Technology and Informatics*, *114*, 18–22. PMID:15923756

KEY TERMS AND DEFINITIONS

eGovernment: The use of ICTs in the public service delivery frameworks.

eHealth: Refers to the use of information and communication technologies (ICT) for health.

eHR: Refers to a digital version of a patient's paper chart.

GDN: Acronym standing for government data network.

ICT: Acronym standing for Information and Communication Technology which include platforms used to manage both static and dynamic information.

IPMS: Acronym for an electronic medical record system standing for Integrated Patient Management System. Botswana's electronic medical record system for attaining a single patient health record.

Low Resource Setting: In health, this refers to areas characterized by a lack of funds to cover health care costs, on individual or societal basis, resulting in limited access to medication, equipment, supplies, and devices.

mHealth: Use of mobile phones and other wireless technology in medical care.

Telemedicine: The use of telecommunication technologies and ICTs to provide clinical health care from a distance.

This research was previously published in Health Information Systems and the Advancement of Medical Practice in Developing Countries edited by Kgomotso H. Moahi, Kelvin Joseph Bwalya, and Peter Mazebe II Sebina, pages 129-148, copyright year 2017 by Medical Information Science Reference (an imprint of IGI Global).

Chapter 51
The Applications of Simulation Modeling in Emergency Departments:
A Review

Soraia Oueida
American University of the Middle East, Kuwait

Seifedine Kadry
Beirut Arab University, Lebanon

Pierre Abichar
American University of the Middle East, Kuwait

Sorin Ionescu
Politehnica of Bucharest, Romania

ABSTRACT

A recent study carried out an empirical investigation of the quality of healthcare delivered to adults and found out that only 54.9±0.6% adult received recommended care. Huge variation in the quality of care depends on patient's condition. In fact, the literature on healthcare is laden with articles like these that emphasize on the importance of the systems view of healthcare problems. Healthcare is a very vast and complex system where different departments interact with each other in order to deliver a certain service to arriving patients. Emergency departments (EDs) are the busiest units of healthcare. Existing problems and their cascading effect will be highlighted by a literature review of a bunch of researches. The purpose of this work is to study, in specific, the emergency department of a hospital with the existing problems and how simulation modeling can interfere in order to solve these problems, increase patient satisfaction and reduce cost. Simulation has emerged as a popular decision support in the domains of manufacturing and services industries.

DOI: 10.4018/978-1-5225-3926-1.ch051

INTRODUCTION

The medical sector has been growing largely over the last decade and healthcare services became more complex and costly, amplified by a poor healthcare delivery system. Healthcare is a highly interconnected dynamic environment where individuals and teams contribute in order to serve patients' demand. The main focus of this study is to discuss this revolution and take care of the whole medical community not only illness, but also improving patient safety, quality, and effectiveness of the healthcare system. This can be achieved by developing new methodologies to improve the health care systems available nowadays.

Many methodologies were presented over the literature in order to study healthcare problems. Some of them are listed as follows (Ceglowski, 2006):

- Patients are grouped by clinicians under several cases; where similar cases should be treated alike and should share the same type of resources every time the same case arises (see Palmer, 1996). This approach can be valuable only in case of few available cases such as in clinics not in large complex systems like ED.
- Time and motion studies were used by industrial engineering analysts in order to introduce enhancement to healthcare (see Hoffenberg et al., 2001).
- Prevention of high patient waiting times and ambulance diversions were discussed over the years and simulation was introduced in order to alleviate this risk (see Jun et al., 1999; Preater, 2002).
- The flow of data in the ED was studied by information science analysts in order to design a computer system that supports the doctors and nurses in their roles (see Nelson et al., 2004).
- ED data inspection for better knowledge of information retrieved.

As a result of the above, the first area to focus on in order to develop an efficient and effective healthcare system is developing systems perspective, where simulation modeling can be generated and a review can be achieved. Simulation modeling can be a solution to tackle this complexity and valuable in providing predictions to forecast the outcome of a change in strategies or policies. The computer simulation is a decision making technique that allows management to conduct experiments with models representing the real system of interest. Busy and complex healthcare systems provide big challenges to managers and decision makers who should be able to serve the high demands constrained by limited budget and high costs of healthcare services. The highest number of patients should be cared of within a limited period of time in order to insure patient satisfaction (reduce waiting time) and increase hospital's revenue (reduce cost).

The delivery of healthcare quality can vary depending on patient's conditions, affecting the recommended care and leading sometimes to urgent and critical health conditions. This huge variation opens the eye on the importance of reviewing the healthcare systems' problems and improving them.

Emergency department (ED) is the most complex, critical and busy unit of a hospital, where medical facility treatment is provided to patients without prior appointment. Other reasons for ED to be a complex system and chosen, specifically, for this study are the high increase in patients' number, the 24/7 operation of the ED, and the open facility to all type of illness and all level of patients. EDs interact with the majority of other departments of the healthcare system. Table 1 shows this interaction. A patient arriving to the ED may be transferred to any other unit of the hospital depending on the diagnosis (such as requiring extra facilities: laboratory, imaging, etc., admission to hospital, referring to surgery

Table 1. ED and interacting departments

	ED	Anesthetics	ICU	Surgery	Cardiology	Radiology	ENT	Genecology/Maternity	Pediatric	Laboratory	Hematology	Microbiology	Neonatal	Nephrology	Neurology	Oncology	Ophthalmology	Orthopedics	Physiotherapy	Dentistry	Dermatology	Gastroenterology	Nutrition	Pharmacy	Admission & Discharge
ED		x	x	x	x	x	x	x	x	x	x	x	x	x	x	x	x	x	x	X	x	x	x	x	x
Anesthetics	x		x	x																					
ICU	x	x		x						x														x	x
Surgery	x		x			x				x									x						x
Cardiology	x			x		x				x														x	x
Radiology	x																							x	
ENT	x			x		x				x														x	x
Genecology/ Maternity	x									x									x					x	x
Pediatric	x									x														x	
Laboratory	x																								
Hematology	x									x														x	
Microbiology	x			x						x															
Neonatal	x							X		x														x	x
Nephrology	x			x						x														x	x
Neurology	x		x	x		x				x														x	x
Oncology	x			x		x				x														x	x
Ophthalmology	x			x																				x	x
Orthopedics	x			x		x													x					x	x
Physiotherapy	x					x																		x	
Dentistry	x																							x	
Dermatology	x																							x	
Gastroenterology	x					x				x															
Nutrition	x																							x	
Pharmacy	x																								x
Admission& Discharge	x		x																						

Figure 1. Patient journey in the ED

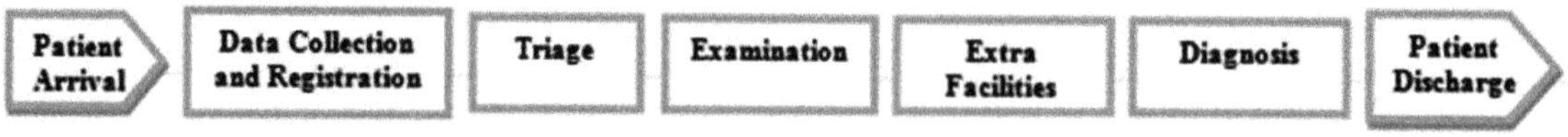

Patient Arrival → Data Collection and Registration → Triage → Examination → Extra Facilities → Diagnosis → Patient Discharge

unit if a surgery is scheduled, referring to pediatric unit in case the patient arriving is a kid/baby, etc.). Moreover, the flow of patient in the ED varies from patient to patient depending on the case and the type of patient. Once arrived to the ED, the patient follows certain assessments before taking the appropriate decision (such as triage, waiting for consultation or directly assigned to a doctor, etc.). However, some essential steps the patient must follow during his journey at the ED are: arrival, consultation, diagnosis, interpretation and decision and finally the process outcome (whether discharged or admitted to the hospital). The patient journey in the ED can be represented in Figure 1.

Due to this complexity and unplanned nature of patient surge, simulation modeling is proven by many researchers to be very effective in order to study the necessary changes needed for better performance. Therefore, predictive modeling, using simulation, is very useful and effective for achieving better results like controlling system costs, responding to new regulations and enhancing patient experience. Figure 2 presents a literature survey from 1997-2010 on the breakdown of the use of simulation. Most of the earlier simulation projects highlighted facility specific issues. Based on the papers reviewed and researches done before, only five percent dealt with multi-facility modeling (Gunal & Pidd, 2010).

Huge data amount will be resulting from the ED simulated system. New techniques should be developed in order to understand this data, and thus leading to the right and efficient information needed for improving the system. Data mining techniques are key factors used by many researchers and proved to be successful in healthcare (see Cullen, 2001; Chae, et al., 2003; Begg et al., 2006). These techniques also help researchers in identifying key measure variables and investigate the data available in hospital databases in order to understand the information that can be useful for the simulation. Since the data collected can be huge and classified under "data rich but information poor" (Han et al., 2001), data mining can be applied to improve the knowledge of important patterns and discover meaningful measures

Figure 2. Simulation survey breakdown

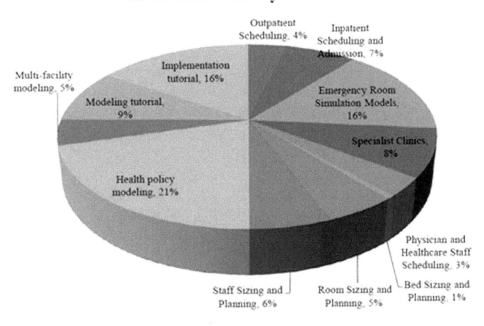

1017

within the data that may lead to a better understanding of the information resulted from the simulation, and thus efficient enhancement can be proposed for the system.

The following section provides a literature review on the different problems facing the ED and how many researchers approached them in order to enhance the quality of care, and thus improve patients' satisfaction. Section III presents a discussion over this literature in order to highlight the main solutions that can alleviate a certain problem in ED and how science management can interfere. Finally, Section IV presents a conclusion and future vision.

LITERATURE REVIEW

The healthcare is a very vast and complex system, where all departments interact with each other to offer care and service for patients. In this literature review, ED is the focus of our research, where complexity arises and prediction is highly needed. Improving EDs may lead to improving various services of the healthcare system and increasing revenue. The different problems studied by different researchers are presented along with some proposed solutions based on simulation modeling. At the end of this section a clear overview based on existing problems versus existing solutions can be achieved and discussed in section 3; leading to a chosen direction in order to improve the healthcare system as a future work.

An ED is the most complex unit of a hospital, where patients appear without any prior appointment, either by their own means or by ambulance. A patient suffering from an accident or a sudden injury, for example, will be directly addressed to the ED. Some of these appearing patients can be with critical cases and need immediate care and others may need a simple treatment. Once arrived to the ED, a patient should be observed before being admitted to the hospital or referred to another unit, like imaging, laboratory, etc. This scenario leads to overcrowding at some peak times and causing a large waiting time thus leading to dissatisfaction. Figure 3 shows an example of an ED.

There are several types of resources in an ED: Staff (doctors, nurses, physicians, and technicians), static resources (triage rooms, examination rooms, x-ray room) and equipment. The process includes in

Figure 3. Emergency Department (ED)

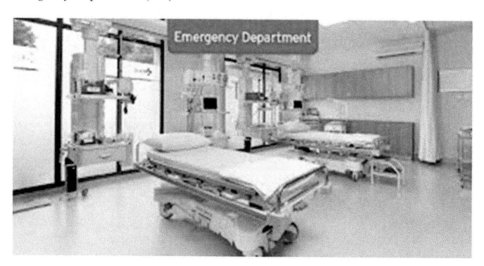

general: arrival to ED, registration, triage, examination, discharge/admission/tests; tests include blood tests or imaging. EDs usually lack sufficient resources in order to serve the unpredictable patient flow.

Most studies and surveys for the past years showed that EDs have a great impact on the healthcare system performance and quality of care. As EDs are linked to many other departments of the hospital, more attention should be addressed here. Thus, improving healthcare needs a recommended improvement in EDs, where patient flow should be monitored, waiting times and length of stay (LoS) should be reduced (to satisfy patient) and revenue should be increased (to satisfy management). The most efficient way in order to approach these problems and find the optimal solution is to use simulation modeling.

Garcia et al. (1995) focused in their simulation modeling on the reduction of waiting time in ED for a hospital in Miami. Baesler F. et al. (2003) built a simulation model using Arena 4.0 in order to estimate the maximum increment rate of ED demands, a specific hospital in Chile could absorb it. The behavior of the variable patient's time in the system was predicted and the minimum number of human resources to serve this demand was defined. Nevertheless, the system should not exceed an acceptable waiting time level. The main focus of the hospital here was to understand the maximum extra demand their ED could absorb without facing problems, considering the patients waiting time, human resources limitations and maintaining the quality of service.

Samaha et al. (2003) studied the operation of a healthcare institution using the Arena simulation modeling. The main purpose of the model was to study the current operation and compare it to some suggested alternative scenarios that can reduce the length of stay patient spends in the ED. Each activity in the ED during a seven-day period, 24 hours a day was evaluated and used as input data to the constructed model. As a result, considerable time was saved without any additional costs. Alternative scenarios are suggestions proposed by the department staff in order to solve the issue of waiting time. Each scenario was implemented into the model in order to validate the output and study its efficiency. The main goal of the model was evaluating patient time, measuring patient throughput, evaluating resource utilization and determining queue sizes; these performance measures are essential in order to assess the effectiveness of the proposed scenarios. They are collected from the output of the model where it should be analyzed; leading to a clear decision on the optimal solution for the problem. Using this simulation model, the hospital improved its service without any unnecessary expenses by testing the proposed solutions via the model before implementing them in the actual running system (ED) (Centeno et al., 2003; Kelton et al.,2002).

Some physicians refer risky and urgent patients to EDs instead of providing care in their clinics (Berenson et al., 2003). As the 24/7 operation and the unneeded appointment make the ED the best option for medical care. Boarding or holding admitted patients until a bed is available, increases the percentage of crowding as well as the waiting time to see a physician; which restrict the system to respond to a patient surge in case of a disaster event. Boarding patients require monitoring, care and critical care procedures. A study about boarding patients considers them as a negative impact on other patient safety. Overcrowding can also cause ambulance diversion. Hospitals spending some time on diversion procedures urge patients to wait for a longer time for evaluation and treatment (Lewin Group, 2005).

Jacobson et al. (2006) presented an overview of DES (Discrete Event Simulation) modeling applications for healthcare clinics. Kolb et al.(2008) proved that the major cause of overcrowding of an ED is the waiting time patients spend in the emergency room waiting for in-patient assistance; which can block important ED resources. They improved patient and staff satisfaction through their design in this study. The design consisted of a discrete event simulation model for testing buffer alternatives in the patient flow. Park et al. (2008) proposed a forecasting model to predict patients' arrival to ED. Papers on treatment delays for high acuity patients (Schull et al., 2004; McCArthy et al., 2002), patient and staff dissatisfaction (Rowe et al., 2006; Abu-Laban (2006), patients left without being seen were reported over the years (Bullard et al., 2009).

Moreover, studies showed that to prevent this overcrowding and access block, many strategies and solutions can be followed; it requires a system level change by changing health policies. Access block, shown in Figure 4, is the delay waiting time that the patient suffers from once being admitted to the ED until he/she gains access to a dedicated bed. Jayaprakash (2009) studied the crowding of EDs in Europe. Access block is one of the main reasons of ED overcrowding and poor quality of care outcomes. Many studies from the UK, US, Canada and Australia have proven this (Forero et al., 2010; Sun et al., 2013).

Gunal and Pidd (2010) presented a literature review for DES models in healthcare where a number of important conclusions were drawn about simulation modelings such as issues faced during modeling from unit specific and facility-specific considerations. Paul et al. (2010) presented also a systematic review of ED simulation literature from 1970 to 2006. As a conclusion of their study, patient's perspective, environmental features and the role of information technology should be also incorporated in future simulation efforts in order to develop solutions to ED overcrowding.

Many solutions were suggested over the years in order to alleviate the overcrowding and access block in EDs and some are presented in the sections below. Solutions were classified under three general categories: modifying a process behavior in the ED, changing staffing levels and schedules and assessing the effect of external variables on the ED. These three categories are supported by simulation modeling techniques and optimization tools in order to find the optimal solution and guarantee the best performance of the ED.

Figure 4. Access block in ED

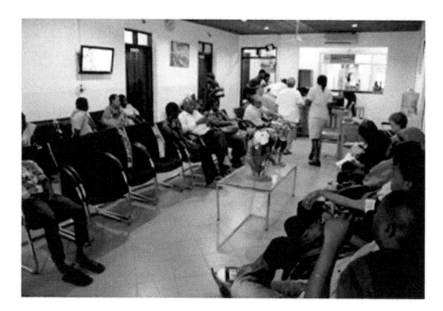

Resource and Operational Rules Management

Reengineering and resource management of the ED consists of changing its aspect by adding specialized units responsible for specific tasks, relocating some equipment, beds, units and changing some hospital operation rules such as introducing the early discharge of patients, etc.

ED Re-Engineering

43% of hospital admissions originate in the ED, therefore the correlation between EDs and the several units of a hospital. A research linked America's ED overcrowding to hospitals restructuring, as a cause of financial pressures (Schull et al., 2001). Redesign or re-engineering of EDs including unit layout changes were presented by Miller et al. (2004), Mould et al. (2013), and Rado et al. (2014); other solutions were also studied by some researchers such as opening new units (Hannan et al., 1974) or expanding the ED capacity (Wiinamaki & Dronzek, 2003).

Kuo et al., 2016, proposed and analyzed the effect of relocating the ED in order to improve operation. They used simulation with Arena to build the system and apply the suggested changes.

Increasing Bed Capacity

Richmond et al. (1990) focused on the effect of bed capacity reduction into waiting times and explore the causes for these observed delays. The complex system was simulated using a dynamic model constructed on iThink software. The model studied the effect of policies changes on the performance of the system (such as controlling the roistering of ED doctors). The shortage in bed numbers may affect the elective admissions by increasing the number of cancellations. A research, proved that only 15-20% of patients arriving to ED require admission and the use of hospital beds (Audit Commission, 1996).

Bagust et al. (1998) used discrete-event stochastic simulation model in order to identify the dynamics of bed usage in emergency admissions. This study examined the relation between the available bed capacity and the unpredictable demand during an ED admission. The insufficient capacity for patients diagnosed for immediate admission may lead to a crisis. Statistics and analysis show that this trend will continue in the future, which indicates a significant increase in demands for beds. This fluctuation in emergency demand will affect the quality and efficiency of care in the hospital. Therefore, a deep understanding of these effects is required in order to apply the needed operational interventions and planning services for avoiding sudden problems leading to crisis. Lane et al. studied the impact of emergency demand on hourly basis emphasizing on the problem of waiting time for admissions (Lane et al., 2000). In this paper, an additional effect was taken into consideration; the random nature of the emergency demand admission affects the use of bed stock, that's why a discrete-event stochastic simulation modeling was used in order to investigate the complex system subject to this random effect. A relation was created between the fluctuating demands for emergency admission and the available in-patient bed capacity. The key output measures of system performance were:

1. Percentage rate of new arrivals to ED that cannot be admitted because of a lack of available beds;
2. Percentage rate of number of days in a year where a critical admission could not be accommodated (crisis day arises here);
3. Bed occupancy rates.

A possible intervention to alleviate the impact of rising emergency admission rates is a better management of existing resources and introducing early discharges which help in raising the bed availability rate. Other interventions can be by avoiding admission if it is not necessary or finding alternatives to admission (treating a patient in ED dedicated room, for example, without the need for hospital admission). As the emergency admissions are difficult to predict, this stochastic modeling proved that spare beds are essential for emergency admissions; where efficiency and a low level of patient risk are the goals.

Lane et al. study focused on the main factors behind the long waiting times for admission in an ED (Lane et al., 2000). Two significant insights, based on policy changes, were found: addition of resources reduce delays to patient demands and reduction in bed numbers do not increase the waiting times for emergency admissions. Bed shortage delays admission to the hospital and also causes cancellations of non-emergency admissions leading to additional future emergency cases.

One of the most significant factors affecting overcrowding is the bed shortage, where patients to be admitted should wait for hospital's bed availability (Derlet & Richards, 2000; Miro et al., 2003). In the UK, this bed shortage can affect even patients who are discharged from the hospital leading to patient dissatisfaction and bad economic events (Schneider et al., 2003). Derlet et al. (2001) met ED directors to define the crowding and evaluate the factors associated with this problem. This study highlights the link between overcrowding problems and nurse shortages. In their perspective, crowding is related to increase patient acuity, shortage in hospital's beds, insufficient space, laboratory/radiology delays, and examination delays, nursing/staff shortage and increasing ED volume. If waiting time spent by the patient in the ED exceeds the time taken to make a decision to admit a patient, then the clinical outcomes will be badly affected (Richardson, 2006; Cameron, 2006). McCarthy et al. (2008) presented a valid performance measure for crowding; which is the ED occupancy rate. This rate refers to the total number of patients divided by the total number of licensed beds.

More studies on this subject proved that modeling methods can improve the flow of patients in an ED by defining the peak times and key factors causing the access block and overcrowding. These models should take into consideration input data based on daily or weekly peak times in order to be able to distribute the admissions evenly across the week and to avoid any expected congestion (Moskop, 2009). Some techniques to be considered are the patient flow systems and bed capacity management. Martin et al. (2011) found that the waiting interval time of a patient from the time of admission request until the exit from ED to be admitted is the main cause of delay in patient flow. The best logical solution to avoid access block and emergency overcrowding is to increase the bed capacity in the hospital and dedicate the corresponding staff needed. When all solutions fail, the management should look upon this solution of increasing the capacity of the healthcare system. In order to alleviate the access block, government can also target some performance measures for the hospitals by introducing a strategy rule that must be followed by all healthcare organizations. Here, the bottleneck of the ED will be the whole organization's problem that must be solved and not just an ED issue. In this way, the emergency care is prioritized; which lead to a more efficient whole healthcare system since the ED interact with many other departments of the healthcare system as discussed earlier.

Hospital Specialization

The problem of ED overcrowding and patient boarding can be also alleviated by a proper assessment of the demographic needs including population age/density, historical trauma, emergency medicine trends and disaster preparedness. Care, is another valuable factor to ED problems, ad it should be provided based on specialization and not to depend on attracting the most number of patients. Therefore, hospitals should compete based on what they can do best. Medical outcomes were proved to be increased and cost to be reduced especially in the case of critical situations (Hillner et al., 2000).

Fast Track System

Yoon et al. (2003) suggested an efficient solution to the congestion problem by introducing the fast-track service in the EDs which is also cost-effective, safe and satisfactory for patients. In the UK, since 2002, this system was deployed under the principle of "see and treat" (Cooke et al., 2004). Chan et al. (2015) classified this problem into two categories: strategies addressing the ED overcrowding and strategies addressing access blocks. As per this study, solutions to these two main problems were, by introducing new concepts or strategies to the healthcare system. The fast-track service discussed here can be introduced in a dedicated area of the ED with a dedicated and efficient number of staff. It was proven to play a great role in alleviating the overcrowding problem. This concept can decrease the overall waiting time, eliminate the wastes and improve the patient flow. By decreasing the waiting time and shortening the length of stay in EDs, congestion issue can be reduced or even solved. Some studies in this area showed that also the rate of unseen patients was reduced. The key principal for this service to succeed is to have the competent and designated staff.

Triage System

Another initiative for reducing patient's complaints and increase satisfaction was conducted by Cooke et al. (2004), where an arriving patient follows the process of assessment at the triage stage, and then he/she will be directed to the appropriate service and staff based on the necessary needs. Therefore, triage system is also a significant way to reduce overcrowding. The triage system refers to a clinical assessment of the patient's medical status upon arrival to the ED; assessed by a primary triage nurse/physician (Robertson-Steel, 2006).

O'Shea (2007) adopted the ED crisis of America's hospitals where factors are attributed to many reasons. In Maryland for example, non-urgent patients occupy over 40% of ED visits. A study showed that visits to EDs increased around 18%. One proposed solution can be by moving out non-emergency patients from emergency rooms leaving the space to urgent patients to be treated, thus decreasing overcrowding and misuse of ED facilities (Maryland Healthcare Commission, 2007).

Duguay and Chetouane (2007) also adopted a simulation model using Arena in order to improve the current operation of an ED by reducing patient waiting times and improving overall service delivery and system throughput. Resource availability is directly linked to patients waiting time. Key resources such as physicians, nurses, examination rooms are considered as control variables. Some features were taken into consideration while building the model such as the random flow of patients (seasonal illness or incident, fluctuates depending on days of the week and patient arrivals may increase during a specific peak time of a given day). Triage codes are a highly considered feature for the modeling system; where an arriving patient receives a triage code based on the severity of his case after being assessed by the triage nurse. The input data collected for model design and validation are based on time durations collected at different stages of the process in the ED. Time durations can be classified under the time spent by a patient during two consecutive activities (waiting duration) and the necessary time to complete an activity (activity duration). The time from registration to available exam room, was observed to be the largest waiting time in this system and therefore considered the main focus of this study. Based on the collected data observation, several alternative resource scenarios were proposed and studied in order to choose the best option to improve this time and apply it for this unit. These scenarios were designed in a way to increase staff/room capacity and decrease the waiting time within budgetary constraints and considering what-if analysis.

The 4-Hours and 3-Hours Rule

The UK NHS in 2004 introduced the 4-hour rule to be applied among all hospitals. The Department of Health launched a health service plan that states a clear policy which imposes an ED not to have a patient total waiting time more than four hours. The application of this policy was not easy, and many struggles were faced to achieve this target. The output of this policy was positive and major changes were resulted as per Cronin and Wright (2006). Munro et al. (2006) achieved a reduced waiting time in his study by applying this policy. Banerjee et al. (2008) stated "long waits in the ED are a thing of the past on the UK". Many factors were attributed to the overcrowding of ED, all leading to the same result of adverse clinical outcomes, patient dissatisfaction. Therefore, to figure out the best scenario and best solution, first the root of the problem should be determined not to affect the entire hospital operation based on the needs of individual regions.

All patients should be observed, admitted, discharged or transferred to another unit within the 4 hours only as presented by Letham and Gray (2012). A study was performed in this area in order to look at some performance measures on emergency overcrowding, access block and mortality rates by using as inputs: hospital data and patient data. This study showed results for pre and post introducing the 4-hours strategy. The results proved that sometimes patient care can be compromised in order to meet the time targets (Geelhoed & de Klerk, 2012).

Another 3-hours rule was suggested by some researchers in improve the total length of stay of the patient since he arrives until his departure from the ED. Discrete event simulation modeling was approached and many what-if scenarios were followed in order to reach this goal. As a result, 30% improvement of patient LoS was proven following this approach (Oh et al., 2016).

Due to the complexity of healthcare systems and the variation of systems from one country to another, the discussed solutions for reducing the overcrowding and access block cannot be applicable in some hospitals or can be less practicable. Nevertheless, the strategies and management approaches discussed above were developed and applied by many hospitals for many years with a proven evidence of efficiency and successful results. Therefore, more investigations and improvements should be taken into consideration on these solutions depending on the place and the type of system.

Early Discharge of In-Patients

Avoiding ED overcrowding and access block, can be achieved by early discharging in-patients; leading to an available bed capacity for new admitted patients. Usually, access block can increase the clinical risk of patients waiting for their turn to be admitted, that is why clinicians and managers should predict, categorize the levels of risks to discharge in-patients earlier and study the consequences behind this step when a sudden large bed capacity is demanded.

Kelen et al. (2006) described the process of discharging in-patients earlier by the "reverse triage", where patients should be safely selected with the lowest risk of consequences. Discharge lounges should be then dedicated for patients to wait for their discharge arrangements and some administrative paper work leading to a saving in bed hours and reduceing the length of stay (Cowdell et al., 2002). This reverse triage system was fully described by an anecdotal report in 2012, putting in evidence the effective use of this system during an unexpected demand for beds (Satterthwaite & Atkinson, 2012).

Holding Units

The access block can be addressed to insufficient bed capacity, inefficient inpatient discharge and inefficient patient flow. In the US, reviews have proven that introducing holding units can reduce the access block and overcrowding by reducing the need for boarding or ambulance diversion (Institute of Medicine Committee, 2006). A study in Spain showed that providing a 16-bed observation unit in the ED of a 900-bed hospital improved the access block (Gómez-Vaquero et al., 2009). Holding units can also be referred as observation units or clinical decision units where the patient arriving to the ED can be examined and treated without the need for admission.

Moreover, a special observation unit should be dedicated for patients showing with low acuity symptoms such as chest pain, stomach ache etc. who may not need any hospital admission. A dedicated person should be assigned for the task of admission/discharge and responding to real-time demands for inpatients.

Other studies showed that the benefits of these holding units were not very efficient comparing to other hospital without any holding units (Schull et al., 2012); therefore, a carefully clinical management plan and adequate support staff should be incorporated in order to achieve a successful approach. Chan et al. (2015) also suggested these holding unit allowing early discharge and increasing capacity using political actions.

Human Resource Management

Resource management consists of adjusting the level of resources needed and capable of serving the maximum number of patients, assigning the appropriate resource to a certain task and editing resource schedules; thus leading to an increase in care demand and a reduction in the patient waiting time.

Optimizing the GP Role

Rieffe et al. (1999) proved that bypassing the general practitioner (GP) can lead to overusing the ED for minor complaints. This will decrease the service quality and increase the ED cost. Lee at al. (1999) conducted a study on ED attendees and found out that 57% were only primary cases. These primary cases can consult a GP instead of using the ED and thus causing additional patient flow. A study conducted by Van Uden et al. (2003) showed that a good way to optimize the GP role is to add after-hours services so they can be always available for primary care patients; thus reducing the inappropriate referrals to the ED.

Staffing Schedules

As discussed in many papers, researchers reached a conclusion where staff resources schedules can highly affect the operations of the ED and have great impact on many factors causing an ED crisis. Preparing these schedules are a complex task since large number of rules should be taken into consideration; such as number of consecutive shifts and weekly hours, conflicting timings, weekends, holidays, individual preferences (sick leaves, special occasions).

Rosetti et al. (1999) proposed a simulation model using Arena in order to determine an optimal attending physician staffing schedules. Since efficient allocation of staff resources is a common problem facing EDs in any hospital. A computer simulation was suggested in order to test alternative ED attending physician staffing schedules and then analyzing the results on the patient throughput and resource utilization. The suggested simulation can help even detecting any inefficiency in the actual system where patient flow, resources, layout and staffing changes can add a noticeable effect. It is agreed that the utilization of ED nurse and physician resources has a significant impact on patient throughput and system performance; therefore, an analysis was performed to reduce the staff idle time and operating expenses, and increase the resource utilization taking into consideration a constant patient quality of care. This can be done by looking at the patient showing up at ED as a function of hours/day, where peak times can be determined. Four different approaches were suggested and analyzed leading to the selection of the best approach where the overall waiting time of patient was significantly decreased as a daily/weekly basis. The approach focused on changing an existing double coverage shift of a current schedule by considering the patient arrival rates for the ED and assigning peak times during a day. Due to the complexity of the ED system and the understaffing, this procedure may increase the level of errors caused by overworked nurses and doctors. As a future work, a quality control analysis could be conducted before and after the implementation of this strategy to determine the problems and any potential solution. This improvement could be achieved by evaluating patient flow and layout designs in parallel with the suggested staff scheduling changes.

Hung (1995) presented a literature review on nurses scheduling using simulation modeling. Other researchers proved the success of these models in nurse scheduling problems using optimization techniques (Berrada, 1993; Weil et al., 1995; Jaumard et al., 1998; Komashi & Mousavi, 2005). Beaulieu et al. (2000) approached a mathematical programming to ensure a feasible performance of this task. The model constructs schedules for all staffing resources within a short period of time and less effort and proposes the best schedules since it takes into account all possible rules. Two major objectives should be considered while modeling: maximizing personnel satisfaction and minimizing salary cost.

Carter and Lapierre (2001) and Sinreich and Jabali (2007) adopted a simulation model to improve the ED operations by studying scheduling policies for physicians. Azadeh et al. (2013) applied fuzzy logic techniques in order to propose the optimal nursing scheduling. Centeno et al. (2003) also used simulation to help ED decision makers in their staff scheduling. The author of this paper presented a procedure that helps in efficiently estimating required parameters for model input data in case assumptions are needed (could not obtain sufficient data for simulation). This is for the reason that, while developing the simulation model for studying and improving the operations of the ED, two challenges were faced: the highly time-varying rate of the arrivals and data paucity (shortage of data). One of the model outputs implicated that by adding an extra doctor and adjusting shifts hours, the average waiting time of patients' consultations can be reduced by 10%. Using different what-if scenarios, that can be simulated using this model, to help hospital managers in taking their decisions for improving the quality of service (such as reducing waiting times) and to assure best allocation of resources. Wang et al. (2009) also focused in their study on the concept of resource allocation. Jerbi and Kamoun (2009) proposed a doctor's shift rescheduling.

Laroque et al. developed a simulation approach that analyzes how resource allocation can impact patient's journey in an ED. Based on some financial restrictions, hospital management cannot assure that resources are always available to fulfill service quality. Therefore, valuable resources (such as doctors and nurses) should be fully utilized. Another factor that should be highlighted is the non-urgent patients who may visit the ED. Increase of patient flow for routine consultation may increase the waiting times, and thus decreasing the quality of service and patient's satisfaction. Authors of this paper developed a simulation model in order to evaluate the impact of staffing and resource scheduling on patient demands, and to achieve insights about ED staffing policies.

Medical Resource Is the Driver

In most researches, the focus to improve the ED operation was the patient itself. Hay et al. (2006) proved that, in the contrary, the patient should not be the driver, but the medical resource should be considered as the main entity of study. It demonstrates the importance of assigning the appropriate doctor to a certain task (patient) along with the corresponding waiting time. Simulation modeling was used in this new approach highlighting three elements: the care paths (models including process and decision), operating priority (which is the clinical priority of the showing case and the waiting time of patient until the process is executed) and the skill sets (where the senior doctor can perform all tasks that a junior doctor can perform, but should not be called for simple tasks). Whenever a patient joins a queue, the operating priority gradually increases relatively to the waiting time. Choosing the right resource for a certain task depends on the severity of the patient's condition, waiting time of the patient and how busy is the hospital. Arena simulation was used with an integrated excel interface for easy configuration.

Subash et al., (2004) and Gunal and Pidd, (2006) classified patients in their study under three categories: "life-threatening", "Major" and "Minor". They studied the effect of junior/senior doctors in consulting patient. Senior doctors are experienced consultants who can spend less time with a patient to reach a clinical decision thus shortening the examination time, laboratory time, assessment time, radiology, discharge time; also, the total waiting time spent in the ED.

Part-Time Jobs and ENPs

The overcrowding can be related to the inappropriate usage of ED utilities by the primary care attendees. In the past several years, part time jobs were offered by some hospitals to general practitioners to serve ED low acuity type of cases leading to a congestion reduction. Theses general practitioners can also refer to senior doctors in the ED for an advice or discussion on the treatment which assure a high quality of care. Low acuity patients are those having minor injuries or minor illness and they constitute the majority of the ED crowding. Other studies showed that using emergency nurse practitioners (ENPs) may increase efficiency since patients will be more satisfied with the quality of care delivered. Carter and Chochnov (2007) performed a systematic review of ENPs working in the ED, concentrating on the outcome measures of this approach; which is the waiting time reduction, higher patient satisfaction, cost-effectiveness and high quality of care which can be equivalent to the same care provided by a junior doctor.

Alternative Staff Distribution

Ahmed and Alkhamis (2009) designed a decision support system simulation combined with optimization in order to determine the optimal number of resources needed to serve an ED in Kuwait taking into consideration management budget restrictions, maximum patient throughput and minimum patient waiting time in the system. The study was made for a public hospital in Kuwait, where decision makers should maximize resources (doctors, nurses, lab technicians) utilization and minimize the waiting time while maintaining the same level of care and a standard patient satisfaction rate. The current staff distribution was studied, and resources limitation was highlighted to figure out an alternative staffing distribution that can improve the ED and reach the target. Patients were classified into different categories based on the severity of their case and transferred to the required service accordingly. This simulation/optimization model focuses on the problem of how to choose the right distribution of resources based on the type of service and taking into consideration the constraints imposed by the system limitations. Many other researchers before Ahmad et al. highlighted the same problem using the simulation/optimization techniques over the past decades, like Swisher et al. (2001), Blasak et al. (2003) and Sinreich and Marmor (2005). These researchers reproduced the behavior of a healthcare system to evaluate its performance and analyze the outcome of different scenarios. Beaulieu et al. (2000) followed a mathematical programming approach in order to schedule doctors for an emergency room. Baesler et al. (2003) adopted a simulation model based on experiments to estimate the maximum capacity for an emergency room. Ahmed and Alkhamis (2009) method differs from all other models since it is not dealing with the mathematical model of the actual system, but by combining simulation with optimization. A complex stochastic objective function represents the optimization model which is subject to some stochastic constraints set by the management; these values can never be analytically evaluated and need simulation intervention. As a future author intention, an interface linkage between excel worksheet and SIMISCRIPT simulation software is intended. Input data for the simulation program will be taken from the excel sheets and accordingly necessary simulation analysis can be achieved. The number of receptionists, doctors, nurses, and lab technicians (etc.) are some of the input data required for evaluation purposes. The output of the simulation program are used for performance measures which includes staff cost, system throughput and average waiting time in the system along with detailed information about the queues formed for each type of service.

Marmor (2010) discussed the complexity of the ED of a hospital and pointed at the operational managerial challenges faced. For this reason, a simulation framework is necessary for realistic tracking of the EDs.

Considering External Factors

External factors such as requesting extra facilities from other units of the hospital, considering different insurance coverage types, predicting strain situations and forecasting disaster conditions affect the operation of the ED and may cause overcrowding or large waiting times. Patients arriving to the ED may be classified into different types of insurance coverage (private insurance, public health insurance, etc.). Also, some patients are uninsured and showed up to the ED for free diagnosis; even if they have a low severity case.

Most of the times, patients arriving to the ED are referred to other units in order to go through extra tests such as imaging or laboratory. These extra facilities help the doctor to come up with an accurate diagnosis and a final decision (whether a patient needs admission or no or whether to be referred to another unit in the hospital such as surgery, etc.). These referrals should be considered in the model for adequate results since patients may be accessing the corresponding units at the same time, thus leading to overcrowding and high waiting times in the ED. Moreover, predicting strain situations and forecasting disaster conditions are essential metrics for a successful ED operation. Thus, care demand can be predicted and the corresponding resource needs (material or human) can be forecasted for optimal operation of the ED during those peak times.

Considering the Lab Tests/Imaging Effect

During the last decade, most studies found in literature, impose an increase in the actual care process (Saunders et al., 1989; Komashie & Mousavi, 2005) or the size and operation of the ED (Samaha et al., 2003; Ruohonen et al., 2006) in order to reach the desired service level (throughput) and reduce waiting times. Saunders et al. (1989) considered in his model, built with Siman/Cinema, several features such as lab tests, triage priorities, teaching aspects, communication delays and physicians' collaboration. Blood tests/results and patients were considered flowing entities in the modeling system; that means the turnaround time of these tests has direct effect on the patient throughput.

Komashie and Mousavi (2005) main objective was to determine the effect of key resources (beds, nurses, doctors) on key performance measures (waiting times, waiting queues and throughput). The Arena model designed was depending on variable service times that can vary depending on the case of the patient. In this study, several essential elements that may affect the process were not taken into consideration (lab tests, triage codes, imaging, etc.). Ruohonen et al. (2006) used Medmodel simulation software in order to evaluate, plan and redesign the healthcare systems. In his study, he introduced a new idea of adding a doctor with the nurse at the triage stage. Therefore, the lab tests can be ordered and medical diagnosis can be performed during the early stage of the process leading to an improvement in waiting times and system throughput. This method allows fast priority recognition and accurate treatment referral. The model adopted lab tests and resource shifts as flowing entities.

Emergency radiology has great impact on waiting time especially in case of trauma patients. Radiology results are needed for patient assessment and discharge. Delays in radiology can lead to unnecessary use of ED beds, increase in length of stay and an increase in patient dissatisfaction (Miele, 2006). Eskandari et al. (2011) proposed considering ED patients using other facilities in the hospital (such as MRI, CT scan etc.) as priority over non-ED patients along with adding financial personnel and five mobile inpatient beds. Paul and Lin (2012) related the long waiting times in EDs to the long waits in triage, delays in tests and receiving results, waiting for a physician or a shortage in nursing staff.

Considering Uninsured Patients

Another factor causing overcrowding can be the increase in the rate of uninsured patients since federal laws implicit any ED to adopt an urgent uninsured patient who lack access to regular primary care even if he is not able to pay the fees. Strunk and Cunningham (2002) highlighted additional factors contributing in the ED rising demand such as capacity constraints for private physicians and scheduling appointments, managed-care restrictions and some low insurance reimbursement rates.

Financial constraints and hospital profit also raise a good factor for ED crowding where some hospitals prefer to reserve a bed for an elective inpatient that is surely paying the necessary fees rather than referring it to an ED patient whose payment is uncertain. One solution presented was to urge a tax deduction for health insurance allowing families and individuals to purchase personal health insurance (Butler & Owcharenko, 2007). Private health plans limits patient showing up to the ED to those having emergency situations only; thus, improving outcomes and reducing costs.

Forecasting Disaster Conditions

More factors should be taken into consideration like managing unexpected catastrophic events discussed by other researchers as well (such as terrorist attacks, natural disasters, pandemic diseases). The Institute of Medicine, a branch of the National Academy of Sciences, recently announced America's emergency medical system to stretch beyond capacity, and thus lack preparedness to accommodate disaster events (Institute of Medicine, 2006).

The disaster events are linked to abnormal conditions that may disturb the normal life in society such as floods, volcanic eruptions, earthquakes, etc. Patvivatsiri (2006) presented a computer simulation model that analyzes patient throughput, assesses resources utilization, evaluates the effect of a terrorist attack and determines necessary staffing level for a corresponding scenario. Paul and Hariharan (2007) studied disaster event impact on ED capacity plan during a terrorist attack. Al Kattan (2009) developed two models to represent ED operations in both normal and disaster conditions. ED operations in earthquake disaster event were studied in Yi et al. (2010). In Joshi and Rys (2011), disaster events patient's arrival patterns and time durations were evaluated using Arena simulation and related to the ability of ED to treat these patients. Xiao et al. (2012) also focused on the optimization of work flow in EDs during extreme events using a DES framework.

Gul and Guneri (2015) carried out a literature review study on simulation modeling used for EDs in both normal and disaster conditions. The literature in this area is vast and expanding with time, but most published studies were based on daily normal conditions only and targeting ED KPIs (Key Performance Indicators) such as length of stay, resource utilization and patient throughput. The best DES model used by many researches in this area was Arena. As a future vision, many suggestions were presented such as considering the financial effects when developing simulation scenarios for improving the ED service or considering disaster times not only the normal period. Few studies only highlighted the costs control of an ED. Immediately after a disaster, the complexity of the ED grows dramatically therefore the need of simulation modeling to forecast the physical and human resources that will be needed. Using the simulation modeling, many scenarios can be proposed, evaluated, comparison and what-if analysis and optimization can be performed.

Considering Big Data Research

The complexity of the ED imposes sharing big data between different departments of the healthcare system in order to assess overcrowding. Halevy and al. showed that the more data provided as input to a simulation system the more scenarios can be conducted and predictions can be accurate; leading to decision making for an optimal solution, improving health service quality, efficiency and cost (Halevy et al., 2009). Big data research approach is proposed to manage the complexity and big volume of the healthcare existing data (Diebold et al., 2012). The increasing data storage capacity and diversity of data types are the main components of this research where healthcare services can be improved depending on the multiplicity of this data. The adoption of insights gained from big data analytics has the potential of saving lives, improve the care delivery process, align payment with performance and expand access to healthcare details (Belle et al., 2015).

In majority of emergency departments' simulations, the model is built upon incomplete data (such as missing arrival time, service times, etc.). Collecting reliable data for the system is a hard task which may often lead to invalid simulations. This problem can be solved by simulation optimization where the unavailable service time durations can be predicted through proposing new algorithms (Guo et al., 2016).

Predicting Strain Situations

As emergency departments have become the immediate and essential medical care unit in a hospital, efficient management of patient flow and predicting resources demand are urgent issues to focus on. Kadri et al. (2014) studied in their research patient flow in the pediatric ED of a hospital in France using Arena simulation modeling taking into consideration strain situations and ED states (normal, degraded, critical) which was not defined in literature before 2012. Strain situations are defined as disequilibrium in the ED where care load flow and care production capacity exceed certain thresholds. To handle this patient influx, EDs require enough human and material resources which are at peak times limited; leading to ED overcrowding and strain situations. The purpose of this study is to build a simulation-based decision support system that takes as input data from the hospital database and based on interviews with healthcare staff in order to predict the strain situations. Inputs are information such as number of patient arrivals, means of arrival, arrival time, types and duration of each treatment, additional examinations, and destination after leaving the ED as well as information regarding the strain situations. Simulation output will help hospital management specifying strain situations, examine the relationship between them, propose correction actions and improve the service at ED. The main strain situations observed from the data collected were the influx of patients, long waits before receiving care, shortage in nursing staff, waiting for doctors, delays in additional examinations and the inability to transfer admitted patients. The simulation model was designed for every day of the week and Sundays were observed to be the most critical day where different scenarios were proposed as solutions, such adding a human resource (nurse/doctor) and material resources (adding an examination room with a doctor or/and a nurse). Results were examined and best scenario was chosen after deep analysis of waiting time reduction and decreasing in length of stay.

Adopting Simulation Techniques

Due to the complexity of the ED, simulation modeling was proven over the years to be a key solution to improve operations. Optimization techniques can be also integrated with simulation, and thus leading to an optimal solution for the arising and studied problem.

Using Queuing System Modeling

Siddharthan et al. (1996) presented a queuing policy in order to reduce the waiting times. Komashie and Mousavi (2005) investigated policy and decision making of an ED, where capacity was adopted by Baesler et al. (2003). Lim, Nye et al. (2012) and Lim, Worster et al. (2012) used mathematical modeling techniques-queuing models, DES, SD (System Dynamics) and ABS (Agent Based Simulation) in order to develop twenty nine scenarios for evaluating waiting time reduction. Abbas B. K. (2014) suggested a simulation model using different scenarios. This model studies the complexity of the ED in a hospital and assesses the patient's time interval process since his arrival to the ED until he receives the needed care. The minimum waiting time can be reached by considering a queuing system modeling. An arriving patient enters the system through the waiting room, shown in Figure 5, where he should pick a number

Figure 5. ED waiting room

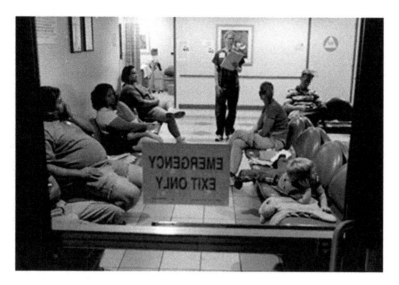

and waits until nurse calls his name and transfers him into the screening room to assess his case (blood pressure, fever, etc.). Based on the patient case, he will be transferred to the examination room to receive the necessary care. Priority discipline should be taken into consideration; patients arriving by ambulance have to receive a priority and urgent care based on the severity of their case.

Integrating Optimization Tools With Simulation Modeling

Recently some studies proved that integration of other simulation method along with the simulation modeling is optimal to find the best solution (like using Opt Quest tool for optimization). Rico et al. (2007), Ahmed and Alkhamis (2009), and Weng et al. (2011) integrated the simulation modeling with optimization (Opt Quest tool) in order to reach the optimal solution. Balanced Scorecard (BSC) was integrated by Ismail, Abo-Hamad and Arisha (2013) with their simulation model to study the ED performance.

Medeiros et al. (2008), Jerbi and Kamoun(2009), Brenner et al. (2010), Taboada et al. (2011), Kuo et al. (2012), and Izady and Worthington (2012) studied staff scheduling in order to optimize the workload and cover patient demand. Morgareidge et al. (2014) demonstrated the advantage of using SSA with DES modeling for facilitating decision making regarding design, reducing costs and improving the ED performance.

INTERPRETATION

As ED is the most complex entity of the healthcare system, the most overcrowding unit and the main focus of our study. Table 2 presents a list of some problems that may affect the ED and some proposed solutions; which researchers should approach in order to alleviate the risk. This table is the result of the literature survey competed in section 2. Note that, due to the high interaction of the ED with several other departments in the hospital, the majority of the problems can lead to the same patient dissatisfaction

Table 2. Some ED overcrowding problems/solutions

Problems	Bed shortage	Admission issues	Resource shortage (Doctors, Nurses, etc.)	Long Waiting times in queues	Admission & Discharge Process	Laboratory & Radiology	Different Insurance Coverage
Solutions	Add extra beds	Predict strain situations	Add resources	Introduce the Triage Category System	Add discharge lounges	Add resources in these units	Improve payment services
	Apply the rule of patient early discharge	Forecast disaster conditions and peak times	Change Staffing Schedules/ Shifts	Introduce the process of Fast-Track System	Add extra administrative staff	Add extra equipment for x-ray, CT-scan, MRI, etc.	Introduce tax deduction by law to push families to purchase private health insurance
	ED re-engineering (such as adding additional units, etc.)	Increase bed capacity	Increase resource utilization	Add Physicians	Hospital Physical Structure Change	Add rooms for extra capacity for these facilities	Limitation of insurance plan to emergency situations
	Introducing new operational rules	Consider Hospital Specialization	Assign part time jobs resources for low acuity patients	Assign the appropriate resource to the right patient			
		Add observation units	Add after-hours GPs/ ENPs for low severity cases	Apply the 4-hours rule			

factor, i.e.: long waiting times and high LoS in the ED. Therefore, the choice of the appropriate solution depends on the type of the problem, type of patients arriving to the ED (age, severity level, etc.), resource utilization levels and scheduling, budget constraints and management constraints.

For example, bed shortage in a hospital can directly affect a patient waiting in the ED for bed availability. Also, a patient referred to another unit for extra tests will have to wait in the ED until the results are ready and, then only, the doctor can finalize his diagnosis and decide whether to treat the patient in the ED, admit him to the hospital or discharge him. Predicting and forecasting peak times can alleviate the risk of overcrowding. Introducing new operation rules and adding new units can improve also the process. New systems, like triage, fast track and assigning the right resource to the right arriving patient can accelerate the process of examination.

All these solutions, proposed earlier, should be integrated into a simulation modeling software in order to build a system close to the real ED and propose enhancement without the need of freezing the operation of the real system. Data mining algorithms can be applied to understand the huge amount of data resulted from the simulation. Moreover, optimization tools such as Opt Quest in Arena simulation software can be very efficient to reach the optimal solution for the best performance of the ED.

CONCLUSION

Healthcare is a large, dynamic and complex system where different units, teams, resources and patients interconnect to serve an activity. This inter-connection of facilities requires a multi-paradigm, flexible simulation modeling methodologies to capture this complexity and present a clear view on how to predict critical events and then reach an optimal decision making.

An ED is a medical treatment facility specializing in emergency medicine, the acute care of patients who present without prior appointment; either by their own means or by that of an ambulance. Most problems affecting the healthcare system are derived from the ED since patient flow is based on prediction without any prior appointment. This department is the biggest interacting unit within the hospital which makes it the most complex system as per the literature review. Studying the cascading effects and their direct link to the ED should be performed using a simulation platform.

As a result from this study, a future vision is deducted such as building a multi-facility platform, using simulation modeling, where the complex system is divided into simpler problems by creating a module for each queue or stage in the process and then combining all together to form the ED system.

Experimentation is the process of improving the system by applying some new changes or suggesting new rules. Three different aspects, discussed earlier in this study, will be the core of this experimentation (see Paul et al., 2010). One scenario can be achieved by changing staffing schedules and assessing the performance of the ED due to this change. Another scenario is modifying a process behavior in the ED (such as adding a new unit or proposing a new operation rule) or assessing the effect of external variables on the ED.

Using a simulation model, the whole complex system representing the real system of the ED will be built and then different scenarios will be created in order to validate this model. The proposed changes can be imposed on the modeled system without affecting the real system in process, and thus predictive analysis can be performed in order to evaluate the performance measures and find the optimal solution for any arising problem. Note that problems affecting ED may be different depending on the region, season, patient age, patient mentality, etc. From these several scenario runs, the optimal solution can be chosen, taking into consideration patient satisfaction (by decreasing waiting times) and increasing management revenue (by decreasing costs, increasing staff utilization, reducing hospital resources use). Therefore, the minimum number of resources required to serve the maximum demand should be predicted.

The computer simulation of the complex ED system will result in massive amount of data generation; where the information needs to be interpreted and analyzed in order to gain better knowledge of the system before experimentation can be suggested and applied. Therefore, efficient system knowledge can be achieved using data mining techniques. Approaching a certain data mining algorithm, useful information in the data collected can be potentially extracted for different processes in the system (Bruballa et al., 2014). Thus, prediction can be easily applied especially in peak times and disaster conditions.

To sum up, for a successful implementation of ED systems, simulation modeling should encourage multi-facilities investigations in order to cover up the complexity of these systems. A very common way to do so is to develop each facility separately (such as arrival, triage, radiology, examination, etc.) and then combine them together using a simulation model and therefore covering up the whole ED system model. This concept proposed earlier in Gunal and Pidd (2007), will be the focus of our research and it will be discussed in details in future work along with developing the required simulation and platform algorithms. Moreover, Majority of the studies reviewed in literature did not focus on the financial effects of the scenarios tested and approached only the normal periods without considering epidemic and disaster times (availability of sufficient medical staff). Therefore, our platform will aim to improve EDs considering as well both cost and epidemic periods during performance measuring.

After reviewing this large number of papers in the literature related to ED operations, Arena was found to be the most powerful simulation modeling tool which is used by majority of researchers, especially during disaster conditions. Most of these papers aim on reducing the waiting times and length of stay in all stages of the ED process, improving resource utilization, maintaining the quality of care either by suggesting different staffing schedules, hiring new staff, proposing new unit re-design; but the majority did not take into consideration the financial impact of these proposed scenarios which can be a highlighted point for our future study. Moreover, for studies of ED at the time of disasters, more focus should be related to the triage state where a new fast track strategy should be developed for patients with high acuity (victims). Studies showed that the impact of other departments of the hospital is worth to be taken into consideration while designing an ED simulation model (such as Mould et al., 2013, Ashour and Kremer, 2013, and Kang et al., 2014).

REFERENCES

Abbas, A. L. B. K. (2014). Simulation Models Of Emergency Department In Hospital. *Journal of Engineering and Development, 18*(2).

Abo-Hamad, W., & Arisha, A. (2013). Simulation-based framework to improve patient experience in an emergency department. *European Journal of Operational Research, 224*(1), 154–166. doi:10.1016/j.ejor.2012.07.028

Abu-Laban, R. B. (2006). The junkyard dogs find their teeth: Addressing the crisis of admitted patients in Canadian emergency departments. *Canadian Journal of Emergency Medical Care, 8*(06), 388–391. doi:10.1017/S1481803500014160 PMID:17209487

Ahmed, M. A., & Alkhamis, T. M. (2009). Simulation optimization for an emergency department healthcare unit in Kuwait. *European Journal of Operational Research, 198*(3), 936–942. doi:10.1016/j.ejor.2008.10.025

Al-Kattan, I. (2009). Disaster recovery plan development for the emergency department-Case study. *Public Administration and Management, 14*(1), 75.

Ashour, O. M., & Kremer, G. E. O. (2013). A simulation analysis of the impact of FAHP–MAUT triage algorithm on the Emergency Department performance measures. *Expert Systems with Applications, 40*(1), 177–187. doi:10.1016/j.eswa.2012.07.024

Audit Commission. (1996). By accident or design Improving A& E services in England and Wales. London: HMSO.

Azadeh, A., Rouhollah, F., Davoudpour, F., & Mohammadfam, I. (2013). Fuzzy modelling and simulation of an emergency department for improvement of nursing schedules with noisy and uncertain inputs. *International Journal of Services and Operations Management, 15*(1), 58–77. doi:10.1504/IJSOM.2013.053255

Baesler, F. F., Jahnsen, H. E., & DaCosta, M. (2003, December). Emergency departments I: the use of simulation and design of experiments for estimating maximum capacity in an emergency room. *Proceedings of the 35th conference on Winter simulation: driving innovation*, 1903-1906.

Bagust, A., Place, M., & Posnett, J. W. (1999). Dynamics of bed use in accommodating emergency admissions: Stochastic simulation model. *BMJ (Clinical Research Ed.)*, *319*(7203), 155–158. doi:10.1136/bmj.319.7203.155 PMID:10406748

Banerjee, A., Mbamalu, D., &Hinchley, G. (2008). The impact of process re-engineering on patient throughput in emergency departments in the UK. *International Journal of Emergency Medicine*, *1*(3), 189-192.

Beaulieu, H., Ferland, J. A., Gendron, B., & Michelon, P. (2000). A mathematical programming approach for scheduling physicians in the emergency room. *Health Care Management Science*, *3*(3), 193–200. doi:10.1023/A:1019009928005 PMID:10907322

Begg, R., Kamruzzaman, J., & Sarkar, R. (2006). Neural Networks in Healthcare: Potential and Challenges. Idea Group Publishing.

Belle, A., Thiagarajan, R., Soroushmehr, S. M., Navidi, F., Beard, D. A., &Najarian, K. (2015). *Big Data Analytics in Healthcare*. BioMed Research International.

Berrada, I. (1993). *Planificationd'horaires du personnel infirmierdansunétablissementhospitalier* (Doctoral dissertation). Departement d'' Inforrnatique et de RechercheOpe'rationnelle, Université de Montreal.

Blasak, R. E., Starks, D. W., Armel, W. S., & Hayduk, M. C. (2003, December). Healthcare process analysis: The use of simulation to evaluate hospital operations between the emergency department and a medical telemetry unit. *Proceedings of the 35th conference on Winter simulation: driving innovation*, 1887-1893.

Brenner, S., Zeng, Z., Liu, Y., Wang, J., Li, J., & Howard, P. K. (2010). Modeling and analysis of the emergency department at University of Kentucky Chandler Hospital using simulations. *Journal of Emergency Nursing: JEN*, *36*(4), 303–310. doi:10.1016/j.jen.2009.07.018 PMID:20624562

Bruballa, E., Taboada, M., Cabrera, E., Rexachs, D., & Luque, E. (2014, August). Simulation and Big Data: A Way to Discover Unusual Knowledge in Emergency Departments: Work-in-Progress Paper. In *Future Internet of Things and Cloud (FiCloud), 2014 International Conference on* (pp. 367-372). IEEE. doi:10.1109/FiCloud.2014.65

Bullard, M. J., Villa-Roel, C., Bond, K., Vester, M., Holroyd, B. R., & Rowe, B. H. (2009). Tracking emergency department overcrowding in a tertiary care academic institution. *Healthcare Quarterly*, *12*(3), 99–106. doi:10.12927/hcq.2013.20884 PMID:19553772

Butler, S. M., &Owcharenko, N. (2007). *Making Health Care Affordable: Bush's Bold Health Tax Reform Plan*. Heritage Foundation.

Cameron, P. (2006). Hospital overcrowding: A threat to patient safety?. *The Medical Journal of Australia*, *184*(5), 203–204. PMID:16515426

Carter, A. J., & Chochinov, A. H. (2007). A systematic review of the impact of nurse practitioners on cost, quality of care, satisfaction and wait times in the emergency department. *Canadian Journal of Emergency Medical Care, 9*(04), 286–295. doi:10.1017/S1481803500015189 PMID:17626694

Carter, M. W., & Lapierre, S. D. (2001). Scheduling emergency room physicians. *Health Care Management Science, 4*(4), 347–360. doi:10.1023/A:1011802630656 PMID:11718465

Ceglowski, A. (2006). *An investigation of emergency department overcrowding using data mining and simulation* (Doctoral dissertation). Monash University.

Centeno, A. P., Martin, R., & Sweeney, R. (2013, December). REDSim: A spatial agent-based simulation for studying emergency departments. In *Simulation Conference (WSC)* (pp. 1431-1442). IEEE. doi:10.1109/WSC.2013.6721528

Centeno, M. A., Giachetti, R., Linn, R., & Ismail, A. M. (2003, December). Emergency departments II: a simulation-ilp based tool for scheduling ER staff. *Proceedings of the 35th conference on Winter simulation: driving innovation,* 1930-1938.

Chae, Y. M., Kim, H. S., Tark, K. C., Park, H. J., & Ho, S. H. (2003). Analysis of Healthcare Quality Indicators Using Data Mining and Decision Support System. *Expert Systems with Applications, 24*(2), 167–172. doi:10.1016/S0957-4174(02)00139-2

Chan, S. S., Cheung, N. K., Graham, C. A., & Rainer, T. H. (2015). Strategies and solutions to alleviate access block and overcrowding in emergency departments. *Hong Kong Medical Journal, 21*(4), 345–352. PMID:26087756

Cooke, M., Fisher, J., Dale, J., McLeod, E., Szczepura, A., Walley, P., & Wilson, S. (2004). *Reducing attendances and waits in emergency departments: A systematic review of present innovations.* Academic Press.

Cowdell, F., Lees, B., & Wade, M. (2002). Discharge planning. *Armchair fan. The Health Service Journal, 112*(5807), 28–29. PMID:12073514

Cronin, J. G., & Wright, J. (2006). Breach avoidance facilitator–managing the A&E 4-hour target. *Accident and Emergency Nursing, 14*(1), 43–48. doi:10.1016/j.aaen.2005.11.005 PMID:16377191

Cullen, P. (2001). *Feature Selection Methods for Intelligent Systems Classifiers in Healthcare (PhD Dissertation).* Chicago: Loyola University of Chicago.

Derlet, R. W., & Richards, J. R. (2000). Overcrowding in the nations emergency departments: Complex causes and disturbing effects. *Annals of Emergency Medicine, 35*(1), 63–68. doi:10.1016/S0196-0644(00)70105-3 PMID:10613941

Derlet, R. W., Richards, J. R., & Kravitz, R. L. (2001). Frequent overcrowding in US emergency departments. *Academic Emergency Medicine, 8*(2), 151–155. doi:10.1111/j.1553-2712.2001.tb01280.x PMID:11157291

Diebold, F. X., Cheng, X., Diebold, S., Foster, D., Halperin, M., Lohr, S., & Schorfheide, F. (2012). *A Personal Perspective on the Origin (s) and Development of "Big Data".* The Phenomenon, the Term, and the Discipline.

Eskandari, H., Riyahifard, M., Khosravi, S., & Geiger, C. D. (2011, December). Improving the emergency department performance using simulation and MCDM methods. *Simulation Conference (WSC) Proceedings*, 1211–1222.

Forero, R., Hillman, K. M., McCarthy, S., Fatovich, D. M., Joseph, A. P., & Richardson, D. B. (2010). Access block and ED overcrowding. *Emergency Medicine Australasia*, 22(2), 119–135. doi:10.1111/j.1742-6723.2010.01270.x PMID:20534047

García, M. L., Centeno, M. A., Rivera, C., & DeCario, N. (1995, December). Reducing time in an emergency room via a fast-track. *In Simulation Conference Proceedings, 1995. Winter* (pp. 1048-1053). IEEE. doi:10.1109/WSC.1995.478898

Geelhoed, G. C., & de Klerk, N. H. (2012). Emergency department overcrowding, mortality and the 4-hour rule in Western Australia. *The Medical Journal of Australia*, 196(2), 122–126. doi:10.5694/mja11.11159 PMID:22304606

Gómez-Vaquero, C., Soler, A. S., Pastor, A. J., Mas, J. P., Rodriguez, J. J., & Virós, X. C. (2009). Efficacy of a holding unit to reduce access block and attendance pressure in the emergency department. *Emergency Medicine Journal*, 26(8), 571–572. doi:10.1136/emj.2008.066076 PMID:19625552

Gul, M., & Guneri, A. F. (2015). A comprehensive review of emergency department simulation applications for normal and disaster conditions. *Computers & Industrial Engineering*, 83, 327–344. doi:10.1016/j.cie.2015.02.018

Gunal, M. M., & Pidd, M. (2006, December). Understanding accident and emergency department performance using simulation. *In Simulation Conference, 2006. WSC 06. Proceedings of the Winter* (pp. 446-452). IEEE. doi:10.1109/WSC.2006.323114

Gunal, M. M., & Pidd, M. (2010). Discrete event simulation for performance modelling in healthcare: A review of the literature. *Journal of Simulation*, 4(1), 42–51. doi:10.1057/jos.2009.25

Guo, H., Goldsman, D., Tsui, K. L., Zhou, Y., & Wong, S. Y. (2016). Using simulation and optimisation to characterise durations of emergency department service times with incomplete data. *International Journal of Production Research*, 54(21), 6494–6511. doi:10.1080/00207543.2016.1205760

Halevy, A., Norvig, P., & Pereira, F. (2009). The unreasonable effectiveness of data. *IEEE Intelligent Systems*, 24(2), 8–12. doi:10.1109/MIS.2009.36

Han, J., & Kamber, M. (2001). *Data Mining: Concepts and Techniques Morgan Kaufmann*. San Francisco: International Thomson.

Hannan, E. L., Giglio, R. J., & Sadowski, R. S. (1974, January). A simulation analysis of a hospital emergency department. In *Proceedings of the 7th conference on winter simulation* (vol. 1, pp. 379-388). ACM. doi:10.1145/800287.811199

Hay, A. M., Valentin, E. C., & Bijlsma, R. A. (2006, December). Modeling emergency care in hospitals: a paradox-the patient should not drive the process. In *Simulation Conference, 2006. WSC 06. Proceedings* (pp. 439-445). IEEE.

Hillner, B. E., Smith, T. J., & Desch, C. E. (2000). Hospital and physician volume or specialization and outcomes in cancer treatment: Importance in quality of cancer care. *Journal of Clinical Oncology*, *18*(11), 2327–2340. doi:10.1200/JCO.2000.18.11.2327 PMID:10829054

Hoffenberg, S., Hill, M. B., & Houry, D. (2001). Does Sharing Process Differences Reduce Patient Length of Stay in the Emergency Department? *Annals of Emergency Medicine*, *38*(5), 533–540. doi:10.1067/mem.2001.119426 PMID:11679865

Hung, R. (1995). Hospital nurse scheduling. *The Journal of Nursing Administration*, *25*(7-8), 21–23. doi:10.1097/00005110-199507000-00010 PMID:7636569

Institute of Medicine. (2006). *Emergency Medical Services: At the Crossroads*. Washington, DC: National Academies Press.

Institute of Medicine Committee on the Future of Emergency Care in the United States Health System. (2007). *Hospital-based emergency care: At the Breaking Point*. Washington, DC: National Academies Press. Available from: http://www.nap.edu/catalog/11621.html

Izady, N., & Worthington, D. (2012). Setting staffing requirements for time dependent queueing networks: The case of accident and emergency departments. *European Journal of Operational Research*, *219*(3), 531–540. doi:10.1016/j.ejor.2011.10.040

Jacobson, S. H., Hall, S. N., & Swisher, J. R. (2006). Discrete-event simulation of health care systems. In Patient flow: Reducing delay in healthcare delivery (pp. 211-252). Springer US. doi:10.1007/978-0-387-33636-7_8

Jaumard, B., Semet, F., & Vovor, T. (1998). A generalized linear programming model for nurse scheduling. *European Journal of Operational Research*, *107*(1), 1–18. doi:10.1016/S0377-2217(97)00330-5

Jayaprakash, N., O'Sullivan, R., Bey, T., Ahmed, S. S., &Lotfipour, S. (2009). Crowding and delivery of healthcare in emergency departments: the European perspective. *Western Journal of Emergency Medicine*, *10*(4).

Jerbi, B., & Kamoun, H. (2009). Using simulation and goal programming to reschedule emergency department doctors shifts: Case of a Tunisian hospital. *Journal of Simulation*, *3*(4), 211–219. doi:10.1057/jos.2009.6

Joshi, A. J., & Rys, M. J. (2011). Study on the effect of different arrival patterns on an emergency department capacity using discrete event simulation. *International journal of industrial engineering. Theory Applications and Practice*, *18*(1), 40–50.

Jun, J. B., Jacobson, S. H., & Swisher, J. R. (1999). Application of Discrete-Event Simulation in Health Care Clinics: A Survey. *The Journal of the Operational Research Society*, *50*(2), 109–123. doi:10.1057/palgrave.jors.2600669

Kadri, F., Harrou, F., Chaabane, S., & Tahon, C. (2014). Time series modelling and forecasting of emergency department overcrowding. *Journal of Medical Systems*, *38*(9), 1–20. doi:10.1007/s10916-014-0107-0 PMID:25053208

Kang, H., Nembhard, H. B., Rafferty, C., & DeFlitch, C. J. (2014). Patient flow in the emergency department: A classification and analysis of admission process policies. *Annals of Emergency Medicine, 64*(4), 335–342. doi:10.1016/j.annemergmed.2014.04.011 PMID:24875896

Kelen, G. D., Kraus, C. K., McCarthy, M. L., Bass, E., Hsu, E. B., Li, G., & Green, G. B. et al. (2006). Inpatient disposition classification for the creation of hospital surge capacity: A multiphase study. *Lancet, 368*(9551), 1984–1990. doi:10.1016/S0140-6736(06)69808-5 PMID:17141705

Kelton, W. D., Sadowski, R. P., &Sadowski, D. A. (2002). *Simulation with ARENA.* McGraw-Hill, School Education Group.

Kolb, E. M., Schoening, S., Peck, J., & Lee, T. (2008, December). Reducing emergency department overcrowding: five patient buffer concepts in comparison. *Proceedings of the 40th conference on winter simulation,* 1516-1525. doi:10.1109/WSC.2008.4736232

Komashie, A., & Mousavi, A. (2005, December). Modeling emergency departments using discrete event simulation techniques. *Proceedings of the 37th conference on Winter simulation,* 2681-2685. doi:10.1109/WSC.2005.1574570

Kuo, Y. H., Leung, J. M., & Graham, C. A. (2012, December). Simulation with data scarcity: Developing a simulation model of a hospital emergency department. *Simulation Conference (WSC) Proceedings,* 1–12.

Kuo, Y. H., Rado, O., Lupia, B., Leung, J. M., & Graham, C. A. (2016). Improving the efficiency of a hospital emergency department: A simulation study with indirectly imputed service-time distributions. *Flexible Services and Manufacturing Journal, 28*(1-2), 120–147. doi:10.1007/s10696-014-9198-7

Lane, D. C., Monefeldt, C., & Rosenhead, J. V. (2000). Looking in the wrong place for healthcare improvements: A system dynamics study of an accident and emergency department. *The Journal of the Operational Research Society, 51*(5), 518–531. doi:10.1057/palgrave.jors.2600892

Laroque, C., Himmelspach, J., Pasupathy, R., Rose, O., & Uhrmacher, A. M. (2012). Simulation with data scarcity: developing a simulation model of a hospital emergency department. *WSC '12 Proceedings of the Winter Simulation Conference.*

Lee, A., Lau, F. L., Hazlett, C. B., Kam, C. W., Wong, P., Wong, T. W., & Chow, S. (1999). Measuring the inappropriate utilization of accident and emergency services? *International Journal of Health Care Quality Assurance, 12*(7), 287–292. doi:10.1108/09526869910287558 PMID:10724572

Letham, K., & Gray, A. (2012). The four-hour target in the NHS emergency departments: A critical comment. *Emergencias, 24*(1), 69–72.

Lewin Group. (2005). *TrendWatchChartbook 2005: Trends Affecting Hospitals and Health Systems.* American Hospital Association.

Lim, M. E., Nye, T., Bowen, J. M., Hurley, J., Goeree, R., & Tarride, J. E. (2012). Mathematical modeling: The case of emergency department waiting times. *International Journal of Technology Assessment in Health Care, 28*(02), 93–109. doi:10.1017/S0266462312000013 PMID:22559751

Lim, M. E., Worster, A., Goeree, R., & Tarride, J. E. (2012). PRM28 physicians as pseudo-agents in a hospital emergency department discrete event simulation. *Value in Health*, *15*(4), A163. doi:10.1016/j.jval.2012.03.884

Marmor, Y. (2010). *Emergency-departments simulation in support of service-engineering: Staffing, design, and real-time tracking* (Doctoral dissertation).

Martin, M., Champion, R., Kinsman, L., & Masman, K. (2011). Mapping patient flow in a regional Australian emergency department: A model driven approach. *International Emergency Nursing*, *19*(2), 75–85. doi:10.1016/j.ienj.2010.03.003 PMID:21459349

Maryland Healthcare Commission. (2007). *Use of Maryland Hospital Emergency Departments: An Update and Recommended Strategies to Address Crowding*. Author.

McCarthy, M. L., Aronsky, D., Jones, I. D., Miner, J. R., Band, R. A., Baren, J. M., & Shesser, R. et al. (2008). The emergency department occupancy rate: A simple measure of emergency department crowding? *Annals of Emergency Medicine*, *51*(1), 15–24. doi:10.1016/j.annemergmed.2007.09.003 PMID:17980458

McCarthy, M. L., Zeger, S. L., Ding, R., Levin, S. R., Desmond, J. S., Lee, J., & Aronsky, D. (2009). Crowding delays treatment and lengthens emergency department length of stay, even among high-acuity patients. *Annals of Emergency Medicine*, *54*(4), 492–503. doi:10.1016/j.annemergmed.2009.03.006 PMID:19423188

Medeiros, D. J., Swenson, E., & DeFlitch, C. (2008, December). Improving patient flow in a hospital emergency department. *Proceedings of the 40th Conference on Winter Simulation*, 1526-1531. doi:10.1109/WSC.2008.4736233

Miele, V., Andreoli, C., & Grassi, R. (2006). The management of emergency radiology: Key facts. *European Journal of Radiology*, *59*(3), 311–314. doi:10.1016/j.ejrad.2006.04.020 PMID:16806785

Miller, M. J., Ferrin, D. M., & Messer, M. G. (2004, December). Fixing the emergency department: A transformational journey with EDSIM. In *Simulation Conference, 2004. Proceedings of the 2004* (Vol. 2, pp. 1988-1993). IEEE. doi:10.1109/WSC.2004.1371560

Miro, O., Sanchez, M., Espinosa, G., Coll-Vinent, B., Bragulat, E., & Milla, J. (2003). Analysis of patient flow in the emergency department and the effect of an extensive reorganisation. *Emergency Medicine Journal*, *20*(2), 143–148. doi:10.1136/emj.20.2.143 PMID:12642527

Morgareidge, D., Hui, C. A. I., & Jun, J. I. A. (2014). Performance-driven design with the support of digital tools: Applying discrete event simulation and space syntax on the design of the emergency department. *Frontiers of Architectural Research*, *3*(3), 250–264. doi:10.1016/j.foar.2014.04.006

Moskop, J. C., Sklar, D. P., Geiderman, J. M., Schears, R. M., & Bookman, K. J. (2009). Emergency department crowding, part 2—barriers to reform and strategies to overcome them. *Annals of Emergency Medicine*, *53*(5), 612–617. doi:10.1016/j.annemergmed.2008.09.024 PMID:19027194

Mould, G., Bowers, J., Dewar, C., & McGugan, E. (2013). Assessing the impact of systems modeling in the redesign of an Emergency Department. *Health Systems*, *2*(1), 3–10. doi:10.1057/hs.2012.15

Munro, J., Mason, S., & Nicholl, J. (2006). Effectiveness of measures to reduce emergency department waiting times: A natural experiment. *Emergency Medicine Journal, 23*(1), 35–39. doi:10.1136/emj.2005.023788 PMID:16373801

Nelson, R., & Millet, I. (2004). *Data Flow Diagrams Versus Use Cases – Student Reactions*. Paper presented at the Tenth Americas Conference on Information Systems, New York, NY.

O'Shea, J. S. (2007). *The Crisis in America's Emergency Rooms and What Can Be Done*. Heritage Foundation.

Oh, C., Novotny, A. M., Carter, P. L., Ready, R. K., Campbell, D. D., & Leckie, M. C. (2016). Use of a simulation-based decision support tool to improve emergency department throughput. *Operations Research for Health Care, 9*, 29–39. doi:10.1016/j.orhc.2016.03.002

Palmer, G. (1996). Casemix Funding of Hospitals: Objectives and Objections. *Health Care Analysis, 4*(3), 185–193. doi:10.1007/BF02252878 PMID:10162141

Park, E. H., Park, J., Ntuen, C., Kim, D., & Johnson, K.Cone Memorial Hospital. (2008). Forecast driven simulation model for service quality improvement of the emergency department in the Moses H. Cone Memorial Hospital. *Asian Journal on Quality, 9*(3), 1–14. doi:10.1108/15982688200800024

Patvivatsiri, L. (2006, December). A simulation model for bioterrorism preparedness in an emergency room. *Proceedings of the 38th conference on Winter simulation*, 501-508. doi:10.1109/WSC.2006.323122

Paul, J. A., & Hariharan, G. (2007, December). Hospital capacity planning for efficient disaster mitigation during a bioterrorist attack. In *Proceedings of the 39th conference on Winter simulation: 40 years! The best is yet to come* (pp. 1139-1147). IEEE Press.

Paul, J. A., & Lin, L. (2012). Models for improving patient throughput and waiting at hospital emergency departments. *The Journal of Emergency Medicine, 43*(6), 1119–1126. doi:10.1016/j.jemermed.2012.01.063 PMID:22902245

Paul, S. A., Reddy, M. C., & DeFlitch, C. J. (2010). A Systematic Review of Simulation Studies Investigating Emergency Department Overcrowding. *Simulation, 86*(8-9), 559–571.

Paul, S. A., Reddy, M. C., & DeFlitch, C. J. (2010). A systematic review of simulation studies investigating emergency department overcrowding. *Simulation, 86*(8-9), 559–571.

Preater, J. (2002). A Bibliography of Queues in Health and Medicine. *Health Care Management Science, 5*(4), 283. doi:10.1023/A:1020334207282

Rado, O., Lupia, B., Leung, J. M., Kuo, Y. H., & Graham, C. A. (2014). Using simulation to analyze patient flows in a hospital emergency department in Hong Kong. In *Proceedings of the International Conference on Health Care Systems Engineering* (pp. 289-301). Springer International Publishing. doi:10.1007/978-3-319-01848-5_23

Richardson, D. B. (2006). Increase in patient mortality at 10 days associated with emergency department overcrowding. *The Medical Journal of Australia, 184*(5), 213. PMID:16515430

Richmond, B. M., Vescuso, P., & Peterson, S. (1990). *iThink™ Software Manuals*. Academic Press.

Rico, F., Salari, E., & Centeno, G. (2007, December). Emergency departments nurse allocation to face a pandemic influenza outbreak. In *Simulation Conference* (pp. 1292-1298). IEEE. doi:10.1109/WSC.2007.4419734

Rieffe, C., Oosterveld, P., Wijkel, D., & Wiefferink, C. (1999). Reasons why patients bypass their GP to visit a hospital emergency department. *Accident and Emergency Nursing*, *7*(4), 217–225. doi:10.1016/S0965-2302(99)80054-X PMID:10808762

Robertson-Steel, I. (2006). Evolution of triage systems. *Emergency Medicine Journal*, *23*(2), 154–155. doi:10.1136/emj.2005.030270 PMID:16439754

Rowe, B. H., Bond, K., Ospina, M. B., Blitz, S., Friesen, C., & Schull, M. (2006). *Emergency department overcrowding in Canada: what are the issues and what can be done?* [Technology overview no 21]. Ottawa: Canadian Agency for Drugs and Technologies in Health.

Ruohonen, T., Neittaanmaki, P., & Teittinen, J. (2006, December). Simulation model for improving the operation of the emergency department of special health care. *In Simulation Conference, 2006. WSC 06. Proceedings of the Winter* (pp. 453-458). IEEE. doi:10.1109/WSC.2006.323115

Samaha, S., Armel, W. S., & Starks, D. W. (2003, December). Emergency departments I: the use of simulation to reduce the length of stay in an emergency department. *Proceedings of the 35th conference on winter simulation: driving innovation*, 1907-1911.

Satterthwaite, P. S., & Atkinson, C. J. (2012). Using reverse triageto create hospital surge capacity: Royal Darwin Hospitals response to the Ashmore Reef disaster. *Emergency Medicine Journal*, *29*(2), 160–162. doi:10.1136/emj.2010.098087 PMID:21030549

Saunders, C. E., Makens, P. K., & Leblanc, L. J. (1989). Modeling emergency department operations using advanced computer simulation systems. *Annals of Emergency Medicine*, *18*(2), 134–140. doi:10.1016/S0196-0644(89)80101-5 PMID:2916776

Schneider, S. M., Gallery, M. E., Schafermeyer, R., & Zwemer, F. L. (2003). Emergency department crowding: A point in time. *Annals of Emergency Medicine*, *42*(2), 167–172. doi:10.1067/mem.2003.258 PMID:12883503

Schull, M. J., Szalai, J. P., Schwartz, B., & Redelmeier, D. A. (2001). Emergency department overcrowding following systematic hospital restructuring trends at twenty hospitals over ten years. *Academic Emergency Medicine*, *8*(11), 1037–1043. doi:10.1111/j.1553-2712.2001.tb01112.x PMID:11691665

Schull, M. J., Vermeulen, M., Slaughter, G., Morrison, L., & Daly, P. (2004). Emergency department crowding and thrombolysis delays in acute myocardial infarction. *Annals of Emergency Medicine*, *44*(6), 577–585. doi:10.1016/j.annemergmed.2004.05.004 PMID:15573032

Schull, M. J., Vermeulen, M. J., Stukel, T. A., Guttmann, A., Leaver, C. A., Rowe, B. H., & Sales, A. (2012). Evaluating the effect of clinical decision units on patient flow in seven Canadian emergency departments. *Academic Emergency Medicine*, *19*(7), 828–836. doi:10.1111/j.1553-2712.2012.01396.x PMID:22805630

Siddharthan, K., Jones, W. J., & Johnson, J. A. (1996). A priority queuing model to reduce waiting times in emergency care. *International Journal of Health Care Quality Assurance, 9*(5), 10–16. doi:10.1108/09526869610124993 PMID:10162117

Sinreich, D., & Jabali, O. (2007). Staggered work shifts: A way to downsize and restructure an emergency department workforce yet maintain current operational performance. *Health Care Management Science, 10*(3), 293–308. doi:10.1007/s10729-007-9021-z PMID:17695139

Sinreich, D., & Marmor, Y. (2005). Emergency department operations: The basis for developing a simulation tool. *IIE Transactions, 37*(3), 233–245. doi:10.1080/07408170590899625

Strunk, B. C., & Cunningham, P. J. (2002). *Treading water: Americans' access to needed medical care, 1997-2001.* Academic Press.

Subash, F., Dunn, F., McNicholl, B., & Marlow, J. (2004). Team triage improves emergency department efficiency. *Emergency Medicine Journal, 21*(5), 542–544. doi:10.1136/emj.2002.003665 PMID:15333524

Sun, B. C., Hsia, R. Y., Weiss, R. E., Zingmond, D., Liang, L.-J., Han, W., & Asch, S. M. et al. (2013). Effect of emergency department crowding on outcomes of admitted patients. *Annals of Emergency Medicine, 61*(6), 605–611. doi:10.1016/j.annemergmed.2012.10.026 PMID:23218508

Swisher, J. R., Jacobson, S. H., Jun, J. B., & Balci, O. (2001). Modeling and analyzing a physician clinic environment using discrete-event (visual) simulation. *Computers & Operations Research, 28*(2), 105–125. doi:10.1016/S0305-0548(99)00093-3

Van Uden, C. J. T., Winkens, R. A. G., Wesseling, G. J., Crebolder, H. F. J. M., & Van Schayck, C. P. (2003). Use of out of hours services: A comparison between two organisations. *Emergency Medicine Journal, 20*(2), 184–187. doi:10.1136/emj.20.2.184 PMID:12642541

Wang, T., Guinet, A., Belaidi, A., & Besombes, B. (2009). Modelling and simulation of emergency services with ARIS and Arena. Case study: The emergency department of Saint Joseph and Saint Luc Hospital. *Production Planning and Control, 20*(6), 484–495. doi:10.1080/09537280902938605

Weil, G., Heus, K., Francois, P., & Poujade, M. (1995). Constraint programming for nurse scheduling. *Engineering in Medicine and Biology Magazine, IEEE, 14*(4), 417–422. doi:10.1109/51.395324

Weng, S. J., Cheng, B. C., Kwong, S. T., Wang, L. M., & Chang, C. Y. (2011, December). Simulation optimization for emergency department resources allocation. *Simulation Conference (WSC) Proceedings,* 1231–1238.

Wiinamaki, A., & Dronzek, R. (2003, December). Emergency departments I: using simulation in the architectural concept phase of an emergency department design. *Proceedings of the 35th conference on Winter simulation: driving innovation,* 1912-1916.

Xiao, N., Sharman, R., Rao, H. R., & Dutta, S. (2012). A simulation-based study for managing hospital emergency departments capacity in extreme events. *International Journal of Business Excellence, 5*(1-2), 140–154. doi:10.1504/IJBEX.2012.044578

Yi, P., George, S. K., Paul, J. A., & Lin, L. (2010). Hospital capacity planning for disaster emergency management. *Socio-Economic Planning Sciences, 44*(3), 151–160. doi:10.1016/j.seps.2009.11.002

Yoon, P., Steiner, I., & Reinhardt, G. (2003). Analysis of factors influencing length of stay in the emergency department. *Canadian Journal of Emergency Medical Care*, 5(03), 155–161. doi:10.1017/S1481803500006539 PMID:17472779

KEY TERMS AND DEFINITIONS

Arena: A discrete event simulation software which helps the modeler in building an experiment model that is similar to the real system and perform experimentation where improvements can be suggested without any interruption of the currently working system.

Data Mining: The fact of dealing with big data where new information can be generated from pre-existing databases.

Experimentation: The process of improving the system by applying new rules and suggesting new operations.

Overcrowding: The fact of having excessive numbers of patients needing or receiving care.

Patient Flow: The process that a patient follows, from the time he enters the system until he is discharged. Patient flow includes both medical and administrative processes.

Patient LoS: The length of stay of a patient spends in the system.

Queuing Analysis: A method used in order to improve patient throughput.

Simulation Modeling: A model designed using a simulation software for a process or system over a period of time.

Waste: A non-added value activity that a certain process may encounter. Customers usually are not willing to pay for wasted activities.

What-If-Analysis: The simulation of several scenarios by applying some changes to the inputs and analyzing the outcome of the outputs.

This research was previously published in the Handbook of Research on Data Science for Effective Healthcare Practice and Administration edited by Elham Akhond Zadeh Noughabi, Bijan Raahemi, Amir Albadvi, and Behrouz H. Far, pages 94-125, copyright year 2017 by Medical Information Science Reference (an imprint of IGI Global).

Chapter 52
Integrated Smart TV-Based Personal E-Health System

Laura Raffaeli
Università Politecnica delle Marche, Italy

Susanna Spinsante
Università Politecnica delle Marche, Italy

Ennio Gambi
Università Politecnica delle Marche, Italy

ABSTRACT

This paper discusses the design and experimental implementation of an integrated system for the delivery of health related services, based on different technologies and devices. The idea is to create a unique point of access for the user, towards both a cloud-based remote service for the consultation of medical reports, and a personal local service that allows to collect and display data from biomedical sensors, to manage user's reminders for medicines, and to monitor the patient's dietary habits. The proposed system employs suitable technologies to simplify the user interaction, such as Near Field Communications enabled devices, and a smart TV equipment. By this way, it is possible to effectively deliver telehealth services also to users who may be less familiar with technological equipments, such as older adults, or people living in rural communities. The experimental implementation proves the feasibility of the proposed service, and the possibility to gain users' adherence and compliance, through proper design criteria.

INTRODUCTION

Developed countries around the world are facing the need to apply dramatic changes to traditional healthcare paradigms, pushing for a rapid shift from in-hospital care, to more advanced home healthcare solutions, according to new, de-centralized models. These changes are driven by several and differentiated factors, either economical, social, and technological ones. In the economic perspective, the global economic crisis puts a big pressure on the welfare and healthcare-related national systems, causing a strong reduction of the available financial resources, against a growing demand of healthcare services and

DOI: 10.4018/978-1-5225-3926-1.ch052

facilities. The demand increases because of an increased incidence of elderly population, and changed life styles, leading to a longer life duration but also a stronger impact of chronic diseases. In the social perspective, most of the developed countries are experiencing a demographic shift (United Nations, 2013); as an example, the life expectancy for males and females in Europe has increased from 45.7 and 49.6 to 75.0 and 79.9 years, respectively, in less than a century. Demographic changes affect a wide range of economic and social fields, as well as policies concerned with health, social welfare, housing, and many other issues. Further, overall problems regarding healthcare services are emerging in many developed countries, such as: the demand for increased availability of care services outside hospitals and medical institutions, and into patients' own premises; the need for improved efficiency of the services, to maintain acceptable quality despite reduced financial resources; the difficulties and costs in recruiting personnel specialized in elderly care, especially to deliver assistance at home (Klersy, De Silvestri, Gabutti, Raisaro, Curti, Regoli & al., 2011).

Telehealth (also known as telemedicine, or remote health) in general refers to a number of technologies, systems, and applications that may be adopted to provide remote support of health care at home. Such a support requires the availability of a set of basic functionalities, like remote consultation and diagnosis, as well as the possibility of collecting data for the monitoring of health parameters and vital signs (e.g. blood pressure, heart rate, and seizure risk). Suitably designed (i.e. compliant, user-friendly, safe) devices for remote patient monitoring have been shown to increase the patients' role in the management of their own health, improve chronic disease management, and reduce the incidence of acute episodes (Spinsante, Antonicelli, Mazzanti & Gambi, 2012). By using a variety of integrated or standalone devices, up-to-date information on patients' chronic disease and/or post-acute care status (including vital signs, heart rate, blood glucose levels, medication management, mental health, physical and cognitive fitness), and even other data (such as patient's location, or ambient parameters that may condition their health status) can be transmitted to family caregivers, providers, or third parties in charge of patients monitoring. Clinicians, or properly trained individuals, can then intervene with coaching actions, or by adjusting the course of treatment.

To ensure patients' adherence and compliance, it is of basic importance to adopt technologies and devices that improve the user experience and make it as easier as possible. The project presented in this paper fulfils these requirements, by providing the experimental implementation of an integrated system to offer a set of health-related services, both remote and local, accessible through a unique interface represented by a smart TV platform. A Cloud-based service enables the remote consultation of personal medical records by the citizens, while the local service supports the self-monitoring of some health-related parameters collected from NFC (Near Field Communication) enabled medical devices, the management of user's reminders for drugs and medicines, and the monitoring of diet habits.

The development of the proposed work is an extension of a previous project by the same authors (Raffaeli, Gambi & Spinsante, 2014), motivated by the idea of implementing a more complete e-health system, including both a remote service for online consultation of medical reports and a service for local self-monitoring and storage of some health-related parameters. The purpose of the study herein presented is to show, by experimental implementation, the feasibility of an innovative way to access health-related services, by means of new devices, such as smart TVs. The experimental outcomes show that the smart TV is a suitable tool of user interaction, both for accessing remotely generated information (managed by a cloud infrastructure) and for the local (i.e. at home) collection and processing of data gathered by the user, by means of classic biomedical devices or new wearable sensors.

The paper is organized as follows: first, a description of the system, its main components and the technologies adopted is provided. Secondly, the two components of the system, i.e. the remote consultation service and the local healthcare service, are described. Finally, the use of the system and related tests are presented before concluding the paper.

BACKGROUND

Related Works

The different technological components encompassed by the proposed system have been separately presented and discussed in the literature, to cover different aspects of healthcare services delivery.

Referring to the literature, an application of cloud computing in the healthcare ecosystem is presented by Bahga & Madisetti (2013). They describe the advantages of a cloud-based EHR system (Electronic Health Records) that aims to provide interoperability, data integration and security, and compare it with the traditional one used in the United States. The project involves the entire healthcare system and offers several benefits to all the stakeholders. In the case proposed by the authors, instead, the service is at its first stage of development: data integration between different laboratories is not achieved yet, and the cloud interface towards the citizens is considered, which represents a first prototype service. The service at issue deals with the remote consultation of medical reports, that is available through a cloud platform provided by the local regional Public Administration. The deployment of this cloud-based solution has been described in detail by Spiga et al. (2014). Biswal et al. (2014) propose another cloud based application to improve the traditional paper-based healthcare system. The developed architecture leans on three tiers: patient, doctor and administrative applications. In addition to offering a set of medical services, the "eHealth Cloud" enables to store and to manage large amounts of electronic medical reports. These data represent a key resource to be analyzed for knowledge extraction regarding benefit, cost and feedback. About this, Chauhan and Kumar (2013) briefly summarize the main advantages and, on the other hand, the challenges for the adoption of cloud services in the healthcare field.

As for other projects that employ the smart TV in social and health applications, Sorwar & Hasan (2012) discuss an integrated tele-monitoring framework that exploits the smart TV platform for both physiological and environmental health monitoring. They only define a theoretical architecture proposal and a possible application scenario, no experimental implementation is presented. Other papers (Alaoui & Lewkowicz, 2013; de Abreu et al, 2011; López-de-Ipiña, Blanco, Laiseca & Díaz-de-Sarralde, 2011) describe projects of smart TV applications designed for elderly people. The development on a smart TV platform aims to improve its usage, thanks to the familiarity of almost everyone with this device.

NFC technology is not designed to transfer large amounts of data, but rather to provide a quick and easy-to-implement type of wireless communication, which can serve as a bridge between already existing services, or may allow the creation of new type of services, specifically designed on NFC communication. The use of NFC to simplify user interaction and management of more complex procedures, such as pairing of Bluetooth devices, has been already addressed in the literature covering several fields of application (Ceipidor et al, 2013; Vergara, Daz-Helln, Fontecha, Hervas, Sanchez-Barba, Fuentes & Bravo, 2010; Zhang & Li, 2011). For example, Puma et al. (2012) list some NFC applications in the healthcare field: patients' identification, control of medications, data acquisition and storage for remote monitoring.

Our proposal, detailed in the following sections, aims at integrating the technologies discussed above in a unique design.

Technology Overview

This subsection provides a brief description of two basic technological elements of the proposed system, i.e. the smart TV and the NFC technology.

A smart TV platform is basically an electronic equipment that provides, as its peculiar feature, the integration in the television set of functions and services linked to the Internet. In particular, the TV set may access online applications enabling an increased level of interaction between the web and the user. As happened for smart phones, smart TVs exhibit advanced multimedia and interaction capabilities, with respect to previous devices (Lee, Sohn, Kim, Kim & Kim, 2013; Park, Jang, Kim & Kim, 2013); they may be integrated into the TV set, or provided by means of external Set Top Boxes.

There is no industry standard for smart TV: different vendors feature different design solutions and approaches, and may provide specific services and applications. To realize this project, a Samsung smart TV has been adopted. This brand provides all the tools to develop applications, such as Eclipse SDK with custom extensions, a TV emulator for PC, Application Program Interface (API) and documentation. The selected platform is equipped with a Linux-based operating system and a TV-based browser engine that enables the execution of interactive applications. An application designed for the smart TV environment is a web-based software component that exploits the smart TV embedded browser to be executed and shown on the TV screen. A generic application is organized as a set of scenes, i.e. web pages, that include HTML elements to contain text, images, default visual components (such as buttons, scroll bars, pop-up windows). The HTML language is used to describe the graphic appearance of the page, integrated by Javascript to include sequences of instructions, and a style sheet (CSS) for page formatting. So, for each scene, at least an HTML file, a CSS file, and a Javascript file are necessary. Further, an application project developed by means of the SDK must also include a configuration file (usually an XML file), and an index file, that represents the point of access to the application.

NFC is a set of standards for smartphones and similar devices to establish radio communication with each other by touching them together, or bringing them into close proximity. The NFC is based on the Radio Frequency Identification (RFID) principle and takes place through an inductive coupling between the devices that have to exchange information. The NFC protocol distinguishes among three operational modes, i.e. active, passive and card emulation. In our system, the passive communication mode is employed: the tag placed in the medical devices or in the drug boxes does not generate its own magnetic field. In contrast, the NFC reader generates a magnetic field that is amplitude-modulated by the passive tag. Such variations can be detected, to collect the corresponding data.

NFC provides a range of benefits owing to his main features, such as those indicated by the NFC Forum (NFC Forum, 2014).

- **Intuitive:** NFC interactions require just a simple touch.
- **Versatile:** NFC is ideally suited to the broadest range of industries, environments, and uses.
- **Open and Standards-Based:** The underlying layers of NFC technology follow universally implemented ISO, ECMA, and ETSI standards.
- **Interoperable:** works with existing contactless card technologies.

- **Technology-Enabling:** NFC facilitates fast and simple setup of wireless technologies, such as Bluetooth, Wi-Fi, etc.
- **Inherently Secure:** NFC transmissions are short range (a few centimeters).
- **Security-Ready:** NFC has built-in capabilities to support secure applications.

NFC brings simplicity and convenience to many aspects of daily life, so it has many fields of application. Moreover, especially in a healthcare application, it is important to ensure an easy user interaction that can be provided by the NFC technology.

SYSTEM DESCRIPTION

Figure 1 represents the architectural model of the proposed healthcare system. The smart TV application links together all the services and represents the user interface to the entire system, that may be separated in two main sub-systems:

- The remote service: concerns the connection between the TV application and the remote data center, for the delivery of the personal reports consultation service;
- The local service: consists of the network involving the NFC-enabled medical devices, the NFC reader, the smart TV and the database, for the local self-monitoring of health parameters.

Cloud Based Remote Healthcare Service

Figure 2 is a representation of the architecture on which the consultation service is based. Several laboratories for medical analyses and examinations are equipped with local servers, that are used as repositories to store the users' examination records. A wired network infrastructure connects the laboratories to the regional data centers, across which a cloud based infrastructure is implemented. According to this archi-

Figure 1. System architecture, including remote consultation service and local healthcare services

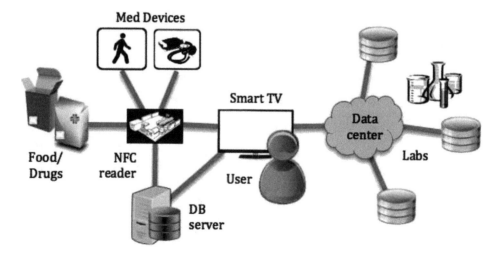

Figure 2. Main elements of the service for remote consultation of personal medical reports

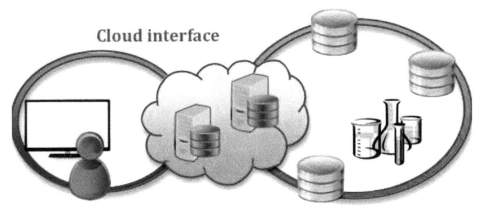

tecture, a request issued by a user is processed by the data center in the cloud. The data center queries each local repository at the medical laboratories, collects and properly formats the received data, and replies to the client application in charge of delivering the information to the final user. A basic element in the design of a remote service relying on a modular architecture is related to the definition of the data formats that will be accepted and exchanged by each actor involved in the process. In the specific case under study, users' medical reports are collected from the laboratory repositories by means of a REST-based paradigm: data are exchanged between clients and servers over HTTP or HTTPS connections, and formatted as JSON (JavaScript Object Notation) objects. A JSON object comprises a number of key-value couples, even in a nested structure. The remote services, each one addressed through a specific URL (Universal Resource Locator), are able to provide the following data:

- List of points of sampling at which patients may perform medical examinations;
- Patient's personal information;
- List of reports available for the patient who performed the log-in;
- Single report containing a set of outcomes.

Local Service for User's Data Management

Figure 3 shows a representation of the network and the technologies employed in the local sub-system for health self-monitoring, for the communication among the involved devices.

The medical devices used are commercial products by A&D Medical, specifically a blood pressure meter and a pedometer (additional products information may be found in the corresponding manuals (AND, 2014; AND, 2014)), both supporting NFC technology. The measured values saved in memory may be acquired by means of an NFC reader, which provides the wired Ethernet connection to a database. Data can be extracted later by the application running on the smart TV that is connected to the same network via Ethernet or Wi-Fi. The repository can be also accessed through a remote connected PC, for example by an authorized doctor or a caregiver. The same NFC reader is also able to read the passive tags placed in the boxes of foods and drugs, and send the corresponding message to the smart TV ap-

Figure 3. Devices and communication technologies in the local sub-system for health self-monitoring

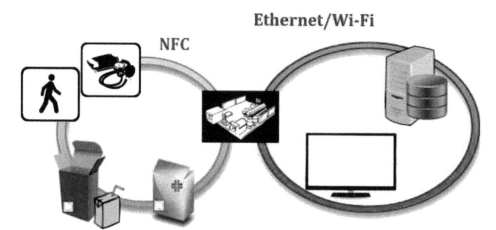

plication. The message contains a code used to identify the product, and to search for the corresponding information in the database.

In the project, an open-source relational database management system (RDBMS) is used, that runs as a server providing multi-user access to several databases. The local database is composed by 3 tables corresponding to user's measurements and reminders have been created ad-hoc for the specific cases. They are structured as in Tables 1, 2 and 3.

The values ''max - min - pulse'' indicate the systolic and diastolic pressure, and the heart rate measured by the BPM, ''steps - aw - cal'' represent the number of steps, active walk (which indicates the distance covered expressed in kilometres), and calorie consumption measured by the pedometer. Two more tables containing nutritional values of food and instructions for medicines have been imported from external sources. One contains the amounts of carbohydrate, protein, salt, vitamins, etc. for hundreds of foods. Drugs information instead may be obtained from free-access databases (a sort of official ''drug index''). This database provides a lot of information, which is redundant for the purposes of this application, so only 4 fields are extracted for each drug: name, instructions, contraindications and dosage.

Table 1. Blood pressure monitor table fields

userID	date	time	max	min	pulse

Table 2. Pedometer table fields

userID	date	steps	aw	cal

Table 3. Reminders table fields

medicine	quantity	time

REMOTE SERVICES FOR MEDICAL RECORDS MANAGEMENT

Interactions between the smart TV client application and the cloud server are performed using the AJAX (Asynchronous Javascript and XML) technology and XMLHttpRequest (XHR), which defines a set of APIs for client/server data transfer. Due to the privacy requirements, communications take place according to the HTTPS protocol, and by the use of SSL (Secure Socket Layer) certificates. All the remote services provide a code and a textual response to each request, that is shown in a pop-up window on the TV screen. Error messages generated by the remote server include, for example:

- **Internal Error:** Due to problems in the execution of the remote server operations;
- User login failed, user password expired;
- Irregular request, when a medical report is available, but not yet ready for remote consultation.

User authentication requires the username and the password issued by the laboratory at the time of medical examination, that are specific for that laboratory. For this reason, the name of the remote laboratory at which the examination took place must also be selected when accessing the application. The insertion of username and password in the proper text input elements is performed by means of the graphic *QWERTY* keyboard shown on the TV screen. The arrow keys of the TV remote controller are used to select characters from the keyboard. In order to simplify and improve the selection of the specific laboratory through the application interface, a function similar to text auto-completion is implemented. The insertion of the first two letters of the laboratory name generates a reduced list of potential candidates, among which the user may choose the right name, in a better and easier way. The laboratories list is downloaded from the server to the client smart TV, at the first user access, stored in a text file in the TV and possibly updated, when new labs are added to the list.

After the authentication step, a specific medical report may be requested among all those available. Each report is composed of several examination outcomes and each one has to be processed according to the specific formatting operations required by the corresponding data type. One of the requirements for the design of the service, was to keep it as much as possible identical to the traditional one. When the medical report includes numerical and textual information, they are properly organized in a table structure, and shown on the TV screen. If it contains an antibiogram examination, it is provided in a different table, in which the number of rows and columns depends on the amount of values to display. Finally, if it includes an electrophoresis examination, the numerical values are collected and, from them, a graphical representation is provided.

The user can access the service for password management through a dedicated page of the TV application. He has to type old and new credentials and a request is sent to update his information in the remote server.

LOCAL SERVICE FOR SELF-MONITORING

The prototype NFC reader has been implemented on a microcontroller board, equipped with Ethernet and NFC interface modules. From the user's point of view, measures may be stored in the database and visualized on the TV simply by getting the NFC reader near to the medical device. The application implemented on the board executes the workflow represented in Figure 4.

After the reading, it is necessary to identify the medical device by means of the product code included in the received bits, in order to choose the appropriate protocol for data mining. The manufacturer has supplied documentation about the communication protocols supported by the medical devices. The measures have to be coupled with the corresponding user so, before collecting the value measured, this information is added by reading another tag that contains the ''user ID''. Referring to the transmission to the smart TV, the resulting messages have the following structure: "code - userID - date - time - max - min - pulse" and "code - userID - date - steps - aw - cal". The two-digit ''code'' has been included to identify the service. Once the information is processed, the application implements two operations:

- Queries the database to create new records and insert the measured values;
- Sends messages (formatted as strings) to the smart TV to notify the presence of new measures.

As concerns the food and drug information, the user may read on the TV screen the nutritional values of food that he is going to eat, or instructions about drugs, for example the dosage. The message recorded in the tag is composed of two digits (the first and the second) representing the type, i.e. food or drug, and a variable-length code to identify the specific product. For medicines, the expiry date is also included. Messages structure is: ''code - id'' and ''code - expiryDate - id''. The board has to read the tag, convert the values to a string and forward it to the smart TV application, which queries the database and displays the results. In this case the workflow is reduced to a few steps, indicated in Figure 5.

Figure 4. Operations implemented by the NFC board: acquisition, processing, connection to server and to smart TV

Figure 5. Workflow executed by the NFC board

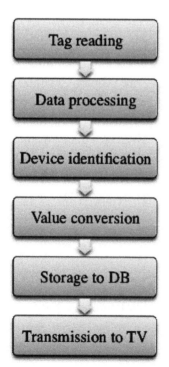

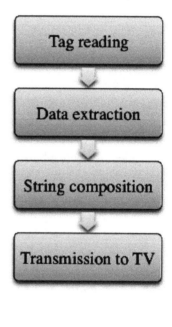

The communication between the board and the smart TV takes place by means of the HTTP protocol. Several requests are needed for the interaction between the application running on the NFC reader and the smart TV application: the first one to initiate the connection, in which client has to provide some headers, then a request for each message to be sent, and the last for disconnection. To manage the requests, the TV application is able to recognize different status and events and to associate them to the corresponding functions defined by the application developer, in order to execute the appropriate operation. Specifically, this application implements the following actions:

- Detects the connection of a device;
- Identifies the device by means of the *DeviceName* included in the request headers;
- Detects the message receiving event and extracts the content;
- Processes the message in the proper way depending on its content.

Information requests from the smart TV to the database server are performed by using HTTP protocol and AJAX technology, and data are given back in the form of JSON objects. Figure 6 represents the procedure for data request and response between the smart TV, the server and the database. The described process is performed in the following situations:

- In case of user's requests for measures display or reminders management;
- Automatically, if a message is received from the NFC reader, both when a new measure has been acquired, and when a tag has been read from a food or drug box;
- Periodically, to realize the reminder function.

The last functionality offered by the local service allows displaying pop-up messages in the bottom-right area of the screen while the user is watching TV. In order to show the reminders pop-up at the appropriate time, the current system time is compared with the times foreseen for the intake of all the medicines the user needs, which are saved in the database. In case of matching, all the parameters of the reminder are shown on the screen. Thanks to specific functions implemented by the smart TV application, users can access the list of elements already saved in the database, insert, delete or modify a reminder by means of the remote control.

Figure 6. Sequence of steps for data exchange between database and smart TV

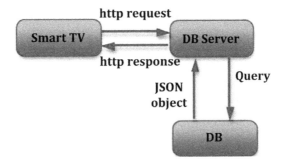

SYSTEM USAGE AND TESTING

As explained in the Introduction, this paper describes an improvement of an existing system implemented by the same authors. Its capabilities were already verified and discussed in the previous work: therefore, this section is going to run over them and mainly refers to the services for request and display on the TV screen of nutritional values and drug instruction leaflets, and to their integration in the system.

Using the System Functionalities

The use of NFC technology in the procedure of measures collection makes easy the user's interaction with the medical devices, so it may be accomplished by means of two simple stages: user tag reading and measure reading. The operations of data storage and transmission are performed automatically. Information request for food and drugs is even easier and faster, since it just requires to tap the box near to the reader.

When the Smart TV application is launched, a small red icon appears in a corner of the screen: this just activates the memo functionality, so the user can go on watching the TV program. Figure 7 illustrates an example of a reminder that appears on the screen at the time of intake of a medicine. The grey box shown in Figure 7 appears on the bottom-right angle of the screen, and does not prevent the user from watching the TV program. If the user needs to activate the other services, he can access the application menu through the *RED* key of the remote control. The available services are listed in the "Home" page: when one of the items is selected, the application switches to the corresponding page.

Figure 8 illustrates the blood pressure monitor page: on the right there is a list of the measures saved in the database sorted by date, while their values are placed on the left. The activity monitor page looks similar, but contains different parameters. If no measures were found on the database, a pop-up window appears to notify this condition.

By accessing the reminders section, users can see a page containing the list of saved reminders and three buttons to perform insertion, modification or removal of a reminder. To insert or modify a reminder, another page is loaded to allow text input functionality. The application notifies the user about the outcome of these procedures by means of pop-up messages.

Pages reporting food nutritional values and medicines instruction leaflets are automatically shown after the tag reading action, by means of the procedure described previously. Figure 9 is an example of an instruction leaflet. Items on the left may be selected by using the arrow keys of the remote control and the corresponding text is shown within the boxes on the right.

Figure 7. Example of a medicine reminder

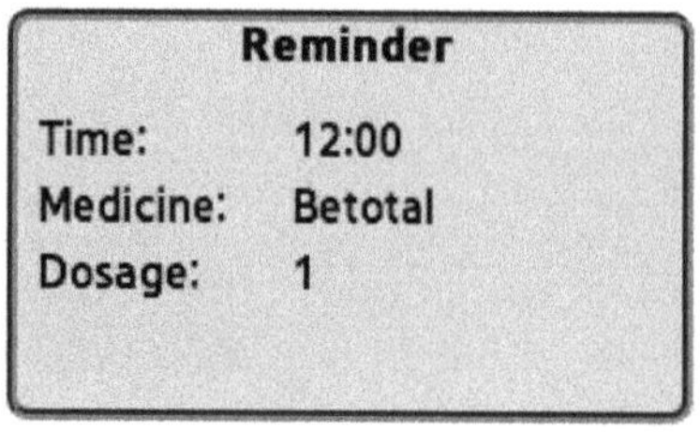

Reminder	
Time:	12:00
Medicine:	Betotal
Dosage:	1

Figure 8. Page showing blood pressure values

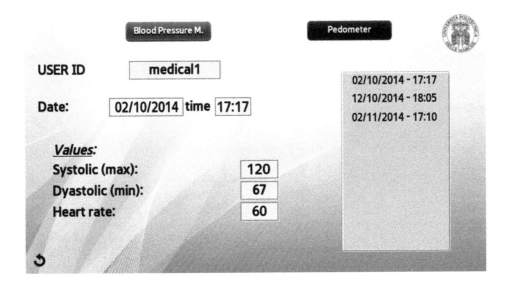

Figure 9. Smart TV application page showing the drug name from the leaflet information

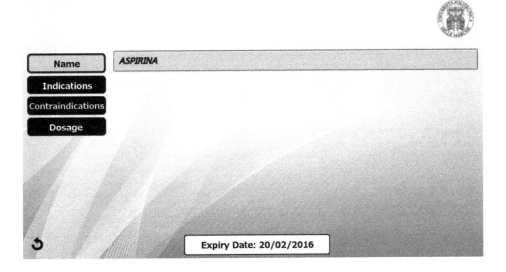

By accessing the service for consultation of medical reports, the application starts loading the login page (Figure 10), including the virtual *QWERTY* keyboard to allow user's credentials insertion. If the login is performed correctly, the user can display the list of available medical examinations and select the one of interest. After the selection, the medical report is transferred from the remote data center to the smart TV, which properly formats and displays it on the TV screen, as shown in Figure 11. If one of the parameters included in the medical report is out of the regular range, it is displayed in red colour in the table, in order to capture the user's attention. The classification of the parameter value as ''in range''

Figure 10. Login page showing the QWERTY keyboard

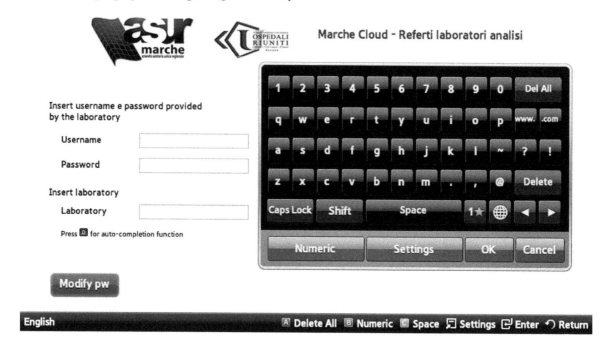

Marche Cloud - Referti laboratori analisi

Insert username e password provided
by the laboratory

Username

Password

Insert laboratory

Laboratory

Press **D** for auto-completion function

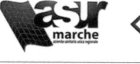

English   Ⓐ Delete All   Ⓑ Numeric   Ⓒ Space   ⧉ Settings   ⤶ Enter   ↻ Return

Figure 11. Table of outcomes

Marche Cloud - Referti laboratori analisi

Examination date: 22/11/2012 Code: 40250
Patient code: 00154431
Lab: RECANATI

Alfa 2	10,7%	
Beta	11,2%	
Gamma	15,8%	
Note:		
EMOCROMO COMPLETO		
GLOBULI BIANCHI	11,52 mila x mmc	4,00 / 10,00
GLOBULI ROSSI	4,81milioni x mmc	4,50 / 5,50
EMOGLOBINA	16,3gr/dL	12,5 / 17,0
EMATOCRITO	45,3%	40,0 / 50,0
MCV	94,1femtolitri	80,0 / 98,0
Contenuto medio Hgb (MCH)	33,9 picogrammi	27,0 / 31,0
Conc.Corp.Media Hgb (MCHC)	36,0 gr/dL	31,5 / 34,5
RDW	13,4%	11,5 / 16,0
HDW	3,0gr/dL	2,2 / 3,2
PIASTRINE	161mila/mmc	150 / 450
NEUTROFILI	64,3%	40,0 / 70,0
LINFOCITI	24,0%	20,0 / 48,0

Il referto, consultabile in forma autenticata ed anonima, ha natura di mera comunicazione di dati tra la struttura sanitaria e
l'interessato, effettuata su specifica richiesta di quest'ultimo e nel rispetto delle disposizioni sul trattamento dei dati personali ex artt.
75-81 d. lgs. 196/2003 e del Provvedimento del Garante Privacy del 19 dicembre 2009 (Linee guida in tema di referti on-line).

or ''out of range'' is performed by the laboratory, and saved into the medical report; the application only provides a different text colour to display the value.

From each service page, the *RETURN* key allows users to go back to the application menu page, and then from it to the standard vision of TV programs.

Experimental Tests

The smart TV application has been tested on real devices in the Telecommunications Laboratory providing satisfactory results, as all the functionalities foreseen in the design phase have been successfully implemented, and their correct execution verified. At the same time, the application is robust against possible user's errors during interaction and browsing of the contents, as well as with respect to possible network connection problems. The whole system presented in this paper has been implemented in experimental setup, and its capabilities have been verified by using a complete set of demo data. In the case of the remote consultation service, an anonymous user has been set up, with his own credentials and reports. These data are coherent with the real ones that are treated in the regional laboratories, as obtained by true reports. In the case of the sub-system for home health monitoring, instead, several measurements have been acquired from the medical devices and stored in the database, and a table of reminders has been populated.

As concerns the consultation of medical reports, approximately 150 points of sampling in the Italian Marche region are already enrolled in the project and offer the possibility of remote consultation of personal reports. When taking a blood sample, the lab personnel give the patient a label, reporting the personal credentials needed to access the consultation service. According to the local health regulations, the lab report is made available after the expected co-payment (by the patient) has been processed. If the patient is exempted from co-payment, or it occurs at the time of sampling, the remote consultation service turns out to be really efficient, as it avoids the need for the patient to get back to the lab, just to pick up his report. The application developed to enable the remote consultation of medical reports through the smart TV is available to general users since December 2012 (Public web server, 2014). From an analysis performed on the data of the first year of availability, the service has been accessed on average 17.8 and 20.8 times daily, respectively, during the first and second semester. The number of accesses varies widely over time, as citizens usually consult reports during daytime of working days. Moreover, it has emerged that the laboratories near the most populous cities have more accesses than those serving small towns.

When dealing with the development of an interface between users and a set of services, it is necessary to provide a tool of interaction easy to use and which has a good impact on them also at first sight. To this aim, the main guidelines for the design of graphic interfaces have been considered (Chorianopoulos, 2008; Nielsen, 1990). As for the interaction by means of the remote controller, a comparative study on TV interface types (Youngjae, Jaekyu, Jung, Chung, Taeil, Kwangsoo & Seunghun, 2012) has been taken into account, which discusses the "general" and the "motion" control methods. The remote controller is more suitable for actions of selection and navigation among the application pages, while the motion control is better in smart applications, such as games and multimedia contents.

The system has been tested in the Laboratory by people not involved in the project and with no previous experience with a smart TV. They were able to effectively use the application and browse the functionalities available. Moreover, in order to assess the usability of the interfaces, an evaluation form has been produced, addressed to persons who do not know the project. The short questionnaire consists of five key points, in addition to the indication of suggestions and problems, as can be seen in Figure 12.

Figure 12. Application evaluation form

APPLICATIONS EVALUATION FORM

Date	
Qualification (student, professor, ...)	
Age	

Application evaluation	Select a value between 1 (min) and 10 (max)									
Look and feel: clarity, first impact, coherence among the different sections	1	2	3	4	5	6	7	8	9	10
Intuitive operation: easy to use and learn how to interact with the application	1	2	3	4	5	6	7	8	9	10
Immediate detection of features, ease of navigation through the contents	1	2	3	4	5	6	7	8	9	10
Efficiency: level of user control, ability of reaching the goals	1	2	3	4	5	6	7	8	9	10
Feedback on user's decisions, notifications, error handling	1	2	3	4	5	6	7	8	9	10

Suggestions/tips (interface, functions, usability, ...)	
Any problems encountered	

The survey has been conducted in the Telecommunications Laboratory on 15 users among students and technical staff, who rated the application and provided some useful suggestions to improve it. The results can be considered very good, as the average score is between 8.1 and 9.2 for all the five main features, and few marginal problems have been reported, that however do not affect the correct operation of the application.

People who tested the system also easily accomplished the procedure of measure acquisition by means of the NFC reader, since it just requires the reader getting close to the specific area on the medical device.

CONCLUSION AND FUTURE WORK

This paper presented the prototype implementation of an integrated system for the delivery of healthcare services, that encompasses several technologies and devices. The service for remote consultation of personal health reports at home builds upon the new paradigm of Cloud Computing, and exploits a familiar, but at the same time new, interface, given by the smart TV. The same device also acts as a point of connection to the locally delivered service of health monitoring, based on biomedical devices equipped with NFC interface. The experimental implementation of the system, encompassing both the remote and the local services, has proved the feasibility of the integrated approach, in which the smart TV acts as the entry point for the user, supporting an easy and friendly interaction.

The proposed architecture meets the emerging trend of integrated healthcare that, whatever the approach, aims at ensuring that the most appropriate and effective care is provided, where and when it is needed, thus offering the potential of achieving better health outcomes and controlling costs, at the same time. The systematic application of Information and Communication Technologies (ICT) in healthcare gives rise to the so-called *connected health* paradigm, that leverages ICT to facilitate the accessing and sharing of information, as well as to allow subsequent analysis of health data across healthcare systems. Electronic medical records and other clinical applications, data repositories and analytic tools, connected biomedical devices and telehealth collaboration technologies all enable connected health, to support communication and collaboration among the various stakeholders involved (Accenture, 2012). The system presented in the paper suggests a possible connected health architecture, open to future extensions related, as an example, to the addition of wearable devices as new sensors to monitor the user's health conditions.

Moving from the Cloud based service, that was implemented at first, the additional and locally executed functionalities have been successfully integrated, and their co-existence does not cause any malfunctions. Both the applications running on the NFC reader and on the smart TV have been properly organized, in order to provide a simplified interface towards the user, from which all the services are seamlessly available and easily accessible. At the moment, the smart TV application has been tested only in a laboratory environment, and not by general users in real life situations, but its availability on public servers will make it possible to collect relevant feedback from the users and improve possible weaknesses. In fact, planned future work includes testing the application in real life situations, with real users (i.e. out of a laboratory environment), and investigating the further integration of the proposed system with existing institutional healthcare services. The experimental system demonstrated the feasibility of an easy-to-use and accessible service for the delivery of healthcare assistance at home, designed and targeted to users who may not have enough skills or experience to use other devices, such as mobile equipment, smart phones or tablets.

REFERENCES

Accenture. (2012). Connected Health: the Drive to Integrated Healthcare Delivery. Retrieved from www.accenture.com/connectedhealthstudy

Alaoui, M., & Lewkowicz, M. (2013). A LivingLab Approach to Involve Elderly in the Design of Smart TV Applications Offering Communication Services. *Proceedings of the 5th International conference, OCSC 2013, Held as Part of HCI International 2013, Las Vegas, NV, USA*. doi:10.1007/978-3-642-39371-6_37

AND. (2014). Activity Monitor and Digital Blood Pressure Monitor Instruction Manuals. Retrieved from http://www.aandd.jp/products/manual/medical/uw101nfc.pdf and http://www.aandd.jp/products/manual/medical/ua767nfc.pdf

Bahga, A., & Madisetti, V. K. (2013). A Cloud-based Approach for Interoperable Electronic Health Records (EHRs). *IEEE Journal of Biomedical and Health Informatics*, *17*(5), 894–906. doi:10.1109/JBHI.2013.2257818 PMID:25055368

Biswas, S., Anisuzzaman, Akhter, T., Kaiser, M.S. & Mamun, S.A. (2014). Cloud based healthcare application architecture and electronic medical record mining: An integrated approach to improve healthcare system. *Proceedings of the 17th International Conference on Computer and Information Technology* (pp. 286-291). doi:10.1109/ICCITechn.2014.7073139

Ceipidor, U. Biader, Medaglia, C.M., Volpi, V., Moroni, A., Sposato, S., Carboni, M. & Caridi, A. (2013). NFC technology applied to touristic-cultural field: A case study on an Italian museum. *Proceedings of the 5th International Workshop on Near Field Communication (NFC)* (pp.1-6). doi:10.1109/NFC.2013.6482445

Chauhan, R., & Kumar, A. (2013). *Cloud computing for improved healthcare: Techniques, potential and challenges. E-Health and Bioengineering Conference.* EHB; doi:10.1109/EHB.2013.6707234

Chorianopoulos, K. (2008). User interface design principles for interactive television applications. *International Journal of Human-Computer Interaction, 24*(6), 556–573. doi:10.1080/10447310802205750

de Abreu, J. F., Almeida, P., Afonso, J., Silva, T., & Dias, R. (2011). Participatory Design of a Social TV Application for Senior Citizens – The iNeighbour TV Project. *ENTERprise Information Systems Communications in Computer and Information Science, 221*, 49–58. doi:10.1007/978-3-642-24352-3_6

ForumN. F. C. (2014). Retrieved from www.nfc-forum.org

Klersy, C., De Silvestri, A., Gabutti, G., Raisaro, A., Curti, M., Regoli, F., & Auricchio, A. (2011). Economic impact of remote patient monitoring: An integrated economic model derived from a meta-analysis of randomized controlled trials in heart failure. *European Journal of Heart Failure, 13*(4), 450–459. doi:10.1093/eurjhf/hfq232 PMID:21193439

Lee, S. H., Sohn, M. K., Kim, D. J., Kim, B., & Kim, H. (2013). Smart tv interaction system using face and hand gesture recognition. *Proceedings of the IEEE International Conference on Consumer Electronics* (pp. 173-174). IEEE Publisher.

López-de-Ipiña, D., Blanco, S., Laiseca, X., & Díaz-de-Sarralde, I. (2011). ElderCare: An Interactive TV-based Ambient Assisted Living Platform. *Activity Recognition in Pervasive Intelligent Environments Atlantis Ambient and Pervasive Intelligence, 4*, 111–125. doi:10.2991/978-94-91216-05-3_5

Nielsen, J. (1990). Traditional dialog design applied to modern user interfaces. *Communications of the ACM, 33*(10), 109–118. doi:10.1145/84537.84559

Park, J. S., Jang, G. J., Kim, J. H., & Kim, S. H. (2013). Acoustic interference cancellation for a voice-driven interface in smart TVs. *IEEE Transactions on Consumer Electronics, 59*(1), 244–249. doi:10.1109/TCE.2013.6490266

Public web server to download the application. IP address: 193.205.130.247. (n. d.). Related guide. Retrieved from http://www.tlc.dii.univpm.it/blog/wp-content/uploads/2014/02/InstallationGuide.pdf

Puma, J. P., Huerta, M., Alvizu, R., & Clotet, R. (2012). Mobile Identification: NFC in the Healthcare Sector. *Proceedings of the Andean Region International Conference (ANDESCON) VI*, Cuenca, Ecuador (pp.39-42). doi:10.1109/Andescon.2012.19

Raffaeli, L., Gambi, E., & Spinsante, S. (2014). Smart TV Based Ecosystem for Personal e-Health Services. *Proceedings of the 8th International Symposium on Medical Information and Communication Technology* (pp. 1-6). IEEE Publisher. doi:10.1109/ISMICT.2014.6825208

Sorwar, G., & Hasan, R. (2012). Smart-TV Based Integrated E-health Monitoring System with Agent Technology. *Proceedings of the 26th International Conference on Advanced Information Networking and Applications Workshops (WAINA)*. doi:10.1109/WAINA.2012.155

Spiga, D., Bilei, G. M., Riahi, H., Storchi, L., Fattibene, E., Manzali, M., . . . Settimi, D. (2014). A Cloud-based solution for Public Administrations. The experience of the Regione Marche. *Proceedings of the 2014 International Conference on Collaboration Technologies and Systems* (pp. 493-499). IEEE Publisher. doi:10.1109/CTS.2014.6867614

Spinsante, S., Antonicelli, R., Mazzanti, I., & Gambi, E. (2012). Technological Approaches to Remote Monitoring of Elderly People in Cardiology: A Usability Perspective. *International Journal of Telemedicine and Applications*, 2012. PMID:23365567

United Nations, Department of Economic and Social Affairs, Population Division. (2013). *World Population Ageing 2013*. ST/ESA/SER.A/348. Retrieved from http://www.un.org/en/development/desa/population/publications/pdf/ageing/WorldPopulationAgeing2013.pdf

Vergara, M., Díaz-Hellín, P., Fontecha, J., Hervás, R., Sánchez-Barba, C., Fuentes, C., & Bravo, J.(2010). Mobile Prescription: an NFC-based proposal for AAL. *Proceedings of 2nd International Workshop on NFC* (pp. 27-32). IEEE Publisher. doi:10.1109/NFC.2010.13

Youngjae, L., Jaekyu, P., Jung, E. S., Chung, D. H., Taeil, K., Kwangsoo, C., & Seunghun, L. (2012). Comparative Study on Advanced TV Interface Types in the Smart Media World. *Proceedings of the 9th International Conference on Ubiquitous Intelligence & Computing and Autonomic & Trusted Computing (UIC/ATC)*.

Zhang, H., & Li, J. (2011). NFC in Medical Applications with Wireless Sensors. *Proceedings of the International Conference on Electrical and Control Engineering (ICECE)* (pp. 718-721). doi:10.1109/ICECENG.2011.6057534

This research was previously published in the International Journal of E-Health and Medical Communications (IJEHMC), 7(1); edited by Joel J.P.C. Rodrigues, pages 48-64, copyright year 2016 by IGI Publishing (an imprint of IGI Global).

Index

A

Acceptability 72, 349, 351, 412, 448, 536, 576, 694, 962, 974, 1093, 1109, 1119, 1339

Accessibility 26, 87, 149, 206, 251, 269, 271-272, 288, 290, 303-304, 306, 308, 310, 314, 323, 334, 382, 404, 505, 519, 545, 566, 656, 673, 717, 754, 770, 775-778, 780, 782, 855, 871, 874, 876, 884, 888, 942, 962, 1069, 1189, 1330, 1400, 1412-1413, 1507-1508, 1520, 1522, 1534-1535

Accountable Care 226, 360-365, 369, 556

Actants 306-308, 310-312, 314, 548, 605, 778-779, 782, 787

Action Research 89, 102

Active Citizenship Network 1170, 1204, 1219

Active RFID 402, 419, 743, 844, 867

Actor-Network Theory 541-542, 547, 599-600, 604-605, 607, 775-776, 778-779

Actors 28, 55, 66, 72, 144-152, 154-155, 157, 163, 172, 181, 202, 220, 247, 249-251, 258-261, 282, 303, 305, 307-312, 318, 491, 493-498, 504-505, 508-510, 516, 522, 547-548, 550, 602, 605-606, 647, 650, 653, 775-778, 780-784, 786-788, 841, 912, 1123, 1125, 1130-1132, 1135-1136, 1145, 1199, 1228, 1281, 1295, 1298, 1301-1302, 1315, 1328, 1367-1368, 1469

Actual Urgency (AU) 400

Adherence 12, 52, 67, 73, 76, 114-115, 121, 156-157, 162, 184, 188, 292, 298-299, 344-346, 351, 371, 482, 526-529, 531, 533, 535, 538, 572, 576, 582, 628-631, 639, 657, 794, 815, 892, 907, 955, 1046-1047, 1102, 1110, 1112-1113, 1119, 1148, 1189, 1251, 1258-1260, 1266, 1370, 1403-1404, 1461, 1485, 1580-1584, 1586-1591, 1596

Administrators 85, 89-90, 95, 148, 304, 409, 543, 605, 702, 706-707, 709-710, 776, 794, 869, 872, 874-875, 877, 883, 999, 1007, 1246, 1254, 1281, 1283, 1287, 1297-1298, 1391, 1457, 1459, 1463, 1487, 1489-1490, 1494, 1573

Advance Care Planning 154-156, 158, 162, 169-172, 181-182, 188, 190, 192, 1248

Affordability 87, 309-310, 412, 765, 781-782, 942, 959, 962, 1264

Africa 145, 148, 150, 271-272, 279-281, 294, 318, 504-508, 511, 520, 997, 1001, 1277, 1281, 1284, 1287-1288, 1369, 1372-1374, 1392, 1403, 1454, 1460

Ageing Population 1064, 1308, 1310, 1323, 1532, 1548

Agent 93, 144, 236, 307, 310, 315-317, 319, 322-326, 331-332, 334, 511, 580, 582, 628, 631-633, 638, 640, 693-694, 704-706, 710, 713-714, 778, 782, 970, 1031, 1529

Aging 71, 338-341, 354-355, 420, 470, 552, 622, 650, 657-658, 792, 914, 1100, 1160, 1239, 1310, 1366

Aging in Place 338-340, 354

Ambulatory Care Services 438

Analytics 87, 104-105, 108-111, 115, 118, 120, 123, 126-127, 129-130, 133, 136, 205, 226-227, 231-232, 241, 246, 424, 443, 456, 649, 661, 667-672, 897, 1030, 1086, 1089, 1099, 1247-1248, 1254-1255, 1398, 1450-1451, 1453-1464, 1468, 1581, 1588-1589

Android 107-108, 115, 317, 324-326, 328-329, 334, 628, 631, 636-638, 1008, 1068, 1261, 1265

Apollo Hospital 102

Aravind Hospital 102

Architecture 54, 97, 103, 129-133, 224, 232-233, 290-292, 315-318, 322, 327, 329-330, 334, 466, 503, 526, 532, 540, 553-556, 561, 564-565, 628, 630, 632, 640, 656, 660, 669-670, 691, 693, 695-699, 768, 784, 828, 833-834, 966, 972, 1048, 1050-1051, 1061, 1069, 1075, 1133, 1159, 1187, 1537, 1561-1562

Arena 36, 530, 970, 1019, 1021, 1023, 1026-1027, 1029-1031, 1033, 1035, 1045, 1135, 1202, 1461

Artificial Intelligence 319, 421, 669, 694, 927, 966, 1246, 1312-1313, 1596

Asset Light 962

D

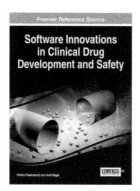
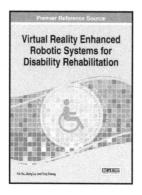
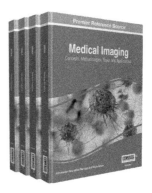
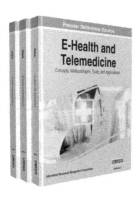
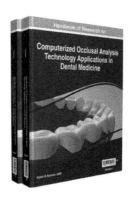
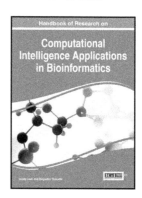
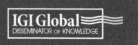 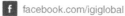

Stay Current on the Latest Emerging Research Developments

Become an IGI Global Reviewer for Authored Book Projects

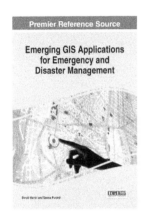

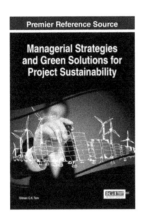

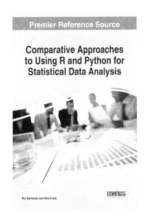

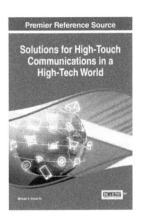

The overall success of an authored book project is dependent on quality and timely reviews.

In this competitive age of scholarly publishing, constructive and timely feedback significantly decreases the turnaround time of manuscripts from submission to acceptance, allowing the publication and discovery of progressive research at a much more expeditious rate. Several IGI Global authored book projects are currently seeking highly qualified experts in the field to fill vacancies on their respective editorial review boards:

Applications may be sent to:
development@igi-global.com

Applicants must have a doctorate (or an equivalent degree) as well as publishing and reviewing experience. Reviewers are asked to write reviews in a timely, collegial, and constructive manner. All reviewers will begin their role on an ad-hoc basis for a period of one year, and upon successful completion of this term can be considered for full editorial review board status, with the potential for a subsequent promotion to Associate Editor.

If you have a colleague that may be interested in this opportunity,
we encourage you to share this information with them.

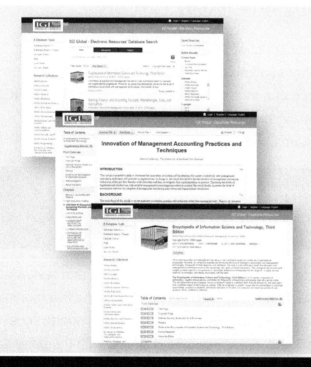
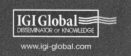

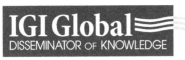
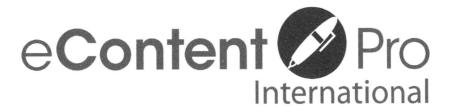
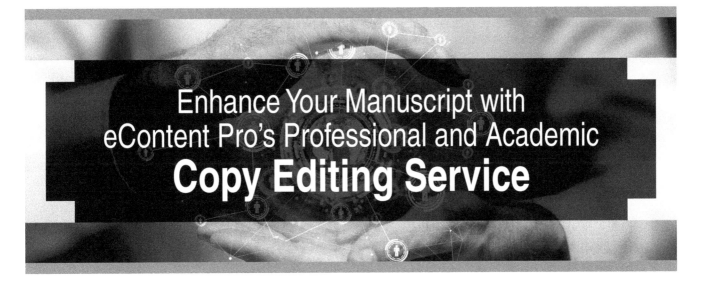

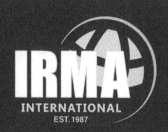
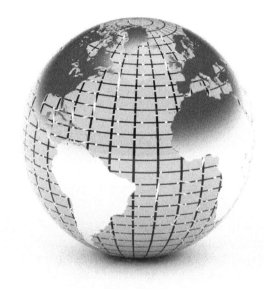

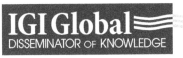
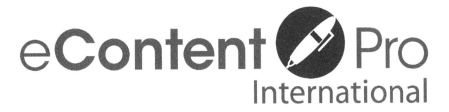
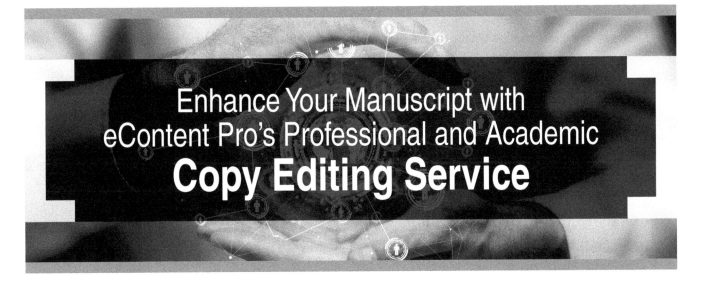

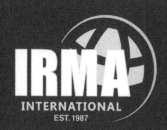

Information Resources Management Association

Advancing the Concepts & Practices of Information Resources Management in Modern Organizations

Become an IRMA Member

Members of the **Information Resources Management Association (IRMA)** understand the importance of community within their field of study. The Information Resources Management Association is an ideal venue through which professionals, students, and academicians can convene and share the latest industry innovations and scholarly research that is changing the field of information science and technology. Become a member today and enjoy the benefits of membership as well as the opportunity to collaborate and network with fellow experts in the field.

IRMA Membership Benefits:

- **One FREE Journal Subscription**

- **30% Off Additional Journal Subscriptions**

- **20% Off Book Purchases**

- Updates on the latest events and research on Information Resources Management through the IRMA-L listserv.

- Updates on new open access and downloadable content added to Research IRM.

- A copy of the Information Technology Management Newsletter twice a year.

- A certificate of membership.

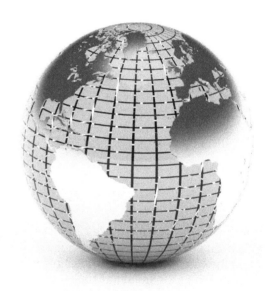

IRMA Membership $195

Scan code or visit **irma-international.org** and begin by selecting your free journal subscription.

Membership is good for one full year.

CPSIA information can be obtained
at www.ICGtesting.com
Printed in the USA
BVHW01*0054131117

500018BV00004B/14/P

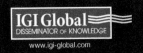

Available to Order Now

Order through www.igi-global.com with **Free Standard Shipping**.

The Premier Reference for Information Science & Information Technology

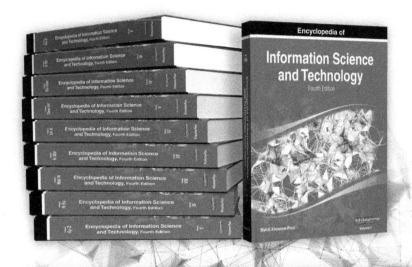

100% Original Content
Contains 705 new, peer-reviewed articles with color figures covering over 80 categories in 11 subject areas

Diverse Contributions
More than 1,100 experts from 74 unique countries contributed their specialized knowledge

Easy Navigation
Includes two tables of content and a comprehensive index in each volume for the user's convenience

Highly-Cited
Embraces a complete list of references and additional reading sections to allow for further research

Included in:

InfoSci®-Books

Encyclopedia of Information Science and Technology **Fourth Edition**
A Comprehensive 10-Volume Set

Mehdi Khosrow-Pour, D.B.A. (Information Resources Management Association, USA)
ISBN: 978-1-5225-2255-3; © 2018; Pg: 8,104; Release Date: July 2017

For a limited time, receive the complimentary e-books for the First, Second, and Third editions with the purchase of the *Encyclopedia of Information Science and Technology, Fourth Edition* e-book.**

The **Encyclopedia of Information Science and Technology, Fourth Edition** is a 10-volume set which includes 705 original and previously unpublished research articles covering a full range of perspectives, applications, and techniques contributed by thousands of experts and researchers from around the globe. This authoritative encyclopedia is an all-encompassing, well-established reference source that is ideally designed to disseminate the most forward-thinking and diverse research findings. With critical perspectives on the impact of information science management and new technologies in modern settings, including but not limited to computer science, education, healthcare, government, engineering, business, and natural and physical sciences, it is a pivotal and relevant source of knowledge that will benefit every professional within the field of information science and technology and is an invaluable addition to every academic and corporate library.

Scan for Online Bookstore

Pricing Information

Hardcover: **$5,695**   E-Book: **$5,695***   Hardcover + E-Book: **$6,895***

Both E-Book Prices Include:
- *Encyclopedia of Information Science and Technology, First Edition E-Book*
- *Encyclopedia of Information Science and Technology, Second Edition E-Book*
- *Encyclopedia of Information Science and Technology, Third Edition E-Book*

* Purchase the Encyclopedia of Information Science and Technology, Fourth Edition e-book and receive the first, second, and third e-book editions for free. Offer is only valid with purchase of the fourth edition's e-book. Offer expires January 1, 2018.

Recommend this Title to Your Institution's Library: www.igi-global.com/books